Postgraduate Paediatric Orthopaedics

The Candidate's Guide to the FRCS (Tr & Orth) Examination

Examination

Second Edition

Postgraduate Paediatric Orthopaedics

The Candidate's Guide to the FRCS (Tr & Orth) Examination

Second Edition

Edited by

Sattar Alshryda MBChB MRCP (UK) MRCS SICOT EBOT FRCS (Tr & Orth) MBA MSc PhD

Consultant Trauma and Paediatric Orthopaedic Surgeon
Al Jalila Children's Specialty Hospital, Dubai Academic Health Corporation, Dubai UAE
Former Consultant Trauma and Paediatric Orthopaedic Surgeon, Royal Manchester Children Hospital, UK
Adjunct Associate Professor, Mohammed Bin Rashid University of Medicine and Health Sciences, Dubai, UAE

Stan Jones FRCS MBChB, MSc Bio Eng, FRCS (Tr & Orth)

Consultant Orthopaedic Surgeon
Al Ahli Hospital, Qatar

Paul A. Banaszkiewicz FRCS (Glas) FRCS (Ed) FRCS (Eng) FRCS (Tr & Orth) MClinEd FAcadMEd FHEA

Consultant Orthopaedic Surgeon
Queen Elizabeth Hospital and North East NHS Surgical Centre (NENSC), Gateshead, UK
Visiting Professor, Northumbria University, UK
British Orthopaedic Association Council Trustee

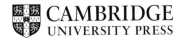
CAMBRIDGE
UNIVERSITY PRESS

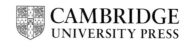

Shaftesbury Road, Cambridge CB2 8EA, United Kingdom

One Liberty Plaza, 20th Floor, New York, NY 10006, USA

477 Williamstown Road, Port Melbourne, VIC 3207, Australia

314–321, 3rd Floor, Plot 3, Splendor Forum, Jasola District Centre, New Delhi – 110025, India

103 Penang Road, #05–06/07, Visioncrest Commercial, Singapore 238467

Cambridge University Press is part of Cambridge University Press & Assessment, a department of the University of Cambridge.

We share the University's mission to contribute to society through the pursuit of education, learning and research at the highest international levels of excellence.

www.cambridge.org
Information on this title: www.cambridge.org/9781108970617

DOI: 10.1017/9781108989879

First Edition 2014
Second Edition 2024

Printed in the United Kingdom by TJ Books Limited, Padstow Cornwall

A catalogue record for this publication is available from the British Library.

A Cataloging-in-Publication data record for this book is available from the Library of Congress.

ISBN 978-1-108-97061-7 Paperback

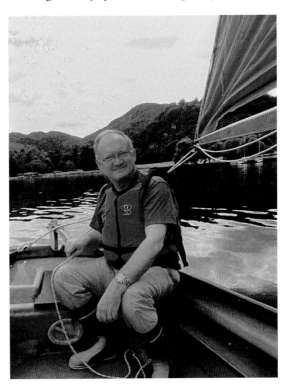

Eighteen months ago, Richard Montgomery kindly agreed to foreword the Second Edition of our Postgraduate Paediatric Orthopaedic book.

All the Postgraduate Orthopaedic forewords for each book published are very carefully chosen. The surgeons we ask are inspirational, widely respected and have influenced practice nationally and internationally.

Richard was very kind and helpful to us as junior consultants, always offering expert advice and guiding us. He was never critical, always encouraging and a mentor to us. Unfortunately, at the time of completing 1st proof corrections, he passed away suddenly. He will be a greatly missed colleague, teacher, and friend.

Contents

Additional videos can be found at www.cambridge
.org/alshryda

Contributors

Alwyn Abraham BSc MBChB FRCS (Tr & Orth)
University Hospitals of Leicester NHS Trust, Leicester, UK

Akinwande Adedapo MBBS FRCS (Eng) FRCS (Glas)
James Cook University Hospital, Middlesbrough, UK

Mubshshar Ahmad MBBS FRCS (Tr & Orth)
University Hospital of North Durham, UK

Tahani Al Ali BSc MSc
Al Jalila Children Speciality Hospital, Dubai Academic Health Corporation, Dubai, UAE

Khalid Alawadi MBBCh Facharzt (Plastic) EBOPRAS FESSH (Hand Surgery) Diploma
Rashid Hospital, Dubai Academic Health Corporation, Dubai, UAE

Ehab Aldlyami MBChB FRCS (Tr & Orth)
Kings College London, Dubai, UAE

Farhan Ali FRCS (Tr & Orth)
Sidra Medicine, Doha, Qatar

Fazal Ali FRCS (Tr & Orth)
Chesterfield Royal Hospital, Chesterfield, UK

Talal Al-Jabri MBBS BSc (Hons) MRCS (Eng) MSc (Surg) FRCS (Tr & Orth)
Imperial College, London, UK

Mohammed Al-Maiyah MBChB FICMS FRCS MSc (Orthop) FRCS (Tr & Orth)
Croydon University Hospital, London, UK

Sattar Alshryda MRCS FRCS (Tr & Orth) MBA MSc PhD
Al Jalila Children Speciality Hospital, Dubai Academic Health Corporation, Dubai, UAE

Tony Antonios BSc MBBS PGCertHBE MSc FRCS (Tr & Orth)
Ashford and St Peter's Hospitals NHS Foundation Trust, Ashford, UK

Simon L. Barker BSc (Hons) MD FRCS (Tr & Orth)
Royal Children's Hospital, Aberdeen, UK

Paul A. Banaszkiewicz FRCS (Glas) FRCS (Ed) FRCS (Eng) FRCS (Tr & Orth) MClinEd FAcadMEd FHEA
Queen Elizabeth Hospital, Gateshead, UK

Dean E. Boyce MB BCh FRCS FRCSEd FRCSPlast MD
The Welsh Centre for Burns and Plastic Surgery, Swansea, UK

Lee M. Breakwell MSc FRCS (Tr & Orth)
Sheffield Children's Hospitals, Sheffield, UK

Rachel Buckingham MB ChB FRCS (Tr and Orth) CTS
Oxford University Hospitals, Oxford, UK

Vittoria Bucknall MBChB BMSc MFSTEd FRCS (Tr & Orth)
Alder Hey Children's Hospital, Liverpool, UK

Clare Carpenter BSc MBBCh MRCS (Eng) Pg Dip Sports Med FRCS (T & Orth) MD
Noah's Ark Children's Hospital, Cardiff, UK

Ashley A. Cole BMedSci BMBS FRCS (Tr & Orth)
Sheffield Children's Hospital, Sheffield, UK

Anthony Cooper BSc MBChB MRCS FRCS (Tr & Orth)
BC Children's Hospital, Vancouver, Canada

John Davies MB ChB MSc (Eng) FRCS (Tr & Orth)
Leeds Teaching Hospitals NHS Trust, Leeds, UK

Gavin DeKiewiet MBChB FRCS RCPS (Glas) FRCS (Ed) FRCSOrth
Sunderland Royal Infirmary, Sunderland, UK

Thomas Dehler FA T&O Germany
Sunderland Royal Hospital, Sunderland, UK

Sara Dorman MBChB BMSc (Hons) MRCS MSc FRCSEd (Tr & Orth) MFSTEd
Sheffield Children's Hospital, Sheffield, UK

Sean Duffy FRCS (Tr & Orth)
Bristol Children's Hospital, Bristol, UK

Deborah M. Eastwood MBBS FRCS
Great Ormond St Hospital and the Royal National Orthopaedic Hospital, London, UK

James A. Fernandes MS (Orth) DNB (Orth) MCh (Orth) FRCS (Tr & Orth)
Sheffield Children's Hospital, Sheffield, UK

Gregory B. Firth MBBCh FCS (Orth) MMed (Orth)
Royal London Hospital, London, UK

Richard Gardner MBBS MRCS FRCS (Tr & Orth)
CURE Ethiopia Children's Hospital, Addis Ababa, Ethiopia

Mark Gaston MB BChir MA (Cantab) FRCSEd (Tr & Orth) PhD
The Royal Hospital for Sick Children (Sick Kids), Edinburgh, UK

Sandeep Gokhale MBBS MRCS (Edinburgh) MS Orthopedics (India)
Noah's Ark Children's Hospital, Cardiff, UK

Sevan Hopyan MD PhD FRCSC
University of Toronto, Toronto, Canada

Richard Hutchinson MBChB MRCS MSc (Dist) Orth (Eng) FRCS (Orth)
Royal Victoria Infirmary, Newcastle, UK

Stan Jones FRCS MB ChB MSc Bio Eng FRCS (Tr & Orth)
Al Ahli Hospital, Qatar

Syed Kazmi MSOP MHA
Al Jalila Children Speciality Hospital, Dubai Academic Health Corporation, Dubai, UAE

Simon Kelley MBChB FRCS (Tr & Orth)
The Hospital for Sick Children, Toronto, Canada

Mohamed Kenawey Consultant Paediatric and Orthopaedic surgeon
Royal Manchester Children Hospital, Manchester, UK

Om Lahoti MS (Orth) Dip N B (Orth) FRCS (Orth) FRCS (C)
King's College Hospital, London, UK

Bavan Luckshman MBBS BSc (Hons) MRCS
Oxford University Hospitals, Oxford, UK

Ben Marson FRCS (Tr & Orth)
Nottingham University Hospital, Nottingham, UK

Ibrar Majid, Consultant Paediatric and Orthopaedic surgeon
Al Jalila Children's Specialty Hospital , Dubai Academic Health Corporation, Dubai, UAE

Fergal Monsell MBBCh MSc PhD FRCS (Orth)
University Hospitals Bristol, Bristol, UK

Nick Nicolaou BSc (Hons) MBBS MSc (Tr & Orth) MRCS (Eng) FRCS (Orth)
Sheffield Children's Hospital, Sheffield, UK

Matt Nixon MD FRCS (Tr & Orth)
Royal Manchester Children's Hospital, Manchester, UK

Kathryn Price BMedSci MMedSci FRCSEd (Tr & Orth)
Nottingham University Hospital, Nottingham, UK

Manoj Ramachandran BSc (Hons) MBBS (Hons) MRCS (Eng) FRCS (Tr & Orth)
Barts NHS Trust, London, UK

Anish P. Sanghrajka MBBS MRCS FRCS (Tr & Orth)
Norfolk and Norwich University Hospitals, Norwich, UK

Gino R. Somers MBBS PhD FRCPA
Hospital for Sick Children, Toronto, Canada

Joanna Thomas MBBS MSc FRCS (Tr & Orth)
University Hospital Southampton NHS Foundation Trust, Southampton, UK

Jennifer Walsh BEng PGDip Stat PhD
Astley Ainslie Hospital, Edinburgh, UK

Foreword to the First Edition

Since 1998, I have convened an annual core curriculum lecture course in paediatric orthopaedics at Alder Hey Children's Hospital. Over the years, we have frequently been asked to recommend books that succinctly cover all of the necessary information and I now believe that we have found such a book in Postgraduate Paediatric Orthopaedics: The Candidate's Guide to the FRCS (Tr & Orth) Examination. As the title suggests, the text is targeted toward trainees sitting the FRCS (Tr & Orth) examination but the book would also be useful for those who seek to enhance or maintain their paediatric orthopaedic knowledge base, including practicing orthopaedic surgeons, GPs, paediatricians and specialist physiotherapists. The text is much more than lecture notes and covers all of the major subjects with sufficient information to keep the reader interested, while still delivering the required facts to an examination candidate as quickly as possible. I congratulate the editors and the authors for producing such a useful text.

Colin E. Bruce
Consultant Children's Orthopaedic Surgeon
Alder Hey Children's Hospital
Liverpool, UK
President of the British Society of Children's Orthopaedic Surgery (BSCOS)

Foreword to the Second Edition

As a past paediatric orthopaedic examiner and Chair of the Intercollegiate Specialty Board for the FRCS Trauma & Orthopaedics exam, I was very interested to see drafts of the text and was honoured to be asked to write this foreword.

I have known Sattar, Paul and Stan and also several of the other distinguished contributors for many years. They are some of the most able, enthusiastic and industrious medical educators that I have met. Their long experience in assisting candidates to prepare for the exam is obvious in this book.

When candidates are preparing for the exam there is a tendency to cram in knowledge in as many fields as possible. However, if that knowledge is not structured, it may be difficult to recall it and to present it to the examiners in a logical way. Recalling the facts, and being able to present them to the examiner in a logical way is vital to exam success.

What the authors provide in this book is a distillation of the key facts and classifications as well as a structure for organizing knowledge about paediatric orthopaedic conditions. I wish it had been available when I was training!

Prof. Richard Montgomery MB, BS, FRCS(Ed), FRCS(Eng)
Hon. Consultant Trauma & Orthopaedic Surgeon,
Middlesbrough & Newcastle upon Tyne
Visiting Professor, School of Health & Social Care,
University of Teesside
Past Chair, Intercollegiate Specialty Board in T&O Surgery,
for the FRCS T&O examination
Past President of the British Limb Reconstruction Society

Preface

Why another exam-related FRCS (Tr & Orth) book? Don't we cover paediatrics in the chapters of the other *Postgraduate Orthopaedics* books?

We always felt the need for a more definitive guide to the paediatric component of the FRCS exam.

We were never entirely happy that the FRCS (Tr & Orth) paediatric syllabus was particularly well written or developed in a number of orthopaedic books. Most lacked the specific subject focus that candidates needed to pass the FRCS (Tr & Orth) exam.

General orthopaedic books tended to scratch the surface of a difficult area of orthopaedics that needs to be learnt well for the exam. Specialized books in paediatrics meant you could lose all focus of the subject's relevance and end up not extracting out the relevant/specific detail required to pass the exam. Moreover, you could end up spending a lot of unnecessary time and effort drowning in these specialized textbooks and not have enough time left to read the basic science, trauma, or hands sections.

Our aim with this book was to make it all-encompassing, so that it covers everything you need to know to pass the FRCS (Tr & Orth) section of the exam, without having to cross-reference from other larger textbooks – a tall order, but one which we hope we manage to succeed in doing.

We were careful not to make the book too detailed, so it ends up being like a subspecialty book in paediatrics. At the same time, we didn't want it to become too flimsy, such that you felt you were missing something and you needed to repeatedly go to the bigger specialized textbooks of paediatric orthopaedics.

Special mention about the unusual time of Covid-19 that occupied a large part of the book writing process. Whilst some authors may say the extra time in lockdown gave them the opportunity to complete tasks, they were unlikely to have done otherwise this wasn't particularly applicable to us. Despite the extra time of lockdown with elective surgery cancelled extra time doesn't always equate with productive efficient time usage.

As with all the *Postgraduate Orthopaedics* book series, we make no claim for the originality of the material contained in the text. This material is available in the larger orthopaedic community. We have simply distilled and focused this knowledge down into something that will hopefully get you through the exam.

We hope you find this book useful in preparing for the exam and we wish you every success. We hope that in some small (or large) way the book will make the difference between you passing and failing the exam

Sattar Alshryda
Stan Jones
Paul A. Banaskiewicz

Acknowledgements

Special thanks to all the authors involved with the *Postgraduate Orthopaedics* book series over the years. Without your input, no book would be possible.

Special thanks to Jessica Papworth and Beth Sexton at Cambridge University Press for their help, guidance, and patience with this second edition of *Postgraduate Paediatric Orthopaedics*.

Special thanks to our medical artist Biswa Prakash Sahoo from India who did a great job of drawing the book illustrations.

Great appreciation for Anthony Michael Rex (Consultant Spine Surgeon), Metwally Sayed Ahmad(Consultant Orthopaedic Surgeon,Kuwait) Karim Khalil (Paediatric Orthopaedic Specialist) and Yasir Adil Al-Humairi (T&O Resident) for their help in the proofreading. Thanks to Faizan Jabbar for coordinating our website structure and to our web designer Farrakh, who has helped us develop and progress our website through the years.

Special thanks to Kath McCourt CBE, Nick Caplan and Dianna Ford at Northumbria University for their help and support through the years.

As ever, thanks to Jo McStea who keeps the whole PGO setup rolling along.

Thanks to James Coey,Assistant Dean Basic Sciences St. George's University for photography,inspiration and just being there to help and guide.

Special thanks to all of our orthopaedic trainers who helped guide and nurture our development through the many years of our own orthopaedic training.

Interactive Website

www.postgraduateorthopaedics.com

This website accompanies the textbook series *Postgraduate Orthopaedics*.

It includes:

- *Postgraduate Orthopaedics: The Candidate's Guide to the FRCS (Tr & Orth) Examination*, 3rd edition
- *Postgraduate Orthopaedics: Viva Guide for the FRCS (Tr & Orth) Examination*
- *Postgraduate Paediatric Orthopaedics*
- *Postgraduate Orthopaedics. SBAs for the FRCS (Tr&Orth) Examination.*

The aim is to provide additional information and resources in order to maximize the learning potential of each book.

The book comes with 20 educational videos. More videos will be added regularly on the accompanying YouTube channel https://www.youtube.com/@ChildrenOrthopaedics.

Additional areas of the website provide supplementary orthopaedic material, updates, and web links. *Meet the Editorial Team* provides a profile of authors who were involved in writing the books. Details of up-and-coming courses are provided. Details of the next diet of exams are provided.

There are many single best answer questions that are exam focused along with case-based discussions, podcasts and webinars.

It is very important our readership gives us feedback. Please e-mail us if you have found any errors in the text that we can correct.In addition, if we have not included an area of orthopaedics that you feel we should cover, please let us know. Likewise any constructive suggestions for improvement would be most welcome.

There is also a list of Postgraduate Orthopaedics courses available for candidates to fine-tune their examination skills.

Abbreviations

AA	anatomical axis		Ca	calcium
AAOS	American Academy of Orthopaedic Surgeons		cAMP	cyclic adenosine monophosphate
ABC	aneurysmal bone cyst		CAPTA	Child Abuse Prevention and Treatment Act
AC	acromioclavicular		CCBS	congenital constriction band syndrome
ACA	acquired coxa vara; axis of correction of angulation		CCV	congenital coxa vara
ACL	anterior cruciate ligament		CDH	congenital dislocation of the hip
ADI	anterior atlanto-dens index		CDK	congenital dislocation of the knee
ADM	abductor digiti minimi		CEA	centre edge angle
ADTA	anterior distal tibial angle		cEDS	classic Ehlers–Danlos syndrome
AER	apical ectodermal ridge		CFD	congenital femoral deficiency
AFO	ankle foot orthosis		CFL	calcaneofibular ligament
AHA	Assisting Hand Assessment		CI	confidence interval
AI	acetabular index		CKD	chronic kidney disease
AIIS	anterior inferior iliac spine		CMCJ	carpometacarpal joint
AIS	adolescent idiopathic scoliosis		CMT	Charcot–Marie–Tooth
aLDFA	anatomical lateral distal femoral angle		CNP	C-type natriuretic peptide
ALP	alkaline phosphatase		COMP	cartilage oligomeric matrix protein
ALPSA	anterior labral periosteum sleeve avulsion		CORA	centre of rotation of angulation
AMC	arthrogryposis multiplex congenita		CP	cerebral palsy
aMPFA	anatomical medial proximal femoral angle		CPIP	Cerebral Palsy Integrated Pathway
AOFAS	American Orthopedic Foot and Ankle Score		CRP	C-reactive protein
			CSVL	Central sacral vertical line
AP	anteroposterior		CtE	Commission through Evaluation (trial)
ASIA	American Spinal Injury Association		CTEV	congenital talipes equinovarus
ASIS	anterior superior iliac spine		CV	coxa vara
ATD	articulotrochanteric distance		CVS	chorionic villus sampling
ATFL	anterior talofibular ligament		CVT	congenital vertical talus
ATiFL	anterior tibiofibular interosseous ligament		DCV	developmental coxa vara
ATLS	Adult Trauma Life Support		DDH	developmental dysplasia of the hip
ATR	angle of trunk rotation		DEXA	dual-energy X-ray absorptiometry
AVN	avascular necrosis		dGEMRIC	delayed gadolinium-enhanced MRI of cartilage
BD	Blount's disease			
BMD	bone mineral density		DIPJ	distal interphalangeal joint
BMP 2	bone morphogenetic protein 2		DMAA	distal metatarsal articular angle
			DMD	Duchenne muscular dystrophy

DRUJ	distal radioulnar joint
ECU	extensor carpi ulnaris
EDF	elongation, derotation, and flexion
EDS	Ehlers–Danlos syndrome
EI	extensor indicis
EMA	epiphyseal–metaphyseal angle; European Medicines Agency
EMG	electromyogram
EMI	extended matching item
EPB	extensor pollicis brevis
EPL	extensor pollicis longus
ERT	enzyme replacement therapy
ESIN	elastic stable intramedullary nail
ESR	erythrocyte sedimentation rate
EXT	exostosin
FAI	femoroacetabular impingement
FCU	flexor carpi ulnaris
FD	fibrous dysplasia
FDA	Food and Drug Administration
FDP	flexor digitorum profundus
FDS	flexor digitorum superficialis
FES	functional electrical stimulation
FFCD	focal fibrocartilaginous dysplasia
FGF-23	fibroblast growth factor 23
FGFR-23	fibroblast growth factor receptor 23
FMDA	Femoral–metaphyseal–diaphyseal angle
FPA	foot progression angle
FTR	femoral: tibial ratio
GA	general anaesthesia
GABA	gamma-aminobutyric acid
GLAD	glenolabral articular disruption
GMC	General Medical Council
GMFCS	Gross Motor Function Classification System
GMFM	Gross Motor Function Measure
GRAFO	ground reaction ankle foot orthoses
HA	hydroxyapatite
HAGL	humeral avulsions of the glenohumeral ligament
HEA	Hilgenreiner epiphyseal angle
HKAFO	hip, knee, ankle, and foot orthosis
HLH	haemophagocytic lymphohistiocytosis
HSCT	haematopoietic stem cell transplant
HSMN	hereditary sensorimotor neuropathy
HVA	hallux valgus angle
IIS	infantile idiopathic scoliosis
IL-6	interleukin-6

IMA	intermetatarsal angle
IP	interphalangeal
IPA	interphalangeal angle
IPJ	interphalangeal joint
IT	iliotibial
ITFJ	inferior tibiofibular joint
JCIE	Joint Committee on Intercollegiate Examinations
JIS	juvenile idiopathic scoliosis
JLCA	joint line convergence angle
JOL	joint surface line
JRA	juvenile rheumatoid arthritis
JSCFE	Joint Surgical Colleges Fellowship Examination
KAFO	knee–ankle–foot orthosis
kEDS	kyphoscoliotic Ehlers–Danlos syndrome
KFS	Klippel–Feil syndrome
LADI	lateral atlanto-dens index
LCL	lateral collateral ligament
LCPD	Legg–Calvé–Perthes disease
LFCA	lateral femoral circumflex artery
LLD	limb length discrepancy
LRS	Limb Reconstruction System
MA	metatarsus adductus; mechanical axis
MACS	Manual Ability Classification System
MAD	mechanical axis deviation
MCL	medial collateral ligament
MCP	metacarpophalangeal
MCPJ	metacarpophalangeal joint
MD	Madelung deformity
MDA	metaphyseal–diaphyseal angle
MED	multiple epiphyseal dysplasia
MFCA	medial femoral circumflex artery
mLDFA	mechanical lateral distal femoral angle
mLDTA	mechanical lateral distal tibial angle
mLPFA	mechanical lateral proximal femoral angle
mMPTA	mechanical medial proximal tibial angle
mPFL	medial patellofemoral ligament
MPJ	metatarsophalangeal joint
MPS	mucopolysaccharidoses
MRA	magnetic resonance arthrography
MTPJ	metatarsophalangeal joint
NAI	non-accidental injury
NF	neurofibromatosis
NF1	neurofibromatosis type 1
NICE	National Institute for Health and Care Excellence

NIPT	non-invasive prenatal test
NMD	neuromuscular disorder
NSA	neck shaft angle
NSAID	non-steroidal anti-inflammatory drug
OBPI	obstetric brachial plexus injury
OCD	osteochonditis dissecans
OR	odds ratio
PA	popliteal angle
PADI	posterior atlanto-dens index
PASTA	partial articular supraspinatus tendon avulsion
PCL	posterior cruciate ligament
PCT	procalcitonin
PFFD	proximal femoral focal deficiency
PFJ	patellofemoral joint
PHHA	posterior humeral head articulation
PHV	peak height velocity
PIPJ	proximal interphalangeal joint
PIS	pinning in situ
PLS	Paediatric Life Support
PMN	polymorphonuclear
PO_4	phosphate
PPA	patellar progression angle
PSA	posterior sloping angle
PSACH	pseudoachondroplasia
PSIS	posterior superior iliac spine
PTFL	posterior talofibular ligament
PTH	parathyroid hormone
PTiFL	posterior tibiofibular ligament
RANK	receptor activator of nuclear factor kappa B
RMI	Reimer's migration index
ROD	renal osteodystrophy
ROM	range of motion; range of movement
RVAD	rib–vertebra angle difference
SAC	space available to the cord
SAPHO	synovitis, acne, pustulosis, hyperostosis, and osteitis
SAR	structures at risk
SBA	single best answer
SCFE	slipped capital femoral epiphysis
SCH	supracondylar humerus fracture
SCIWORA	Spinal cord injury without radiological abnormality
SD	standard deviation; skeletal dysplasia
SDR	selective dorsal rhizotomy
SED	spondyloepiphyseal dysplasia

SEDC	spondyloepiphyseal dysplasia congenita
SEDT	spondyloepiphyseal dysplasia tarda
SEMLS	single event multilevel surgery
SER	supination–external rotation
SH	Salter–Harris
SHORDT	shortening osteotomy realignment distal tibia
SHUEE	Shriners Hospital Upper Extremity Evaluation
SMA	spinal muscular atrophy
SMO	supramalleolar foot orthosis
SPNBF	subperiosteal new bone formation
SRT	substrate reduction therapy
SUFE	slipped upper femoral epiphysis
SUPERankle	systematic utilitarian procedure for extremity reconstruction
SWASH	Sitting, Walking, And Standing Hip (brace)
TAMTA	transmalleolar thigh angle
TAR	thrombocytopenia absent radii
TB	tuberculosis
TCA	talocalcaneal angle
TEN	titanium elastic nail
TFA	thigh–foot angle; tibiofemoral angle
TGF	transforming growth factor
TLSO	thoracic, lumbar, and sacral orthosis
TMA	transmalleolar thigh angle; tarsometatarsal angle
TMDA	tibial–metaphyseal–diaphyseal angle
TSF	Taylor Spatial Frame
TTTG	tibial tuberosity trochlear groove
UBC	unicameral bone cyst
UCL	ulnar collateral ligament
UV	ultraviolet
VACTERL	vertebral defects, anal atresia, cardiac defects, tracheo-oesophageal fistula, renal anomalies, and limb abnormalities
VDRO	varus and derotation osteotomy
vEDS	vascular Ehlers–Danlos syndrome
VMO	vastus medialis obliquus
WBC	white blood cell count
WCC	10
WES	whole exome sequencing
WGS	whole genome sequencing
ZPA	zone of polarizing activity
ZPC	zone of provisional calcification

Introduction and General Preparation

Paul A. Banaszkiewicz

Introduction

The same sentiments still apply from our first edition's chapter that general FRCS (Tr & Orth) exam guidance material can become a little dull and tedious to most candidates. We again have tried to avoid any unnecessary repetition of material, concentrating on the important details vital for exam success.

Since we wrote the introduction chapter for the first edition book several years ago, candidate preparation for the FRCS (Tr & Orth) exam has significantly altered in two major ways. The first is the established use of WhatsApp groups for exam preparation, and the second is an even bigger more widespread reliance on being part of a study group for exam preparation.

One of the major concerns for most candidates is to know the most likely paediatric viva questions that regularly appear in the exam. Equally important is to be aware of any unusual clinical cases that have unexpectedly appeared in the Section 2 exam. This is especially important for the intermediate cases as a difficult, unusual condition can sink your day.

Facioscapulohumeral muscular dystrophy is a fairly rare case that, for most candidates, is off their radar for the clinical exam. In several consecutive diets of exams, this disorder ended up as an intermediate case. Candidates who had no clue about the condition almost invariably failed badly, whilst those in the know usually performed very well. There was usually a large discrepancy in performance between the two types of candidates. A candidate's performance on this particular intermediate case could be the defining feature of whether a candidate passed or failed their entire exam.

In the last five years, there has been widespread normalization in the use of WhatsApp groups for exam preparation. At its most basic level, this involves candidates listing their own exam experiences almost immediately after their exam is completed. As such, questions are widely circulated and freely available for both trainees and non-trainees to digest.

The problems that existed with the 'candidate accounts' that floated around on the Internet still exist with the WhatsApp accounts. Most 'candidate experiences' are all written in a very similar vein and after reading the first two or three, very little extra new material is then uncovered. Also these accounts become just an endless list of topics without a structured answer to the question being provided.

Study groups are now more than ever vital for exam success, with many groups scheduling 1–2 hours of exam discussion and practice on the Internet most nights.

The aims of the exam are to see if you have enough knowledge to practise safely as a day-one orthopaedic consultant in a district general hospital in the generality of orthopaedics. The exam is not set out to test you in microscopic detail about trivial irrelevancies. The exam is not even designed to test for subspecialty interest. The other quoted analogy that is often used by Royal Colleges is that the exam should be viewed as a mature conversation between two consultant colleagues. I have never bought into this comparison but you will equally find many who accept this metaphor.

The first day you are on call as a consultant, your registrar may phone you up about a child with a painful hip in casualty. A child with knock knees may have been wrongly referred to your adult knee clinic. Your trauma practice may cover children and you may worry about risks of growth arrest with particular fracture patterns.

The History of the FRCS (Tr & Orth) Exam

In the late 1970s, the old-style FRCS ceased to mark the end of training and had become the entry into higher surgical training. The only exam in Britain devoted exclusively to orthopaedics was the MChOrth from the University of Liverpool. To take this exam, you generally had to work in or around the Mersey Deanery.

The situation was clearly unsatisfactory and, under the guidance of the Royal College of Surgeons in Edinburgh, a Specialty Fellowship exam in orthopaedics was introduced in 1979. This exam was optional but soon became established as a benchmark of completion of training and a quality assurance measure. It was an entirely clinical exam with a viva voce format. The standard was high, and the pass mark variable. It was not an easy exam to pass, but it became accepted that recognition of the standard of higher surgical training by assessment in the form of an exam is essential in orthopaedics. This is, in fact, applicable to all surgical specialties, not just orthopaedics.

In time, the exam was accepted by all four Royal Colleges, and in 1990, a new intercollegiate exam was introduced. This originally took place twice a year in each of the colleges in turn. This exam became a requirement for accreditation, together with the satisfactory completion of training in an approved programme that had been inspected and approved by the Specialist Advisory Committee.

For many years, it was difficult to get hold of any valuable exam guidance. The exam appeared to be surrounded in secrecy. Despite a curriculum and syllabus, many candidates entered the exam not really knowing what to expect. The usual line was that if you had undertaken good clinical work, read the appropriate literature and had a sound grasp of basic sciences, you would be expected to pass.

It was generally difficult to get useful information and tips from previous candidates, such as the expected standard or the questions likely to be asked. Another fact – now easily forgotten – was that the Internet was in its infancy and there simply was not the candidate support network that there is today.

There were not a large number of courses available to guide a candidate on the expected standard, and some courses set the level far too high. The idea was that you were panicked into hitting the books, as you perceived that your knowledge was not up to the required standard. This was fine if you had a year or so to go before the exam and you could plan a more intensive schedule of revision, but not so good if your exam was sooner.

The situation began to change around the turn of the millennium. A number of candidates began writing down their own experiences as a revision tool for the next wave of candidates sitting the exam. A small select number of candidates in larger training programmes began to form study groups. These study groups acquired, and circulated, these candidate accounts among themselves to help with exam preparation. The deal was that once you had passed, you wrote your own account for those candidates coming after you to use for their preparation. In time, these candidate experience reports began to circulate more freely in a wider domain.

Today there are numerous websites containing candidates' exam experiences. These include the British Orthopaedic Trainee Association, various regional training programme sites, and lastly individual accounts from successful candidates. The major problem with many candidate experiences is that they deal with specific viva or clinical questions in a rather superficial way, mainly with bullet point headings. Also, we have yet to see an unsuccessful candidate's experience posted on the Internet. Candidates generally learn more from what went wrong than if only successful accounts are presented. WhatsApp groups and Telegram are now replacing the Internet as means for trainees to quickly communicate to each other exam tips and tricks or to discuss difficult learning points.

The standard of FRCS (Tr & Orth) exam courses has, by and large, significantly improved and, in general, candidates are much more informed and have a better idea of what types of question tend to get asked. So one of the most major changes with the FRCS (Tr & Orth) exam in the last 10 years is that the mystery surrounding it has completely evaporated away.

The old-style viva with a variable number of questions is definitely a thing of the past. The viva is now standardized for candidates, with similar questions being asked for each topic covered. This leads to a much fairer exam, with much less potential for any discrimination.

Exam Format

The current FRCS (Tr & Orth) exam encompasses two sections: Section 1 is a written exam, and Section 2 the clinical and oral exams. For further information, and to make sure that your information is up to date, we suggest that you carefully review the Intercollegiate Specialty Board website (www.jcie.org.uk).

Section 1

Section 1 is the written component of the Intercollegiate Examination in Trauma and Orthopaedic Surgery. In 2018, the Joint Committee on Intercollegiate Examinations (JCIE) agreed to phase out extended matching item (EMI) questions. When compared to single best answer (SBA) questions, EMI questions were less able to differentiate between candidates and were difficult to construct. EMI questions have not featured in the FRCS (Tr & Orth) examinations from January 2021 onwards.

Section 1 exam will consist of two papers as follows:

Paper 1 (2 hours and 15 minutes)

SBA – 120 questions

Paper 2 (2 hours and 15 minutes)

SBA – 120 questions

Total 4 hours and 30 minutes – 240 questions.

Candidates will have a two-year period from their first attempt to pass the Section 1 exam, with a maximum of four attempts with no re-entry. Details are available on the JCIE website (www.jcie.org.uk). Candidates with proven dyslexia may be eligible for the Section 1 examination times to be extended and this should be highlighted in advance of the exam.

There is no negative marking; therefore, all questions should be attempted. Sample questions can be viewed on the JCIE website. Experienced examiners perform a formal process of standard setting to decide the final pass mark for each paper. SBA questions are subject to quality assurance procedures, including feedback from both examiners and candidates. Difficulty level, content, discrimination index, and internal consistency are analysed. Ambiguous questions, or those deemed insufficient to differentiate between candidates, are removed through this process.

SBA questions consist of an introductory theme, a question stem, and five possible responses (listed as A to E), of which one is the most appropriate answer. SBA questions are exactly what the name suggests: candidates choose the best from five possible answers. It is important to note that this is not a 'single correct answer', but a 'single best answer'. Moreover, all five possible answers could be considered correct, but candidates are asked which is best, or most appropriate, given the information provided. As questions are designed to test higher-order thinking, this could mean that limited or irrelevant information is provided. Questions require a judgement based on interpretation of the available evidence. Questions that candidates later complain about, for example 'there was more than one correct answer' or that a question was 'too ambiguous', can often prove the best performing questions.

For more detailed information on the dynamics of the Section 1 paper, candidates should read Chapters 1 and 2 of *SBAs for the FRCS (Tr&Orth) Examination: A Companion to Postgraduate Orthopaedics Candidate's Guide.*

Section 2

This underwent major changes in 2020. For some time, the General Medical Council (GMC) had been keen to remove altogether the clinical examination component from the Section 2 exam. There were considerable ongoing discussions and disagreement among the GMC, the four Royal Colleges, and various stakeholders. A compromise was reached in that although the short cases would be replaced by short case clinical examination technique vivas, the intermediate cases involving patients would remain. There would be four intermediate cases, with one of them being simulated.

The introduction of this new Section 2 clinical exam was significantly disrupted with the Covid-19 pandemic, with several exam diets being cancelled. There was an urgent need to begin examining a large backlog of trainees to prevent the orthopaedic training system from grinding to a halt. It was therefore decided to temporarily hold the clinical component without direct patient involvement using iPads. Six short case examination vivas were introduced, along with the temporary use of simulated intermediate cases, both showing candidates a series of clinical photographs on iPads on which questions were based. When the pandemic settles, it is expected that patient involvement with the intermediate cases will resume.

The clinical component was often viewed as the most difficult part of the whole exam to pass and these changes had a major impact on how candidates prepare for the exam. Although the Royal Colleges remain positive and upbeat, a significant number of consultants are disappointed with the changes. If you are an educationalist, you are likely to follow the party line and state that the exam assessment will remain as robust as ever. In practice, there is a huge difference in skills, professionalism, and knowledge required to examine a patient with a rotator cuff tear, and elicit and interpret positive clinical signs, as opposed to just describing how you would go about examining for this in a viva situation. If you have prelearnt the talk and gone through some practice runs in your study group, you should be more than halfway towards passing the viva.

The short case clinical examination technique viva involves candidates being shown a clinical case and describing how they would go about examining that patient – for paediatrics, it could be a picture of a young child with a unilateral pes planus deformity, perhaps an obvious tarsal coalition – and describing their approach to that particular patient.

Superficially, this viva is similar to the oral topics viva, but the Joint Surgical Colleges Fellowship Examination (JSCFE) Committee are at great pains to point out that the clinical short case vivas are very different. There are no questions on management of the condition and the specific aim of the viva is to work through clinical examination. Be prepared to be grilled in detail about how you perform a particular clinical test, and the theory behind it. More important than how you perform a particular test is how the test will change your management of the condition. For example, if the Coleman block test demonstrates that the hindfoot is rigid, how will this change your management of the pes cavus deformity?

A decision has been reached to minimize the use of radiographs or scans in this viva, as this will avoid steering the conversation on to management.

Candidates' feedback for the paediatric short case clinical vivas suggests that these are particularly difficult to answer. Previously, unless the exam was being held near a paediatric tertiary centre, the amount of complex paediatric cases brought into the exam hall was usually limited. Now a photograph of a very rare paediatric condition can be shown and candidates may struggle to piece together a structured examination format to satisfy the examiners. Added to this, the general unfamiliarity of this new exam format means that stress levels are much greater in paediatric clinicals than was ever the case.

Clinicals

The clinicals are divided into six five-minute clinical examination technique vivas, including upper and lower limb, as well as spine, vivas.

At present, there are four intermediate cases, 15 minutes each (five-minute history, five-minute clinical examination, five-minute discussion). These involve patients.

Orals

The oral component is divided into four 30-minute viva sections:
- Basic science
- Trauma, including spine
- Adult elective orthopaedics, including spine
- Paediatric orthopaedics and hand surgery, including shoulder and elbow.

Paediatric Section

The paediatric oral section is combined with the hands and upper limbs section. The examiners have to introduce themselves to the candidate and remind the candidate which oral he or she is about to be examined on, to allow the candidate time to settle. Feedback is given where appropriate such as: 'OK, let's move on' or 'We have covered this area, let's go on'. Examiners are encouraged to avoid remarks such as 'Excellent', 'Well done', 'That's great', or 'Fantastic'.

Props, such as radiographs, pictures, and charts, are usually used to lead into a question.

Three paediatric topics are discussed – these usually cover a trauma-type question, one big (A-list) topic, and a less obvious clinical topic.

Hammering on when a candidate could not answer a question used to be a common candidate complaint, but examiners are now actively dissuaded from this practice.

All candidates are treated in exactly the same manner and marks are based on performance only. Examiners are instructed to allow for candidates' nervousness and are told not to respond to inappropriate behaviour by a candidate. Inappropriate behaviour would include rudeness or sarcastic remarks to the examiners, impoliteness, and bad-mannered or derogatory comments about facilities or organization issues.

A significant change is that viva questions are now more clinically orientated and relevant to the types of situation that may present to a consultant orthopaedic surgeon in clinical practice. For this reason, potential exam questions are now significantly more scrutinized than previously, before being approved by the exam committee for inclusion in the exam.

When to Sit the Exam

It is generally accepted that you will need about one full year of preparation before you will feel confident to sit the exam.

In theory, it should be relatively easy for you to decide if you have enough experience and have prepared in sufficient detail to sit the exam. In practice, a multitude of competing issues usually complicate this decision.

If you are a trainee, you will have been sitting the UK In-Training Exam for the last three or four years and should know your annual scores. Many training programmes also have yearly mock clinical and viva exams, and will not let you sit the real exam unless you have achieved a good enough pass in these mock tests.

In the past, you may have had a charitable training programme director who was willing to take a chance with you, but this is now less likely, as it may have a direct bearing on the number of trainees allocated to a region.

As a general rule, do not use up an attempt if you are underprepared and unlikely to pass, as you have only four attempts at the exam and you are essentially throwing away one opportunity. The old advice that it would be good practice and allow you to sail through the second attempt is a wrong tactic, and is out-of-date advice from a different time.

Study Groups

A key factor for your success will be the formation of a study group that meets regularly, discusses various topics, and arranges practice viva sessions.

Study groups now more than ever are very important and the key to successfully and as painlessly as possible passing the exam. They offer support and help to an otherwise long, lonely and difficult exam journey. Just as important is the opportunity that study groups allow for individuals to talk through and conceptualize difficult topics. A large part (but not all) of the exam is about how well you can communicate to the examiners. The more practice you get, the more skilled you will be with this.

There are a number of factors that will contribute to a study group's success and also some aspects that you should avoid. The group should comprise 3–4 candidates who all need to get along well with each other and should not be too far apart from one another in terms of knowledge. If there are significant rivalries and petty jealousies within the group, with trainees trying to score points off each other, the group is not going to work out. Be careful of candidates who think that they are too good for the group; they are likely to let you down near the end and do their own thing.

Also, be careful with candidates who are unlikely to pass the exam first time round and who are just too far behind with their studies to contribute significantly to group discussions. Give these candidates the benefit of the doubt, as surprises do happen, but be concerned if you draw repeated blanks with large gaps in core knowledge. Politely sideline such candidates if the extra input is significantly affecting the group's performance. In general, do not include candidates who are a few months, or perhaps a year, off sitting the exam. They are unlikely to have sufficient motivation and drive at this stage in their revision.

Study groups have refined their study techniques in that there is more savvy use of the Internet late at night and at weekends to have in-depth discussions of topics and viva practice. Particularly with some like-minded trainees working in various parts of the country, they may organize regular Zoom meetings to go through topics.

Some trainees arrange to meet up with each other for 2–3 days before the actual exam to practise their own viva exam approach.

Covid-19 and Webinars

With the Covid-19 pandemic, there has been a huge explosion in the amount of online webinars available to candidates. A substantial number are directed towards the FRCS (Tr & Orth) exam. As a resource for learning, webinars are controversial and have had a mixed response. Some trainees definitely prefer this learning medium and believe that it is the way forward for the future. Others view the whole thing as passive learning, with trainees at home, with their feet up on a couch, not really actively involved with the process.

Webinars can be presented live or be pre-recorded. Prerecorded webinars allow the lecture to be broadcast at a later date and means that the lecture can be redone a few times until it is fit for purpose. Live is more spontaneous, but mistakes can occur in delivery and there are always some delays with screen sharing. It is also possible to have breakout groups and smaller group teaching sessions.

Some accounts are free but usually have limited facilities available, whilst to stream professionally can be very expensive. Quality can vary, depending on Internet connectivity and whether a professional webcam is used.

The four Royal Colleges have recorded many webinars, which are now available on their website, as an educational resource. With so many different webinars available, candidates need to be focused and efficient in their use of study time.

There are also large sources of YouTube videos and podcasts available to trainees. Some sources are excellent, and others less so, but it is important that trainees are ruthless in weighing up whether to use that particular source and the benefit it will provide.

Last-Minute Preparation

In the last 2–3 weeks leading up to the exam, try not to panic and attempt to go over all your revision again. This will not work and will just lead to you getting even more stressed and irrational. Use this time for quick, focused revision.

Attending a last-minute revision course as a sort of dry run a couple of weeks before the real exam is becoming more popular. This only really works if you are not too far away from the required standard and the dry run is used to iron out, finetune, and rehearse your performance. Hoping to get lucky with a sort of quick revision before the real exam, but with significant knowledge gaps, is unlikely to be successful.

Exam Tactics

Dress sensibly: no loud ties, short shirts, or Vivienne Westwood high heels. Everything straight down the line. Do not stand out. Do not smell of cigarettes, as this is very off-putting for most people. A bit of cologne is OK, but unless you have a body odour problem, be careful not to use too much, as this may also be offputting to examiners.

If you tend to sweat a lot under your armpits, get yourself a strong proven deodorant to avoid this. We see a small number of candidates in the exam where their armpits are covered in huge wet patches of sweat. This must be uncomfortable for candidates and off-putting to patients. In simple terms, although this should not affect your mark, it just does not look good.

If you are one of a small number of candidates who are significantly affected by exam stress, it may be reasonable to get some professional help. The scenario during the exam would be extreme nervousness, difficulty focusing on what question is being asked, wet armpits, and sweat pouring off your face. This situation is very uncomfortable and will affect your performance. A beta-blocker will probably have no significant physiological affect but psychologically may help to calm you down and improve your overall exam performance. We would suggest speaking to your GP for advice.

Book a hotel fairly near the exam venue, preferably within walking distance, although this may not always be possible.

Allow plenty of time to arrive promptly at the exam. We know the arguments of turning up too early and getting freaked out by other candidates talking too much and winding you up. This is irritating, but a fair amount less stressful than leaving your arrival to the last minute and risking that you get caught up in traffic and turn up late.

Keep Your Distance

A piece of advice that we keep repeating is to get away from other exam candidates as quickly as possible after completing the various exam sections. It is extremely questionable whether anything useful can be gained by hanging around to chat to other candidates after completing the clinicals or vivas.

At best, this will unnerve you and can make you feel uncomfortable; at worst, it will put you off for the remaining parts of the exam. Even worse, you may end up in a bar afterward, drowning the sorrows of a perceived poor performance and ruin any chances of that last-minute brush-up of key topics you had planned for later that evening.

Stay focused during the exam period. Don't let your guard down; don't relax, and don't be fooled into a false sense of security.

At the same time, and in equal measure, don't get paranoid, edgy, and uptight, as this is just as counterproductive. You need to come across as relaxed and professional, as someone who is in control and who can be relied on. This mindset is much easier to achieve if you stay clear of other candidates. Perhaps the only exception should be candidates in your study group; you could chat to them for a few minutes after each exam section.

Suggested Reading

Which orthopaedic paediatric books to use for preparation for the paediatric section of the FRCS (Tr & Orth) exam is very much a matter of personal preference and choice. However, some books are more suited and better to use than others.

[1] Practice of Pediatric Orthopaedics

The numerous illustrations are first class, and the book has excellent recommendations and reviews. It is easy to read and fairly comprehensive. In view of the changes in the clinicals with the introduction of short case examination vivas, the large volume of pictures are especially useful to help with pattern recognition and spot diagnoses.

[2] Joseph's Paediatric Orthopaedics

We were a little guarded in our previous review of the first edition, but the book has gone onto a second edition, so perhaps we were being too harsh with our criticisms. Overall, it is an excellent book to borrow from a library, and perhaps buy if you can get a discounted copy, rather than having to buy the more expensive hardback edition.

The book is targeted at higher surgical trainees and younger consultants. It is written by paediatric orthopaedic surgeons from four different continents. Although this gives the book a truly international flavour, in the highly focused world of FRCS (Tr & Orth) exams, this can be a drawback.

It is firmly emphasized on treatment, allowing trainee orthopaedic surgeons to make an informed contribution during their time in the paediatrics department and to speak confidently about the approach to individual patients during their specialty exams.

[3] Pediatric Orthopaedic Secrets, 3rd ed

By and large, the Secrets series has improved greatly in recent years. Some of the material in the paediatric book does not particularly match the FRCS (Tr & Orth) syllabus and the format is only loosely applicable to the exam. That said, we have come across a number of candidates who swear by the Secrets series. We advise that you borrow one from the library before buying. It has good reviews. The book has not been updated since 2007 but does not feel out of date just yet. It has a question-and-answer format that some candidates may find useful.

[4] Oxford Textbook of Trauma and Orthopaedics, 2nd ed

This is more of a reference book with a fairly detailed paediatric section. Reducing the three-volume first edition into a single volume in the second edition was a masterstroke and makes the book much easier to read.

[5] Miller's Review of Orthopaedics

This has a reasonably good paediatric section. As the text is listed, the section is probably best suited for revision for Section 1 of the FRCS (Tr & Orth) exam.

[6] AAOS Comprehensive Orthopaedic Review

This book is similar in style to Miller's, but more comprehensive. It has excellent reviews and is recommended for FRCS (Tr & Orth) exam preparation. The biggest drawback is the price.

[7] Paediatric Orthopaedics in Clinical Practice

This book is great, but whilst reading, a candidate may get an uneasy feeling that there are more focused paediatric FRCS (Tr & Orth) exam-related books that should be taking priority. It is a broad-based book that can be used by a number of different doctors dealing with paediatric orthopaedics.

[8] Pediatric Orthopedics in Practice

This is a comprehensive book that is very well written and easily digestible. It is expensive and has a European slant, so it is unlikely to be many candidates' first choice of book to buy. Worth a look-through if you need a slightly different approach to that hard-to-understand topic with which you may be struggling.

[9] Paediatrics for the FRCS (Tr + Orth) Examination

This is a great book written for the FRCS (Tr & Orth) exam. Lots of hidden gems within and exam-orientated viva questions to keep you occupied. Highly recommended.

[10] Core Knowledge in Orthopaedics: Pediatric Orthopaedics

We bought this book several years ago, and it was a reasonable book at the time to use as a guide for a number of different paediatrics-related projects with which we were involved. The book is beginning to date and one to perhaps pass over, as there are

[11] Pediatrics (Orthopaedic Surgery Essentials Series)

This is a great series that include many fantastic subject titles such as basic science and lower limb arthroplasty. The book is written by American authors so is not well suited to the UK FRCS (Tr & Orth) exam. The book does need to be updated. One to buy second-hand if going for a bargain on Amazon.

[12] Orthopaedic Knowledge Update: Pediatrics

Some candidates like these books. We have used this series in the past but have become a bit indifferent to it. It does have its moments and candidates may find some chapters useful for consolidation purposes. An American book that is expensive to buy whilst attempting to create a monopoly on education.

References

1. Diab M, Staheli LT. (2015) *Practice of Pediatric Orthopaedics*, 3rd ed. Philadelphia, PA: Lippincott Williams & Wilkins.

2. Joseph B, Nayagam S, Loder R, Torode I. (2009) *Paediatric Orthopaedics: A System of Decision-Making*. London: Hodder Arnold.

3. Staheli LT, Song KM. (2007) *Pediatric Orthopaedic Secrets*, 3rd ed. Philadelphia, PA: Elsevier Saunders.

4. Bulstrode C, Wilson-MacDonald J, Eastwood D, *et al.* (2017) *Oxford Textbook of Trauma and Orthopaedics*, 2nd ed. Oxford: Oxford University Press.

5. Miller MD. (2012) *Review of Orthopaedics*, 6th ed. Philadelphia, PA: Saunders.

6. Lieberman JR. (2009) *AAOS Comprehensive Orthopaedic Review*. Rosemont, IL: American Academy of Orthopaedic Surgeons.

7. Aresti NA, Ramachandran M, Paterson M, Barry M. (2016) *Paediatric Orthopaedics in Clinical Practice*, 1st ed. London: Springer.

8. Gelfer Y, Eastwood D, Daly K. (2018) *Pediatric Orthopaedics in Practice*, 1st ed. Oxford: Oxford University Press.

9. Gelfer Y, Eastwood D, Daly K. (2018) *Paediatrics for the FRCS (Tr + Orth) Examination*, 1st ed. Oxford: Oxford University Press.

10. Dormans JP. (2005) *Core Knowledge in Orthopaedics: Pediatric Orthopaedics*, 1st ed. St Louis, MO: Mosby.

11. Cramer KE, Scherl SA, Einhorn TA, Tornetta P. (2003) *Pediatrics (Orthopaedic Surgery Essentials Series)*, 1st ed. Boston, MA: Lippincott Williams and Wilkins.

12. Martus JE. (2003) *Orthopaedic Knowledge Update: Pediatrics 5*. Rosemont, IL: American Academy of Orthopaedic Surgeons.

Chapter 2

Clinical Assessment

Stan Jones and Sattar Alshryda

Introduction

Assessing a child with orthopaedic problems is more challenging than assessing adults. Children are poor historians and parents are usually emotional. Establishing a rapport during the first visit (and in the exam) is essential – although not always easy or possible. It gets easier with experience though.

The initial contact with the child and family involves introducing oneself to all the family members, including the child. This should be carried out in a professional, yet friendly, manner. The cultural background of the family should be considered and it is important to conform to gender order for introductions. Whenever possible, the discussion should be held with the child, whilst allowing the parents to add any relevant details or clarify some ambiguity.

The next stage of the assessment should aim to allay the anxiety/fear of the child. This can be done in a variety of ways and depends on the age of the child. In a younger child, the introduction to toys may be all that is required, whilst in the older child, it may involve talking about friends, sports, movies, school, or a piece of clothing.

History
Presenting Complaint

The three main complaints that bring children to a clinic (and exam) are:

1. Pain
2. Deformities (including physiological and pathological ones)
3. Altered functions (including gait abnormalities).

Ten relevant questions should be asked about the main complaint:

1. Duration of symptoms
2. Severity
3. Mode of onset
4. Any history of any injury or provoking factors
5. Frequency and timing of symptoms
6. Aggravating and relieving factors, and progression
7. Any functional impairment
8. Impact on carers, school, sports, and social life
9. Previous investigations and results
10. Treatment received and their effects.

It is also important to consider the presenting complaints in relation to the age of the child; for example, Perthes disease has to be considered as a differential in a young child (4–8 years of age) with a history of hip and knee pain, whereas in an adolescent with similar complaints, one has to think of slipped upper femoral epiphysis (SUFE).

Normal variants, including in-toeing, out-toeing, bowed legs, knocked knees, and flat feet, are common 'deformities' that trigger consultation. These must be confidently differentiated from similar pathological deformities such as Blount's disease, congenital vertical talus, and tarsal coalition.

Deformity that is unilateral, or asymmetric or progressive, is often pathological. Severe deformities (more than two standard deviations (SDs) to what is accepted for the same age and gender), associated short stature, overweight, or syndromes could be pathological.

Children's functions improve naturally as they get older (see Table 2.1 for key motor and social skills). Regression should trigger search for progressive neurodegenerative diseases and Rett's syndrome. Delayed milestones should trigger a thorough history and neurological examination before reassuring parents as within normal. Hand preference during the first two years of life is a sign of hemiplegic cerebral palsy (CP).

Table 2.1 Normal developmental milestones

Age	Motor skills	Social skills
3 months	Lifts head up when prone	Smiles when spoken to
6 months	Sits with support, head steady when sitting	Laughs and smiles spontaneously
9 months	Sits without support	Waves 'bye-bye', vocalizes 'ma-ma' or 'da-da'
1 year	Walks with one-hand support	Starts cooperating with dressing
2 years	Runs forward	Uses three-word sentences, matches colours
3 years	Jumps in place	Dresses oneself, puts on own shoes
5 years	Hops	Names four colours; counts 10 objects correctly
6 years	Skips	Does small buttons on shirt; ties bows on shoes

Birth History and Developmental Milestones

A history of antenatal problems, such as bleeding during pregnancy, maternal diabetes, and premature and/or difficult labour, is common in children with CP. Reduced fetal movements during late pregnancy has been associated with arthrogryposis. First pregnancy, breech presentation, and oligohydramnios have been linked to developmental dysplasia of the hip (DDH). Nowadays, club foot and major congenital limb deformities are diagnosed during antenatal fetal ultrasound.

Enquire about developmental milestones, for example when the child first sat and walked. In a third of late walkers, the cause is pathological, for example CP [1].

Family History

A number of genetic or non-genetic orthopaedic conditions run in some families. DDH and club foot are common in families who have first-degree members with the same condition. Multiple bony exostoses and osteogenesis imperfecta are genetic diseases and therefore are common among relatives.

Finally, a history of past illnesses and hospitalizations completes the history.

Clinical Examination

Examination of a child commences as soon as the child and the family enter the consulting room. The child must continue to be observed, whilst the history is taken, as valuable clues can be gained.

The child should be undressed appropriately, but with their cooperation, and must be kept warm at all times. The modesty of the older child should always be respected, that is, by providing a gown.

The infant can be examined on the parent's lap.

Examination should be focused and relevant to the presenting complaint. A systematic approach is important, but this can be modified according to the child's preference or the situation. The examination generally involves:

- General assessment/screening
- Functional assessment (walking, running, sitting, standing, picking objects, writing, turning keys, etc.)
- Specific assessment of joints or parts (the 'look, feel, move, and special tests' approach).

General Assessment/Screening

1. Inspection of the child's (or parents') face may reveal the following:

   a. Typical features such as in trisomy 21 (flat face with upward and slanted palpebral fissures or epicanthic folds, high-arched palate). Recognized dysmorphic features suggestive of a syndrome or skeletal dysplasia such as achondroplasia (average-sized trunk, short upper arms and thighs, large head with prominent forehead) (Figure 2.1)

   b. Plagiocephaly and congenital torticollis are signs of packaging disorders; check for hip dysplasia (Figure 2.2)

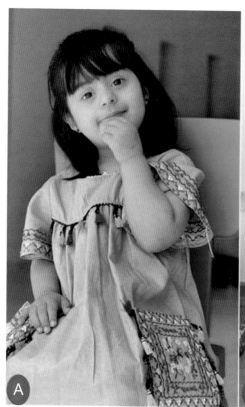
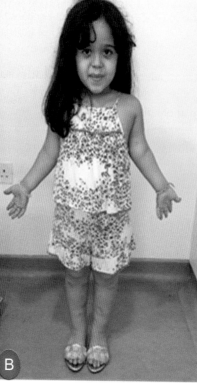

Figure 2.1 A typical facial appearance can give a clue for the underlying diagnosis and problems. (A) shows a child with trisomy 21, and (B) shows a child with achondroplasia.

c. Blue eyes – a parent with blue eyes may clinch the diagnosis of osteogenesis imperfecta (see Chapter 25, Figure 25.11)

d. Facial asymmetry, large (asymmetric) tongue – may suggest Beckwith–Wiedemann syndrome (Figure 2.3)

e. Observe for wheelchairs, walking aids, orthoses, and shoes

f. Look for skin changes, café-au-lait spots, axillary freckling, and neurofibromas (see Chapter 24, Figure 24.4) – are suggestive of neurofibromatosis; vascular

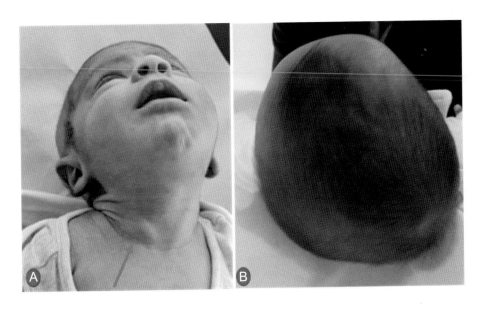

Figure 2.2 (A) Congenital torticollis with typical sternomastoid tumour (blue arrow – not always present). (B) Positional plagiocephaly. Both signs have been associated with DDH. It is important to differentiate the latter from craniosynostosis, which is a premature closure of one of the skull sutures. In positional plagiocephaly, both fontanelles are open, and posterior and anterior head flattening is parallel and usually gets better quickly over a few weeks. If in doubt, refer to neurosurgery.

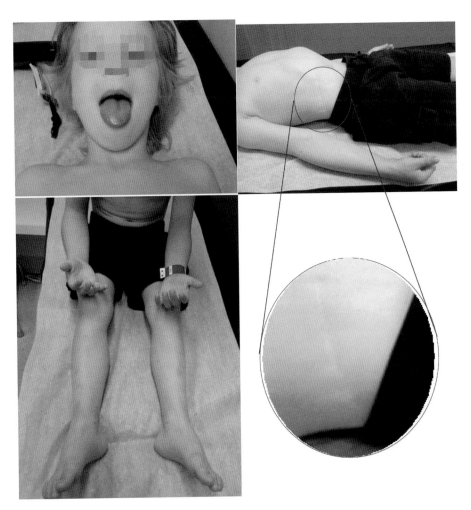

Figure 2.3 A child with Beckwith–Wiedemann syndrome. There is hemihypertrophy of the right side of the body, including the face and tongue. There is a right lower abdominal scar from a previous nephrectomy.

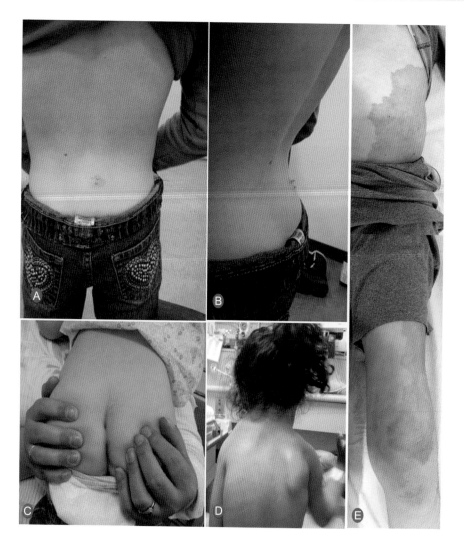

Figure 2.4 Useful signs on general inspection of the back. (A) and (B) show skin tag and fatty swelling in a patient with lipomeningocele (see also Chapter 18, Figure 18.25 which shows the feet of the same patient). (C) shows a sacral dimple in an infant with developmental dysplasia of the hip; be wary of spinal cord tethering. (D) shows a patient with Klippel–Feil syndrome and Sprengel's shoulder associated with vertebral fusion. (E) shows vascular malformation associated with several syndromes such as Klippel–Trenaunay–Weber syndrome.

marking (haemangiomas) – may suggest Klippel–Trenaunay–Weber syndrome; hairy patches, skin tags, or sacral dimples – may indicate underlying spinal pathology (Figure 2.4); nail abnormalities in ectodermal dysplasia and nail–patella syndrome (Figure 2.5).

2. Screening for height and weight of the child and parents, paying attention to asymmetry in body proportions; for example, disproportion between the truncal height and limb lengths may suggest a skeletal dysplasia. These measurements are usually performed by nursing staff before the consultation and should be entered into age- and gender-specific charts.

Functional Assessment

This is the second part of children's orthopaedic examination. It is less intimidating than the third part and can reveal a substantive amount of information.

Ask the Child to Stand

Whilst the child is standing, inspection is carried out from the front, sides, and back, assessing:

- The standing posture and curvature of the spine
- The level and contour of the shoulders
- The level of the anterior superior iliac spines
- For any evidence of genu valgum or varus (intermalleolar and intercondylar distance)
- For calf hypertrophy (myopathy) or muscular wasting
- For surgical or other scars
- For hindfoot alignment – valgus or varus
- For evidence of tiptoeing, flat foot, or cavus deformity.

The Gowers' test is carried out if a myopathy is suspected. Gowers' sign is positive if a child, on rising from sitting on the floor, uses his hands to climb up his thighs for support (Figure 2.6).

Ask the Patient to Walk

Gait and gait abnormalities are fully covered in Chapter 18c. However, a quick summary relevant to this chapter is presented here.

The child is then asked to walk in a straight line. Whilst doing so, observe from the feet upward:

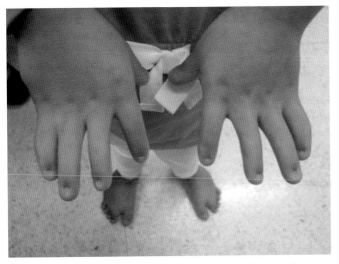

Figure 2.5 Absent nails. Nail abnormalities can be a manifestation of, or associated with, several orthopaedic conditions such as nail–patella syndrome and ectodermal dysplasia.

- Feet – is there heel strike? What is the foot progression angle? Is there a problem with clearance?
- Knee extension on heel strike and knee flexion in swing – is the patella pointing inwards or outwards?
- Hips – flex for 45° on heel strike and extend fully on toe-off (pre-swing)
- Trunk – should move smoothly on the weight-bearing side without excessive shift (no Trendelenburg gait)
- Upper limb swing
- Explore any evidence of a limp (asymmetrical movement of the lower limbs).

Table 2.2 summarizes the commonest types of gait that we encounter in a paediatric orthopaedic clinic.

Ask the Patient to Run

This will uncover spasticity (which is speed-dependent hypertonia) and distract children from performing their best gait.

Table 2.2 Commonest types of gait encountered in a paediatric orthopaedic clinic

Types	Description
Antalgic	The stance phase of the affected limb is hurried, with a quick swing phase of the opposite limb. This is usually caused by a painful condition of the affected limb
Trendelenburg	Normally, during stance phase, the hip abductors of the standing leg keep the opposite part of the body upward. A Trendelenburg gait is caused by failure of the hip abductor mechanism. The opposite pelvis dips down, instead of rising, during the stance phase of gait. Often there is a compensatory lurch of the body to the affected side to bring the body's centre of gravity to the centre of the standing leg, for example, dislocated hip, short femoral neck, weak hip abductors
Short limb	As the name implies, this gait is observed in children with a short limb. The shoulder on the side of the shorter lower limb dips down during the stance phase of gait
High stepping	This gait pattern is usually observed in children with a foot drop or an equinus deformity. A lack of sufficient ankle dorsiflexion during the swing phase results in increased knee flexion to facilitate clearance of the foot
Toe walking	This is observed when a child's initial contact is with the forefoot, and not with the hind foot. This is covered in more detail in Chapter 25
Ataxic	This gait pattern is broad-based (like a drunk's!). Seen in cerebellar conditions

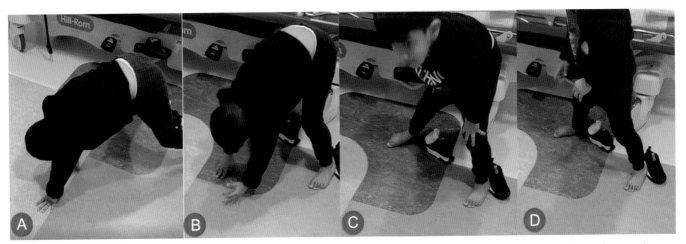

Figure 2.6 (A-D) A child with a positive Gowers' sign. The child uses his hands on his knees to support his trunk muscles to be able to stand. He is known to have Duchenne muscular dystrophy.

Upper Limb Functions

Given the functional importance of the hands and upper limbs, patients are usually referred to the occupational therapist for comprehensive assessment and documentation. However, a quick screening for the ability to pick objects from a table, turning keys in doors, writing, washing the face, and brushing hair or teeth is clinically useful and relevant.

Specific Assessment of Joints or Parts

This part of the assessment should be tailor-made to where the problem is and the nature of the problem. As in the adult, the 'look, feel, move, and special tests' approach is recommended. Many relevant findings are shown in the corresponding chapters of this book. However, we describe some useful tests and techniques in this section to complement knowledge in the subsequent chapters.

Hip Joint

'Look and feel' may not yield much information as the hip is a deep-seated joint, although scars may be observed. Assess active, before passive, joint range of motion (ROM) in all directions (flexion and extension; abduction and adduction; internal and external rotations). If active ROM is full, assessing passive ROM is not required. It is imperative to stabilize the pelvis during ROM testing to ensure that hip, and not pelvic, movements are measured.

Internal and external rotations are often examined in the prone position (with the hip fully extended). Again, the pelvis and trunk must be stabilized to prevent the body from rocking during examination which could produce errors in measurements.

Fixed flexion deformity is measured using the Thomas' test and is often used as a surrogate for hip extension. However, true hip extension can be measured in the prone position using the Staheli method (Figure 2.7).

Knee Joint

Contrary to the hip joint, inspection of the knee joint can reveal lots of information (Figure 2.8). Genu varum and genu valgum deformities are usually obvious, but procurvatum and recurvatum are usually less obvious (do not miss them!). Swelling around the knee may be localized or generalized. Localized swelling may be:

1. Anterior over the tibial tubercle (Osgood–Schlatter disease)
2. Posterior (popliteal cyst)
3. To the sides (bony exostosis or meniscal cyst).

Generalized swelling may be due to a large effusion or inflammatory synovitis.

Whilst the child is seated on a couch, with the limbs hanging freely, the position of the patella (alta or baja) and the way it tracks should be noted. Palpate for skin temperature and tenderness. The site of tenderness usually points to the underlying diseased parts.

Active ROM should be 0° (full extension) to 150° of flexion. Any limitation must be noted.

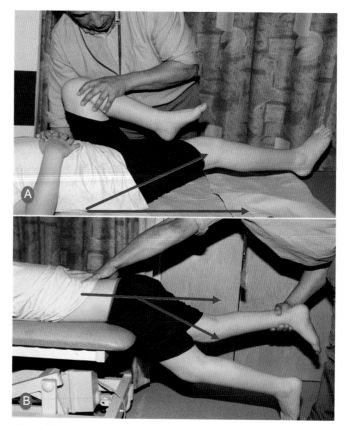

Figure 2.7 (A) The Thomas' test. The child is asked to flex both hips maximally, with the knees flexed. The examiner places a hand under the lumbar region to ensure that the lumbar spine is flat (i.e. the pelvis is neutral, with no anterior or posterior tilt) and any lumbar lordosis is eliminated. Next the tested side is allowed to extend on the examination couch, and the angle between the couch and the leg is measured as the fixed flexion deformity of the hip. Any potential for the pelvis to tilt can be minimized by flexing the opposite leg to stabilize the pelvis. In the presence of a fixed flexion deformity of the knee, it is advisable to allow the limb to extend over the side of the couch, thus enabling a true measurement of the hip flexion deformity. (B) The Staheli test. This measures the degree of hip extension (and not just the fixed flexion deformity) and is performed prone. The lumbar spine must be straight, and the pelvis in neutral. The examiner extends the thigh until this stops or the pelvis starts to rise. The horizontal thigh angle is the amount of hip extension. The above child has approximately 20° of fixed flexion deformity.

The medial and lateral collateral ligaments are assessed by applying valgus and varus stress, respectively, with the knee in extension and with 30° of flexion. The anterior cruciate ligament (ACL) and posterior cruciate ligament (PCL) are assessed using the anterior and posterior drawer tests. A modified McMurray's test is used to assess for a painful torn meniscus.

Foot and Ankle

Examination of the feet should be undertaken whilst the patient is standing, seating, and walking. Any scars, swellings, or deformities should be noted.

Localized tenderness may be observed over the second or third metatarsophalangeal joint (MPJ) in Freiberg's disease, on either side of the heels in Sever's disease, and over the navicular bones in accessory navicular bone of Kohler's disease (Figure 2.9).

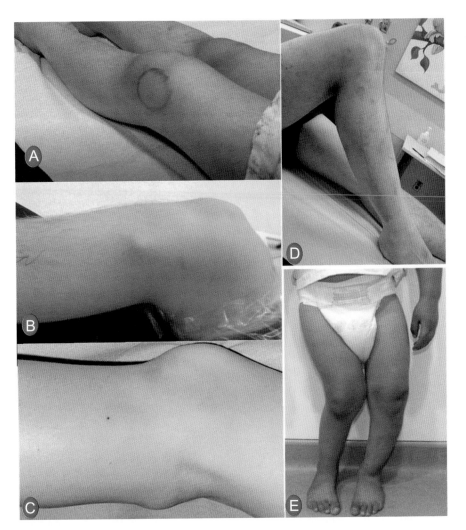

Figure 2.8 Knee inspection can reveal several abnormalities. (A) shows a generalized swelling (knee effusion). The circular mark is where the EMLA cream was applied for a later aspiration. The diagnosis is juvenile rheumatoid arthritis. (B) shows a bony swelling over the proximal tibia that was caused by osteochondroma. (C) shows a popliteal cyst. (D) shows a child with recurvatum. This child had lower limb trauma and posterior cruciate ligament (PCL) rupture. Notice the longitudinal scar of a previous fasciotomy for compartment syndrome. (E) shows a child with genu valgus deformity secondary to metabolic bone disease.

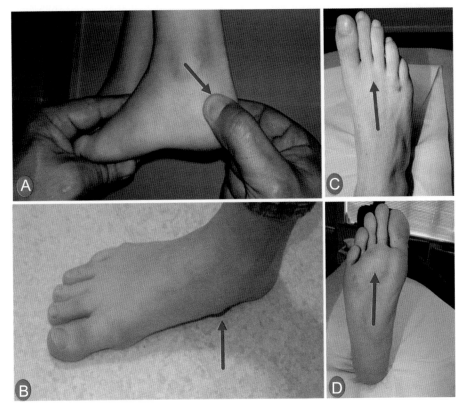

Figure 2.9 The sites of tenderness (red arrows) give a clue to the underlying diagnosis. (A) shows the squeeze test in Sever's disease where there is tenderness on either side of the calcaneal apophysis. (B) shows a prominent accessory navicular bone, which causes highly localized bony tenderness. (C) and (D) show the sites of tenderness in Freiberg's disease.

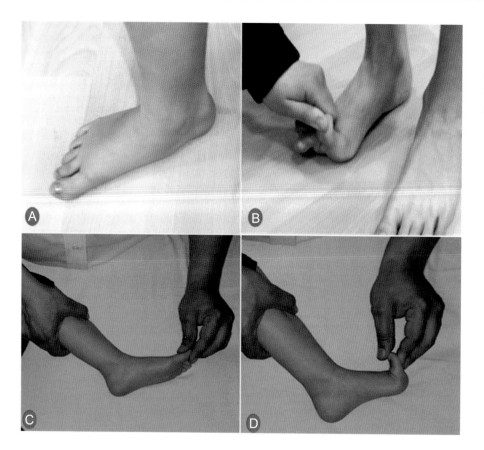

Figure 2.10 The Jack's test can be useful in assessing the flexibility of flat feet in children who cannot stand on their tiptoe or cannot stand at all. The images show two techniques of how to perform the Jack's test (A,C). The principle is that dorsiflexion of the big toe reconstitutes the medial arch through the windlass mechanism of the plantar fascia (B,D).

Most children have flexible flat feet where the heels are in slight valgus and the medial arches are flat. However, on tiptoeing, the heels move into a varus position and the medial arches form (see Chapter 3, Figure 3.12). This will not be the case in a pathological flat foot such as tarsal coalition (see Chapter 8, Figure 8.12). The **Jack's test** can be used in children who cannot stand on their toes for whatever reasons (Figure 2.10).

Pes cavus, by contrast, is almost always pathological. A thorough search for any possible cause is essential before going ahead with any planned surgical correction. This condition is fully covered in Chapter 8. In pes cavus, the medial (sometimes even the lateral) arch is high, the heel in varus, the first ray flexed, and the toes clawed. These deformities are flexible initially but become fixed over time. The **Coleman block is an important test**, as it ascertains whether the varus heel is fixed or still flexible. This influences management in that if fixed, calcaneal osteotomy is usually indicated for deformity correction (Figure 2.11).

Joint ROM should be assessed and recorded systematically, that is, ankle, subtalar, mid-tarsal, metatarsophalangeal, and interphalangeal joints. Reduced joint ROM in children is often caused by joint contractures (soft tissue contractures) rather than by intra-articular pathologies. Loss of ankle dorsiflexion is often caused by tightness in the gastrocnemius and/or soleus muscles. The Silfverskiöld test can distinguish which muscle is the predominant cause of equinus.

Spine

The child is undressed appropriately, and the spine is assessed from the back and sides, with particular attention to any visible abnormalities (Figure 2.12). The spine should be straight from the back. From the side, there is lordosis in the neck and lumbar areas, and kyphosis in the thoracic (and sacrococcygeal) area. The shoulders should be at the same level, and both waists are symmetrical.

The Adam forward bending test would reveal a rotational deformity and make scoliosis more pronounced (see Chapter 10, Figure 10.12). The fingertips should reach the floor on forward bending. If not, there may be tightness in the hamstring muscles (commonest) or reduced spine ROM.

Shoulder

Look at the shoulder from the back, side, and front (without being intimidating!). Pay attention to the contour of the shoulder. Is there Sprengel's shoulder, neck webbing, or low-lying hairline? Observe for the presence of the pectoralis muscles. Feel for hotness, tenderness, or lumps. The shoulder is a common site for osteochondroma.

Check for ROM – active, then passive. Children with obstetrical brachial plexus injury (OBPI) are good exam cases. They commonly have internal rotation contractures, weak external rotation, and abduction movement (see Chapter 12).

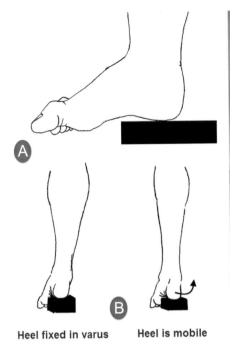

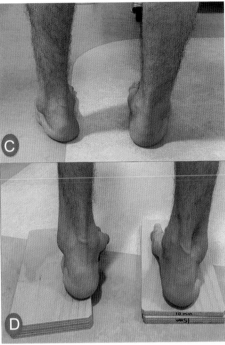

Heel fixed in varus   Heel is mobile

Figure 2.11 The Coleman block test (A) and (B). The tripod theory of pes cavus suggests that sometimes the heel is pushed in varus to accommodate for fixed plantar flexion of the first ray, and the converse also applies (C). Therefore, if the first ray is allowed to drop off the edge of a wooden block, this would remove its push on the heel and the heel should correct to its normal neutral or to a slight valgus position (D). However, if the heel is fixed in varus, this does not happen and corrective osteotomy is required. This is demonstrated on images C & D, where the left foot heel did not correct even when the first ray is allowed to drop down on the edge of wooden boards.

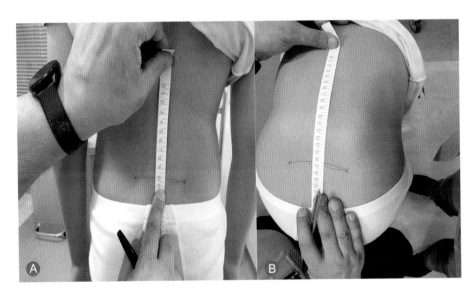

Figure 2.12 The Schober test. A line is drawn across the posterior superior iliac spine (PSIS) dimples. A tape measure is held against the lumbar spine, 10 cm higher (A). The patient is asked to bend forwards as if attempting to touch their toes (B). The distance should increase by at least 5 cm (the line reaches 16 cm, as in B) when the lumbar spine motion is normal.

Elbow

Elbow varus or valgus deformities are often immediately visible; however, rotational deformities are often less obvious. Use the Yamamoto test to demonstrate any associated internal rotation deformity in a child presenting with a gunstock deformity.

Pronation and supination ROMs are included in the elbow examination. Restriction may be caused by radioulnar synostosis, a neglected Monteggia fracture, or a malunited forearm fracture.

Children with hemiplegic CP often have a pronation contracture. It is useful to know whether there is any active supination or not. If there is active supination, release or lengthening will be useful; however, if there is no supination, pronator teres transfer to the supinator is more beneficial.

Wrist and Hand

Wrist and hand examination in children is as complex as that in adults. However, it should be kept simple.

- Look: swellings (such as ganglions) and deformities (Madelung deformity or ulnar and flexion deformity in CP). Look for the thumb position and finger postures. Thumbs in hand deformity and Swan neck deformity of the fingers are common. Scars are often hard to spot in the hand and surprisingly, some extra digits or missing digit are overlooked during the examination!
- Feel: for any hotness, tenderness, fluctuation of any swelling, or thickening of the synovium.
- Move: assess whether observed deformities are flexible or rigid. Do they change when the joint above or below is flexed or extended (this means that structures crossing both joints are tight)?

A full neuromuscular examination completes the examination of any joint.

Limb Length Discrepancy

Limb length discrepancy (LLD) can be assessed using a tape measure or the block test. The latter is the preferred method. The child is made to stand, with the short leg on blocks of varying heights, till the pelvis appears level to the examiner's eye (Figure 2.13). It is important that the hips and knees are kept extended.

In a child with a fixed flexion deformity of the hip or knee, or an adduction or abduction deformity of a limb, an assessment of LLD will have to be performed, with the child supine and the normal limb held in a position comparable to the deformed limb. Measurements using a tape measure are then undertaken.

It is important to note that adduction deformities of the hip produce apparent shortening, whereas the opposite is true for abduction deformities.

Once an LLD is established, the Galeazzi test is undertaken to determine whether the shortening is above or below the knee (Figure 2.14).

Radiological measurements complement the clinical examination and can be deceptive if they are not correlated with the clinical examination findings.

Rotational Profile

Several children present with in-toeing and out-toeing. These could be normal variants (see Chapter 3) or part of a pathological process. Therefore, it is important to assess the rotational profile of the limbs.

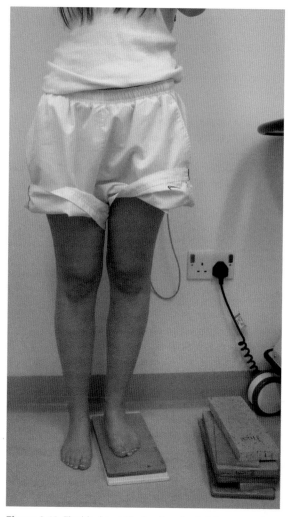

Figure 2.13 The block test. Blocks of varying heights are used to equalize the legs and level the pelvis. This is a better way to estimate the height of a shoe raise or insole.

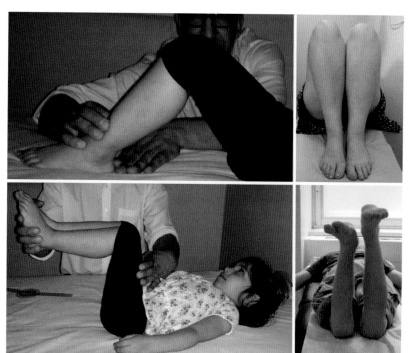

Figure 2.14 The Galeazzi test. These clinical photographs show various modifications of the Galeazzi test to identify the site of the LLD, whether in the femur or in the tibia.

The rotational profile assessment starts whilst assessing the gait by observing the foot (FPA), knee, and patellar (PPA) progression angles (Figure 2.15). On the couch, the rotational profile is best undertaken with the child lying prone [2] and with the knee flexed, and the examiner's palm applied to the back of the child to keep the pelvis level. The degree of internal and external rotations of the hip joint is noted (normal range of external rotation is 45–70°, and internal rotation 10–45°).

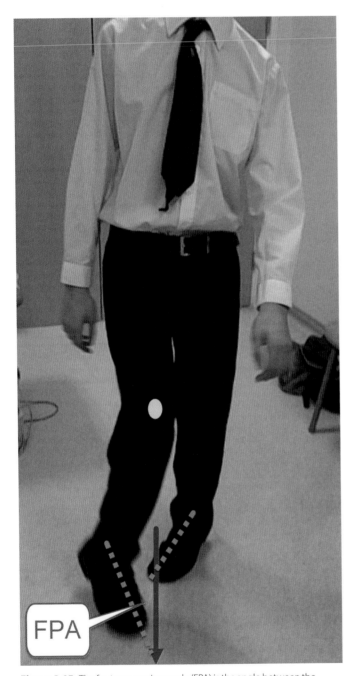

Figure 2.15 The foot progression angle (FPA) is the angle between the longitudinal axis of the foot (dashed blue line) and the direction of walking (red arrow). Normal FPA ranges between −5° and +20°, with − meaning internal. The patellar progression angle (PPA) refers to where the patella is pointing to (usually internal, neutral, or external). If the FPA and PPA both point inwards, torsion comes from above the knee. If the FPA is inwards and the PPA is outwards, then the rotation comes from below the knee.

The presence of excessive internal rotation and limited external rotation would imply excessive femoral neck anteversion (Figure 2.15).

The Gage test (also known as the Craig's test or Ryder's method) is then undertaken to confirm the degree of femoral anteversion (FAV). This is noted by measuring the angle between the long axis of the leg and an imaginary vertical line when the greater trochanter is most prominent (Figure 2.16). At birth, the femoral anteversion is about 40° and by age 16 years is approximately 16°. Figure 2.17 shows the relationship between the FPA and FAV.

Tibial torsion is assessed by measuring the thigh–foot angle (TFA) and the transmalleolar thigh angle (TMA). The TFA is the angle between the long axis of the thigh and a line bisecting the sole of the foot in its resting position (Figure 2.18). A normal angle is 0–20° of external rotation. The TMA is the angle formed by the thigh axis and the line perpendicular to the transmalleolar line. Because the lateral malleolus is normally posterior to the medial malleolus, the TMA is more externally rotated than the FTA by about 10° (Figure 2.18). The TMA is a better measurement for tibial torsion, but it is more difficult to measure. The TFA is a good measurement for tibial torsion if the foot is normal; however, foot deformities, such metatarsus adductus or abductus, result in wrong findings.

Foot contributions to rotational profile abnormalities are assessed by using either the heel bisector line or the lateral border. Both are addressed in Chapter 3 (Figure 3.4).

Generalized Joint Laxity

The Beighton score is a simple system to quantify joint laxity and hypermobility. It is a nine-point score where the higher the score, the higher the laxity. The threshold for joint laxity in a young adult ranges from 4 to 6. It is usually practical after the age of eight (Figure 2.19).

Special Tests in Children with Cerebral Palsy

Several tests are used to assess patients with CP to complete an orthopaedic neuromuscular examination chart (see Chapter 18a, Table 18a.3; a snapshot is shown in Figure 2.24), which is essential when planning treatment [3]. These tests cover joint ROM, strength of key muscles, and degree of spasticity. Some of these tests are summarized below; the rest are covered in Chapter 18a. Most of these tests are best performed by two practitioners, usually physiotherapist.

The Foot

Check for deformities (usually planovalgus or cavovarus) – is the deformity fixed or flexible? It is essential to test for individual muscle strength to understand how any deformity was caused, especially if planning tendon transfer.

The Ankle

The gastrocnemius muscle becomes tighter than the soleus muscle because it crosses more growth plates. This can be tested

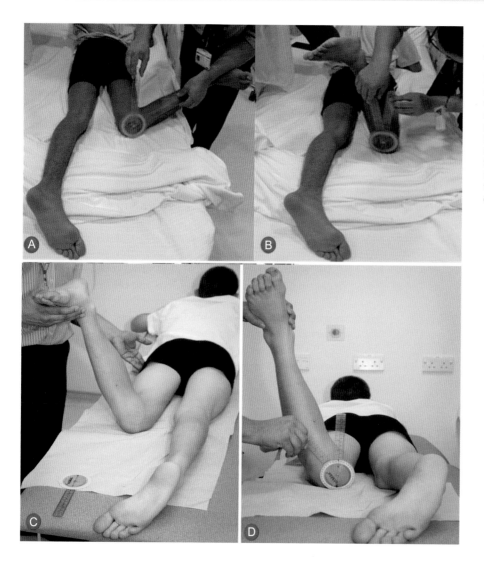

Figure 2.16 Rotational profile of the femur. (A) and (B) show measurements of internal rotation and external rotation of the hip, respectively. Based on the age of the child, the difference between the measurements represents femoral anteversion. Femoral anteversion can be formally checked using the Gage test (C, D). (C) The examiner feels where the greater trochanter is most prominent and holds the leg. (D) The angle between the long axis of the leg and an imaginary vertical line is measured. Notice any rise in the ipsilateral hemipelvis on flexing the knee (Duncan–Ely test), which indicates tightness in the rectus femoris – a useful test in children with cerebral palsy.

using the Silfverskiöld test. The degree of ankle dorsiflexion is measured with the knee flexed and extended. Flexing the knee relaxes the gastrocnemius muscle only and therefore tests for any tightness in the soleus. A minimum of 20° is required for normal walking (Figure 2.20).

The Knee

Knee contracture is common in CP. Normal knee ROM is 0–150°. Knee extension should be measured with the hip extended (which relaxes the hamstring muscles) and gives the true fixed flexion deformity of the knee, which is usually caused by the capsule (or bony deformity). Knee flexion contracture reduces step length and gait efficiency. Also the position of the patella should be checked. Patella alta is very common in children with CP and this is surgically correctable, with important functional gains.

The popliteal angle (PA) is a measure for hamstring tightness and their impact on the step length. It is performed with the child supine, and the hip flexed at 90° and the contralateral

hip extended. The knee is then extended. The angle between the vertical line and the tibia is the PA (normally <20°) (Figure 2.21).

Measuring the PA with the hip flexed to 45°, rather than to 90° (mimicking hip flexion in normal gait), is clinically more relevant. This modified PA measurement should be 0°. Anything more would reduce the step length.

An anterior pelvic tilt tightens the hamstring muscles and increases the PA. Flexing the contralateral hip to correct any anterior pelvic tilt is performed in the hamstring shift test and this will give a more accurate measurement of true hamstring tightness.

The Hip

The Thomas' and Staheli tests are covered earlier (Figure 2.7). The Thomas' test is easier to perform; however, it cannot measure the amount of hip extension, which is rarely relevant.

Adduction contracture is a risk factor for hip dislocation. The pelvis needs to be stabilized to measure the amount

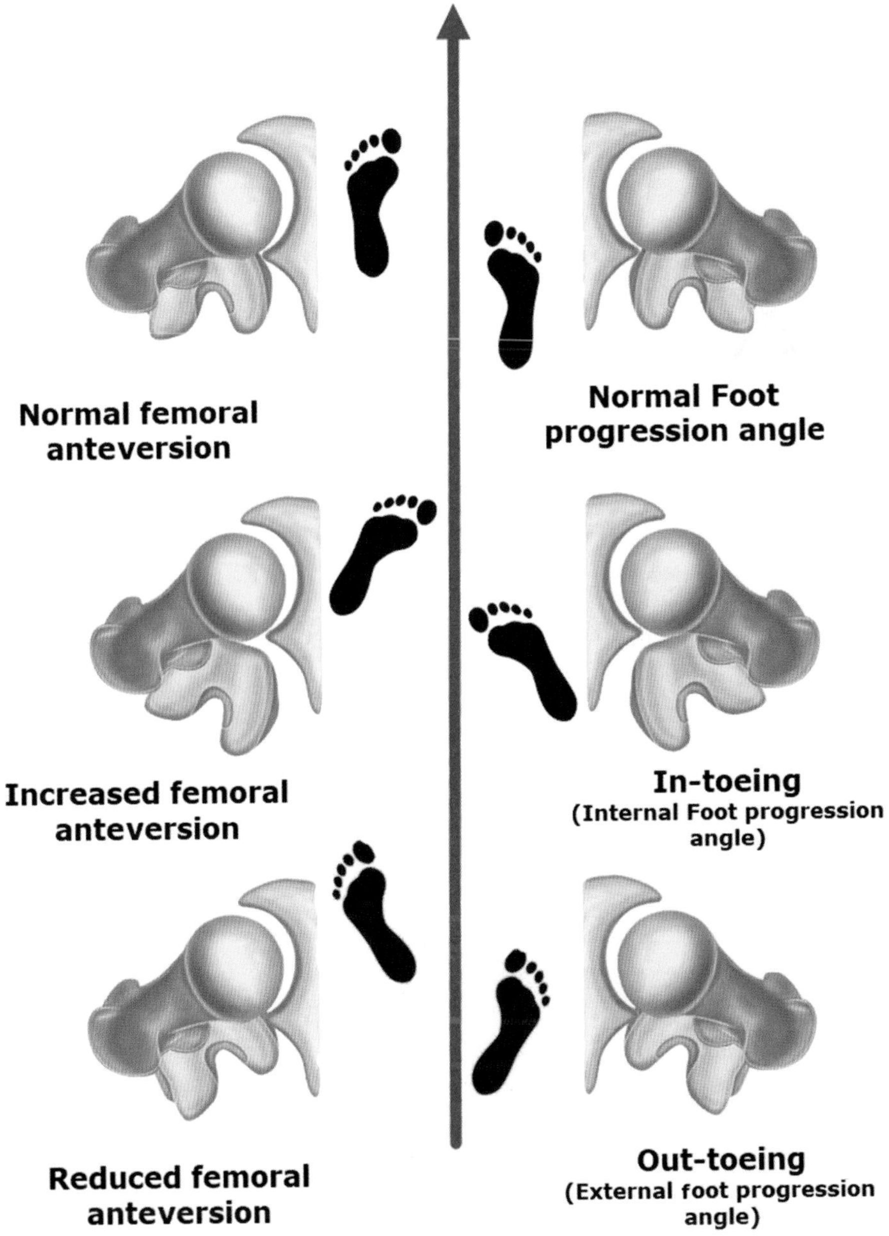

Figure 2.17 The relationship between the foot progression angle and femoral anteversion.

Normal femoral anteversion

Increased femoral anteversion

Reduced femoral anteversion

Normal Foot progression angle

In-toeing
(Internal Foot progression angle)

Out-toeing
(External foot progression angle)

of hip abduction – either unilateral or combined. Hip abduction of <30° poses a risk of hip dislocation. Tight muscles must be treated with focused physiotherapy, abduction braces, and Botox injections or muscle lengthening.

Hip adduction contracture can be caused by medial hamstring muscles (often as they cross multiple physes) and/or hip adductors. Measuring hip abduction with the knee flexed (relaxing the medial hamstrings) and extended helps to differentiate between the two (**Phelp's test**; Figure 2.22).

The **Ober's test** for abductor contracture includes the iliotibial band. The child is on his/her side, with the spine straight. The knee is flexed to 90°, and the hip to be tested (the uppermost

one) is then brought from flexion to extension. The thigh should normally drop in adduction (towards the examination couch). If there is abduction contracture, the hip cannot be adducted to a neutral position (Figure 2.23).

The **Duncan–Ely test** assesses for rectus femoris contracture. The child is prone and the knee is gradually flexed. The examiner feels for spasticity and resistance of the rectus muscle and observes the elevation of the ipsilateral hemipelvis (Figure 2.16).

It is important to differentiate between a contracted (short) muscle and a spastic muscle. During ROM testing, the first catch during testing is named R1, whereas the maximum ROM with gentle and slow stretching is named R2. A large difference

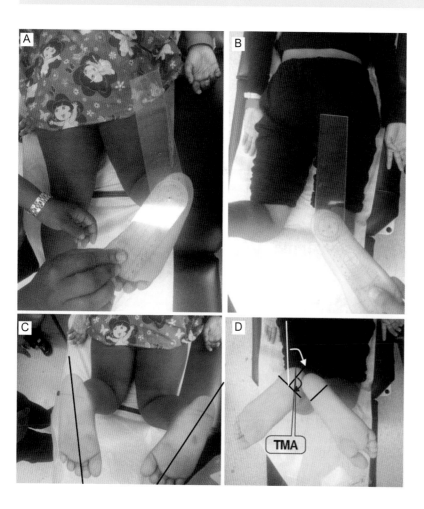

Figure 2.18 The thigh–foot angle and transmalleolar thigh angle. (A) and (B) show the thigh–foot angle in two patients. (A) Tibial in-torsion. (B) Tibial ex-torsion. (C) The heel bisector line passes through the second interdigital space, which is normal. (D) The transmalleolar angle.

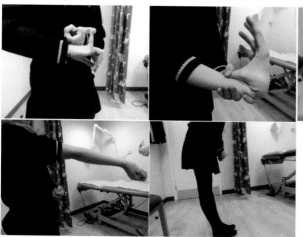

Figure 2.19 Beighton score.

Criteria	Note
Little finger dorsiflexion	1 if >90°, 2 if bilateral
Thumb to forearm (wrist flexion)	1 if thumb tips touch the forearm skin, 2 if bilateral
Elbow extension	1 if hyperextension >10°, 2 if bilateral
Knee extension	1 if hyperextension >10°, 2 if bilateral
Trunk flexion with knees fully extended	1 if palms can rest flat on the floor

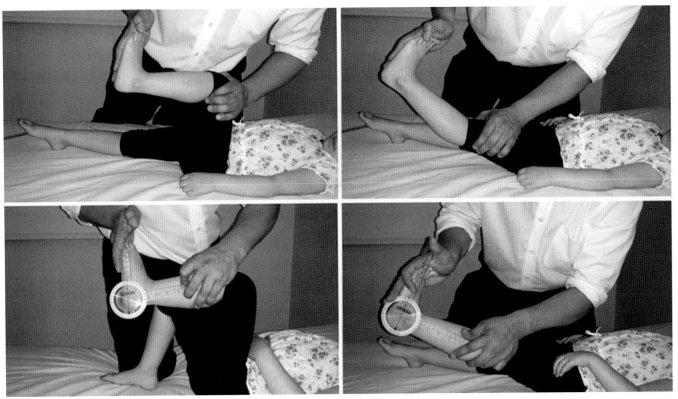

Figure 2.20 The Silfverskiöld test. Flexing the knee relaxes the gastrocnemius and tests the tightness in the soleus. If there is no difference in ankle dorsiflexion, whether the knee is flexed or extended, both muscles or Achilles tendon are tight. If ankle dorsiflexion is less with the knee extended, this indicates a tight gastrocnemius and this needs selective lengthening.

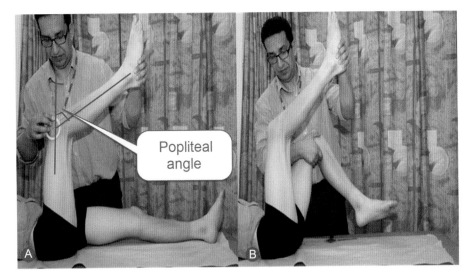

Figure 2.21 (A) Popliteal angle measurement. (B) The hamstring shift test.

between R2 and R1 indicates greater spasticity, and vice versa. Botox injection can improve this difference. Traditionally, Botox is recommended when the difference is >20°. A lesser difference may be of no clinical significance.

Muscle spasticity is graded by using the modified Ashworth scale. This is not required for the exam, but it is mentioned here for completion:

- 0: no increase in muscle tone
- 1: slight increase in muscle tone, with a catch and release or minimal resistance at the end of the ROM when an affected part(s) is moved in flexion or extension
- 1+: slight increase in muscle tone, manifested as a catch, followed by minimal resistance through the remainder (less than half) of the ROM

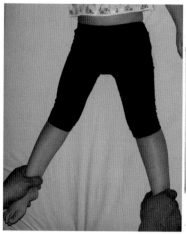
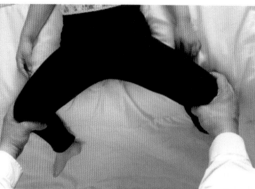

Phelp's test:
Difference in hip abduction with knee extended and flexed

Figure 2.22 The Phelp's test. The medial hamstrings tighten with knee extension, reducing hip abduction.

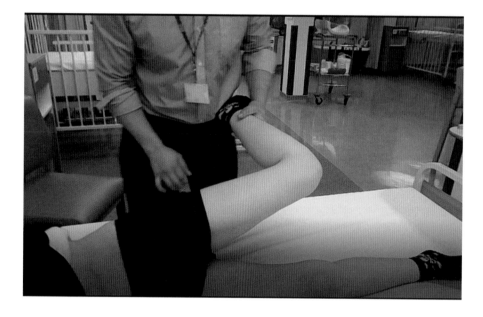

Figure 2.23 A positive Ober's test. The hip remains abducted when it is extended.

- 2: marked increase in muscle tone throughout most of the ROM, but the affected part(s) is still easily moved
- 3: considerable increase in muscle tone and passive movement difficult
- 4: affected part(s) rigid in flexion or extension.

In preparation for the exam, try to practise completing the chart shown in Figure 2.24 for every patient with CP until you become very slick. Video 2.1 will give you guidance and a framework to use if you are asked to examine a patient with CP in your clinicals.

> ▷ **Video 2.1** Cerebral palsy examination.

Key Points: Summary of Children Assessment

- History:
  - Presenting complaint (with the 10 relevant questions)
  - Birth history and developmental milestones
  - Family history.
- Examination:
  - General assessment and screening
  - Functional assessment (relevant)
  - Specific joint/part assessment (guided by suspected diagnosis).
- Investigations:
  - Radiological
  - Biochemical
  - Others.

Date	Joint	Sagittal		R(R1)	L(R1)	Coronal	R	L	Transverse	R	L
	Ankle	Dorsiflexion (Knee 0)		15	-10(0)	Inversion	F	F	HBL	2IDS	2IDS
		Dorsiflexion (Knee90)		20	-5(5)	Eversion	F	F	FTA	15E	15E
		Plantarflexion		F	F	Midfoot break	No	Y	TMTA	NT	NT
		Plantaris		No	No	Hallux valgus	No	No			
	Knee	Extension		F	F						
		Flexion		F	F						
		Popliteal angle	1	60(40)	60(40)	Valgus					
			2			Varus					
			35°	<20	<20						
		Patella alta		No	No						
	Hip	Flexion		F	F	Abduction (Knee0)	45	45	Internal Rotation	65	90
		FFD		No	No	Abduction (Knee90)	50	50	External Rotation	30	0
		Extension		NT	NT	Adduction					
	Ankle	Dorsiflexion		5	4	Inversion					
		Plantarflexion		5	5	Eversion	5	3			
	Knee	Flexion		5	5						
		Extension		5	5						
	Hip	Flexion		5	5	Abduction	5	5			
		Extension		5	5	Adduction	5	5			
	Ankle	Dorsiflexion (Knee 0)		1	2						
		Dorsiflexion (Knee90)		1	2						
	Knee	Hamstring		1	2						
	Hip	Rectus		0	0						

Row groups (left vertical labels): **Range of motions**, **Strength**, **Spasticity**

	LLD= 0 (x-ray 4 mm) Galleazzi test: -Ve Spine: mild scoliosis Confusion test: Negative (good selective control)
Keys	R=Right; L=Left; R=range of motion 2, R1=range of motion 1; F=Full; Knee0= Knee fully extended; Knee90=knee flexed to 90; HBL=Heel Bisector line, FTA=Foot thigh angle, TMTA=Transmalleolar Thigh Angle; NT= not tested, LLD=Leg length discrepancy. Red=worsened; uncoloured=unchanged; green=improved in comparison to last visit

Figure 2.24 A sample of cerebral palsy assessment chart.

References

1. Herring JA. *Tachdjians' Pediatric Orthopaedics*, 4th ed., Vol. 1. Philadelphia, PA: Saunders Elsevier; 2008.

2. Staheli L. *Fundamentals of Pediatric Orthopaedics*, 4th ed. Philadelphia, PA: Lippincott Williams & Wilkins; 2008.

3. Dormans JP. *Pediatric Orthopaedics: Core Knowledge in Orthopaedics*. Philadelphia, PA: Elsevier Mosby; 2005.

Chapter 3

Normal Lower Limb Variants in Children

Manoj Ramachandran and Gregory B. Firth

Background

Normal variants in children are common and include:

1. Angular variants (variation in the coronol plane – genu varum and genu valgum)
2. Rotational variants (variation in the axial plane – in-toeing and out-toeing gait)
3. Flexible flat feet.

Although common, they often cause undue parental anxiety, prompting frequent visits to primary care centres [1–3]. A substantial proportion of referrals to paediatric orthopaedic clinics consist of normal physiological variants in growing children. Careful history and examination, and knowledge of the clinical course of rotational and angular deformities allow accurate assessment of children to exclude pathology and provide reassurance to parents. The aim of this chapter is to highlight areas of normal variation in paediatric orthopaedic practice and to identify abnormal features that require further investigation.

Angular Variants

Angular normal variants tend to be symmetrical and cause no pain. Clinical examination should focus on quantifying the magnitude of the deformity, but also whilst excluding rotational abnormalities and ligamentous laxity, as these can exaggerate the appearance of angular deformities. Children with tibial in-torsion and femoral ex-torsion can present with apparent genu varum.

Salenius and Vankka, in a landmark study of tibiofemoral angles in 1 500 knee X-rays (1 000 normal children), showed that children have genu varum (bow legs) up to the age of 18 months (mean of 15° at birth and 0° at 18 months). Thereafter, a genu valgum (knock knees) alignment ensues (mean of 12° around 4 years of age), which subsequently reduces to the normal value in adults (7–8° of valgus) by the age of 7 years (Figure 3.1) [4]. This study has been replicated in a modern radiological study with more stringent methodology [5].

Besides the physiological causes, several other causes have been recognized for genu varum and genu valgum. These are summarized in Table 3.1 below.

Genu Varum (Bow Legs)

Physiological genu varum is thought to relate to intrauterine positioning, which leads to contracture of the medial knee joint capsule. This, in addition to internal tibial torsion common in this age group, accentuates the deformity when children weight-bear. Therefore, referrals for bow legs are common for children aged between 10 and 14 months, the average age at which children start to stand and ambulate. The knee intercondylar distance is measured with the medial malleoli in contact and the patellae facing forwards, and should be <6 cm in this age group [6].

Table 3.1 Causes of genu varum and genu valgum alignments

Genu varum	Genu valgum
1. Normal variant (physiological)	1. Normal variant (physiological)
2. Blount's disease	2. Primary tibia valga (idiopathic)
3. Trauma	3. Trauma (Cozen fracture)
4. Infection	4. Infection
5. Tumours such as osteochondroma	5. Tumours such as osteochondromas
6. Skeletal dysplasia (achondroplasia, osteogenesis imperfecta, metaphyseal chondrodysplasia)	6. Skeletal dysplasia (pseudoachondroplasia, multiple epiphyseal dysplasia)
7. Metabolic (vitamin D deficiency, fluoride poisoning, osteogenesis imperfecta)	7. Metabolic (renal osteodystrophy and obesity)
8. Focal fibrocartilaginous dysplasia (see Chapter 6, Figure 6.19)	8. Neuromuscular disorders (polio) and tight iliotibial band

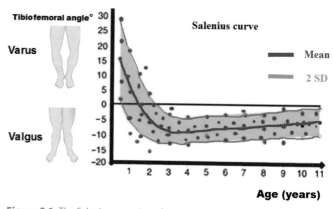

Figure 3.1 The Salenius curve. Leg alignment in the coronal plane (varus and valgus) undergoes a unique pattern of changes from birth until adulthood. Newborn babies have average lower limb varus of 15°. As children start standing and walking, the lower limbs become straight at around 18 months of age. Then they go into progressive valgus, reaching 12° at around 4 years of age. Valgus then gradually decreases, reaching the adult value (7° of valgus) at around age 8. The standard deviation (SD) is 8° (more in boys, 10°; and less in girls, 7°).

The parents of most children with bow legs can be reassured that the natural history of this normal variant will be one of spontaneous improvement. Red flags that should be looked out for include:

1. Unilaterality or asymmetry of >5°
2. Severe (beyond 2 SDs of the mean predicted by the Salenius curve)
3. Genu varum in children aged >3 years
4. Accompanied by short stature
5. Other features (such as family history, delayed milestones, and features of underlying causes mentioned in Table 3.1).

Authors Note: Aetiological Causes for Genu Varum and Genu Valgum Listed in Order of Relative Frequency

Some studies suggest that participation in high-impact sports may predispose to genu varum later in childhood [7, 8]. Genu varum has been shown to occur more frequently in adult football players than in the general population. This, in addition to external tibial torsion, has been similarly shown in several large cross-sectional studies of adolescents participating in a variety of high-impact sports, compared to non-sporting individuals [7, 8]. It is, however, not clear if the demands for intensive practice on the growing skeleton leads to the varus axis, or whether knee varus confers some advantage, resulting in the natural selection of such individuals.

This has important clinical implications, as such angular deformities of the knee are associated with an increased risk of injury [7] and possible osteoarthritis in later life. Abnormal kinetic forces (increased lateral ground reaction force) in children with bow legs during running has been suggested to accelerate the progression of degenerative joint disease [9]. Further studies are required to understand this relationship.

Genu Valgum (Knock Knees)

Referrals for knock knees are common in children over the age of 3 years. Knock knees can be accentuated by, or associated with, obesity, vitamin D deficiency, ligamentous laxity, and flat feet. The association of genu valgum with obesity and flat feet was positively shown in a cohort of 1 364 children between the ages of 3 and 7 years. In addition, torsional deformities, such as femoral anteversion with compensatory external tibial torsion, may make a physiological genu valgum appear more severe. The intermalleolar distance is measured with the child standing and the knees just touching each other, with the patellae facing forwards, and should be <8 cm from 8 years and above (Figure 3.2) [6]. The chance of having genu valgum was increased by over 70 times in obese children in a study by Ciaccia *et al.* who reviewed 1 050 schoolchildren [10].

Red flags that should be looked out for include:

1. Severe (intermalleolar distance >8 cm at age 8 years or older)

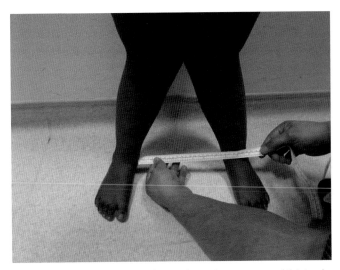

Figure 3.2 Ankle intermalleolar distance. It is easier to measure whilst standing, if the child can stand.

2. Unilaterality or asymmetry of >5°
3. Accompanied by obesity
4. Other features (such as family history, delayed milestones, and features of underlying causes mentioned in Table 3.1).

Key Points: Red Flags for Angular Variants (Genu Varum or Genu Valgum)

1. Unilaterality or asymmetry of >5°
2. Severe:
   a. Tibiofemoral angle is beyond 2 SDs of the mean predicted by the Salenius curve)
   b. Ankle intermalleolar distance >8 cm at 8 years or above
3. Genu varum in children aged >3 years or genu valgum in children aged <2 years
4. Accompanied by short stature or obesity
5. Other features are present (such as family history, delayed milestones, low vitamin D, and other features of underlying causes mentioned in Table 3.1).

Physiological bow legs or knock knees are normal variants that generally require observation and reassurance at 6- to 12-monthly intervals. If progressive or asymptomatic, other causes should be excluded (Table 3.1). Sports should always be encouraged in children, unless the physiological bowing is symptomatic.

If severe, progressive, or symptomatic, the deformity can be corrected using hemi-epiphysiodesis of the distal femoral physis or the proximal tibial physis, or both, depending on where the deformity is coming from. This can be easily measured on the anteroposterior long leg standing radiograph (see Chapter 23).

Close observation post-hemi-epiphysiodesis surgery must be made to avoid overcorrection, recurrence, or rebound phenomena if the plates are removed before skeletal maturity [11–13].

Rotational Variants

The child's lower limb rotational profile is a composite of measurements of the bones and joints. The most obvious manifestation of rotational abnormalities is the position of the feet – commonly referred to as 'in-toeing' or 'out-toeing'. Overall, only 0.1% of rotational deformities persist and may necessitate surgery, if severe, with functional disability in adolescents.

In-Toeing Gait ('Pigeon-Toed' Gait)

In-toeing can be caused by conditions in the spine, pelvis, hip, femur, knee, tibia, ankle, foot, and big toes. It can also be dynamic, caused by overactive muscles such as the gracilis or tibialis anterior muscles. However, the three commonest reasons for in-toeing gait are: metatarsus adductus (MA; foot), internal tibial torsion (tibia), and persistent femoral anteversion (femur).

Metatarsus Adductus

MA is the commonest congenital foot deformity, occurring in 1 in 1 000 births (Figure 3.3). It is defined as an internal angulation of the forefoot (or metatarsals) on a neutral or flexible hindfoot and is not part of another paediatric foot condition (e.g. congenital talipes equinovarus).

Clinically, the foot has a curved lateral border, and the heel bisector line (an imaginary line drawn in the middle of the heel) passes through the second interdigital space. Bleck proposed a clinical classification [14] based on the heel bisector line relationship with the toes (Figure 3.4). There are two recognized types of MA: flexible (can be easily straightened out) and rigid.

Flexible and isolated MA are benign conditions that resolve spontaneously by the age of 5 years (or even earlier). Treatment

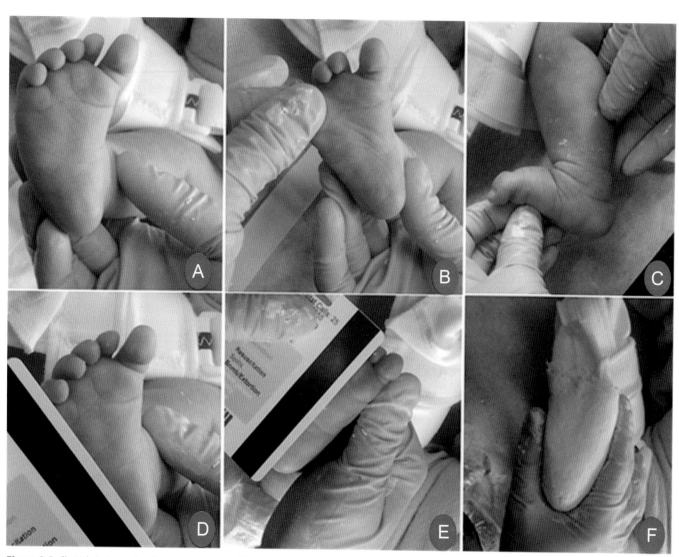

Figure 3.3 Clinical photographs of severe metatarsus adductus (A, D) which was fully correctable (B, E) and treated by serial casting (F). (C) shows a normal hindfoot with no equinus of the heel, an important differentiation from a clubfoot.

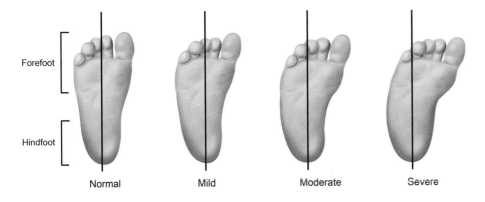

Figure 3.4 Bleck's classification of metatarsus adductus. Normal: the heel bisector line passes through the second and third interdigital spaces; mild: through the third toe; moderate: through the third and fourth interdigital spaces; and severe: through or beyond the fourth and fifth interdigital spaces.

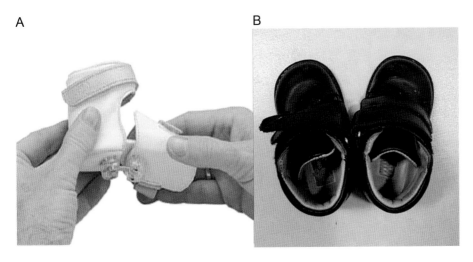

Figure 3.5 Orthoses used in treating metatarsus adductus. (A) Bebax forefoot orthoses. (B) Reverse last shoes.

is rarely indicated. In a study of 379 children with MA, nearly 90% required no treatment [15].

Parental stretching, serial casting, orthoses (including reverse last shoes) (Figure 3.5), and surgery have been recommended as treatment options for persistent, rigid, or symptomatic MA. However, the evidence to support these interventions is weak. Furthermore, there is a lack of specific indications for these interventions in MA.

Eamsobhana and colleagues showed that parental stretching had no effect in 94 newborn feet with MA [16]. Nevertheless, it is still recommended by many to 'treat parents'.

For the rigid type, and cases that do not resolve by 9 months of age, serial casting or orthoses have been recommended and may be of value [16]. Herzenberg and colleagues showed that orthoses (Bebax forefoot orthosis; Figure 3.5) and serial casting are equally effective, although orthosis worked out cheaper than casting, in children with resistant MA [17]. Their inclusion criterion was 'infants who failed home stretching'. The age range was 3–9 months and it is not clear if these patients required any treatment at all [18].

Pentz and Weiner [19] published their experience with 795 patients treated for MA with a straight metal bar and attached reverse last shoe protocol, with a 99% likelihood of obtaining a fully corrected foot. Surgical intervention was deemed necessary in <1% of cases. A lack of control seriously undermines this study and it is not unreasonable to assume that the high success rate of 99% for full correction was attributed to the natural history of MA, and not due to orthotic support.

In neglected or severe cases, Feng and colleagues recommended surgery in children with MA over the age of 6 years. However, these children make up a very small minority of this group and the majority of the literature supports conservative management of this condition [20].

A few surgical techniques have been described to treat resistant MA. These have been used alone or in various combinations, including medial capsulotomy to reorient the first cuneiform metatarsal joint, sectioning of the abductor hallucis brevis, and lateral column shortening (in long feet) and medial column lengthening (in short feet) [21–23]. More details are provided in Chapter 8.

Internal Tibial Torsion

Internal tibial torsion occurs when the tibia turns inwards more than normal. Clinically, the feet are internally rotated, whilst the patella remains in a neutral position (or even in an externally rotated position). This can be measured clinically by the foot–thigh angle (Figure 3.6) or, even better, by the transmalleolar thigh angle (TMTA) when there is an intrinsic foot deformity such as MA or a mid-foot break (Figure 3.7).

The amount of tibial torsion can also be quantified radiologically by measuring the angular difference between the transmalleolar axis of the ankle and the bicondylar axis of the knee on CT scanning (Figure 3.8).

Internal tibial torsion is most apparent when infants first begin to walk and parents may mention that their child trips frequently and appears clumsy. The condition affects both sexes

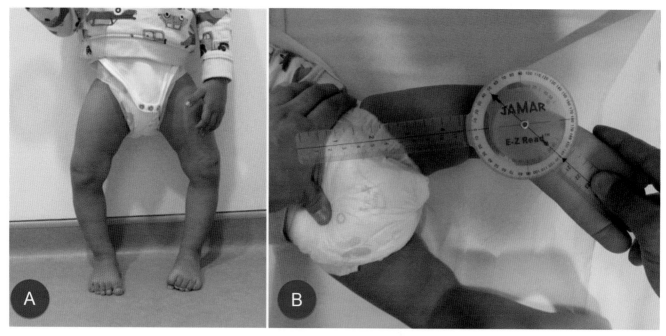

Figure 3.6 A child with bilateral tibial torsion (A). Notice the feet pointing inwards, with the patellae pointing outwards. The foot-thigh angle quantifies the amount of deformity and is less reliable than the transmalleolar thigh angle when there is an intrinsic foot deformity (B).

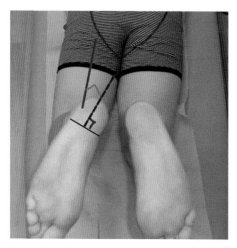

Figure 3.7 The transmalleolar thigh angle (TMTA). The black line connects the medial and lateral malleoli (TML). The TMTA is the angle between the thigh axis (red) and the line perpendicular to the TML (dashed line). Some authors measure the angle between the thigh axis and the TML as the TMTA.

equally; it is bilateral in two-thirds of affected infants and is associated with MA in about a third. Varus at the knee, either physiological or disease-related (such as in Blount's disease), is often associated with internal tibial torsion.

The clinical course is of spontaneous resolution – the transmalleolar axis rotates laterally from 2–4° at birth to 10–20° in adulthood [24]. Resolution is most rapid in infancy. Three per cent of adults show persistence of major internal tibial torsion, although disability is rare. Treatment with orthotic devices is unnecessary and ineffective. In severe cases with functional disability, such as frequent trips and falls, tibial rotational osteotomy may be considered for children older than 10 years of age.

Femoral Anteversion

Femoral version is defined as the angular difference between the axis of the femoral neck and the transcondylar axis of the knee in the axial plane. The natural femoral version has been well

Figure 3.8 Measurement of the amount of tibial torsion on CT scanning where the knee condylar sections are overlapped on both malleoli. A line touching the proximal tibial condyles intersects the transmalleolar lines to form the tibial torsion angle.

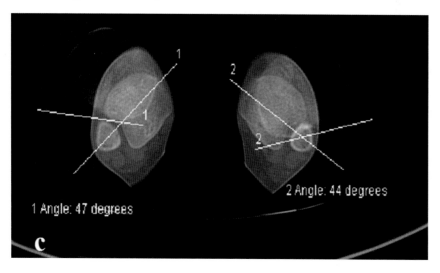

1 Angle: 47 degrees

2 Angle: 44 degrees

documented in a 20-year follow-up study of 1 148 hips. On average, femoral anteversion is 40° at birth, decreasing throughout growth to 16° in adulthood [25].

Femoral anteversion is most pronounced between 4 and 6 years of age. The femoral anteversion angle has been shown with three-dimensional CT to have the greatest improvement in girls under the age of 6 years [26]. It is twice as common in girls and is nearly always symmetrical. It is also often familial. Children sit with their limbs in the 'W' position, walk with an in-toeing gait with the patella pointing inwards ('squinting patella'), and run in an awkward pattern ('egg beater' pattern, with inward rotation of the thighs and outward rotation of the legs and feet in swing phase) (Figure 3.9). The amount of femoral torsion can be quantified using CT measuring the angle between the femoral neck axis and the posterior condylar knee axis (Figure 3.10).

In-toeing typically becomes more pronounced when children are tired. Tripping as a result of crossing feet may occur. Femoral anteversion spontaneously resolves in >80% of affected children by late childhood and parents should be reassured of this [27].

Femoral anteversion was once speculated to cause osteoarthritis of the hip or knee and to impair physical performance; however, this has been disproved by several studies [28]. Various orthotics have been used in the past, but none have shown efficacy [25]. In the rare adolescent who has a major cosmetic deformity, patellar maltracking, or patellofemoral instability, rotational osteotomy of the femur may be considered, although the rate of complications is high (15% overall risk of non-union, malunion, delayed union, or infection), but is not routinely recommended, even in severe cases [29]. Nelitz also highlighted that the level of the osteotomy can affect the coronal alignment of the leg and this should be taken into account before surgery is performed [30].

Out-Toeing Gait

In early infancy, out-toeing is normal and usually resolves by 18–24 months of age. Out-toeing in older children is usually due to external tibial torsion and occasionally due to femoral

retroversion; the latter is more commonly seen in obese adolescents. However, more serious conditions, such as Perthes disease and slipped capital femoral epiphysis, should always be considered in older children, especially if unilateral.

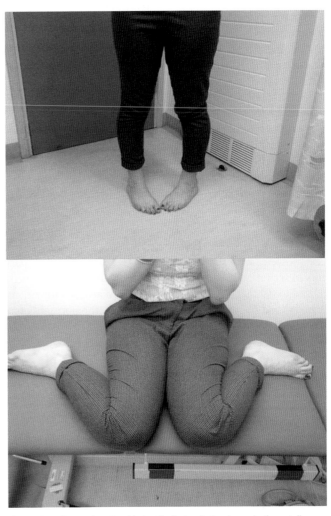

Figure 3.9 Femoral torsion. Notice the feet pointing inwards, the patellae pointing inwards, and the W-sitting position.

Figure 3.10 Femoral torsion: 25° on the right side and 39° on the left side, as measured on CT scanning.

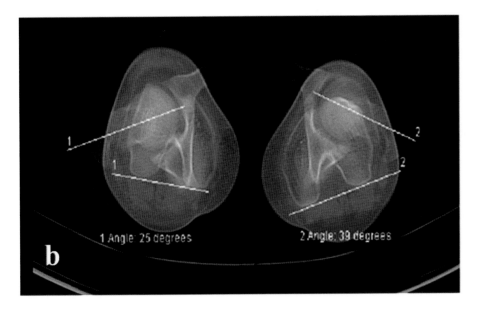

An out-toeing gait is seen less often than in-toeing. At birth, calcaneovalgus may present as out-toeing, with the foot being able to dorsiflex nearly to the shin. This condition is a normal variant and may be confused with congenital vertical talus (CVT). A lateral radiograph of the plantar-flexed foot will differentiate between the two conditions, with the talus in CVT not aligning with the metatarsals.

Calcaneovalgus generally responds quickly to passive plantar flexion stretching exercises, whereas CVT typically requires serial casting or surgical correction [31].

External tibial torsion can cause disability; for example, there is an increased prevalence of patellofemoral instability and patellofemoral pain. It is also thought to develop in compensation to femoral anteversion, which may lead to the 'miserable malalignment syndrome', where there is an increased risk of patella dislocation. Presentation is usually in adolescent girls, with symptoms of anterior knee pain or patellar instability. This area is covered in more details in Chapter 6.

Flexible Pes Planus (Flat Feet)

Feet problems are by far the commonest reason that prompt parents to seek medical advice in children, with 90% of concerns related to flat feet [32]. Flat feet are defined as feet with larger-than-normal plantar contact area; however, the normality has not been defined or agreed on. Several authors tried to quantify flat feet using footprint or plantar contact areas, but these have not been shown to be correlated with symptoms.

All newborns and toddlers have flat feet and the medial arch becomes visible later in life. The prevalence of flat feet inversely correlates with age: about 45% in children aged 3–6 years, decreasing to 15% in older children [33].

Several reasons have been proposed to explain flat feet in children:

1. The presence of a fat pad beneath the medial longitudinal arch
2. The intrinsic laxity of bones and joints in children's feet – most tarsal bones are made of cartilage at birth (Figure 3.11)
3. The lack of neuromuscular control in children starting to stand and walk, resulting in flattening of the foot on weight-bearing – this typically resolves between the ages of 4 and 8 years; the reason for persistence of flat feet in some children is unclear, but some authors have alluded to a deficiency in the anterior facet of the subtalar joint as contributory [34].

Clinically, the heel is in valgus, with sagging of the medial arch. A careful assessment should be made to differentiate a flexible flat foot from a rigid one. A rigid flat foot (<1% of children with flat feet) is usually painful and caused by tarsal coalitions (presentation is typically in adolescence), CVT, or inflammatory disorders (pes planus is a common feature of juvenile idiopathic arthritis). The medial arch of a flexible flat foot reconstitutes on tiptoeing (Figure 3.12) or when the foot is dependent (Figure 3.13). Children rarely have symptoms, with parental concern mainly related to cosmesis or the misconstrued belief that the condition could lead to pain or functional problems in later life [35].

Examination may reveal the flat foot to be severe and causing the shoe to become deformed. We consider flat feet to be severe when the lateral border of the foot is lifted off the floor (Figure 3.14).

Most flexible flat feet are physiological, asymptomatic normal variants, which require no treatment. Other neurological (cerebral palsy), muscular (muscular dystrophy), syndromic (trisomy 21), and connective tissue (Marfan and Ehlers–Danlos syndromes) disorders and tightness in the gastrosoleus muscles should be actively excluded on history and examination. Some cases of flexible flat feet may be painful, with more specific problems after activity.

Key Points: Red Flags of Flat Feet

1. Rigid
2. Painful
3. Severe.

Treatment of paediatric flexible flat feet has been controversial and debate is still ongoing, with no current ideal intervention guidelines. Historically, various devices (e.g. high-top shoes) were used to correct and prevent such deformities.

Kanatli and colleagues found that in a cohort of 45 children with symptomatic flat feet, corrective shoes with increased medial arch support were not effective in the development of the medial arch, when compared to a control group [36]. Wegner

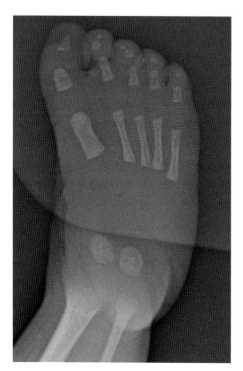

Figure 3.11 X-ray of a newborn child. Notice that only two out of seven tarsal bones are ossified and the rest are made of cartilage, which is soft and pliable.

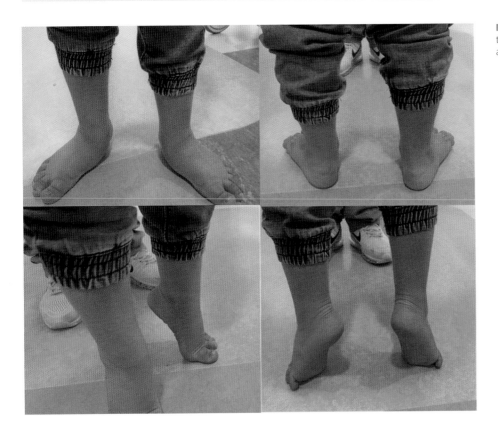

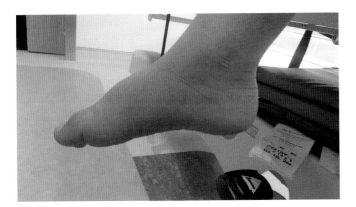

Figure 3.13 Flexible flat feet showing a good longitudinal arch when dangling freely.

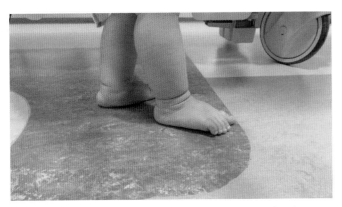

Figure 3.14 Severe flexible flat foot. Notice the lateral border of the foot is lifted off the floor on weight-bearing.

and colleagues performed a prospective study on 129 children to determine whether flexible flat feet in children can be influenced by treatment. Children were randomly assigned to one of four groups: group I, controls; group II, treatment with corrective orthopaedic shoes; group III, treatment with a Helfet heel-cup; or group IV, treatment with a custom-moulded plastic insert. They showed that wearing corrective shoes or inserts for 3 years does not influence the course of flexible flat feet in children [37]. The consensus now is that asymptomatic flexible flat feet are benign and treatment is mainly directed towards symptoms of pain and severity of the deformity. Dars and colleagues in a systematic review of 11 studies (three randomized controlled trials, two case–control studies, five case-series, and one single-case study) concluded that there was still uncertainty on the effectiveness of foot orthoses in treating flexible flat feet in children due to heterogeneity of the included studies, but they indicated that foot orthoses were associated with a reduction in pain and possible improvement in foot posture, gait, and function [38]. A Cochrane review of non-surgical treatment for paediatric flat feet included three trials (305 children) only. Two of these indicated that customized foot orthoses may improve pain and function in children with juvenile idiopathic arthritis and painful flat feet. The third trial did not show a significant difference [33].

Surgery is rarely indicated in treating flexible flat feet. It is reserved for severe cases with intractable pain. Three types of surgical treatment have been in use. These are:

1. Subtalar joint arthroereisis
2. Realignment osteotomies
3. Fusion of joints.

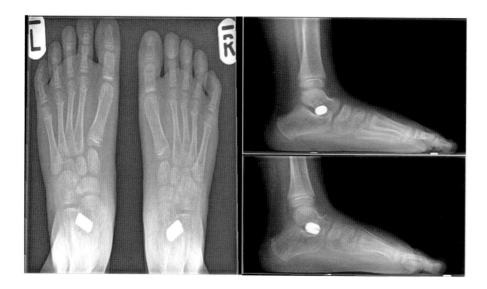

Figure 3.15 Foot X-rays showing bilateral subtalar joint arthroereisis.

Arthroereisis is a surgical procedure that involves placing an implant (which looks like a large conical screw) into the sinus tarsi between the talus and the calcaneus (heel) to limit subtalar joint movement without stopping it completely (Figure 3.15). Although the technique was introduced in the early seventies, it is still controversial, with many authors questioning the indications for its use and long-term outcome [39]. Reported complications rates are up to 19% of cases [40–42]. Indino and colleagues in a recent study of 112 children who had symptomatic flat feet and insertion of an arthroereisis screw, with a mean follow-up of 40 months, found that it significantly improved radiographic parameters, although these scores were not correlated with the clinical scores [43].

Realignment osteotomies involves cutting tarsal (and sometimes metatarsal) bones to align the foot better and create foot arches. It is commonly associated with soft tissue procedures (capsular plication, tendon lengthening, tightening, or transfer). These are covered in more details in Chapter 8.

Suh in a systematic review comparing realignment osteotomies to arthroereisis found that realignment osteotomy achieved more radiographic corrections and more improvements in the American Orthopedic Foot and Ankle Score (AOFAS), in comparison to arthroereisis. Complications were commoner with osteotomies than with arthroereisis, and the reoperation rates were similar [42].

Joint fusion (arthrodesis) procedures are not recommended in children with flexible flat feet due to the risk of adjacent joint disease.

How Are Normal Variants Assessed?

Careful history and examination are mandatory in the evaluation of the lower limbs in children. It is crucial to elucidate the reason for consultation and to identify parental concerns, for example, pain, long-term disability, cosmesis, awkward walking or running, and frequent trips or falls. Occasionally, rotational or angular malalignment is the presenting symptom of underlying disorders; for example, children with mild spastic hemiparesis (cerebral palsy) may present with unilateral intoeing. To manage the problem effectively, it is essential to determine the level of the deformity, as it may occur anywhere between the foot and the hip. Two or more deformities may be additive to, or compensate for, each other. Examination of a child's rotational and angular profiles should therefore proceed in a sequential fashion.

Examination Overview
Musculoskeletal Examination of a Typical Child
- Weight
- Height
- Body mass index (overweight = 20–24.9; obese >25).

Angular Profile in Coronal Plane (Especially in the Presence of Knock Knees or Bow Legs)
- Distance between the knees whilst standing or lying, with the ankles together

---

Key Points: Normal Variant Assessment

- It is crucial to elucidate the reason for consultation and to identify parental concerns.
- It is essential to determine the level of the deformity, as it may occur anywhere between the foot and the hip. Two or more deformities may be additive to, or compensate for, each other.
- Occasionally, rotational or angular malalignment is the presenting symptom of underlying disorders such as in-toeing in cerebral palsy and bowed legs in Blount's disease.
- The presence of obesity, short stature, and vitamin D deficiency should alert the clinician to be able to differentiate normal variants from pathology.

- Distance between the ankles whilst standing or lying, with the knees together (Figure 3.2)
- Tibiofemoral angle, with the patient standing, useful as a baseline to compare with future examinations.

Rotational Profile (Especially if a Child In-Toes or Out-Toes)

- Observe gait and foot progression angle (the angle the child's foot makes with the direction of his or her forward progression) (Figure 3.12)
- Observe the child standing (squinting patella of femoral anteversion; sitting ('W' position; Figure 3.9)), running (to accentuate the problem), and lying down
- Shape of the foot (heel bisector line – normal between the second and third toes) (Figure 3.4)
- Tibial rotation (thigh–foot angle) – prone position, with the knees flexed to 90°, and the angle the foot makes with the thigh is measured (Figure 3.16); although the thigh–foot angle is easier to measure, the TAMTA is more accurate, particularly if there are intrinsic foot deformities such as MA
- Femoral rotation – prone position, with the knees flexed to 90°; hip rotation is generally symmetrical in internal and external rotations (Figure 3.17).

Flat Feet

- Observe the shape of the feet, and the presence and height of the medial arches (with the hind foot in valgus)
- Check for tightness of the gastrocsoleus muscles
- Check for flexibility of the feet (ask to stand on toes; check for subtalar joint movement)
- Hypermobility (see Chapter 2).

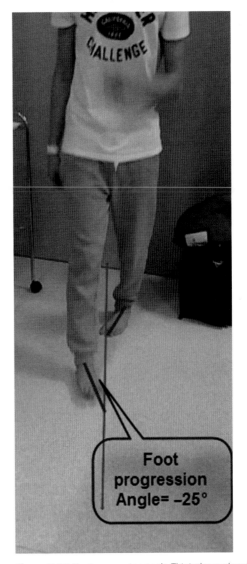

Figure 3.16 Foot progression angle. This is the angle subtended between the straight line along which the patient is walking and the lines drawn through the long axes of the foot.

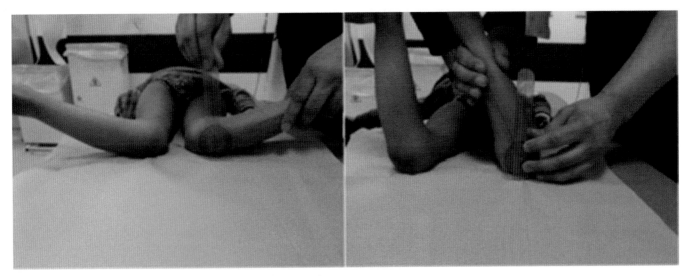

Figure 3.17 Femoral torsion. More internal rotation, compared to external rotation.

Key Points: Normal Variants and Pitfalls

- Take the concerns of the family seriously, providing the parents with information about the clinical course of normal variants and emphasizing that these variants tend to resolve spontaneously and only observation is required.
- Consider risk factors, and treat or advise accordingly (vitamin D deficiency, obesity, sporting activity).
- Think outside the box:
  - Genu varum at any age with an acute deformity centred at the proximal tibia – possible Blount's disease
  - Unilateral or bilateral knee, hip, or thigh pain, or progressive out-toeing in an adolescent, especially if overweight or obese – possible slipped capital femoral epiphysis
  - Unilateral or bilateral knee, hip, or thigh pain in a school-aged child – possible Perthes disease
  - Painful, rigid flat feet, especially in adolescents – possible tarsal coalition
  - Always check for gastrocsoleus tightness when faced with flat feet. Tight gastrocnemius muscles with a mid-foot break are becoming common with the change in lifestyle (see Chapter 7).

References

1. Gunz AC, Canizares M, MacKay C, Badley EM. Magnitude of impact and healthcare use for musculoskeletal disorders in the paediaric: a population-based study. *BMC Musculoskelet Disord*. 2012;13:98.

2. Carli A, Saran N, Kruijt J, Alam N, Hamdy R. Physiological referrals for paediatric musculoskeletal complaints: a costly problem that needs to be addressed. *Paediatr Child Health*. 2012;17(9):e93–7.

3. Blackmur JP, Murray AW. Do children who in-toe need to be referred to an orthopaedic clinic? *J Pediatr Orthop B*. 2010;19(5):415–17.

4. Salenius P, Vankka E. The development of the tibiofemoral angle in children. *J Bone Joint Surg Am*. 1975;57(2):259–61.

5. Sabharwal S, Zhao C, Edgar M. Lower limb alignment in children. *J Pediatr Orthop*. 2008;28(7):740–6.

6. Heath CH, Staheli LT. Normal limits of knee angle in white children – genu varum and genu valgum. *J Pediatr Orthop*. 1993;13(2):259–62.

7. Witvrouw E, Danneels L, Thijs Y, Cambier D, Bellemans J. Does soccer participation lead to genu varum? *Knee Surg Sports Traumatol Arthrosc*. 2009;17(4):422–7.

8. Thijs Y, Bellemans J, Rombaut L, Witvrouw E. Is high-impact sports participation associated with bowlegs in adolescent boys? *Med Sci Sports Exerc*. 2012;44(6):993–8.

9. Jafarnezhadgero AA, Shad MM, Majlesi M, Granacher U. A comparison of running kinetics in children with and without genu varus: a cross sectional study. *PLoS One*. 2017;12(9):e0185057.

10. Ciaccia MCC, Pinto CN, da Costa Golfieri F, *et al.* Prevalence of genu valgum in public elementary schools in the city of Santos (SP), Brazil. *Rev Paul Pediatr*. 2017;35(4):443–7.

11. Woo K, Lee YS, Lee W-Y, Shim JS. The efficacy of percutaneous lateral hemiepiphysiodesis on angular correction in idiopathic adolescent genu varum. *Clin Orthop Surg*. 2016;8(1):92.

12. Farr S, Alrabai HM, Meizer E, Ganger R, Radler C. Rebound of frontal plane malalignment after tension band plating. *J Pediatr Orthop*. 2018;38(7):365–9.

13. Park SS, Kang S, Kim JY. Prediction of rebound phenomenon after removal of hemiepiphyseal staples in patients with idiopathic genu valgum deformity. *Bone Joint J*. 2016;98-B(9):1270–5.

14. Bleck EE. Metatarsus adductus: classification and relationship to outcomes of treatment. *J Pediatr Orthop*. 1983;3(1):2–9.

15. Ponseti IV, Becker JR. Congenital metatarsus adductus: the results of treatment. *J Bone Joint Surg Am*. 1966;48(4):702–11.

16. Eamsobhana P, Rojjananukulpong K, Ariyawatkul T, Chotigavanichaya C, Kaewpornsawan K. Does the parental stretching programs improve metatarsus adductus in newborns? *J Orthop Surg*. 2017;25(1):230949901769032.

17. Herzenberg JE, Burghardt RD. Resistant metatarsus adductus: prospective randomized trial of casting versus orthosis. *J Orthop Sci*. 2013;19(2):250–6.

18. Hossain M, Davis N. Evidence-based treatment for metatarsus adductus. In: Alshryda S, Huntley JS, Banaszkiewicz PA, eds. *Paediatric Orthopaedics: An Evidence-Based Approach to Clinical Questions*. Cham: Springer; 2016. pp. 51–75.

19. Pentz AS, Weiner DS. Management of metatarsus adductovarus. *Foot Ankle*. 1993;14(5):241–6.

20. Feng L, Sussman M. Combined medial cuneiform osteotomy and multiple metatarsal osteotomies for correction of persistent metatarsus adductus in children. *J Pediatr Orthop*. 2016;36(7):730–5.

21. Cahuzac JP, Laville JM, de Gauzy JS, Lebarbier P. Surgical correction of metatarsus adductus. *J Pediatr Orthop*. 1993;2(2):176–81.

22. Knorr J, Soldado F, Pham TT, Torres A, Cahuzac JP, de Gauzy JS. Percutaneous correction of persistent severe metatarsus adductus in children. *J Pediatr Orthop*. 2013;34(4):447–52.

23. Napiontek M, Kotwicki T, Tomaszewski M. Opening wedge osteotomy of the medial cuneiform before age 4 years in the treatment of forefoot adduction. *J Pediatr Orthop*. 2003;23(1):65–9.

24. Staheli LT, Corbett M, Wyss C, King H. Lower-extremity rotational problems in children. Normal values to guide management. *J Bone Joint Surg*. 1985;67(1):39–47.

25. Fabry G, MacEwen GD, Shands AR, Jr. Torsion of the femur. A follow-up study in normal and abnormal conditions. *J Bone Joint Surg Am*. 1973;55(8):1726–38.

26. Kong M, Jo H, Lee CH, Chun S-W, Yoon C, Shin H. Change of femoral anteversion angle in children with intoeing gait measured by three-dimensional computed tomography reconstruction: one-year follow-up study. *Ann Rehabil Med*. 2018;42(1):137.

27. Karol LA. Rotational deformities in the lower extremities. *Curr Opin Pediatr.* 1997;9(1):77–80.

28. Eckhoff DG, Kramer RC, Alongi CA, VanGerven DP. Femoral anteversion and arthritis of the knee. *J Pediatr Orthop.* 1994;14(5):608–10.

29. Staheli LT, Clawson DK, Hubbard DD. Medial femoral torsion. *Clin Orthop Relat Res.* 1980;Jan–Feb (146):222–5.

30. Nelitz M. Femoral derotational osteotomies. *Curr Rev Musculoskelet Med.* 2018;11(2):272–9.

31. Yang JS, Dobbs MB. Treatment of congenital vertical talus: comparison of minimally invasive and extensive soft-tissue release procedures at minimum five-year follow-up. *J Bone Joint Surg Am.* 2015;97(16):1354–65.

32. Rome K, Ashford RL, Evans A. Non-surgical interventions for paediatric pes planus. *Cochrane Database Syst Rev.* 2010;7:CD006311.

33. Evans AM, Rome K. A Cochrane review of the evidence for non-surgical interventions for flexible pediatric flat feet. *Eur J Phys Rehabil Med.* 2011;47(1):69–89.

34. Kothari A, Bhuva S, Stebbins J, Zavatsky AB, Theologis T. An investigation into the aetiology of flexible flat feet. *Bone Joint J.* 2016;98-B(4):564–8.

35. Carr JB, Yang S, Lather LA. Pediatric pes planus: a state-of-the-art review. *Pediatrics.* 2016;137(3):e20151230.

36. Kanatlı U, Aktas E, Yetkin H. Do corrective shoes improve the development of the medial longitudinal arch in children with flexible flat feet? *J Orthop Sci.* 2016;21(5):662–6.

37. Wenger DR, Mauldin D, Speck G, Morgan D, Lieber RL. Corrective shoes and inserts as treatment for flexible flatfoot in infants and children. *J Bone Joint Surg Am.* 1989;71(6):800–10.

38. Dars S, Uden H, Banwell HA, Kumar S. The effectiveness of non-surgical intervention (foot orthoses) for paediatric flexible pes planus: a systematic review: update. *PLoS One.* 2018;13(2):e0193060.

39. Mosca VS. Flexible flatfoot in children and adolescents. *J Child Orthop.* 2010;4(2):107–21.

40. Metcalfe SA, Bowling FL, Reeves ND. Subtalar joint arthroereisis in the management of pediatric flexible flatfoot: a critical review of the literature. *Foot Ankle Int.* 2011;32(12):1127–39.

41. Ford SE, Scannell BP. Pediatric flatfoot. *Foot Ankle Clin.* 2017;22(3):643–56.

42. Suh DH, Park JH, Lee SH, *et al.* Lateral column lengthening versus subtalar arthroereisis for paediatric flatfeet: a systematic review. *Int Orthop.* 2019;43(5):1179–92.

43. Indino C, Villafañe JH, D'Ambrosi R, *et al.* Effectiveness of subtalar arthroereisis with endorthesis for pediatric flexible flat foot: a retrospective cross-sectional study with final follow up at skeletal maturity. *Foot Ankle Surg.* 2020;26(1):98–104.

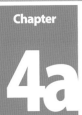

Chapter

4a

Slipped Upper Femoral Epiphysis

Sattar Alshryda and Paul A. Banaszkiewicz

Background

Slipped upper (or capital) femoral epiphysis (SUFE or SCFE, respectively) is not common, with an incidence of 2 in 100 000. Nevertheless, it is a very common exam topic because it has several features that can differentiate poor, average, and excellent candidates.

The name is a misnomer because the femoral head stays in the acetabulum whilst the femoral neck and metaphysis move. In varus SUFE, which is by far the commonest, the neck moves anterosuperiorly (the head becomes posterior and inferior relative to the neck). The so-called 'valgus slip' is rare. It was first described by Müller in 1926 and no more than 50 cases have been reported since [1].

Epidemiology

The incidence of SUFE varies from 1 to 10 per 100 000, depending on:

1. Gender: it is commoner in boys (various ratios are quoted by various studies), with a peak incidence occurring in boys at age of 12–15 years and in girls at age of 10–13 years. Thus, boys tend to have a slip 2 years older than girls. SUFE is rarely reported after the age of 20 years [2]
2. Laterality: it is commoner on the left side (like developmental dysplasia of the hip (DDH)). The reason is unknown; this may be related to the sitting posture of right-handed children whilst writing. It is bilateral in about 20% (half of patients present initially with both hips involved, whilst the other half develop it later, and the majority within 18 months of presentation of the first hip). Younger patients and those with endocrine or metabolic abnormalities are at much higher risk of bilateral involvement
3. Race [3]: commoner in blacks and Polynesians
4. Geographical variation: 0.2 per 100 000 in eastern Japan [4], 2.13 per 100 000 in south-western United States, and as high as 10.08 per 100 000 in north-eastern United States [5]. It is difficult to know how much of this variation is true and how much is secondary to better detection of mild cases
5. Seasonal variations: this is debatable; some studies have shown it is commoner in June and July.

Aetiology

The cause is poorly understood. Anatomical, histological, and mechanical factors have roles in the disease process. Slips occur when shear forces exceed the strength of the growth plate. This happens when the shear force is excessive or the growth plate is weak, or both.

The following features are known to increase the shear forces:

1. Increased weight (>80th centile)
2. Femoral retroversion (>10°)
3. Femoral protrusia
4. More vertical slope of the physis
5. Trauma.

Weakness of the physis may be due to:

1. Renal failure osteodystrophy (95% bilateral)
2. Previous radiation therapy
3. Increased physis height due to widened hypertrophic zone
4. Endocrine disorders (65% bilateral):

   a. Hypothyroidism (usually SUFE is the first presenting feature)
   b. Growth hormone deficiency or excess
   c. Panhypopituitarism
   d. Craniopharyngioma
   e. Hypogonadism
   f. Hyperparathyroidism
   g. Multiple endocrine neoplasia
   h. Turner's syndrome.

The age–weight test has been proposed to identify SUFEs that are caused by underlying conditions such as endocrine and metabolic disorders. The test is negative when the patient's age is between 10 and 16 years and the weight ≥50th centile and positive when these are beyond these boundaries. The probability of a child with a negative test result having idiopathic SUFE is 93%, and that of a child with a positive test result having atypical SUFE is 52%.

Authors Note: The Age–Weight Test

The age–weight test was introduced by Loder and Greenfield in 2001 [6]. They studied the demographics of 433 patients (285 idiopathic, 148 atypical), with 612 SUFEs, and found that weight and age were predictors of atypical SUFE. They recommended using the test to identify atypical SUFE. A negative test corresponds to an age between 10 and 16 years and weight ≥50th centile, and a positive test when outside of these values. For cases with a negative test, 93% were found to have an idiopathic SUFE. For cases with a positive test, 52% were found to have an atypical SUFE.

The test has not been widely adopted because of lack of specificity for atypical slips.

Clinical Presentation

The classical description is of an overweight child presenting with groin, thigh, and/or knee pain (referred pain, obturator nerve) and limping. There may be a history of minor trauma. Age is usually between 11 and 14 years. The child may be able to weight-bear (stable slip) or may not be able to do so even with crutches (unstable).

The leg is short and externally rotated (Figure 4a.1). There is usually restricted flexion, abduction, and internal rotation of the affected hip. Moreover, there is obligatory further external rotation when the hip is flexed more (Figure 4a.2).

Children with SUFE can also present more acutely with inability to walk after a minor trip. On the other hand, some children remain asymptomatic until early adulthood when they present with femoro-acetabular impingement (FAI) or premature arthritis (Figure 4a.3) [7].

Investigations
Radiological Tests

1. Plain radiographs (AP and true lateral views): although most centres use AP and frog lateral views, the latter is not advised particularly in unstable slips, as it may displace the slip further. It is also less precise in assessing the severity of a slip due to variations in positioning of the limbs. Several radiological signs have been described including (Figures 4a.4 and 4a.5):
   a. Trethowan's sign. A line (referred to as Klein's line) drawn on the superior border of the femoral neck in the AP view should pass through the femoral head. In SUFE, the line may pass over the epiphysis or intersect less height of the epiphysis than on the non-slipped side

   b. Decreased epiphyseal height as the head is slipped posteriorly behind the neck
   c. Remodelling changes of the neck with a sclerotic, smooth superior part of the neck and callus formation on the inferior border
   d. Increased distance between the tear drop and the femoral neck metaphysis

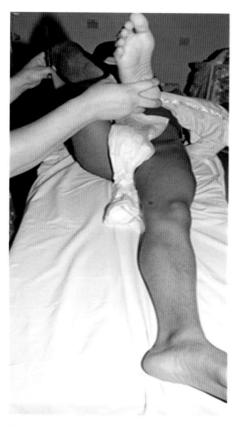

Figure 4a.2 Obligatory passive external rotation during hip flexion (Drehmann sign).

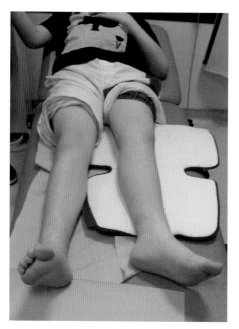

Figure 4a.1 A child with left slipped upper femoral epiphysis. Notice the short and externally rotated left leg (mimics a fractured neck of femur). The patient was able to ambulate (stable slip). He was initially treated with a knee brace because he presented with knee pain before the correct diagnosis of SUFE was made.

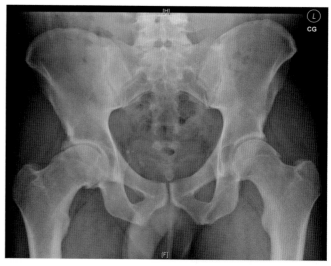

Figure 4a.3 Subclinical slipped upper femoral epiphysis. This 42-year-old electrician presented with right hip pain and stiffness. He recalled hip and knee pain when he was a teenager. He did not seek medical advice as he felt the pain was not severe.

e. Capener's sign: normally on the AP pelvis, the posterior acetabular margin cuts across the medial corner of the upper femoral metaphysis. In SUFE, the entire metaphysis is lateral to the posterior acetabular margin

f. Widening and irregularity of the physeal line (early sign)

g. Steel's blanch sign – a crescent-shaped, dense area in the metaphysis due to superimposition of the neck and head.

2. CT: this is not essential to diagnose and treat SUFE; however, it can be valuable in:

   a. Assessing the anatomical features accurately (such as degree of slip, head–neck angle, retroversion, severity of residual deformity and presence of callus)

   b. Ruling out penetration of the hip joint by metalware

   c. Confirming closure of the proximal femoral physis.

3. Ultrasound: it has been proposed to provide diagnostic and prognostic values in treating SUFE by demonstrating joint effusion and a step between the femoral neck and the epiphysis [8, 9]. However, this has not been adopted widely.

4. MRI:

   a. Useful in assessing equivocal cases at the pre-slip stage when plain radiographs do not show convincing features (Figure 4a.6)

   b. Assessment of avascular necrosis (AVN) of the femoral head

c. Delayed gadolinium-enhanced MRI of cartilage (dGEMRIC) scans have been used to assess for cartilage wear in femoroacetabular impingement (FAI) cases.

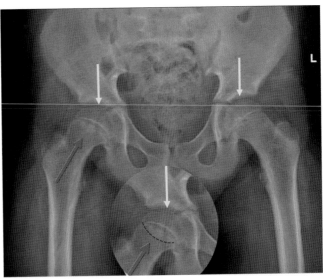

Figure 4a.5 Widened physis, reduced height of the epiphysis, and Steel's blanch sign. One of the earliest signs of slipped upper femoral epiphysis is widening and irregularity of the physeal line (right hip physis). There is decreased epiphyseal height (yellow arrows) as the head is slipped posteriorly behind the neck. The Steel's blanch sign (red arrows) is a crescent-shaped, dense area in the metaphysis due to superimposition of the neck and head (dashed red line in the inset).

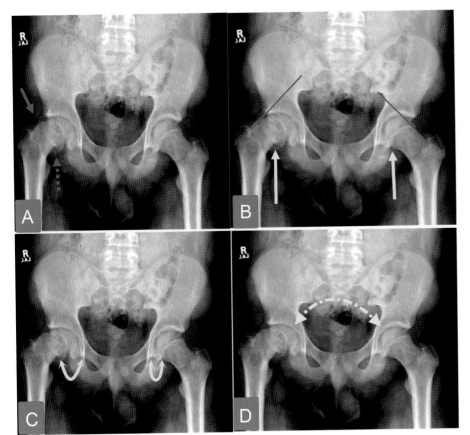

Figure 4a.4 Radiological signs in slipped upper femoral epiphysis. (A) shows the remodelling changes of the neck, with a bent, sclerotic, smooth superior part of the neck (solid purple arrow) and callus formation on the inferior border (dashed purple arrow). (B) shows a positive Trethowan's sign. Klein's line does not intersect the slipped epiphysis drawn on the superior border of the femoral neck in the AP view; it should pass through the femoral head. It also shows Capener's sign (solid yellow arrow) where the posterior acetabular margin cuts across the medial corner of the upper femoral metaphysis on the normal side, but not on the slipped side. (C) shows the increased distance between the tear drop and the femoral neck metaphysis. (D) shows chondrolysis (narrowed joint space), which is an uncommon complication of SUFE.

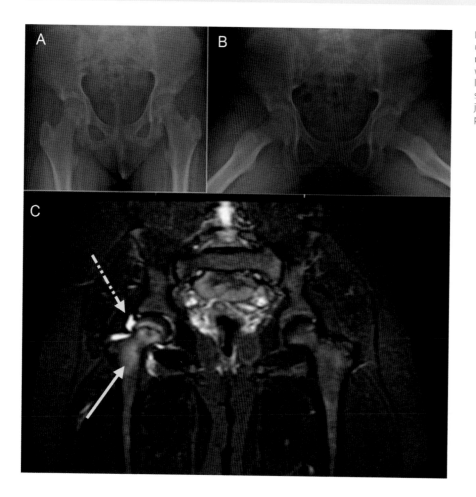

Figure 4a.6 MRI scan demonstrating slipped upper femoral epiphysis in a patient with an almost normal X-ray. (A) and (B) show radiographs of a child who presented with a painful right hip/knee. These look normal. However, the MRI scan in (C) shows high signal around the physis (solid yellow arrow) and joint effusion (dashed yellow arrow), consistent with pre-slip.

Blood Tests

Patients with an atypical SUFE require endocrine and metabolic screening, which is better performed by endocrine or metabolic specialists. Some blood tests may be requested by anaesthetists for safety purposes.

Classifications

SUFE has been classified into the following:

1. Functionally, according to the patient's ability to bear weight (stable or unstable)
2. Chronologically, according to onset of symptoms (pre-slip, acute, chronic, or acute-on-chronic)
3. Morphologically, according to the direction of displacement of the femoral epiphysis relative to the neck (varus or valgus slip).

Functional (Loder's Classification): According to Weight-Bearing Status

1. Stable: the patient is able to ambulate
2. Unstable: the patient is unable to ambulate, even with crutches [10].

In a series of 55 cases of SUFE, Loder showed that AVN developed in 47% of unstable slips, but in none of the stable slips. Several studies showed similar findings [11, 12].

Chronological: Relating to the Onset of Symptoms

1. Pre-slip: the patient has symptoms with no anatomical displacement of the femoral head. There may be useful radiological evidence such as widening of the physis and osteopenia of the pelvis
2. Acute: there is an abrupt displacement through the proximal physis, with symptoms and signs developing over a short period of time (<3 weeks)
3. Chronic: patients with a chronic slipped capital femoral epiphysis present with pain in the groin, thigh, and knee that varies in duration, often ranging from months to years
4. Acute-on-chronic: initially, the patient has chronic symptoms but develops acute symptoms as well following a sudden increase in the degree of slip.

Morphological (Majority of Cases of SUFE)

The epiphysis is displaced posteriorly and inferiorly (also called a varus or posterior slip) relative to the femoral neck. In rare cases, the displacement is either superior or posterior (also called valgus or anterior slip).

Key Points: Stability of Slip

There has been some confusion about Loder's classification of SUFE. Loder considered a slip as stable if walking and weight-bearing were still possible, with or without crutches. Confusion arises when a patient can stand, or even walk, but cannot weight-bear on the affected leg. According to Loder's classification, this is still considered a stable slip.

Kallio and colleagues introduced a different definition for unstable slip [8, 9]. They considered a slip as unstable when there is movement between the epiphysis and the metaphysis, whereas a stable slip corresponds to an adherent physis during weight-bearing, active leg movements or gentle joint manipulation. In their study of 55 cases of SUFE, they found that physeal instability was better indicated by joint effusion and an inability to bear weight. A slip is highly unlikely to be unstable in a child who is able to bear weight and has no joint effusion on ultrasound.

Ziebarth and colleagues [13] introduced the term 'intra-operative stability' for children with SUFE when the physis was not disrupted and had no abnormal movement. This 'intra-operative stability' was then compared to Loder's 'clinical stability' criteria in 82 patients with SUFE treated by open surgery. They found that the sensitivity and specificity of Loder's classification (stable and unstable) to predict physeal disruption (i.e. intraoperative instability) were 39% and 76%, respectively.

Mobility and weight-bearing status are the best current surrogates for slip stability and predictors of AVN, although they may not be the best. Search for better predictors of future AVN is ongoing.

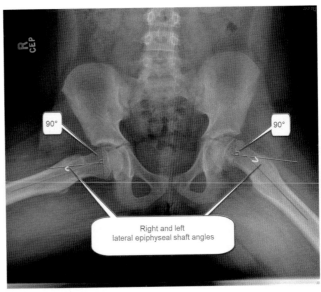

Figure 4a.7 Southwick angle. Angular displacement is measured by the Southwick angle, which is the difference between the lateral epiphyseal shaft angle of the slipped side and that of the non-slipped side. A mild slip (grade I) has an angle difference of <30°; a moderate slip (grade II) has an angle difference of between 30° and 50°, and a severe slip has a difference of over 50°.

reason that Southwick used the difference between the lateral epiphyseal shaft angle of the slipped side and that of the normal side, instead of the lateral epiphyseal shaft angle itself, is to guide the amount of flexion required to match both sides in corrective osteotomy.

Key Points: Classification and Grading of SUFE

In practice, most clinicians tend to use a combination of Loder's classification and Southwick's radiographic classifications. There is some crossover between the classifications, but severe slips are more likely to be unstable [16].

Grading

Grading the severity of the slip is based on radiographic findings – the degree of displacement either by proportion of slip (Wilson) [14] or by angle of slip (Southwick) [15] (Figure 4a.7).

The Wilson grading is based on the proportion of slip:

- Grade I: mild slip – where displacement of the physis as a proportion of the neck width is less than one-third
- Grade II: moderate slip – where displacement is between one-third and one-half of the neck width
- Grade III: severe slip – where displacement is greater than one-half of the neck width.

Angular displacement is measured by the Southwick angle, which is the difference between the lateral epiphyseal shaft angle of the slipped side and that of the non-slipped side:

- Grade I: mild slip – has an angle difference of <30°
- Grade II: moderate slip – has an angle difference of between 30° and 50°
- Grade III: severe slip – has a difference of over 50°.

In bilateral slips, the Southwick angle is calculated by subtracting 12° from the lateral epiphyseal shaft angle.

Most surgeons use the lateral epiphyseal shaft angle and the Southwick angle interchangeably (which is incorrect). The

Treatment

The aim of treatment is to prevent further progression of the slip with the least complications. Although it is tempting to reduce the slip to near-anatomical position, this goal has always been tempered by concerns about the potentially devastating complications of AVN and chondrolysis.

The choice of treatment of SUFE depends on the following factors:

1. Type of slip (stable or unstable)
2. Severity (mild, moderate, or severe)
3. Availability of surgical expertise
4. How soon patients present after symptoms.

Figure 4a.8 summarizes the authors' recommendations. Although controversy is still present on the best treatment options [17], the following approach is the most widely adopted and supported by the latest published evidence.

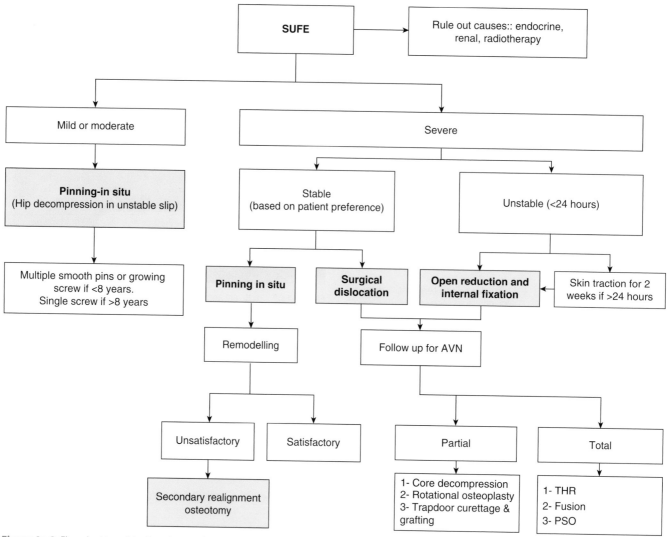

Figure 4a.8 Flow chart to guide slipped upper femoral epiphysis treatment.

Treatment of Stable SUFE

There is an almost universal consensus that treatment of a mild (and, to a lesser extent, moderate) stable slip should be by pinning in situ (PIS). The quoted AVN rate (which is a good surrogate for bad outcome) is 1.5% (slightly higher than what Loder reported in his original series).

How to perform PIS for SUFE is a common end-stage viva question and it is expected that candidates have a thorough understanding of this procedure.

If the slip is severe, PIS can be technically difficult, if not impossible. Closed reduction is often not successful and not recommended because of the risk of AVN. Two options are recommended:

1. Primary corrective osteotomy
2. PIS (if possible) with a future secondary realignment procedure.

Key Points: Pinning In Situ of Slipped Upper Femoral Epiphysis

1. The operation is performed under general anaesthesia.
2. Intravenous antibiotic is given at the time of induction.
3. The patient is positioned supine on the fracture table. The other limb can be placed in a traction boot (without applying traction) and moved gently to maximum abduction or flexed and abducted on stirrup to allow for imaging. In a stable slip, it is possible to perform the operation on a radiolucent table. The lateral view of the hip is obtained by flexing the hip. Regardless of the table used, optimum visualization of the femoral head before the procedure is essential.

4. The trajectory of the screw is identified and marked using a guide wire placed on the skin overlying the proximal part of the femoral neck and head, crossing the physis in a perpendicular fashion in the AP and lateral views (Figure 4a.9).

5. The guide pin is inserted freehand where the drawn lines intersect, then advanced through the soft tissues to engage the antero-lateral femoral cortex. The position and angulations of the guide wire are adjusted under fluoroscopic guidance to obtain a proper alignment, before the guide wire is advanced further into the bone.

6. The entry point is usually anterior (more so than the entry point for neck of femur fracture fixation). For unstable slips, a second guide wire is essential to provide rotational stability whilst inserting the first screw. If the second wire is in the correct place, it can be used for inserting a second cannulated screw, if desired.

7. After the appropriate screw length has been determined, the femoral neck and epiphysis are drilled using the cannulated instruments, whilst periodically checking the guide wire position is not advancing into the hip.

8. A 7.3- or 6.5-mm fully threaded, reversed cutting cannulated screw is then inserted.

9. It is essential to ensure there is no protrusion of the guide wire tip or the screw in the joint, particularly in the blind spot (Figure 4a.10). Three commonly used techniques to do so are: the withdrawal technique, using three-dimensional C-arm (if available), or injecting radiographic dye through the cannulated screw.

   a. The withdrawal technique is a commonly used method and is accurate if it is performed well. This involves moving the femoral head slowly in one direction (e.g. internal rotation). The screw tip appears to come closer and closer to the femoral head edge (but it should not breach the edge); then with further movement in the same direction, the screw tip starts moving away from the edge. The same technique is repeated in the other direction. There must not be any breach in any direction.

   b. The three-dimensional C-arm (mobile CT scanner) is relatively accurate, but it is not widely available and has a higher risk of radiation.

   c. Lehman proposed injecting radiographic dye through the screw cannula for detection and avoidance of pin penetration. The presence of the dye in the joint is an indication of penetration. However, once penetration happens, this method becomes less useful, as it cannot guide as to whether penetration still exists after backing out of the screw [18].

10. The patient can be allowed toe touch weight-bearing or partial weight-bearing, depending on the stability of the slip. This can progress gradually to full weight-bearing over 6 weeks' time.

11. Outpatient follow-up is until physeal closure.

Several primary corrective osteotomies have been practised. Three are worth mentioning: Fish's osteotomy (1984) [19], Dunn's osteotomy (1978) [20], and Ganz surgical dislocation of the hip (2001) [21]. The three techniques correct the slip at the subcapital level (where the deformity is); however, they differ in their surgical approaches.

In Fish's osteotomy, the Smith–Peterson anterior approach to the hip is used and does not involve a trochanteric osteotomy. In Dunn's and Ganz's osteotomies, the patient is positioned on the side, with the affected hip uppermost. The greater trochanter is osteotomized through the growth plate (Dunn's osteotomy) or by flip trochanteric osteotomy (Ganz's technique). In Fish's and Dunn's osteotomies, the femoral head remains in the acetabulum (no joint dislocation) during the procedure, whereas the hip joint is carefully dislocated during Ganz surgical dislocation (Figure 4a.11). The slip is temporarily stabilized with two wires during the process of dislocating the slip.

Ganz surgical hip dislocation has shown superior results to all other realignment procedures, in terms of AVN rates and patient satisfaction, in treating **stable** slips. This has not been the case with unstable slips (see below).

Key Points: Primary Corrective Osteotomy of the Slip

Success of the primary corrective osteotomy approaches is closely related to protecting (and may be restoring) the blood supply to the femoral head, which comes mainly from the posterior portion of the extracapsular anastomotic ring. In a stable slip, there is usually gradual deformity, causing the vessels in the posterior portion of the extracapsular anastomotic ring to shrink in length (Figure 4a.12). Forceful reduction risks tearing these shrunk vessels compromising the femoral head blood supply.

Contrary to the other two osteotomies, Ganz surgical dislocation provides good access to the posterior portion of the capsule, with the potential to remove any callus that is tethering vessels in the posterior portion of the extracapsular anastomotic ring.

A recent systematic review and patient level analysis of 41 studies (2 227 stable SUFEs) showed that PIS was associated with the lowest AVN rate (1.5%). The rates of chondrolysis, FAI, and osteoarthritis were relatively low in patients who underwent PIS. However, these low complication rates were not translated into high patient satisfaction rates among these patients, with only 47% reporting an 'excellent' outcome. This contrasts with Ganz surgical dislocation, for which, although the AVN rate was higher (3.3%), 87% of patients reported an 'excellent' outcome. Furthermore, five of the seven studies which investigated the Ganz surgical hip dislocation reported AVN rates of 0% [11] (Table 4a.1).

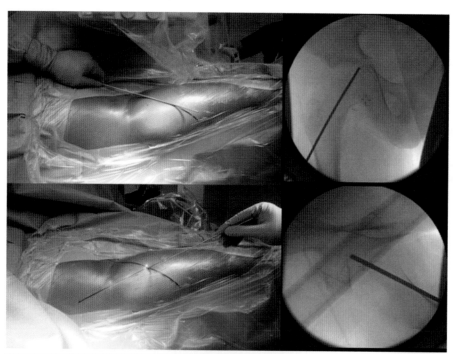

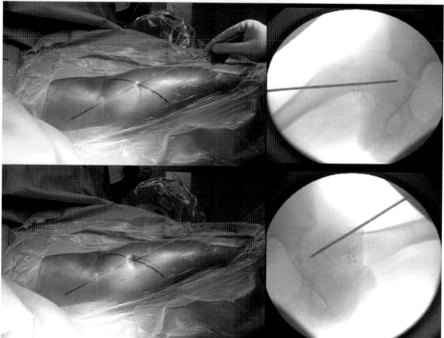

Figure 4a.9 Pinning a slipped upper femoral epiphysis. A guide wire is used to mark the trajectory of the screw on the AP and lateral views, then inserted percutaneously through the neck to the head to create what we call the inverted Umbrella sign (see bottom c-arm image).

Secondary realignment procedures (following PIS and healing of the slip) have been performed at one of four levels:

1. Subcapital level – this can be done using the same procedures that are used for primary corrective osteotomy (namely Ganz's, Dunn's, or Fish's osteotomy) [20–22]
2. The base of the femoral neck level (Kramer and Barmada) [23, 24]
3. The intertrochanteric level (Imhauser osteotomy) [25]
4. The subtrochanteric level (Southwick osteotomy) [15].

The last two (the intertrochanteric and subtrochanteric levels) are often grouped together as subtrochanteric osteotomies.

Anatomical correction can be best achieved by osteotomy at the subcapital level (at the centre of rotation of angulation (CORA)), and least achieved by subtrochanteric osteotomies. However, the risk of AVN is highest with osteotomy at the subcapital level (reported to be 3–11%), less with base of neck osteotomy (2.1%), and lowest with subtrochanteric osteotomy (1.5%) (Table 4a.1).

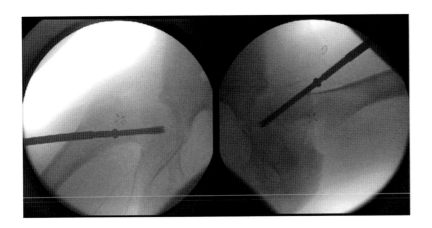

Figure 4a.10 Pinning a slipped upper femoral epiphysis. There is a blind spot where the screw can be protruded into the joint space, yet not visible on the C-arm images due to magnification effect.

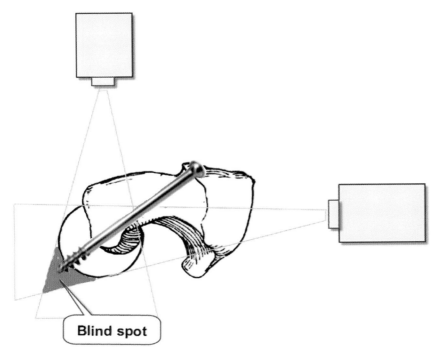

Blind spot

Residual deformity that has not improved naturally by remodelling, or by any of the above procedures, can be further treated with femoral head/neck osteochondroplasty. This can be performed arthroscopically, through a limited anterior arthrotomy, or by surgical hip dislocation.

Table 4a.1 Stable SUFE treatment outcomes

Intervention	Hips	Avascular necrosis	Chondrolysis	Satisfactory patient results[a]
Pinning using single screw	722	11 (1.5%)	15 (2.1%)	113 (47%) excellent 86 (36%) good 19 (8%) fair 10 (4%) poor 11 (5%) failure
Pinning using multiple pins	273	6 (2.2%)	11 (4%)	76 (67%) excellent 19 (17%) good 0 (0%) fair 16 (14%) poor 3 (3%) failure
Physeal osteotomy (Fish's and Dunn's)	615	68 (11.1%)	60 (9.8%)	131 (28%) excellent 210 (45%) good 46 (10%) fair 72 (16%) poor 3 (6%) failure

Table 4a.1 (cont.)

Intervention	Hips	Avascular necrosis	Chondrolysis	Satisfactory patient results[a]
Ganz surgical dislocation	95	3 (3.1%)	2 (2.1%)	52 (87%) excellent 2 (3%) good 0 (0%) fair 5 (8%) poor 1 (2%) failure
Base of neck osteotomy	92	2 (2.1%)	6 (6.5%)	22 (60%) excellent 11 (30%) good 2 (5%) fair 2 (5%) poor
Intertrochanteric osteotomy	336	5 (1.5)	16 (4.8%)	121 (44%) excellent 105 (38%) good 35 (13%) fair 15 (5%) poor

[a] Satisfactory patient results based on closely related ratings such as Heyman and Herndon classification, Harris hip scores, or Iowa hip scores.
Source: Adapted from Naseem *et al.* [11].

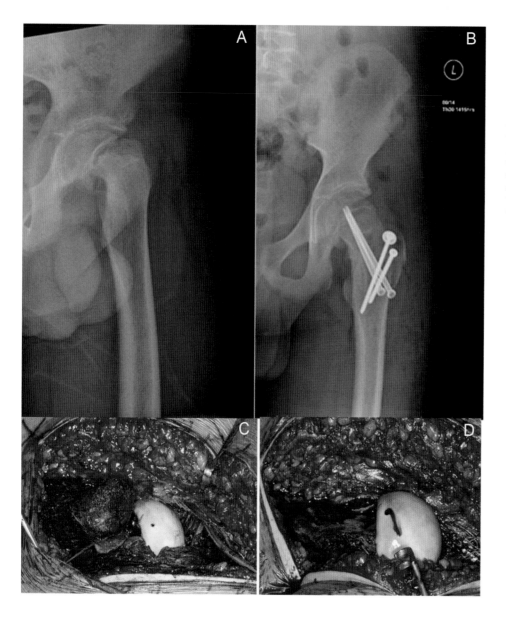

Figure 4a.11 Ganz surgical dislocation. (A) shows an X-ray of a child who presented with a severe, but stable, slip. The remodelling features and callus formation are clues for a stable slip. (C) and (D) are intraoperative pictures of Ganz surgical correction. (C) shows the femoral head carefully peeled off the neck, leaving a flap of tissue where the blood vessels to the head remain intact. The small hole (usually a 2-mm drill hole) shows no bleeding before reduction (kinked vessels), but bleeding resumes spontaneously after reduction. (B) shows the slip was stabilized by two screws (some surgeons use three wires), and the greater trochanter (flip osteotomy) also stabilized by two screws.

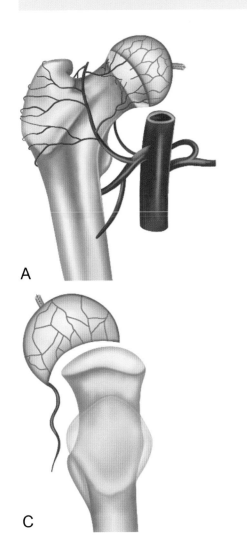

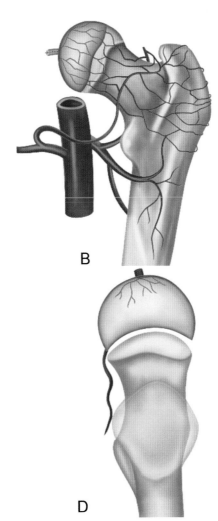

Figure 4a.12 Blood supply to the femoral head. The anterior portion of the extracapsular ring is formed primarily by the lateral femoral circumflex artery (A). The posterior, lateral, and medial aspects of the ring are formed by the medial femoral circumflex artery (B). The greatest volume of blood flow to the femoral head comes through the lateral ascending cervical vessel (the termination of the medial femoral circumflex artery), which crosses the capsule in the posterior trochanteric fossa where it is vulnerable to injury by intramedullary nailing through the piriformis fossa or by osteotomy of the greater trochanter (as in Dunn's osteotomy) (C-D).

Treatment of Unstable SUFE

The principle of treating unstable slips is similar to that of treating stable ones, which is to prevent further progression with the least possible complications. However, there are two important issues to consider:

1. Being unstable, there is an opportunity for spontaneous or unintentional reduction of the severity of the slip
2. The high risk of AVN (47%) and interrelated factors such as timing of surgery, intracapsular pressure, and severity of the slip.

Several techniques and approaches have been recommended and practised in different parts of the world, and even within the United Kingdom. We critically analysed the current techniques by performing a systematic review and patient level data analysis of 25 studies that provided patient level data on 661 patients with unstable slips. The included studies evaluated six different methods, namely:

1. Epiphysiodesis using bone peg
2. PIS (without any attempt of reduction)

3. Closed reduction and pinning (including slips where gentle reduction, positions, and unintentional reduction occurred)
4. Open reduction and internal fixation (86% of the data provided by a single study using the Parsch technique)
5. Physeal osteotomy (Dunn's and Fish's)
6. Ganz surgical dislocation.

The AVN rates were not significantly different among these methods, with one exception (Table 4a.2). The Parsch technique showed a significantly lower AVN rate of 5%, in comparison to other techniques.

Parsch and colleagues described a simple technique of open reduction of unstable SUFEs [26]:

Without any attempt at closed reduction, a Watson Jones approach is used to expose the hip joint. An anterior arthrotomy is performed with a longitudinal capsulotomy. A central K-wire is introduced by a power drill from the greater trochanter into the femoral neck, stopping short of the metaphyseal border of the slip.

With the surgeon's fingertip inside the capsule at the gap between metaphysis and epiphysis that can be palpated. A gentle reduc-

tion maneuver is performed by the assistant joggling the leg into flexion, abduction, and internal rotation, monitored by the finger inside the joint. The gentleness of the maneuver is of paramount importance. The surgeon's finger inside the capsule helps to avoid an undesired abrupt movement.

As soon as the surgeon notices the successful reduction of the metaphysis on the epiphysis, the assistant advances the previously introduced K-wire.

Then two more wires are introduced. The Manchester group added one more step – that of performing a 2-mm hole on the femoral head to confirm bleeding before any manipulation (Figure 4a.13).

Several favourable principles of the Parsch technique may have produced such good outcomes, including:

1. Operation performed as an emergency (within 24 hours)
2. No attempt at closed reduction
3. Emphasis on controlled and gentle reduction guided by the surgeon's finger
4. Decompression of the capsule reduces the intracapsular pressure, which may improve femoral head circulation. This is still controversial. Crepeau and colleagues showed that the average intracapsular hip pressure in the stable SUFE group (13 hips) was 27 mmHg, whereas the average pressure in the unstable SUFE group (15 hips) and normal group (11 hips) was 48.2 and 21.8 mmHg, respectively. There was no significant difference between the normal and stable SUFE groups, but there was a statistically significant difference between the stable and unstable SUFE groups ($P <0.001$) [27]. Ibrahim and colleagues in a systematic review of nine studies reported that the cumulative evidence does not indicate an association between hip decompression and a lower rate of osteonecrosis of unstable SUFE. However, they advised that hip decompression of unstable SUFE remains an option that can potentially decompress the intracapsular hip pressure and optimize blood flow to the femoral head [28]

5. The opportunity to check for femoral head blood supply.

It will be interesting to see whether Parsch's findings will be replicated by other centres. Ganz reported a 0% AVN rate in his series of unstable SUFE [29], but this rate was not replicated by other centres, with pooled AVN rates of 18% (Table 4a.2).

Timing of Surgery

There is increasing evidence that earlier surgery could result in lower AVN rates. Parsch reported three patients with AVN; two were operated on after 24 hours from presentation [26]. However, the rarity of the condition and the difficulty in extracting time to surgery data from published evidence render the current evidence weak.

Table 4a.2 Treatment of unstable SUFE

Interventions	Hips	Avascular necrosis
Epiphysiodesis	64	7 (11%)
Pinning in situ	115	38 (33%)
Closed reduction and pinning	269	71 (26%)
Open reduction and internal fixation (Parsch technique)	84	4 (5%)
Physeal osteotomies (Dunn's or Fish's)	59	10 (17%)
Ganz surgical dislocation	70	13 (18%)
Total	661	143 (22%)

Source: Adapted from Alshryda *et al.* [30].

Key Points: Surgical Procedures to Treat SUFE

Surgical techniques are common viva questions. Candidates would be expected to know full details for some operations (such as pinning in situ), whereas with other procedures, knowledge of the broad principles (such as surgical dislocation and corrective osteotomies) are sufficient.

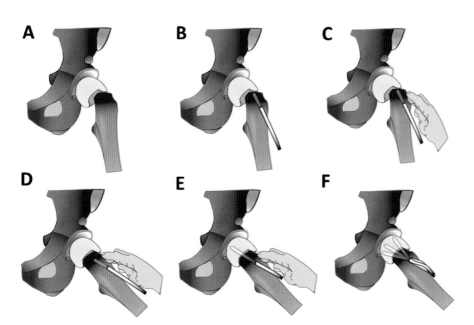

Figure 4a.13 The Parsch technique for treatment of unstable slips. (A) The patient is positioned supine on a radiolucent table. (B) A K-wire is introduced, just short of the metaphyseal border. (C, D) A jogging manoeuvre reduces the unstable part of the slip, controlled by the surgeon's fingertip. (E) The K-wire is advanced after achieving reduction of the unstable slip component. (F) Additional K-wires are added to enhance the stability of fixation. Source: Drawing is courtesy of Dr Jonathan Schoenecker.

The above systematic review and patient level analysis [30] of unstable SUFE reported an AVN rate of 13.3% (28/210) for those hips that were treated within 24 hours, 40% (38/95) for those that were treated between 24 hours and 72 hours, and 14.8% (5/53) for those that were treated after 72 hours.

Other smaller studies showed similar trends [31–33]. Therefore, the current trend is to stabilize unstable SUFE within 24 hours of the event. If this is not possible for whatever reason, surgery could be delayed for about 2–3 weeks to allow the inflammation to subside. A similar phenomenon has been noted in distal tibial pilon and ankle fractures when early operation before swelling starts or delaying surgery until swelling subsides reveal better results. Further research is required to identify the optimal timing of surgery, and the reasons to support it.

Treatment of the Contralateral Non-slipped and Asymptomatic Side

The quoted risk of contralateral slips varies from 18% to 60%, with 20% of slips being bilateral at presentation. The rest might develop a contralateral slip within 18 months from the date of the index slip. The complication rates associated with prophylactic pinning have been reported to be approximately 5%, including AVN and peri-prosthetic fractures (Figure 4a.14) [34–36]. It also affects the femoral neck length, a rarely considered recognized effect. Therefore, complications from prophylactic treatment should be weighed against the potential benefit. Both proponents and opponents have some evidence to support their views [37].

Stasikelis *et al.* [38] performed a retrospective review of 50 children who had unilateral SUFE, to determine parameters that predict later development of a contralateral slip. They found the modified Oxford bone age to be strongly correlated with the risk of development of a contralateral slip; a contralateral slip developed in 85% of patients with a score of 16, in 11% of patients with a score of 21, and in no patients with a score of 22 or more. The modified Oxford bone age is based on the appearance and fusion of the iliac apophysis, femoral capital physis, and greater and lesser trochanters. The relatively complicated way to calculate this score precludes its widespread use.

Phillips and colleagues [39] examined the posterior sloping angle (PSA) (Figure 4a.15) in 132 patients as a predictor for developing a contralateral slip. The mean was 17.2 ± 5.6° in 42 patients who subsequently developed a contralateral slip, which was significantly higher ($P = 0.001$) than the mean of 10.8 ± 4.2° for the 90 patients who did not develop a contralateral slip. If a PSA of 14° was used as an indication for prophylactic fixation, 35 slips (of 42 = 83.3%) would have been prevented and 19 (of 90 = 21.1%) would have been pinned unnecessarily.

We recommend a pragmatic approach for contralateral pinning, with the following factors playing a role in decision-making:

1. Age of the child (<10 years is associated with a higher risk of bilaterality)
2. Slips associated with renal osteodystrophy and endocrine disorders (high incidence of bilaterality)
3. Poor compliance of the child and family

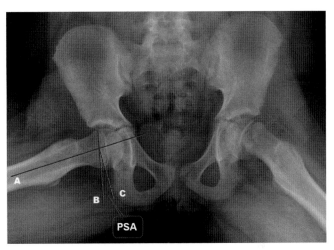

Figure 4a.15 The posterior sloping angle (PSA) predicts a contralateral slip. The PSA is measured by a line (A) from the centre of the femoral shaft through the centre of the metaphysis. A second line (B) is drawn from one edge of the physis to the other, which represents the angle of the physis. Where lines A and B intersect, a line (C) is drawn perpendicular to line A. The PSA is the angle formed by lines B and C posteriorly, as illustrated.

Figure 4a.14 Peri-prosthetic fracture that was treated with open reduction and internal fixation using a proximal femur locking plate.

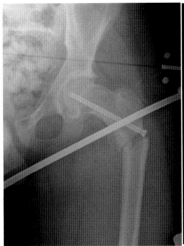
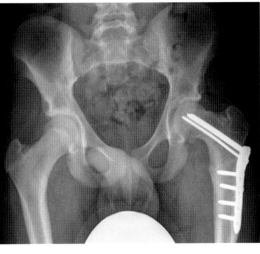

4. The nature of current slip (a very bad slip that occurred over a very short period of time may justify pinning the other side)
5. PSA >14° and/or a modified Oxford score of 16 or less.

Hip Spica and Bone Graft

Hip spica cast was used as the definitive management of SUFEs in the past, but it was associated with high chondrolysis rates (19% of 37 SUFEs) and slip progression after removal of the spica. On the good side, it showed lower rates of contralateral slip (7% of 30 hips). There may be a role for hip spica as an adjunct to PIS, particularly if bone quality is poor or the fixation is not adequate.

Similarly, bone graft (peg) epiphysiodesis was used in the past as the definitive management of SUFEs. However, most authors agree that PIS is a simpler procedure, with less intra-operative blood loss, fewer post-operative complications, and comparable post-operative results. It may be used to support fixation when there is excessive osteolysis and the fixation is at risk of failure [40].

Complications
Avascular Necrosis of the Femoral Head

AVN is a serious complication and closely linked to bad outcomes. It can involve the full femoral head (total) or part of the femoral head (partial). The smaller the extent of AVN, the better the outcome. In the majority of cases, AVN becomes apparent within a year or two, with the patient presenting with increasing stiffness and pain following a period of improvement after stabilization. Infection and loss of fixation should be excluded first, although they are much rarer than AVN.

MRI is the most sensitive and specific test to diagnose and assess the extent of AVN. Involvement of >30–50% of the femoral head indicates an increased risk of articular collapse [41].

Several medical and surgical treatments have been recommended to overcome the symptoms caused by AVN, with variable success rates. Table 4a.3 summarizes these treatments.

Chondrolysis

Chondrolysis is rapid and progressive loss of articular cartilage seen in some SUFEs. The cause is unknown; however, a few theories have postulated an autoimmune phenomenon or some interference with cartilage nutrition. Risk factors leading to chondrolysis include immobilization in a cast, unrecognized pin penetration, and severe SUFE. This may be due to pin penetration or a protruded screw, but it has been reported also in other situations. Clinically, the patient develops increasing pain and stiffness, and the X-ray shows a decrease in the apparent joint space of >2 mm, compared to that of the contralateral hip.

Metalware Removal

Several studies have shown that removing metalware after pinning SUFE was associated with substantive complications, which negates the benefits [42–44]. However, the plate of a corrective proximal femoral osteotomy is strongly recommended to be removed, particularly for cases where the future need for total hip arthroplasty is thought to be high. A plate that is fully covered with bone can pose serious challenges for future hip replacement and could potentially compromise the outcome.

Other Complications

- Residual deformity and FAI – a very common complication of SUFE. Arthroscopic osteoplasty is often inadequate to address the amount of deformity. Secondary corrective osteotomies (alone or combined with arthroscopic or open osteoplasty) are often helpful in improving patients' symptoms
- Osteoarthritis
- Leg length discrepancy – this is usually minor and rarely exceeds 2 cm. Insole is often all that is required.

Table 4a.3 Summary of treatments for avascular necrosis

Medical treatments	Surgical treatments
1. Bisphosphonates	1. Core decompression
2. Bone morphogenetic proteins	2. Rotational osteotomy to move a small necrotic area away from a weight-bearing area
3. Anticoagulants, statins, and vasodilators	3. Curettage and bone grafting with the trapdoor technique
4. Pulsed electromagnetic field	4. Hip arthrodesis (fusion)
5. Extracorporeal shockwave therapy	5. Pelvic support osteotomy
6. Hyperbaric oxygen therapy	6. Total hip arthroplasty (becomes the first choice of treatment for total avascular necrosis)

References

1. Lode RT, et al. Valgus slipped capital femoral epiphysis. *J Pediatr Orthop*. 2006;26(5):594–600.
2. Kelsey JL, Keggi KJ, Southwick WO. The incidence and distribution of slipped capital femoral epiphysis in Connecticut and Southwestern United States. *J Bone Joint Surg Am*. 1970;52(6):1203–16.
3. Loder RT. The demographics of slipped capital femoral epiphysis. An international multicenter study. *Clin Orthop Relat Res*. 1996;322:8–27.
4. Ninomiya S, Nagasaka Y, Tagawa H. Slipped capital femoral epiphysis. A study of 68 cases in the eastern half area of Japan. *Clin Orthop Relat Res*. 1976;119:172–6.
5. Loder RT, et al. Slipped capital femoral epiphysis. *Instr Course Lect*. 2001;50:555–70.
6. Loder RT, Greenfield ML. Clinical characteristics of children with atypical and idiopathic slipped capital femoral epiphysis: description of the age–weight test and implications for further diagnostic investigation. *J Pediatr Orthop*. 2001;21(4):481–7.
7. Lehmann TG, et al. Radiological findings that may indicate a prior silent slipped capital femoral epiphysis in a cohort of 2072 young adults. *Bone Joint J*. 2013;95-B(4):452–8.
8. Kallio PE, et al. Slipped capital femoral epiphysis. Incidence and clinical assessment of physeal instability. *J Bone Joint Surg Br*. 1995;77(5):752–5.

9. Kallio PE, *et al.* Classification in slipped capital femoral epiphysis. Sonographic assessment of stability and remodeling. *Clin Orthop Relat Res.* 1993;294:196–203.

10. Loder RT, Richards BS, Shapiro PS, Reznick LR, Aronson DD. Acute slipped capital femoral epiphysis: the importance of physeal stability. *J Bone Joint Surg Am.* 1993;75(8):1134–40.

11. Naseem H, *et al.* Treatment of stable slipped capital femoral epiphysis: systematic review and exploratory patient level analysis. *J Orthop Traumatol.* 2017;18(4):379–94.

12. Alshryda S, *et al.* Severe slipped upper femoral epiphysis; fish osteotomy versus pinning-in-situ: an eleven year perspective. *Surgeon.* 2014;12(5):244–8.

13. Ziebarth K, *et al.* Clinical stability of slipped capital femoral epiphysis does not correlate with intraoperative stability. *Clin Orthop Relat Res.* 2012;470(8):2274–9.

14. Wilson PD, Jacobs B, Schecter L. Slipped capital femoral epiphysis: an end-result study. *J Bone Joint Surg Am.* 1965;47:1128–45.

15. Southwick WO. Osteotomy through the lesser trochanter for slipped capital femoral epiphysis. *J Bone Joint Surg Am.* 1967;49(5):807–35.

16. Montgomery R. Slipped upper femoral epiphysis. *Orthop Trauma.* 2009;23(3 June):169–83.

17. Thawrani DP, Feldman DS, Sala DA. Current practice in the management of slipped capital femoral epiphysis. *J Pediatr Orthop.* 2016;36(3):e27–37.

18. Lehman WB, *et al.* A method of evaluating possible pin penetration in slipped capital femoral epiphysis using a cannulated internal fixation device. *Clin Orthop Relat Res.* 1984;186:65–70.

19. Fish JB. Cuneiform osteotomy of the femoral neck in the treatment of slipped capital femoral epiphysis. A follow-up note. *J Bone Joint Surg Am.* 1994;76(1):46–59.

20. Dunn DM, Angel JC. Replacement of the femoral head by open operation in severe adolescent slipping of the upper femoral epiphysis. *J Bone Joint Surg Br.* 1978;60-B(3):394–403.

21. Ganz R, *et al.* Surgical dislocation of the adult hip a technique with full access to the femoral head and acetabulum without the risk of avascular necrosis. *J Bone Joint Surg Br.* 2001;83(8):1119–24.

22. Fish JB. Cuneiform osteotomy in treatment of slipped capital femoral epiphysis. *N Y State J Med.* 1972;72(21):2633–40.

23. Kramer WG, Craig WA, Noel S. Compensating osteotomy at the base of the femoral neck for slipped capital femoral epiphysis. *J Bone Joint Surg Am.* 1976;58(6):796–800.

24. Barmada R, *et al.* Base of the neck extracapsular osteotomy for correction of deformity in slipped capital femoral epiphysis. *Clin Orthop Relat Res.* 1978;132:98–101.

25. Imhauser G. [Late results of Imhauser's osteotomy for slipped capital femoral epiphysis (author's transl)]. *Z Orthop Ihre Grenzgeb.* 1977;115(5):716–25.

26. Parsch K, Weller S, Parsch D. Open reduction and smooth Kirschner wire fixation for unstable slipped capital femoral epiphysis. *J Pediatr Orthop.* 2009;29(1):1–8.

27. Crepeau A, *et al.* Intracapsular pressures after stable slipped capital femoral epiphysis. *J Pediatr Orthop.* 2015;35(8):e90–2.

28. Ibrahim T, *et al.* Hip decompression of unstable slipped capital femoral epiphysis: a systematic review and meta-analysis. *J Child Orthop.* 2015;9(2):113–20.

29. Ziebarth K, *et al.* Capital realignment for moderate and severe SCFE using a modified Dunn procedure. *Clin Orthop Relat Res.* 2009;467(3):704–16.

30. Alshryda S, *et al.* Evidence based treatment for unstable slipped upper femoral epiphysis: systematic review and exploratory patient level analysis. *Surgeon.* 2018;16(1):46–54.

31. Lowndes S, Khanna A, Emery D, Sim J, Maffulli N. Management of unstable slipped upper femoral epiphysis: a meta-analysis. *Br Med Bull.* 2009;90:133–46.

32. Peterson MD, *et al.* Acute slipped capital femoral epiphysis: the value and safety of urgent manipulative reduction. *J Pediatr Orthop.* 1997;17(5):648–54.

33. Kalogrianitis S, *et al.* Does unstable slipped capital femoral epiphysis require urgent stabilization? *J Pediatr Orthop B.* 2007;16(1):6–9.

34. Baghdadi YM, *et al.* The fate of hips that are not prophylactically pinned after unilateral slipped capital femoral epiphysis. *Clin Orthop Relat Res.* 2013;471(7):2124–31.

35. Sankar WN, *et al.* What are the risks of prophylactic pinning to prevent contralateral slipped capital femoral epiphysis? *Clin Orthop Relat Res.* 2012;471(7):2118–23.

36. Kroin E, *et al.* Two cases of avascular necrosis after prophylactic pinning of the asymptomatic, contralateral femoral head for slipped capital femoral epiphysis: case report and review of the literature. *J Pediatr Orthop.* 2015;35(4):363–6.

37. Jerre R, *et al.* The contralateral hip in patients primarily treated for unilateral slipped upper femoral epiphysis. Long-term follow-up of 61 hips. *J Bone Joint Surg Br.* 1994;76(4):563–7.

38. Stasikelis PJ, *et al.* Slipped capital femoral epiphysis. Prediction of contralateral involvement. *J Bone Joint Surg Am.* 1996;78(8):1149–55.

39. Phillips PM, *et al.* Posterior sloping angle as a predictor of contralateral slip in slipped capital femoral epiphysis. *J Bone Joint Surg Am.* 2013;95(2):146–50.

40. Herring JA. *Tachdjians' Pediatric Orthopaedics*, 4th ed, Vol. 1. Philadelphia, PA: Saunders Elsevier; 2008.

41. Murphey MD, *et al.* ACR appropriateness criteria osteonecrosis of the hip. *J Am Coll Radiol.* 2016;13(2):147–55.

42. Ilchmann T, Parsch K. Complications at screw removal in slipped capital femoral epiphysis treated by cannulated titanium screws. *Arch Orthop Trauma Surg.* 2006;126(6):359–63.

43. Bellemans J, *et al.* Pin removal after in-situ pinning for slipped capital femoral epiphysis. *Acta Orthop Belg.* 1994;60(2):170–2.

44. Holm AG, Reikeras O, Terjesen T. Long-term results of a modified Spitzy shelf operation for residual hip dysplasia and subluxation. A fifty year follow-up study of fifty six children and young adults. *Int Orthop.* 2017;41(2):415–21.

Legg–Calvé–Perthes Disease

Sattar Alshryda and Paul A. Banaszkiewicz

Introduction

Perthes disease is avascular necrosis (AVN) of the femoral head in a growing child caused by interruption of blood supply to the femoral head. The condition was first described by Waldenström, but he attributed it to tuberculosis. It was then described more accurately by Arthur Legg (American), Jacques Calvé (French), and George Perthes (German) almost at the same time – hence the name Legg–Calvé–Perthes disease (LCPD).

It has an incidence of 1 in 10 000 and commonly affects children aged between 4 and 9 years who are often small with delayed bone age. It is bilateral in 15% of cases, but involvement is usually asymmetrical and never simultaneous, in contrast to multiple epiphyseal dysplasias.

Aetiology

The aetiology is unknown; however, several theories have been put forward.

The Anatomical Theory

Blood supply to the femoral head changes as a child grows (Table 4b.1). At birth, it is supplied by the medial and lateral circumflex arteries, as well as by the artery of the ligamentum teres. Contribution from the lateral circumflex artery diminishes and is taken over by the medial circumflex artery as the child grows. This changeover to the adult pattern may be affected by several factors comprising the blood supply to the femoral head leading to ischaemic necrosis.

The Hydrostatic Pressure Theory

This theory attributes the reduction in blood supply to the femoral head to the increase in intraosseous venous pressure which has been noticed in several cases. Heikkinen *et al.* [1] studied the

venous drainage of the femoral neck in 73 children with LCPD, using intraosseous venography films. Fifty-five contralateral symptomless hips were used as controls. They noted that venous drainage was pathological in 46/55 hips (82%) in the fragmentation phase and in 7/18 hips (39%) in the reossification stage, and normal in the healed stage. Two out of the 55 symptomless hips showed pathological venous drainage. They also noted that disturbances in the venous drainage of the femoral neck seem to correlate with the stage of activity of LCPD. However, this increase in venous hydrostatic pressure may be a cause, rather than an effect.

The Thrombophilic Theory

It is well known that children with haemoglobinopathies, such as sickle cell disease and thalassaemia, commonly have AVN of the femoral head. There is also some evidence of association of LCPD with various forms of thrombophilia. In a study by Balasa *et al.* [2], 72 patients with LCPD were compared to 197 matched health control. The factor V Leiden mutation was commoner in LCPD patients (8/72) than in controls (7/197) ($\chi^2 = 5.7$; $P = 0.017$). A high level of anticardiolipin antibodies was found in 19 of the 72 LCPD patients, compared to 22 of the 197 controls ($\chi^2 = 9.5$; $P = 0.002$). Some studies showed an association of LCPD with protein S and C abnormalities [3, 4], although other studies [5, 6] did not show such an association. With such conflicting evidence, coagulation abnormalities may have some aetiological role in LCPD, but this is to be confirmed.

There are other aetiological and associated factors, but their exact roles have not been delineated yet:

1. Trauma, hyperactivity, and attention deficit disorder – hyperactivity often results in trauma, occluding the blood vessels supplying the femoral head, and thus resulting in femoral head AVN
2. Susceptible child (abnormal growth and development):
   a. Low birthweight
   b. Low socio-economic class
   c. Bone maturation delays
   d. Boys > girls (4/1)
3. Hereditary and familial factors
4. Passive smoking
5. Transient synovitis (controversial) [7].

A recent study of finite element analysis modelling of the blood supply to the juvenile femoral head suggested that the

Table 4b.1 Blood supply to the femoral head

Age	Birth to 4 years	4 years to adult	Adult
Source	Medial and lateral circumflex arteries from profunda femoris artery	Posterosuperior and posteroinferior retinacular arteries from medial femoral circumflex artery	Medial femoral circumflex to lateral epiphyseal artery
	Ligamentum teres from posterior division of obturator artery	Negligible lateral circumflex artery	
		Minimum ligamentum teres	

interruption in blood supply is caused by kinking of the blood vessels. This is facilitated by delayed ossification and soft(er) articular cartilage [8], which could be potentially explained by most of the above factors.

Pathophysiology

The interruption of blood supply results in infarction of part or all of the femoral head. The repair processes start soon after, initially by osteoclastic response to resorb the necrotic bone. However, new bone formation to replace the resorbed trabeculae gets delayed because of a poor initial osteoblastic response [9]. This imbalance between bone resorption and new bone formation renders the bone trabeculae weak and susceptible to collapse.

The AVN associated with LCPD also triggers chronic synovitis [10], which is characterized by perivascular aggregation of lymphocytes and plasma cells [11]. This leads to hypertrophy of both the ligamentum teres and articular cartilage early in the disease and predisposes to the femoral head extruding from under the margin of the acetabulum [12, 13].

Weakened avascular bone of the extruded femoral head cannot withstand the physiological stresses of weight-bearing and irreversible deformation of the femoral head ensues (Figure 4b.1). Extrusion in excess of 20% is associated with a high risk of permanent deformation of the femoral head [14, 15].

Presentation

Patients commonly present with an insidious onset of a limp and anterior thigh or knee pain. Usually, they have activity-related pain, which is relieved by rest. Some children may present with a more acute onset of symptoms. There may be a history of minor trauma.

Examination usually reveals limited hip motion, particularly abduction and internal rotation. Gait is often antalgic and the Trendelenburg test is usually positive. There may be muscle spasm with evidence of thigh, calf and buttock atrophy from disuse. Leg length discrepancy indicates significant femoral head collapse. Evaluation of the patient's overall height, weight and bone age may be helpful to exclude skeletal dysplasias or growth disorders.

Blood tests are helpful in ruling out other conditions (see Differential Diagnosis). In the majority of cases, plain radiographs (AP and frog leg lateral) will confirm the diagnosis. However, in some early cases, radiographs may be normal and an MRI scan is required.

Radiological findings include widening of the joint space, a smaller capital femoral epiphysis, the crescent sign (denotes subchondral fracture) and flattening of the epiphysis (Figure 4b.2).

A bone scan may be helpful in the early stages of the disease, when the diagnosis is in question, particularly if the differential diagnosis is between transient synovitis and LCPD. The most accurate imaging modality for diagnosing early disease is MRI.

Theissen [16] reported a diagnostic accuracy of 97–99% for MRI, compared to 88–93% for plain X-ray and 88–91% for bone scan.

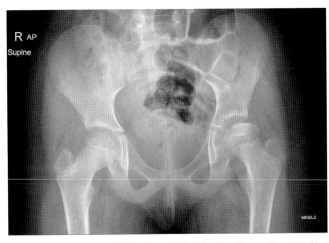

Figure 4b.1 A child with left hip Legg–Calvé–Perthes disease. Hypertrophy of both the ligamentum teres and articular cartilage (seen as increased distance between the femoral head and the teardrop) early in the disease predisposes to the femoral head extruding from under the margin of the acetabulum.

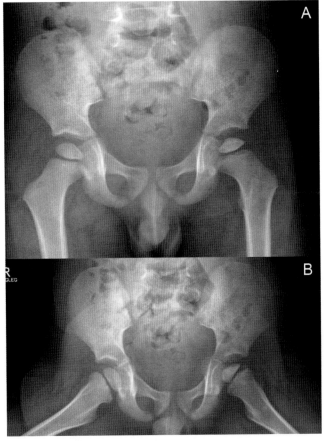

Figure 4b.2 Left hip Legg–Calvé–Perthes disease. (A) is an AP radiograph of the pelvis showing slight sclerosis and flattening of the left femoral head. (B) shows a typical crescent sign (subchondral bone fracture).

Differential Diagnosis

1. Unilateral LCPD:
   a. Septic arthritis (usually the child is unwell, with fever and high levels of inflammatory markers)

b. Sickle cell (history, sickling test, haemoglobin electrophoresis)

c. Eosinophilic granuloma (rare, other lesions including the skull, radiological features of single or multiple osteolytic lesions with cortical erosion, biopsy often needed for diagnosis)

d. Transient synovitis (lack of characteristic radiographic changes).

2. Bilateral LCPD is not common and requires skeletal survey and blood tests to exclude:

a. Hypothyroidism (thyroid function tests)

b. Multiple epiphyseal dysplasia (usually bilateral and simultaneous, other joint epiphyseal involvement) (Figure 4b.3)

c. Spondyloepiphyseal dysplasia (involvement of the spine)

d. Meyer's dysplasia: delayed, irregular ossification of the femoral epiphyseal nucleus. Commoner in males, usually occurs in the second year of life, mostly bilateral and the disorder usually disappears by the end of the sixth year. Bone scans are normal (Figure 4b.4)

e. Sickle cell

f. Mucopolysaccharidoses.

Radiographic Stages

Waldenström classified the evolution of LCPD into four stages, based on radiographic changes (Figure 4b.5).

Initial (Sclerotic/Necrotic) Stage

Ischaemia leads to subchondral bone death and necrosis (dead bone looks dense on plain radiographs). There is joint space widening due to continuous cartilage growth (nutrient from

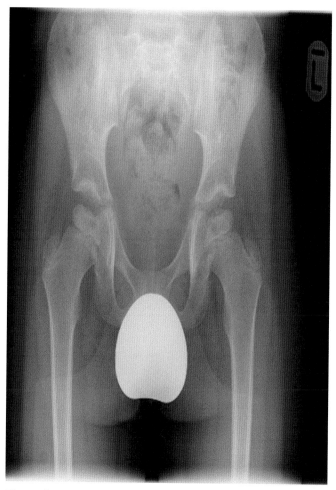

Figure 4b.4 Meyer's dysplasia. There is delayed, but symmetrical, ossification of the femoral epiphyseal nucleus. This usually disappears by the end of the sixth year and femoral heads become fully ossified. Bone scans are normal.

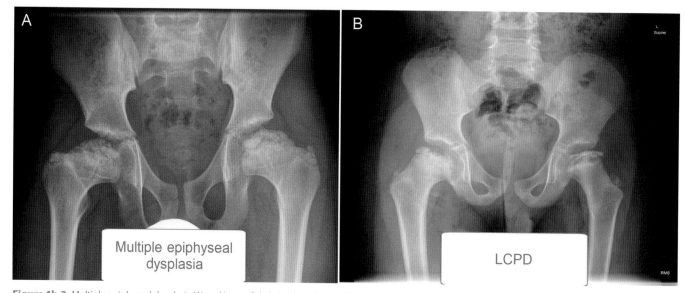

Figure 4b.3 Multiple epiphyseal dysplasia (A) and Legg–Calvé–Perthes disease (B). In multiple epiphyseal dysplasia, femoral head involvement is usually bilateral, simultaneous, and symmetrical. Notice also fragmentation of the greater trochanteric apophyses. In Legg–Calvé–Perthes disease, femoral head involvement is usually asymmetrical and never simultaneous.

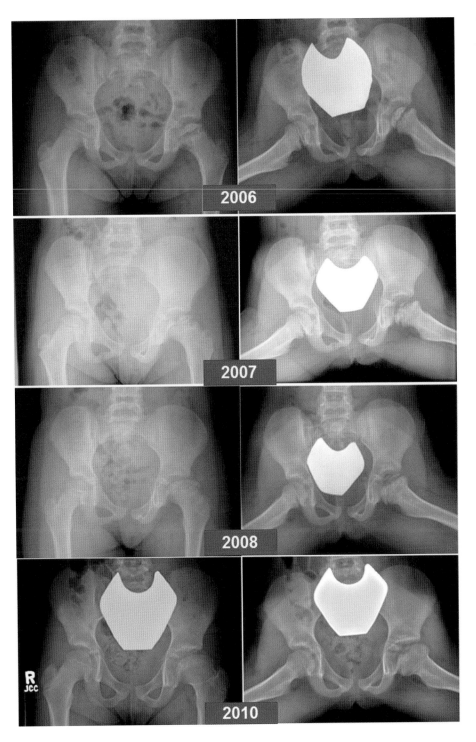

Figure 4b.5 Waldenström radiographic stages. These pelvic X-rays (AP and lateral) belong to a girl who presented with LCPD at the age of 5 years, showing the four stages of the disease (sclerotic stage, 2006; fragmentation phase, 2007; healing stage, 2008; and remoulding stage, 2010). The first three stages are further divided into early (subgroup a) and late (subgroup b) stages.

the synovial fluid) and hypertrophy of the synovium and ligamentum teres. This can be subdivided into early (no loss in epiphyseal height) or late where there is some loss of epiphyseal height, but the epiphysis is still in one piece. This stage lasts 6–12 months.

Fragmentation (Resorption) Stage

In this stage, revascularization has started, recruiting osteoblasts and osteoclasts. The latter remove dead and necrotic bone, causing radiolucent fissures among dead fragments. This stage can be further divided into early (1–2 fissures only) or late when the head is in several fragments. This stage usually lasts from 12 to 24 months.

Reossification (Healing) Stage

Vascular regeneration by the process of creeping substitution leads to reossification of the femoral head. It starts peripherally and progresses centrally. This usually appears as a small and expanding fragment at the lateral part of the epiphysis, marking the beginning of this stage IIIa. This soft bone matures and covers more than a third of the epiphysis in stage IIIb. This stage usually lasts from 6 to 24 months.

It is critical to keep the soft head within the acetabulum for natural moulding in order to maintain its sphericity. If the soft head extrudes (uncontained within the acetabulum), it gets deformed and loses its sphericity. This explains the basis of containment treatment.

Remodelling (Residual) Stage

The head is considered to have healed when there is no avascular bone visible on radiographs (no changes in the density of the femoral head); however, it continues to remodel until skeletal maturity. The head becomes large (coxa magna) and hard. The neck is usually short and wide. The sphericity is variable. The acetabulum also remodels to match the femoral head deformity. The older the child is, the less the remodelling and the poorer the outcome.

Radiographic Classifications

Various classifications have been described to assess the extent of femoral head involvement.

Catterall, 1971

Based on the extent of head involvement at the fragmentation phase, Catterall advised four stages [17] (Figure 4b.6). The lateral part of the femoral head (later named as the lateral pillar) gets affected in stages III and IV.

Salter and Thompson, 1984

Salter and Thompson recognized that Catterall's first two groups and second two groups were distinct and therefore proposed a two-group classification; this is often referred to as modified Catterall's classification:

- Salter and Thompson group A: less than half of the head involved
- Salter and Thompson group B: more than half of the head involved.

As in Catterall's classification, the main difference between these two groups is the integrity of the lateral pillar. In group A, the lateral pillar is intact.

(Herring) Lateral Pillar, 1992

This is based specifically on the integrity of the lateral pillar on the AP film only, at the beginning of the fragmentation phase (Table 4b.2; Figure 4b.7).

Classifications Addressing Outcome

Mose Classification

This system uses a concentric circle technique to compare and classify the final outcome in LCPD at the end of the

Table 4b.2 (Herring) Lateral pillar of Legg–Calvé–Perthes disease

Groups	Description
A	Normal height of the lateral third of the head is maintained. Fragmentation occurs in the central segment of the head
B	>50% of the original lateral pillar height is maintained. There may be some lateral extrusion of the head
C	<50% of the original lateral pillar height is maintained. The lateral pillar is lower than the central segment early on
B/C	<50% of the original lateral pillar height is maintained. The lateral pillar is higher than the central segment

Grade	Description	Diagram
Catterall I	0 - 25 % head involvement. Only anterior epiphysis (therefore seen only on the frog lateral film)	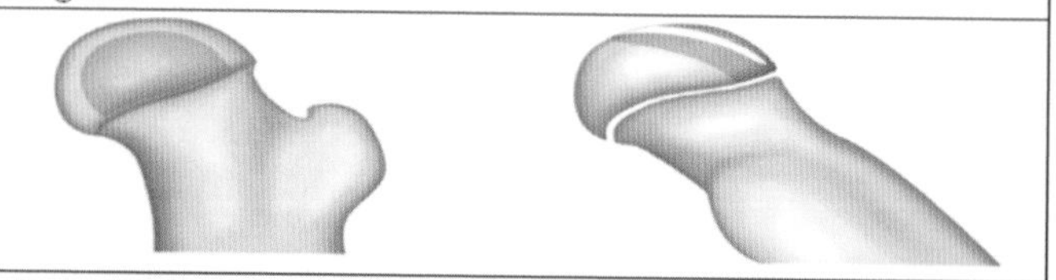
Catterall II	25 - 50 % head involvement. Anterior and central segment - fragmentation (sequestrum). Lateral part / rim is intact (protects the central involved area). Junction - clear. Metaphyseal reaction present - anterior. Subchondral fracture - anterior	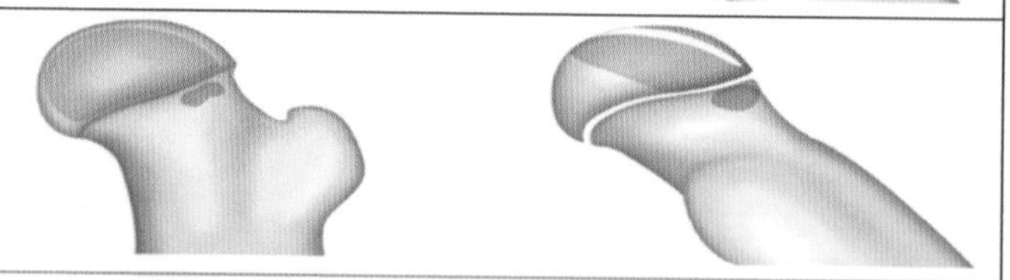
Catterall III	50 - 75 % head involvement. Anterior segment involved. Lateral head - also fragmented. Only the medial portion is spared. Loss of lateral part / support worsens the prognosis. Junction - sclerotic. Metaphyseal reaction present - anterior and lateral	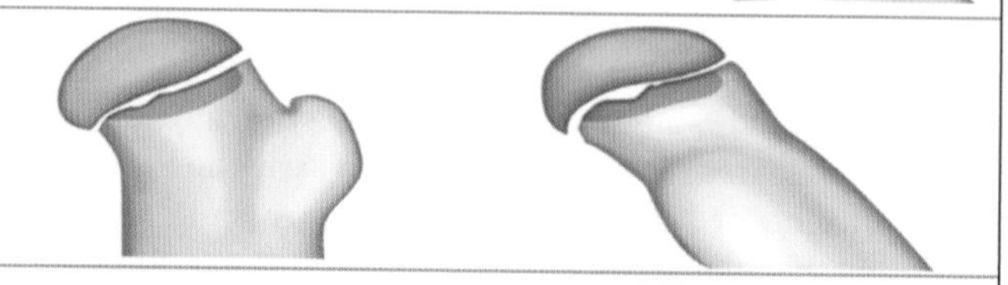
Catterall IV	>75 % head involvement	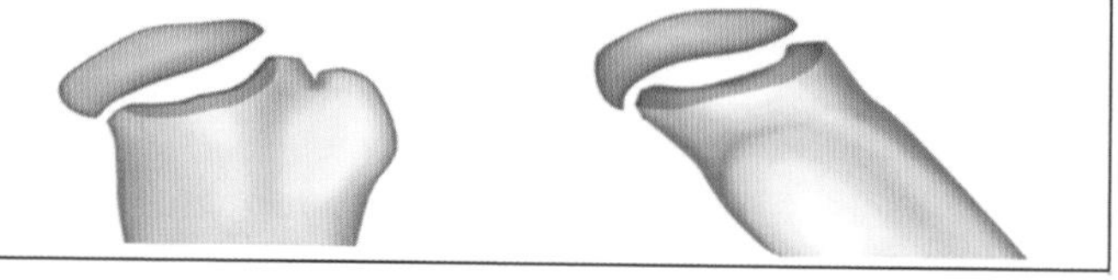

Figure 4b.6 Catterall classification of Legg–Calvé–Perthes disease.

remodelling stage. The final shape of the head is compared to a perfect circle using the Mose template on both AP and lateral images (Figure 4b.8).

Given that a congruous, but aspherical, head can perform well suggests that the Mose criteria are too strict and impractical.

Stulberg Classification

Stulberg *et al.* [18] investigated 88 patients (99 hips) with LCPD over 40 years of follow-up and showed that a lack of sphericity and congruency were both predictors for poor outcome (symptomatic osteoarthritis) (Table 4b.4; Figure 4b.9).

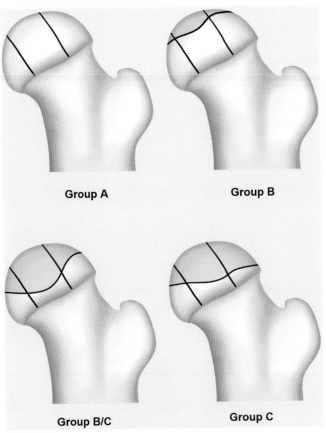

Figure 4b.7 Herring classification of Legg–Calvé–Perthes disease.

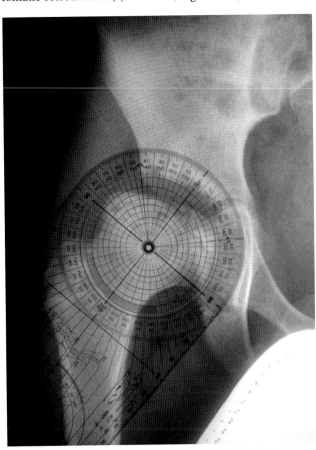

Figure 4b.8 Mose grading of Legg–Calvé–Perthes disease.

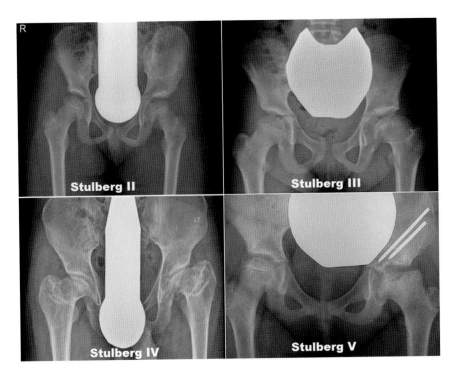

Figure 4b.9 Stulberg grading of Legg–Calvé–Perthes disease outcome.

Table 4b.3 Mose grading of Legg–Calvé–Perthes disease

Outcomes	Description
Good	Aspherical head contour is within 1 mm of a given circle on both views
Fair	Aspherical head contour is between 1 and 2 mm
Poor	Aspherical head contour is >2 mm

Table 4b.4 Stulberg grading of Legg–Calvé–Perthes disease[a]

Head	Class	Description	Risk of future osteoarthritis
Spherical and congruent	I	Normal spherical head	No increased risk of arthritis
	II	Spherical head, coxa magna/breva, steep acetabulum	
Aspherical, but congruent	III	Ovoid- or mushroom-shaped head	Mild to moderate arthritis develops in late adulthood
	IV	Flat head on flat acetabulum (may hinge on abduction)	
Aspherical and incongruent	V	Flat head, but normal acetabulum	Severe arthritis before age of 50

[a] See also Figure 4b.9.

A modified version of Stulberg classification is becoming popular and has a superior interobserver agreement [19] (Figure 4b.10). It consists of three groups: group A hips (Stulberg I and II) have a spherical femoral head; group B hips (Stulberg III) have an ovoid femoral head; and group C hips (Stulberg IV and V) have a flat femoral head.

Table 4b.5 shows recognized clinical and radiological prognostic signs.

Table 4b.5 Poor prognostic signs

Poor clinical prognostic signs (FOOBS)	Poor radiological prognostic signs[a]
Female	Gage's sign (V-shaped lucency at lateral epiphysis
Older age	Horizontal growth plate – caused by growth plate arrest on the lateral side due to excessive pressure
Obesity	Lateral epiphyseal calcification (lateral to the epiphysis – indicates the part of the head has already extruded)
Bilateral	Lateral subluxation – implies loss of lateral support, uncovering of the femoral head >3 mm in excess of opposite side (measured as the horizontal distance between a vertical line through the outer lip of the acetabulum and the lateral edge of the femoral head physis) or >20% of extrusion
Stiffness	Metaphyseal rarefaction/cyst

[a] See Figure 4b.11.

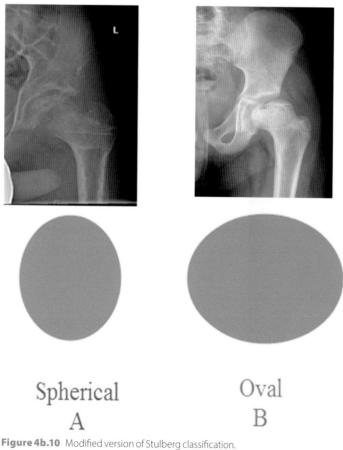
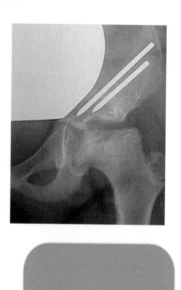

Spherical
A

Oval
B

Flat
C

Figure 4b.10 Modified version of Stulberg classification.

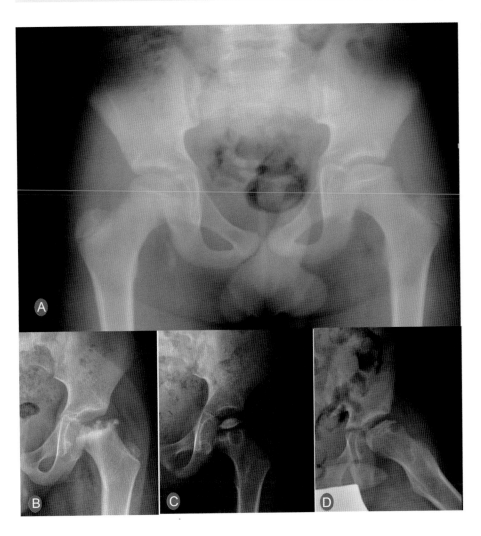

Figure 4b.11 Poor prognostic radiological signs in children with Legg–Calvé–Perthes disease. (A) Horizontal growth plate. (B) Lateral epiphyseal calcification. (C) Large metaphyseal cysts. (D) Gage's sign.

Treatment

Management of LCPD is one of the most controversial in paediatric orthopaedics. Various treatment methods are used to treat LCPD; these vary from long-term non-weight-bearing to months of abduction cast treatment, to combined femoral and pelvic surgical procedures, to ignoring the disease altogether. The following is a summary of various treatments, with the evidence behind them.

Symptomatic Treatments

These include:

1. Rest and lifestyle modification. In the acute phase, when symptoms are bad, complete rest, including a period of skin traction, helps improve symptoms, reduce spasm, and improve range of motion. When symptoms have improved, walking, swimming, and low-resistance cycling are encouraged. Contact and tackling sports are prohibited.

2. Analgesic and anti-inflammatory drugs

3. Physiotherapy plays an important role in improving range of motion.

Key Points: Non-weight-Bearing

There is little evidence to suggest that prolonged non-weight-bearing is effective in preventing femoral head deformity. It can have adverse mental effects. Therefore, striking the right balance between allowing children with LCPD to live as normal as possible and protecting the affected hip is important.

Casting and Bracing

Several types of casting (such as Petri or broomstick casts) and braces (such as Scottish Rite, Birmingham, or SWASH braces) have been advocated to produce containment of the femoral head within the acetabulum. They work by abducting and flexing (and internally rotating) the hip to reposition the femoral head deep in the acetabulum and protect it from collapse until reossification (at least stage IIIb). This may take 2 years or more, making compliance a real issue in this age group. When there is a severe adduction contracture, a period of traction ± adductor tenotomy may be necessary before applying these casts or braces (Figure 4b.12).

A

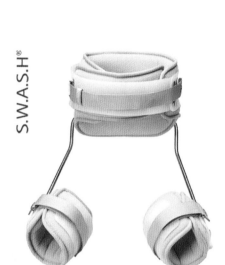

B

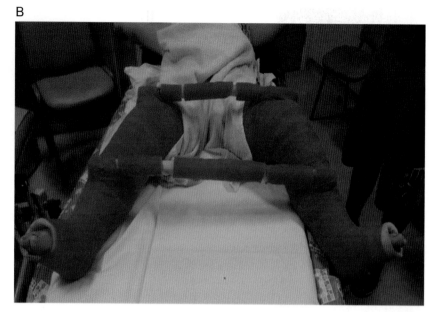

Figure 4b.12 (A) shows a SWASH (Sitting, Walking, And Standing Hip) brace. It is designed to keep the hip abducted and internally rotated during sitting, walking, and standing, to improve containment. (B) shows a Petri cast, which involves two above-knee casts with 10–20° of knee flexion. The broomsticks are positioned to produce 20° of hip internal rotation; they are removable to allow continuous physiotherapy. The former is meant to be worn until the end of the healing stage. The latter is too restrictive to be worn for a long time. It is mainly utilized for around 6 weeks to overcome substantive stiffness.

Surgical Treatments

Based on the stage of the disease and the child's age, surgical treatments can be grouped into containment surgery and salvage surgery.

Containment Surgery

The principle of containment surgery is to protect the soft femoral head from weight-bearing and muscular forces that push it against the acetabular margin. The anterolateral part of the avascular head is usually the most vulnerable to deformation during the early stages of the disease. This can be achieved by 'containment' of the entire femoral head within the acetabulum. Although this can be achieved by braces or casting, there are issues with convenience, tolerance, and compliance [20].

Surgical containment can be achieved by:

1. Femoral varus derotation osteotomy (Figure 4b.13) [21–25] – moderate varus angulation of 20° and external rotation of the distal fragment of 20–30° are often sufficient to achieve satisfactory containment [26]

2. Pelvic osteotomy (Salter osteotomy and triple osteotomy are the most widely used) (Figure 4b.14) [27, 28] – although combining femoral and pelvic osteotomies (Figure 4b.15) were promoted for better results [29–32]; the supporting evidence is insufficient [33]

3. Improved head coverage by shelf acetabuloplasty or Chiari osteotomy [34–37]

4. Articulated (hinged) hip distractor (external fixator) (Figure 4b.16) [38–40].

Key Points: What Osteotomy?

Our preference (which is based on our own personal experience and interpretation of the literature) is to perform (effective) femoral varus derotation osteotomy. By 'effective', we mean that it is good enough to contain the whole femoral head, even if it means excessive varus. Salter osteotomy has a limitation on how much containment can be achieved. Triple osteotomy is more effective than Salter osteotomy in achieving containment, but it is technically more demanding and may affect the birth canal.

Excessive varus often leads to marked limping (Trendelenburg gait). Although some remodelling and improvement in gait can happen, it is seldom adequate in children above 8 years old. That is why some recommend combined pelvic and femoral osteotomies in children above 8 years old. However, we still prefer effective varus osteotomy, even if it means that we may need to do valgus osteotomy when the femoral head is fully healed. We warn patients and parents about this.

We reserve articulated (hinged) hip distractor for a small group of older patients (aged 12 years and above) with substantive hip stiffness. In this group of children, the above containment surgical (femoral and pelvic osteotomies) options are not very effective. Femoral osteotomy does not remodel well and the outcome is usually poor. In patients who tolerate the hip distractor well, the outcome is surprisingly good. However, tolerance is usually poor and rarely can patients tolerate it for >6 months.

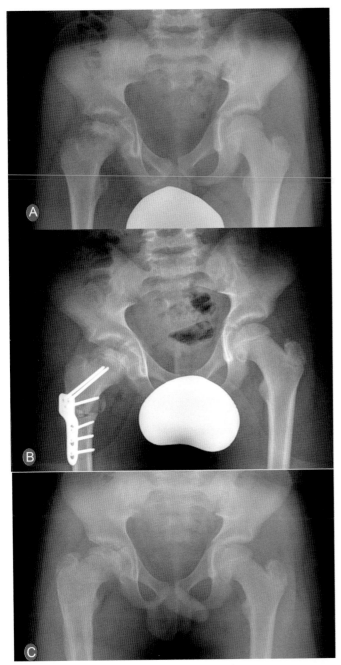

Figure 4b.13 Varus derotation femoral osteotomy for right hip Legg - Calvé - Perthes disease.(A) Pre-op AP radiographs (B) Post op AP radiographs demonstrating Initial plate fixation osteotomy (C) AP radiographs following osteotomy healing and removal of metal work

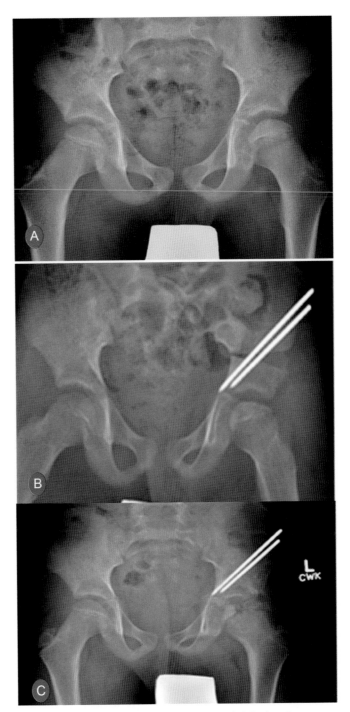

Figure 4b.14 Salter osteotomy for left hip Legg -Calvé -Perthes disease. (A) Pre-op radiographs (B) Post op AP radiograph initial pin fixation Salter osteotomy (C) AP radiograph of healed Salter osteotomy

Indication and Timing of Surgical Containment

There is still no consensus on indication and timing of surgery. However, there is a growing trend, backed by weak evidence, suggesting the following indications:

1. Any age with the head starting extrusion (>20%)

2. Older children (the age cut-off seems to be dropping from 8 years to 6 years) and still in early stages (stages I and IIa).

Children who are younger than 6 years with no femoral head extrusion do not benefit from containment surgery. Children who present late (stage IIb and later) may not benefit from surgical containment.

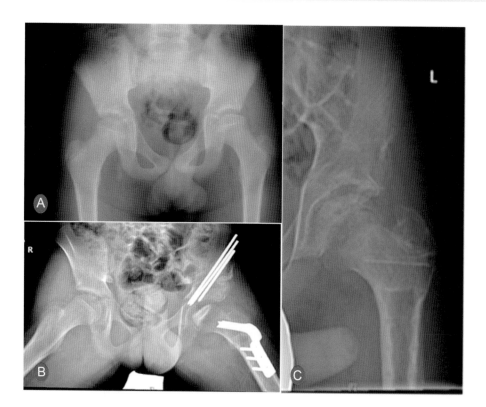

Figure 4b.15 Combined femoral and Salter osteotomies in a 9-year-old child with Legg - Calvé -Perthes disease. (A) Pre op AP radiograph (B) Immediate post op AP radiograph (C) AP radiograph healed osteotomies with metalwork removal

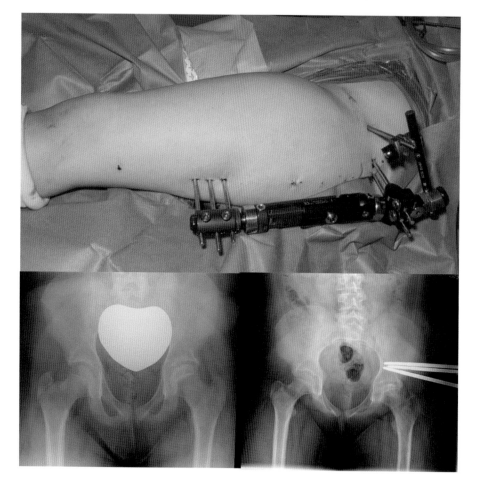

Figure 4b.16 Articulated (hinged) hip distractor in treating Legg–Calvé–Perthes disease.

Key Points: Evidence-Based Practice

Indication and timing of treatments have evolved since the first edition of this book. We previously recommended treatments that were based on age and Herring's pillar classification. For treatment to be effective, it needs to be initiated well before the stage of fragmentation when Herring staging can be identified with some degree of certainty [41]. Therefore, current indications are based on age, stage of the disease and femoral head extrusion. Stiffness precludes containment surgery and should be treated before contemplating containment surgery.

Two well-conducted systematic reviews and meta-analyses of 23 studies, including 1 232 patients and 1266 hips, demonstrated that in **patients younger than 6 years**, operative and non-operative treatments are equally as likely to result in a successful radiographic outcome (odds ratio (OR) = 1.071; P = 0.828; 95% confidence interval (CI), 7.377–32.937).

In **patients older than 6 years**, operative treatment is nearly twice as likely to result in a successful radiographic outcome (OR = 1.754; P <0.0001; 95% CI, 1.299–2.370). Sex had no significant influence on radiographic outcome (OR = 1.248; P = 0.486; 95% CI, 0.670–2.325). The two reviews reached a different conclusion regarding the superiority of pelvic versus femoral osteotomy [42, 43].

Herring *et al.* [44] reported on the results of the Legg Perthes Study Group. Thirty-nine surgeons from 28 centres took part in a prospective study. Each surgeon agreed to apply a single treatment method to each patient who met the study criteria. All patients were between 6 and 12 years of age at the onset of the disease and none had had prior treatment. The treatment groups were no treatment, range of motion treatment in which the patient did exercises once a day, Atlanta brace treatment, femoral varus osteotomy and Salter osteotomy. The study showed that age, lateral pillar grading, and treatment methods were significantly related to outcome.

In group B and B/C hips, with age at onset of >8 years, 73% of the operated hips had a Stulberg I or II result, compared to 44% of the non-operated hips (P = 0.02). In group B hips, with age at onset of 8 years or younger, there was no advantage demonstrated for the surgical group. Group C hips were not shown to benefit from surgical or non-surgical treatments.

Wiig *et al.* [45] reported on a nationwide prospective study. Twenty-eight hospitals in Norway were instructed to report all new cases of LCPD over a period of 5 years. A total number of 368 patients with unilateral disease were included in the study. For patients aged over 6 years at diagnosis with >50% necrosis of the femoral head (n = 152), surgeons from different hospitals had chosen one of three methods of treatment: physiotherapy (55 patients), the Scottish Rite abduction orthoses (26 patients), and proximal femoral varus osteotomy (71 patients). The study showed that the strongest predictor of poor outcome was femoral head involvement of >50% (modified Catterall's classification), followed by age at diagnosis, then by lateral pillar grades. In children aged over 6 years at diagnosis with >50% of femoral head necrosis, proximal femoral varus osteotomy gave a significantly better outcome than orthoses or physiotherapy. There was no difference in outcome after any of the treatments in children aged under 6 years.

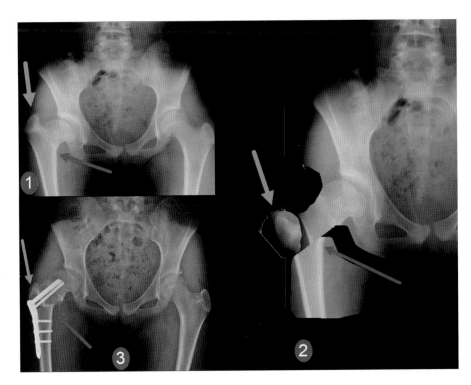

Figure 4b.17 Wagner osteotomy to treat an overgrown greater trochanter and a short femoral neck (1). The greater trochanter (green arrows) is cut just above the junction with the femoral neck. It is essential to protect the femoral head's blood supply which loops at the junction. The femoral shaft is then cut along the lower border of the femoral neck (red arrow) and slid outwards (2). The osteotomized greater trochanter is then placed lateral to the femoral neck and above the femoral shaft, and all fragments are stabilized using a proximal locking plate (3).

Salvage Surgery

Several surgical interventions have been advocated to improve symptoms or outcomes of healed LCPD. These can be summarized as follows:

1. Valgus osteotomy for hips with hinged abduction [46]. This occurs when the femoral head impinges on the acetabular margin in abduction, causing pain and limping. Hip arthrography and examination under general anaesthesia usually confirm the diagnosis when the hip is more congruent in adduction. Valgus osteotomy usually improves symptoms [46–48]
2. Trochanteric growth arrest using drill epiphysiodesis or a screw to prevent overgrowth (still not popular)

3. Advancement of the greater trochanter when it is overgrown
4. Wagner osteotomy to correct an overgrown greater trochanter and a short neck (Figure 4b.17)
5. Surgical treatment for femoroacetabular impingement (arthroscopic or open femoral head acetabuloplasty, including femoral head reduction procedure).

Medical Treatment

Medical treatments using bisphosphonates to slow or prevent femoral head collapse and/or bone morphogenetic protein to stimulate new bone formation are being investigated in animal and human studies [49]. They may have a potential role in preventing or reducing head deformity in LCPD, as sole treatments or combined with containment surgery [50].

References

1. Heikkinen E, *et al.* Venous drainage of the femoral neck in various stages of activity in Perthes' disease. *Rontgenblatter.* 1979;32(1):46–9.
2. Balasa VV, *et al.* Legg–Calvé–Perthes disease and thrombophilia. *J Bone Joint Surg Am.* 2004;86-A(12):2642–7.
3. Thomas DP, Morgan G, Tayton K. Perthes' disease and the relevance of thrombophilia. *J Bone Joint Surg Br.* 1999;81(4):691–5.
4. Hayek S, *et al.* Does thrombophilia play an aetiological role in Legg–Calvé–Perthes disease? *J Bone Joint Surg Br.* 1999;81(4):686–90.
5. Hresko MT, *et al.* Prospective reevaluation of the association between thrombotic diathesis and legg–perthes disease. *J Bone Joint Surg Am.* 2002;84-A(9):1613–18.
6. Gallistl S, *et al.* The role of inherited thrombotic disorders in the etiology of Legg–Calvé–Perthes disease. *J Pediatr Orthop.* 1999;19(1):82–3.
7. Landin LA, Danielsson LG, Wattsgård C. Transient synovitis of the hip. Its incidence, epidemiology and relation to Perthes' disease. *J Bone Joint Surg Br.* 1987;69(2):238–42.
8. Pinheiro M, *et al.* New insights into the biomechanics of Legg–Calvé–Perthes' disease: the role of epiphyseal skeletal immaturity in vascular obstruction. *Bone Joint Res.* 2018;7(2):148–56.
9. Kim HK, Herring JA. Pathophysiology, classifications, and natural history of Perthes disease. *Orthop Clin North Am.* 2011;42(3):285–95, v.
10. Neal DC, *et al.* Quantitative assessment of synovitis in Legg–Calvé–Perthes disease using gadolinium-enhanced MRI. *J Pediatr Orthop B.* 2015;24(2):89–94.
11. Joseph B, Pydisetty RK. Chondrolysis and the stiff hip in Perthes' disease: an immunological study. *J Pediatr Orthop.* 1996;16(1):15–19.
12. Kamegaya M, *et al.* Arthrography of early Perthes' disease. Swelling of the ligamentum teres as a cause of subluxation. *J Bone Joint Surg Br.* 1989;71(3):413–17.
13. Joseph B. Morphological changes in the acetabulum in Perthes' disease. *J Bone Joint Surg Br.* 1989;71(5):756–63.
14. Green NE, Beauchamp RD, Griffin PP. Epiphyseal extrusion as a prognostic index in Legg–Calvé–Perthes disease. *J Bone Joint Surg Am.* 1981;63(6):900–5.
15. Joseph B, *et al.* Natural evolution of Perthes disease: a study of 610 children under 12 years of age at disease onset. *J Pediatr Orthop.* 2003;23(5):590–600.
16. Theissen P, *et al.* The early diagnosis of Perthes disease: the value of bone scintigraphy and magnetic resonance imaging in comparison with x-ray findings. *Nuklearmedizin.* 1991;30(6):265–71.
17. Catterall A. The natural history of Perthes' disease. *J Bone Joint Surg Br.* 1971;53(1):37–53.
18. Stulberg SD, Cooperman DR, Wallensten R. The natural history of Legg–Calvé–Perthes disease. *J Bone Joint Surg Am.* 1981;63(7):1095–108.
19. Wiig O, Terjesen T, Svenningsen S. Inter-observer reliability of the Stulberg classification in the assessment of Perthes disease. *J Child Orthop.* 2007;1(2):101–5.
20. Rich MM, Schoenecker PL. Management of Legg–Calvé–Perthes disease using an A-frame orthosis and hip range of motion: a 25-year experience. *J Pediatr Orthop.* 2013;33(2):112–19.
21. Axer A. Subtrochanteric osteotomy in the treatment of Perthes' disease: a preliminary report. *J Bone Joint Surg Br.* 1965;47:489–99.
22. Axer A, *et al.* Indications for femoral osteotomy in Legg–Calvé–Perthes disease. *Clin Orthop Relat Res.* 1980;150:78–87.
23. Hoikka V, Lindholm TS, Poussa M. Intertrochanteric varus osteotomy in Legg–Calvé–Perthes disease: a report of 112 hips. *J Pediatr Orthop.* 1986;6(5):600–4.
24. Kitakoji T, Hattori T, Iwata H. Femoral varus osteotomy in Legg–Calvé–Perthes disease: points at operation to prevent residual problems. *J Pediatr Orthop.* 1999;19(1):76–81.
25. Copeliovitch L. Femoral varus osteotomy in Legg–Calvé–Perthes disease. *J Pediatr Orthop.* 2011;31(2 Suppl):S189–91.
26. Joseph B, Srinivas G, Thomas R. Management of Perthes disease of late onset in southern India. The evaluation of a surgical method. *J Bone Joint Surg Br.* 1996;78(4):625–30.
27. Salter RB. Legg–Perthes disease: the scientific basis for the methods of treatment and their indications. *Clin Orthop Relat Res.* 1980;150:8–11.
28. Kumar D, Bache CE, O'Hara JN. Interlocking triple pelvic osteotomy in severe Legg–Calvé–Perthes disease. *J Pediatr Orthop.* 2002;22(4):464–70.
29. Lim KS, Shim JS. Outcomes of combined shelf acetabuloplasty with femoral varus osteotomy in severe Legg–Calvé–Perthes (LCP)

disease: advanced containment method for severe LCP disease. *Clin Orthop Surg*. 2015;7(4):497–504.

30. Olney BW, Asher MA. Combined innominate and femoral osteotomy for the treatment of severe Legg–Calvé–Perthes disease. *J Pediatr Orthop*. 1985;5(6):645–51.

31. Javid M, Wedge JH. Radiographic results of combined Salter innominate and femoral osteotomy in Legg–Calvé–Perthes disease in older children. *J Child Orthop*. 2009;3(3):229–34.

32. Kamegaya M, *et al.* Single versus combined procedures for severely involved Legg–Calvé–Perthes disease. *J Pediatr Orthop*. 2018;38(6):312–19.

33. Mosow N, *et al.* Outcome after combined pelvic and femoral osteotomies in patients with Legg–Calvé–Perthes disease. *J Bone Joint Surg Am*. 2017;99(3):207–13.

34. Kruse RW, Guille JT, Bowen JR. Shelf arthroplasty in patients who have Legg–Calvé–Perthes disease. A study of long-term results. *J Bone Joint Surg Am*. 1991;73(9):1338–47.

35. Willett K, Hudson I, Catterall A. Lateral shelf acetabuloplasty: an operation for older children with Perthes' disease. *J Pediatr Orthop*. 1992;12(5):563–8.

36. Daly K, Bruce C, Catterall A. Lateral shelf acetabuloplasty in Perthes' disease. A review of the end of growth. *J Bone Joint Surg Br*. 1999;81(3):380–4.

37. Carsi B, Judd J, Clarke NM. Shelf acetabuloplasty for containment in the early stages of Legg–Calvé–Perthes disease. *J Pediatr Orthop*. 2015;35(2):151–6.

38. Laklouk MA, Hosny GA. Hinged distraction of the hip joint in the treatment of Perthes disease: evaluation at skeletal maturity. *J Pediatr Orthop B*. 2012;21(5):386–93.

39. Aly TA, Amin OA. Arthrodiatasis for the treatment of Perthes' disease. *Orthopedics*. 2009;32(11):817.

40. Segev E, *et al.* Treatment of severe late-onset Perthes' disease with soft tissue release and articulated hip distraction: revisited at skeletal maturity. *J Child Orthop*. 2007;1(4):229–35.

41. Joseph B. Management of Perthes' disease. *Indian J Orthop*. 2015;49(1):10–16.

42. Nguyen NA, *et al.* Operative versus nonoperative treatments for Legg–Calvé–Perthes disease: a meta-analysis. *J Pediatr Orthop*. 2012;32(7):697–705.

43. Saran N, Varghese R, Mulpuri K. Do femoral or Salter innominate osteotomies improve femoral head sphericity in Legg–Calvé–Perthes disease? A meta-analysis. *Clin Orthop Relat Res*. 2012;470(9):2383–93.

44. Herring JA, Kim HT, Browne R. Legg–Calvé–Perthes disease. Part II: Prospective multicenter study of the effect of treatment on outcome. *J Bone Joint Surg Am*. 2004;86-A(10): 2121–34.

45. Wiig O, Terjesen T, Svenningsen S. Prognostic factors and outcome of treatment in Perthes' disease: a prospective study of 368 patients with five-year follow-up. *J Bone Joint Surg Br*. 2008;90(10):1364–71.

46. Bankes MJ, Catterall A, Hashemi-Nejad A. Valgus extension osteotomy for 'hinge abduction' in Perthes' disease. Results at maturity and factors influencing the radiological outcome. *J Bone Joint Surg Br*. 2000;82(4): 548–54.

47. Yoo WJ, *et al.* Valgus femoral osteotomy for hinge abduction in Perthes' disease. Decision-making and outcomes. *J Bone Joint Surg Br*. 2004;86(5):726–30.

48. Choi IH, Yoo WJ, Cho T-J, Moon HJ. Principles of treatment in late stages of Perthes disease. *Orthop Clin North Am*. 2011;42(3):341–8, vi.

49. Young ML, Little DG, Kim HK. Evidence for using bisphosphonate to treat Legg–Calvé–Perthes disease. *Clin Orthop Relat Res*. 2012;470(9): 2462–75.

50. Kumar V, *et al.* Do bisphosphonates alter the clinico-radiological profile of children with Perthes disease? A systematic review and meta-analysis. *Eur Rev Med Pharmacol Sci*. 2021;25(15):4875–94.

Developmental Dysplasia of the Hip

Sattar Alshryda and Paul A. Banaszkiewicz

Background

Developmental dysplasia of the hip (DDH) is a spectrum of disorders of hip development that presents in different forms at different ages and may range from:

1. Hip dysplasia found on ultrasound and radiographs with no clinical abnormalities. If untreated, it may normalize or may progress to frank dislocation

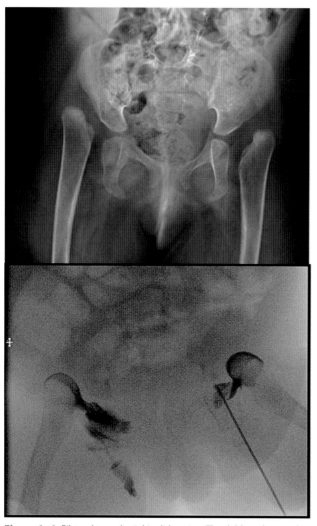

Figure 4c.1 Bilateral teratologic hip dislocation. The child was born with bilateral club feet and hip dislocation. Abduction is minimal and both hips are dislocated; the femoral heads sit high and have created a false acetabulum. Examination under anaesthesia and arthrography (undertaken at the time of club feet tenotomy) confirmed the initial impression that these hips are not reducible. Notice the very tight capsular isthmus with a typical hourglass deformity on the hip arthrogram.

2. Hip instability (dislocatable hip), such that the femoral head can be displaced partially (subluxated) or fully (dislocated) from the acetabulum by an examiner, but relocated spontaneously
3. A dislocated hip that is reducible on examination (reducible hip).
4. Dislocated hip that cannot be reduced during examination (irreducible hip).

Teratologic dislocation of the hip is a distinct form of hip dislocation that usually occurs with other disorders such as arthrogryposis, myelodysplasia and neuromuscular diseases. These hips are dislocated before birth, have limited range of motion and are not reducible on examination (or even by closed reduction under general anaesthesia) (Figure 4c.1).

Klisic in 1989 recommended the term developmental dysplasia of the hip (DDH), instead of congenital dislocation of the hip (CDH), to indicate the developmental nature of the hip disorder in two senses:

1. The hip may be clinically normal at birth
2. The hip may get better or worse as the child develops.

The incidence of DDH is difficult to determine because of the different forms of presentation (as above), the type of examinations used to detect hip abnormalities, the differing skill levels of examiners and the populations being studied (Figure 4c.2). The following is generally accepted

- Ultrasound abnormality (8/100 births)
- Abnormal clinical finding (2.3/100 births)
- Dislocation (1.4/1 000 births).

Aetiology

The causes of DDH are multifactorial involving genetic, intrauterine, and environmental factors. The following are recognized risk factors (7 Fs):

Normal hips	92%	
Radiological abnormalities	8%	5.7%
Dislocatable		2.3%
Dislocated, but reducible		
Dislocated, but not reducible		

Figure 4c.2 The spectrum of newborns' hip state and average incidence.

1. First baby (the uterus is tighter and less elastic)
2. Female (lax ligament by maternal hormone relaxin)
3. Family history (may be a genetic predisposition)
4. Fetal malposition (extended knee breech presentation)
5. Fetal packaging disorders (oligohydramnios, twins, feet metatarsus adductus, and neck torticollis)
6. LeFt side (60% left hip, 20% right hip, and 20% both hips; may be related to fetal position)
7. Other factors:
   a. Geographical and racial factors (commoner in native Americans and Europeans than Asians and Africans)
   b. Social factors (commoner in a population that uses swaddling). The incidence of DDH in Japanese infants prior to 1965 was as high as 3.5%. In 1975, a national campaign on swaddling was introduced and as a result, there was a remarkable reduction in the incidence of DDH to <0.2%, a 17-fold reduction.

A couple of meta-analyses of over a million babies showed that the main independent risk factors are breech presentation, female gender and family history [1, 2].

Pathoanatomy

It is essential to understand normal growth and development of the hip joint, and the pathoanatomy of DDH and its natural history.

The hip joint develops as a cleft in the primitive limb bud at about 7 weeks of gestation. The concave shape of the acetabulum is determined by the spherical-shaped femoral head within the acetabulum. The two bony ends are covered by fully formed cartilage by the 11th week of gestation. Failure at this stage of development leads to proximal femoral focal deficiency.

At birth, the entire proximal femur (femoral head, neck, greater, and lesser trochanters) is a cartilaginous structure. Its development occurs through a combination of appositional growth on the surfaces and physeal growth at the junction of the cartilaginous proximal femur and the femoral shaft. The proximal femur is ossified through three ossification centres. An ossification centre appears in the centre of the femoral head between 4 and 7 months of life. This centre grows until physeal closure between the ages of 14 and 17. The greater trochanter begins to ossify during the fourth year. It joins the shaft approximately

1 year after puberty. The lesser trochanter is the final centre to ossify and fuse at the onset of puberty (Figure 4c.3).

At birth, the acetabulum is composed of hyaline cartilage whose periphery is attached to the fibrocartilaginous labrum. The hyaline cartilage of the acetabulum is continuous with the triradiate cartilages, which interconnect the three bones of the pelvis (the ilium, ischium, and pubis). Most of acetabular development occurs by age of approximately 8 years (Figure 4c.4) [3].

The final contour of the hip socket is further achieved by three acetabular epiphyseal centres, which appear at around the age of 8 years and fused at around the age of 18 years [4]:

1. The anterior epiphyseal centre (os acetabulum) – forms the anterior rim as part of the pubis
2. The superior epiphyseal centre (acetabular epiphysis) – forms along the superior edge of the acetabulum and the anterior inferior iliac spine (AIIS) as part of the ilium
3. The posterior epiphyseal centre (os marginalis) – forms the posterior rim.

The cartilaginous parts of the growing femoral head and the acetabular roof have vascular sinusoids which supply oxygen and nutrients. Too much pressure on these cartilaginous parts during reduction can cause ischaemic necrosis (Figure 4c.5).

In DDH, there are distinct pathological changes which are initially reversible. At or shortly after birth, the affected hip spontaneously slides into and out of the acetabulum, leading to flattening of the anterosuperior rim of the acetabulum. At this stage, the rim is made of hyaline cartilage and the attached fibrocartilaginous labrum. This usually gets deformed and either everted or inverted, depending on the direction of the deforming forces (Ortolani called this deformed rim the neolimbus).

Some of these hips spontaneously reduce and become normal, with complete resolution of the pathological changes. Other hips remain dislocated, leading to secondary pathology.

A fibro-fatty tissue (known as the pulvinar) fills the shallow acetabulum and may impede reduction (this point is controversial). The ligamentum teres becomes stretched and hypertrophied, and presses on the acetabular rim and the lower part of the femoral head. The transverse acetabular ligament is hypertrophic

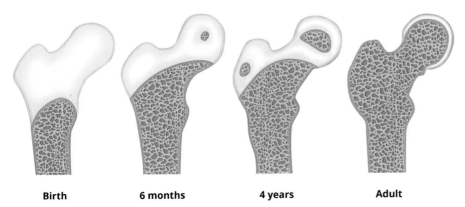

| Birth | 6 months | 4 years | Adult |

Figure 4c.3 Proximal femur development.

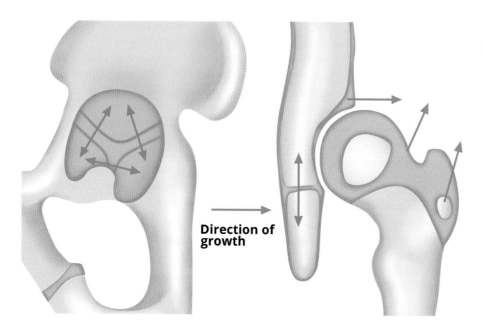

Figure 4c.4 Acetabular development. The blue arrows show the direction of ossification and growth.

Direction of growth

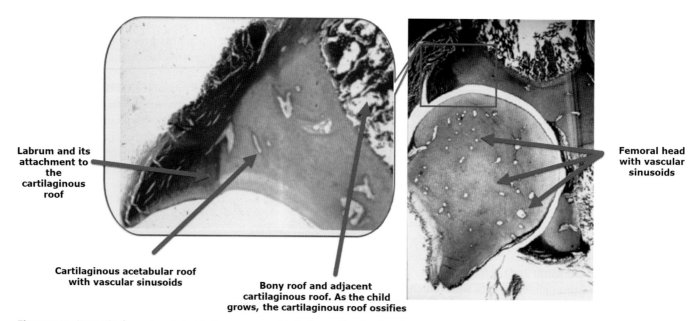

Labrum and its attachment to the cartilaginous roof

Cartilaginous acetabular roof with vascular sinusoids

Bony roof and adjacent cartilaginous roof. As the child grows, the cartilaginous roof ossifies

Femoral head with vascular sinusoids

Figure 4c.5 Sinusoids of a newborn baby hip. These are present in the femoral head and cartilaginous acetabular roof. Excessive pressure during hip reduction can close these sinusoids, leading to avascular necrosis of the femoral head and persistent acetabular dysplasia. Source: Images are courtesy of Professor Reinhard Graf.

and tight, giving the socket a horseshoe shape. Growth of the ace-tabulum and dislocated head leads the joint capsule to assume an hourglass shape with a narrow isthmus which is smaller in diameter than that of the femoral head. The iliopsoas, which is pulled tight across this isthmus, contributes to this narrowing. The capsule isthmus narrows further through a 'Chinese finger-trap' mechanism. There is an associated increase in femoral ante-version and some flattening of the femoral head, as it lies against either the ilium or the abductor muscles (Figure 4c.6).

Clinical Presentations

Clinical findings vary, depending on age.

Neonates and Infants

DDH is usually asymptomatic, with no discomfort or pain. There may be subtle clinical signs such as asymmetrical skinfold (not very specific) and limited abduction of the hip or leg asym-metry (Galeazzi sign) (Figure 4c.7).

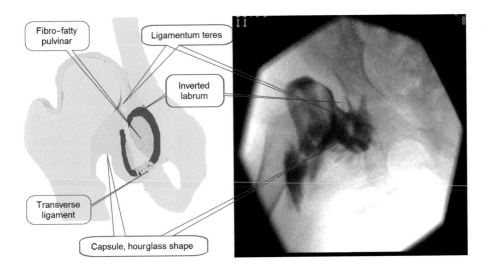

Fibro-fatty pulvinar

Ligamentum teres

Inverted labrum

Transverse ligament

Capsule, hourglass shape

Figure 4c.6 The pathoanatomical changes in developmental dysplasia of the hip.

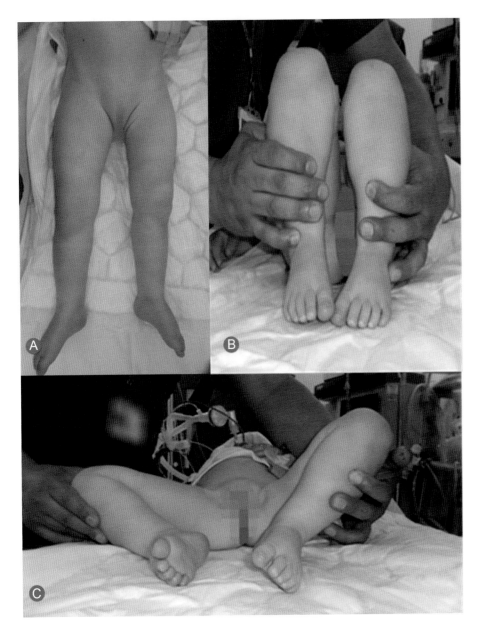

A

B

C

Figure 4c.7 Some common features of unilateral hip dislocation. (A) shows asymmetrical skin crease and a short and externally rotated leg. (B) demonstrates a positive Galeazzi test, and (C) shows limited hip abduction.

The Ortolani and Barlow tests are very important in the early weeks of life, but their values become less as the child gets older. The **O**rtolani test identifies a dislocated hip (**Out**) that can be reduced. Flex the infant's hip and knee to 90°, then gently abduct the thigh. The middle finger is placed over the greater trochanter to feel for the reduction of the dislocated head, as it comes from the dislocated position into the socket. With time, it becomes more challenging to reduce the femoral head into the acetabulum and the Ortolani test becomes negative.

The **B**arlow test is performed by attempting to dislocate the femoral head from within the acetabulum. The hip is adducted and gentle pressure is applied to slide the hip posteriorly. The Barlow test is rarely positive after 10 weeks.

Bilateral limitation of hip abduction, asymmetrical skin crease, and leg length discrepancy (LLD) have low specificity in detecting DDH in the neonate, and many children with normal hips demonstrate this feature.

Unilateral limited abduction has 70% sensitivity and 90% specificity for DDH in infants aged >3 months [5]. The Ortolani and Barlow tests have 60% sensitivity and 100% specificity in expert hands, in comparison to ultrasound which has 90% sensitivity and specificity [6].

In bilateral hip dislocation, there is no asymmetry of abduction and no LLD, making detection more difficult, and children with bilateral hip dislocation are diagnosed late, often after they start walking.

The Klisic test can be used to detect dislocation, especially after 3 months. The index finger is placed on the ASIS, and the middle finger on the greater trochanter. An imaginary line drawn between these two points should point towards or above the umbilicus. When the hip is dislocated, the more proximal greater trochanter causes the line to pass below the umbilicus (Figure 4c.8).

Walking Age

The presenting feature is usually a limp, with the affected limb appearing shorter. The child tends to toe-walk on the affected side to compensate for shortening.

Examination reveals a classical Trendelenburg gait (and a positive Trendelenburg sign), limited abduction on the affected side, and the knees at different levels when the hips are flexed (Galeazzi sign).

As in younger children, bilateral dislocation is more difficult to recognize than unilateral dislocation, as there is no asymmetry of abduction and no LLD. Excessive lordosis due to fixed flexion deformity may be the presenting symptom. Clinical examination will reveal a waddling gait, a bilateral positive Trendelenburg sign, and excessive internal and external rotation of the dislocated hips.

It is essential to examine the child for other potential problems in the neck, spine, and feet.

Investigations

Ultrasound

Ultrasound has become the gold standard for confirming the diagnosis and guiding treatment of DDH. Four different ultrasound techniques have been described and used: **Graf**, **Harcke**,

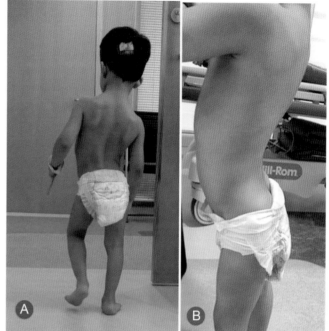
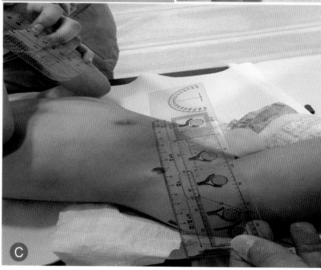

Figure 4c.8 A late-presenting child with bilateral dislocated hips. (A) shows a waddling gait where the child moves all his body to the weight-bearing side to help lift the swinging leg. (B) shows excessive lumbar lordosis, and (C) shows a positive Klisic sign.

Terjensen, and **Suzuki**. The Graf method has been shown to be superior to the other three in terms of reliability, sensitivity, specificity, and reproducibility [7, 8]. How to interpret the hip ultrasound using the Graf method is fully explained in Video 4c.1.

Video 4c.1 How to interpret the infant hip ultrasound.

Graf defined five major types of hip (I, II, D, III, and IV). These are further divided into subtypes, as shown in Table 4c.1. Type I is a normal hip. Type IIa is an immature hip, and the rest are abnormal (Figure 4c.9). Most experts currently recommend treating hips which are Graf type IIb or worse, and to observe those which are type IIa.

Table 4c.1 Graf's sonographic grading for developmental dysplasia of the hip

Type	Alpha angle (α)			Beta angle (β)		Descriptions
I	>60°			<55°	Ia	Normal hip (at any age). This grade is further divided into Ia (β <55°) and Ib (β >55°). The significance of this subdivision is not yet established. The patient does not need follow-up
				>55°	Ib	
II	50–59°	IIa		<77°		If the child is <3 months. This may be physiological and does not need treatment; however, follow-up is required
		IIb		<77°		>3 months, delayed ossification
	43–49°	IIc	Stable	<77°		Critical zone, labrum not everted. This is further divided into stable and unstable by the provocation test
			Unstable			
D	43–49°			>77°		This is the first stage where the hip becomes decentred (subluxed). It used to be called IId, but for the above reason, it is a stage on its own now
III	<43°	IIIa				Dislocated femoral head with the cartilaginous acetabular roof pushed **upwards**. This is further divided into IIIa and IIIb, depending on the echogenicity of the hyaline cartilage of the acetabular roof (usually compared to the femoral head), which reflects the degenerative changes (Figure 4c.9)
		IIIb				
IV	<43°					Dislocated femoral head with the cartilaginous acetabular roof pushed **downwards** (Figure 4c.9)

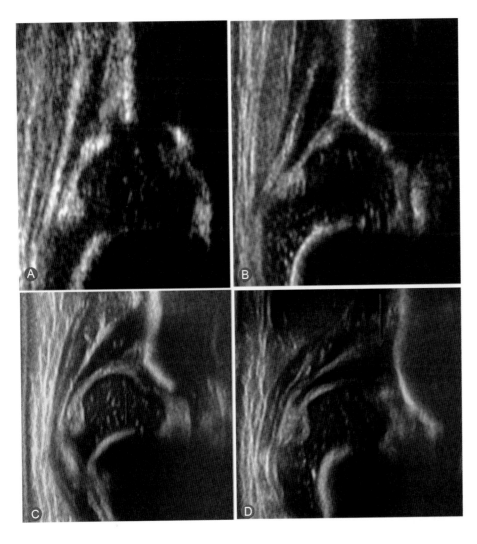

Figure 4c.9 Four distinctive types of hips, according to Graf. (A) shows type I hip, which is normal. The femoral head is centred; the acetabular rim is sharp, and over 50% of the head is covered with the bony roof. If the alpha angle is measured, it will be above 60°. (B) shows a type II hip where the femoral head is centred, but coverage is <50% and the acetabular rim is rounded. (C) shows a type III hip where the femoral head is no longer centred, but the cartilaginous roof and attached labrum are pushed upwards, in contrast to a type IV hip (D) where these are pushed downwards.

However, this recommendation has been contested as a significant number of patients with sonographic abnormalities may correct spontaneously without treatment [9, 10]. Treatment at an earlier age is straightforward, with very low complication rates, and the success rate drops significantly if treatment is initiated after 6 weeks [11, 12].

Universal ultrasound screening for DDH is undertaken in Germany, Austria, and Switzerland. Although universal screening will identify many infants with abnormal findings in the hip that may completely resolve if left untreated, it has resulted in a reduction in late presentation of DDH [12–16]. There is, however, ongoing debate regarding the cost-effectiveness and efficacy of universal screening for DDH.

In the United Kingdom, ultrasound screening is used in high-risk groups (breech presentation, first-degree relatives – scanned within 6 weeks) and neonates with abnormalities detected on clinical examination (scanned within 2 weeks).

In an article in *Journal of Bone and Joint Surgery* in 2009, Mahan *et al.* [17] recommended physical examination screening for all newborns and selective use of ultrasonography for those with positive physical examination, breech delivery, or a positive family history of DDH. Whilst Mahan *et al.* recognized the limitations inherent to the decision analysis process, they thought it represented the best way to balance the risks and benefits of screening for hip dysplasia.

Independent task forces from the United States, Canada, and Australia, as well as a Cochrane review, concluded that 'the evidence is insufficient to recommend routine screening' for hip dysplasia and they were 'unable to assess the balance of benefits and harms of screening' for DDH [18–20].

Radiography

The newborn hip joint is mostly cartilaginous; that is why ultrasonography is better than plain radiographs in assessing early DDH. However, the femoral capital epiphysis ossifies at about 6 months of age, and as it gets bigger, it undermines the value of ultrasonography and plain radiographs become more useful then.

On pelvis radiographs, several landmarks, reference lines, and angles have been shown to be useful when assessing DDH:

1. **H**ilgenreiner's line is a **h**orizontal line through the triradiate cartilages.
2. **P**erkin's line is a vertical line drawn at the lateral margin of the acetabulum **p**erpendicular to Hilgenreiner's line. These two lines create four quadrants. Most of the femoral head normally should lie in the anteromedial quadrant.
3. Shenton's line is a curved line that is drawn from the lesser trochanter, along the inferior femoral neck, to the inferior border of the superior pubic ramus, in contrast to the lateral Shenton's line, which is drawn from the greater trochanter along the superior femoral neck and the ilium (Figure 4c.10). Both lines should have a smooth curve without a break.
4. The acetabular index (AI) is an angle formed by Hilgenreiner's line and a line drawn along the acetabular surface to the lateral edge of the acetabulum (Figure 4c.11).

The mean AI is <30° at birth, 23 at 6 months, and <20° by 2 years of age; however, it is better to compare these to standard charts for males and females, rather than memorizing them.

After triradiate cartilage closure, a horizontal line is drawn from the inferior tip of the teardrop to the lateral edge of the acetabulum; this is called Sharp's angle, which is usually <40°.

5. The AI of the weight-bearing zone, or the sourcil angle (of Tonnis) – typically <15°.
6. Centre edge angle (CEA) of Wiberg. This is usually useful after the age of 6 years (Figure 4c.12):
   a. Anterior CEA (on the AP view): angle between two lines drawn from the centre of the femoral head. One is vertical (parallel to Perkin's line), and the other passes to the lateral acetabular edge. It is >20° by the age of 14 years, and >25° in adults.
   b. Lateral CEA (on the false profile view): angle between a perpendicular line from the centre of the femoral head and the acetabular edge line; normally it is >17°.
7. Teardrop: this is formed by the wall of the acetabulum laterally, the wall of the lesser pelvis medially, and the acetabular notch inferiorly. The teardrop appears between 6 and 24 months of age in a normal hip, and later in a dislocated hip. The appearance of a normal U-shaped teardrop is a good sign; however, its absence, or a widened and V-shaped teardrop, is a bad sign.

Treatment

The principles of treating DDH are:

1. Achieving a concentric reduction
2. Maintaining stability of reduction
3. Promoting normal growth and development of the hip
4. Avoiding or minimizing complications.

Without a good reduction, normal hip growth may not take place, leading to persistent or even worsening dysplasia, which, in turn, leads to either redislocation (when severe) or premature osteoarthritis. Sometimes, even with a perfect reduction, normal hip development does not occur (persistent dysplasia) and this requires timely intervention. We will address the treatment of DDH based on age; however, it is important to remember that chronological age does not always match with biological age and there is overlap among age-based treatment recommendations.

Children from birth up to 6 months

Hip ultrasound, based on Graf methods, has become an integral part of treatment in this age group (Figure 4c.13).

Several devices have been used to treat children in this age group. However, the Pavlik harness is by far the most commonly used worldwide [11] (Figure 4c.14).

The **Pavlik** harness is a reduction, but also a retention, device. It is designed to facilitate hip motion that is essential for reduction and maintaining the reduction. Continuous motion prevents localized excessive pressure on the femoral head, reducing the risk of AVN.

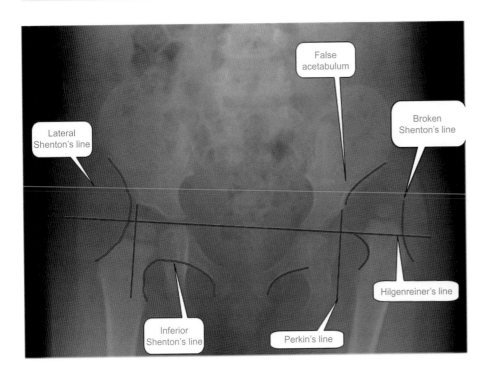

Figure 4c.10 Plain X-ray of the pelvis of a 19-month-old child with a dislocated left hip. Notice the left femoral head is in the upper lateral quadrant and Shenton's lines are broken.

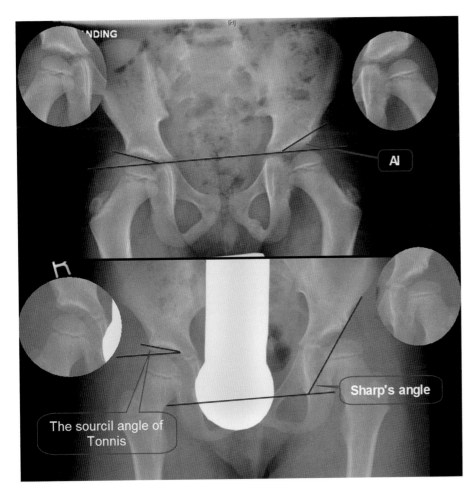

Figure 4c.11 Plain X-rays of the pelvis with left hip residual dysplasia, as shown by a greater acetabular index and Sharp's angles. Notice the lateral subluxation of the left hip by measuring the distance between the medial head border and the acetabular floor.

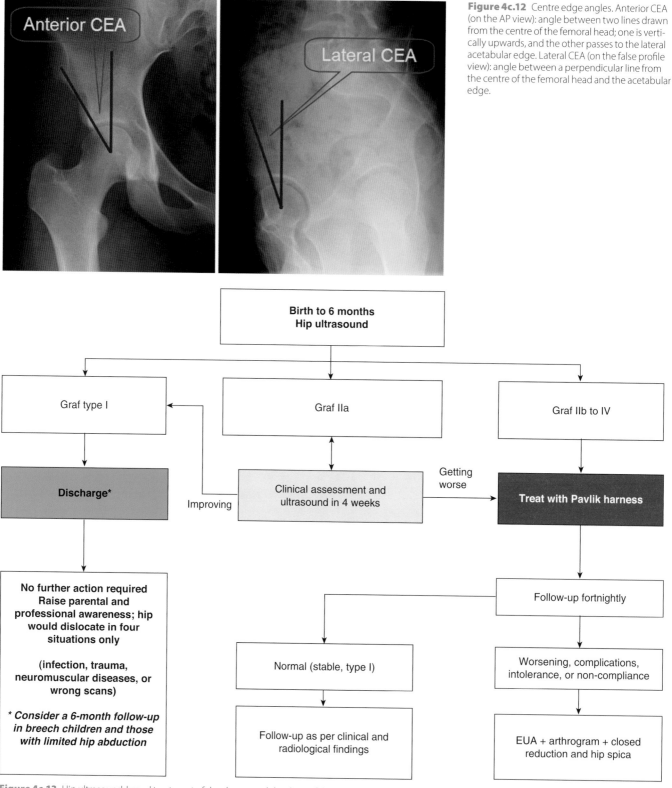

Figure 4c.12 Centre edge angles. Anterior CEA (on the AP view): angle between two lines drawn from the centre of the femoral head; one is vertically upwards, and the other passes to the lateral acetabular edge. Lateral CEA (on the false profile view): angle between a perpendicular line from the centre of the femoral head and the acetabular edge.

Figure 4c.13 Hip ultrasound-based treatment of developmental dysplasia of the hip.

The Pavlik harness has shoulder and leg straps. The anterior leg straps are to keep the hip flexion at around 100°, whereas the posterior leg straps are to keep hip abduction in the safe zone (Figure 4c.15). The harness is sized by measuring the chest circumference.

There are five sizes: premature, small, medium, large, and extra large). Excessive flexion may cause femoral nerve palsy or inferior dislocation, whereas too little flexion may cause the hip to redislocate. Forced abduction may lead to AVN of the femoral head; that is why some new Pavlik harness designs have an extra

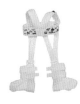 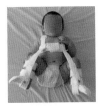 Pavlik harnes

  von Rosen splint

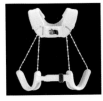 Tubingen brace

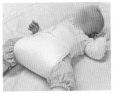 Frejka pillow

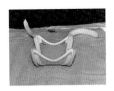 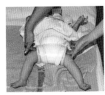 Aberdeen brace

Figure 4c.14 Various devices used to treat DDH in the first 6 months of life. The Pavlik harness is by far the most commonly used worldwide. The Frejka pillow and Aberdeen brace are historical now.

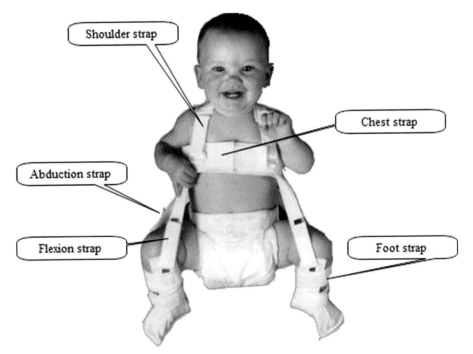

Shoulder strap

Chest strap

Abduction strap

Flexion strap

Foot strap

Figure 4c.15 Pavlik harness. Source: Picture courtesy of Wheaton Brace Company.

optional strap connecting the anterior straps to prevent excessive abduction.

It is essential to check a child with a Pavlik harness frequently (initially weekly, then every 2–4 weeks) for reduction, ultrasound progression, size (as the child may outgrow the harness), and documenting active knee extension (functioning femoral nerve).

Pavlik harness treatment failure is predicted for children older than 6 weeks, bilateral hip dislocation, and irreducible hip (negative Ortolani test).

Complications

1. Failure of reduction (reported success rates varied between 60% and 97%, with an average of 90%)
2. Damage to the posterior acetabular wall when there is a persistent posterior dislocation
3. AVN of the head of the femur (2.4%; range 0–15%)
4. Skin damage
5. Brachial plexus injury
6. Knee dislocation
7. Femoral nerve palsy (2.5%).

Murnaghan and colleagues reported a femoral nerve palsy incidence of 2.5% (30 cases) in 1218 patients treated with a Pavlik harness, with 87% presenting within 1 week of harness application. Femoral nerve palsy was more likely in older, larger patients in whom DDH was of greater severity. Patients whose femoral nerve palsy resolved within 3 days had a 70% chance of having successful treatment with the harness, whereas those who had not recovered by 10 days had a 70% chance of treatment failure. The success rate associated with treatment with a Pavlik harness was 94% in the control group, and 47% in the palsy group [21].

Contraindications of Pavlik Harness

1. Significant muscle imbalance such as myelomeningocele
2. Major stiffness, as in arthrogryposis
3. Ligamentous laxity, such as in Ehlers–Danlos syndrome
4. Severe respiratory compromise (Craig splint may be useful)
5. Irreducible hip
6. Age >6 months (relative).

Children from 6 months to 18 months (or younger who failed treatment with Pavlik Harness)

The goals of treatment are to obtain and maintain reduction of the hip within the safe zones of Ramsey (see below). This can be achieved by either closed or open reduction.

Closed Reduction

This is usually performed under anaesthesia in conjunction with hip arthrography. The hip is manually reduced and the range of motion where the hip remains reduced is noted. The hip is adducted to the point of redislocation and that position is noted. The hip is again reduced and then extended until it dislocates, and the point of dislocation is noted. These arcs represent the safe zone of reduction that was coined by Ramsey and associates [22], and refers to the range of motion in which the hip remains reduced in relation to the maximum range of motion. The wider the range, the better. Two important facts are considered:

1. The average movement of a hip in a spica is 15°, so it is important to keep the hip away from the line of dislocation by ≥20° to reduce the risk of dislocation inside the spica.
2. The risk of AVN increases with the hip put at its maximum range of motion, particularly abduction, so it is safer to keep the hip 20° less than the maximum range of motion.

So the safe zone is within 15–20° of the maximum range of motion and dislocation range. The maximum range of motion can be increased by adductor tenotomy (to increase abduction) and psoas tenotomy (to increase extension). These tenotomies should not be routine but are recommended in the presence of a narrow safe zone (Figures 4c.16 and 4c.17, and Video 4c.2).

The hip is then immobilized in a hip spica, with the position of the limb in the safe zone (typically just over 90° of hip flexion, 45° of hip abduction, and 30° of internal rotation).

 Video 4c.2 Closed reduction of a dislocated hip.

Hip Arthrography

This is performed under general anaesthesia through a medial (or subadductor) approach in children because it is technically easy and, more importantly, extracapsular leak of the dye is less likely to obscure the important structures laterally (femoral head, labrum, cartilaginous part of the acetabulum, and amount of coverage).

The area is prepped and draped to allow easy access to the hip in anticipation of undertaking other procedures such as adductor tenotomy or open reduction. A spinal needle attached to a 10-ml syringe is introduced underneath the adductor tendon towards the hip. This is under X-ray screening. Usually, a 'give' is felt once the needle pierces the joint capsule and is in the joint. Water is injected to fill the capsule. There should be a backflow if the needle is in the right place. One to 2 ml of contrast medium is injected slowly under X-ray control. Then the hip is screened for reduction and stability through the full range of motion (Figures 4c.18 and 4c.19).

Key Points: Closed Reduction of Dislocated Hips in Children

The skills of performing closed reduction of a dislocated hip in children are quick to learn, but take a long time and experience to master. They require a skilful plaster technician to support the surgeon. That is why some surgeons prefer to wait longer and perform an open reduction, instead of a closed reduction. The downside of waiting is missing out on potential hip remodelling, which is highest in the first year of life.

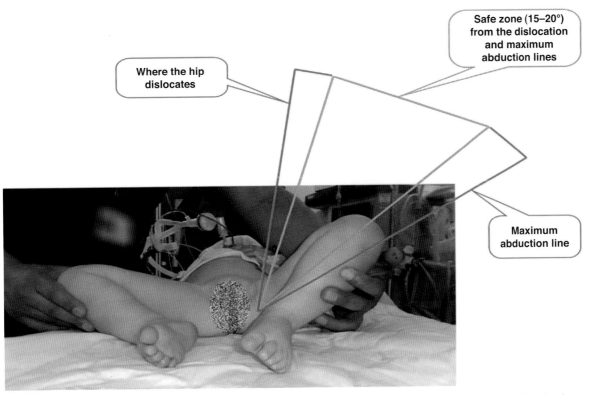

Figure 4c.16 Coronal safe zone. This is the range of motion where the hip is kept reduced, with a lower risk of AVN. It is 15–20° lateral to the point of dislocation, and 15–20° medial to the maximum abduction line.

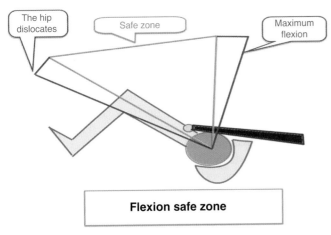

Figure 4c.17 Sagittal safe zone (see text for description).

Open Reduction

This is indicated when:

1. Closed reduction is not possible
2. The hip is reduced but remains unstable, or stability can only be achieved by holding the hip in extreme abduction or internal rotation (this happens when the safe zone is narrow). The former may cause redislocation, and the latter may cause AVN.

Open reduction may be performed from a medial approach (in <1-year olds) or an anterior approach (in older children). There are three described **medial approaches**:

- Anteromedial (Iowa) – anterior to the pectineus and medial to the femoral sheath
- Medial (Ludloff) – uses the interval between the pectineus muscle anteriorly and the adductor longus and brevis muscles posteriorly
- Posteromedial (Ferguson) – uses the interval between the adductor longus and brevis muscles anteriorly and the gracilis and adductor magnus posteriorly.

The disadvantages of the medial approach are a limited view of the hip, possible interruption of the medial femoral circumflex artery (the literature shows higher AVN rates) [23, 24] and inability to perform a capsulorrhaphy. Some centres and surgeons have stopped using the medial approach.

The **anterior hip approach** (Smith–Petersen) utilizes internervous planes between the tensor fascia lata and sartorius (superficial) and the rectus femoris and gluteus medius (deep). The reflected head of the rectus is detached from the anterior lip of the acetabulum to reach the hip joint capsule.

For optimum exposure, the iliac crest apophysis is split and peeled off the inner and outer tables of the iliac bone down to the greater sciatic notch. The psoas tendon is divided over the pelvic brim. The joint capsule is exposed anteriorly, medially, and laterally (270° exposure). A T-shaped capsulotomy is performed to open and visualize the hip. The pulvinar is removed; the ligamentum teres is excised, and the hip joint is reduced and tested. The large, redundant capsule is closed in a T-V fashion (capsulorrhaphy) using non-absorbable sutures (Figure 4c.20; Video 4c.3).

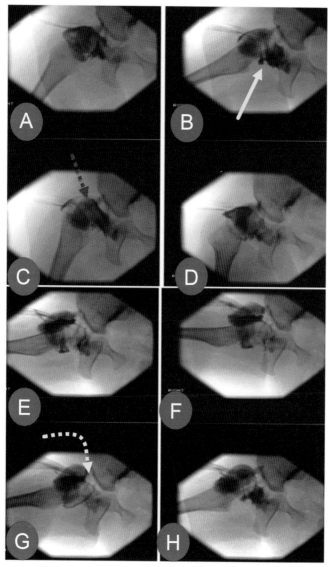

Figure 4c.18 Hip arthrogram showing the outline of the cartilaginous femoral head. (B) and (C) show the hourglass shape of the capsule. They confirm hip dislocation where the head is not sitting in the acetabulum, and there is significant medial dye pooling >7 mm (solid yellow arrow). The ligamentum teres is thickened and elongated (best seen in C) as a lighter band (dashed red arrow). Hip reduction is assessed in different positions: reduced in (E), (F), and (G). (G) and (H) show the effect of rotation on reduction where external rotation in (H) led to dislocation anteriorly, whereas internal rotation did not (G); in fact, the hip became more stable. The curved, dashed yellow arrow shows the cartilage roof, which is expected to ossify to provide more stability to the femoral head.

 Video 4c.3 Open reduction of a dislocated hip.

In most cases, a pelvic osteotomy is then performed (see below). The wound is closed in layers. A hip spica is applied, with the hip in 30° of abduction, 30° of flexion, and 30° of internal rotation. The knee should be flexed to 30° to relax the hamstrings and control rotation in the cast. This is different from the position of the spica in closed reduction, and there may be some variations among different centres.

Pelvic Osteotomies

Two pelvic osteotomies are commonly used to improve joint stability at this stage: either Salter innominate osteotomy or Pemberton osteotomy. These are used because they are designed to increase anterolateral coverage, the commonest type of acetabular dysplasia (deficiency) in children with DDH. Intraoperative indications are:

1. Unstable hip that tends to dislocate anteriorly
2. High AI on fluoroscopy images
3. Suboptimal coverage of the femoral head when the leg is placed in extension and neutral rotation (less than a third of the femoral head should be visible).

Children with recurrent dislocation or those treated for a long time in a Pavlik harness may develop a different pattern of dysplasia that requires a different type of pelvic osteotomy such as Dega or San Diego types of osteotomy (see Chapter 18a).

Salter (Innominate) Osteotomy

This is undertaken through an anterior approach. The innominate bone (ilium) is osteotomized with a Gigli saw, from the sciatic notch to the AIIS. Care must be taken to avoid damage to the neurovascular structures in the sciatic notch. The entire acetabulum, together with the pubis and ischium, is rotated as one piece anteriorly and laterally hinged on the symphysis pubis. The osteotomy is held open anterolaterally by a wedge of bone harvested from the iliac crest and stabilized with two or more threaded pins or wires (Figure 4c.21) [25].

Pemberton Pelvic Osteotomy

Pemberton osteotomy is performed as an incomplete osteotomy from just above the AIIS through both the medial and lateral tables of the ilium, but does not cut through the posterior column. The osteotomy is distracted using a laminar spreader hinging on the posterior limb of the triradiate cartilage to provide increased anterior and lateral coverage (Figure 4c.21). A bone graft is impacted at the osteotomy site to keep the correction, and this is usually stable and does not require fixation.

There are several advantages of the Pemberton technique over Salter osteotomy. The incomplete cut maintains inherent stability and does not usually require supplementary internal fixation. As the posterior hinge is intact, it prevents trans-iliac lengthening (which sometimes occurs in Salter osteotomy). This also guarantees that the distal fragment (acetabulum, pubis, and ischium) rotates, rather than translates, which is essential to achieve anterolateral coverage. One more advantage of Pemberton osteotomy is the ability to fine-tune femoral head coverage (anterior versus lateral coverage) by changing the shape and site of the inside and outside cuts. Therefore, it has reshaping, as well as redirectional, benefits (Figure 4c.21).

Dega and San Diego osteotomies provide good lateral, but limited anterior, coverage. Although they can increase stability by increasing lateral coverage, anterior coverage is not as good as with Salter and Pemberton osteotomies. The clinical significance of less anterior coverage has not been shown to be an issue (yet) (see Chapter 18a, Figure 18a.21).

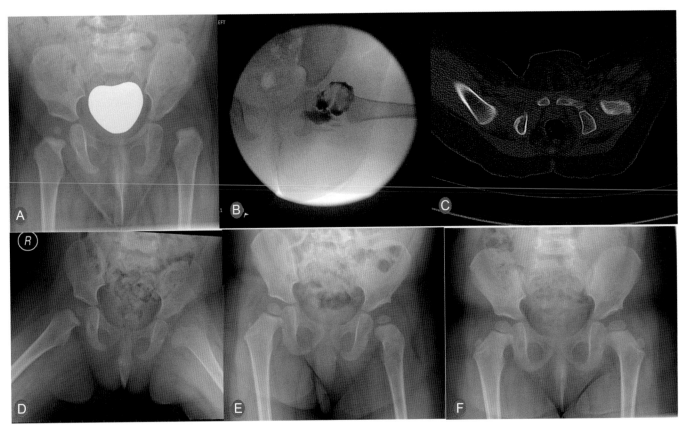

Figure 4c.19 A 1-year-old child with a dislocated left hip (A). He underwent closed reduction and adductor tenotomy. The arthrogram shows a well-reduced hip with acceptable medial pooling (B). The post-operative CT scan shows a well-reduced hip (C). (D) shows an X-ray shortly after the cast was removed. (E) and (F) are annual follow-up X-rays. Note the improvement in hip abduction contracture (common after hip spica), femoral head growth, and improvement in hip acetabular dysplasia to normal values.

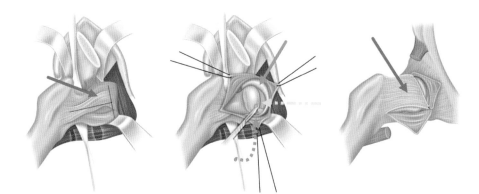

Figure 4c.20 T-V capsulorraphy (red arrows). The capsule is opened in a T-shaped fashion, taking care not to cut the labrum and attached cartilaginous roof (solid green arrow). The ligamentum teres is divided (curved, dashed green arrow) and the pulvinar is cleared (dashed yellow arrow); the joint is reduced, and then the capsule is closed in a V-shaped fashion to reduce redundant supralateral space.

Femoral Osteotomy

A femoral osteotomy (shortening, varus, derotation or a combination thereof) may be required. Shortening should be considered when excessive pressure is placed on the femoral head when it is reduced, particularly in children older than 2 years. The surgeon should be able to distract the joint by a few millimetres without much force; if this is not possible, the reduction is probably tight and shortening is warranted. If the joint remains stable only in wide abduction, a varus osteotomy is indicated. If there is excessive femoral anteversion and the reduction requires significant internal rotation to maintain stability, then a femoral derotation osteotomy is needed.

Children from 18 months to 30 months

Treatment of children in this age group with hip dislocation is more challenging. There is usually a more severe grade of dislocation with the surrounding muscles more severely contracted. They almost always need a pelvic and femoral osteotomy (Figure 4c.22).

Children older than 30 months

The presence of the femoral head inside the acetabulum is essential for the acetabulum to grow bigger. In older children with a dislocated hip, the femoral head is usually larger than

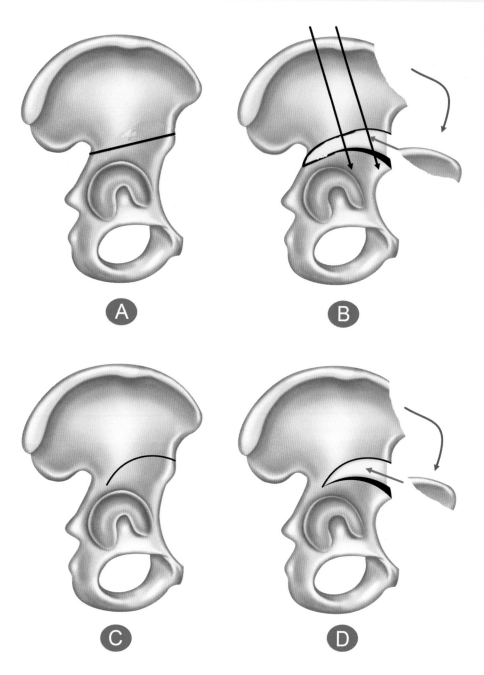

Figure 4c.21 Differenced between Salter and Pemberton pelvic osteotomies. In Salter osteotomy, the ilium is completely divided (A, B), whereas in Pemberton osteotomy, it is not. A small part of the posterior column at the triradiate cartilage level is left uncut (C, D), and the acetabular roof is hinged on this arc to allow anterior or anterolateral coverage. Obvious advantages include greater stability than with Salter osteotomy and no requirement for metal fixation. Rotation, rather than translation, is guaranteed with Pemberton osteotomy because of the posterior uncut hinge. Pembersal osteotomy refers to Pemberton osteotomy when the posterior hinge is cut undeliberately.

the acetabular socket. Forcing a large femoral head into a small socket is likely to damage both and lead to a bad clinical outcome.

There is some debate on the upper age at which a successful reduction can be achieved. Reduction of bilateral dislocations is frequently unsatisfactory in children older than 8 years, whereas reduction of unilateral dislocations should be attempted for children aged up to 9 or 10 years. This is because gait asymmetry and function are more markedly affected in unilateral cases.

Complications

Several complications that are specific to hip reduction surgery have been reported:

1. Residual or persistent dysplasia (likely to be due to AVN of the acetabular ossification centre) (Figures 4c.5 and 4c.23)
2. AVN of the femoral head

3. Redislocation (early or late)
4. Inferior dislocation
5. Fragility fracture (hip spica and immobilization cause bone weakness)
6. Stiffness
7. Spica problems (too tight, too loose, skin damage).

Residual Dysplasia

It is important to follow up children with DDH, as residual or persistent dysplasia is not uncommon. Untreated dysplasia could lead to redislocation or premature osteoarthritis. Surgery is generally indicated if:

1. The AI fails to improve over 18 months (6-monthly pelvic X-rays) or normalize (AI <20°) by the age of 4 years

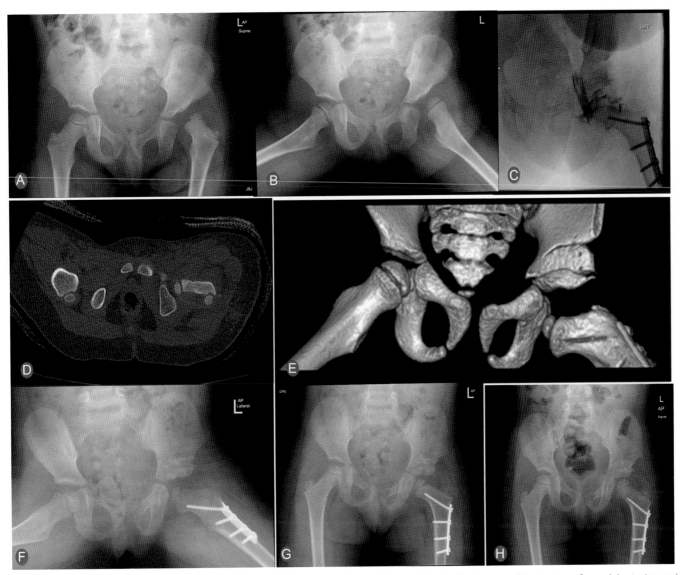

Figure 4c.22 A 2-year-old girl with a dislocated left hip (A, B). She was treated by open reduction of the hip, Pemberton pelvic osteotomy, femoral shortening, and derotation osteotomy. (D) CT showing a well-reduced hip. (E) shows the anatomical features of Pemberton osteotomy where a small part of the posterior column remains uncut (behind the wedged graft on this image). (F), (G), and (H) are annual follow-up images.

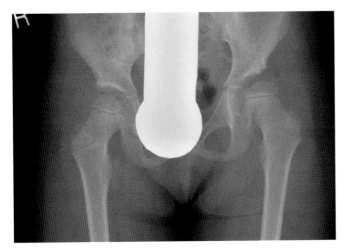

Figure 4c.23 Persistent dysplasia. The radiograph shows a shallow acetabulum on the left side. Although the femoral head is spherical and concentric in the acetabulum, it is not well covered. Her acetabular index is 29° left and 21° right, and 50% of the head is uncovered.

2. Inadequate acetabular coverage (CEA <15°, uncovering >30% after 4 years)

3. Progressive subluxation and instability

4. Pain.

The appropriate procedure should be selected, based on the site of deformity, severity, congruity of the joint, age and available expertise. Table 4c.2 summarizes the current recommended procedures for various types of persistent hip dysplasia [26]. In severe dysplasia, pelvic osteotomy may be combined with femoral osteotomy to achieve an optimal result.

Each osteotomy provides anatomical advantages that may suit a particular clinical and radiological situation better. Below, we provide the main features of each osteotomy to enable a confident discussion about them in the exam.

Pemberton and Salter osteotomies are almost equivalent and can be used interchangeably (see above). They redirect the acetabulum forward and outward, producing anterior and

Table 4c.2 Residual dysplasia treatment

2–6 years		6 years to skeletal maturity		Skeletal maturity	
Concentric reduction achieved + normal-sized acetabulum	Concentric reduction achieved + large acetabulum	Concentric reduction achieved + normal-sized acetabulum	Concentric reduction not possible + small-sized acetabulum	Concentric reduction achieved	Concentric reduction not possible + small-sized acetabulum
Pemberton or Salter osteotomy	Dega or Pemberton osteotomy	Pemberton or Salter osteotomy (<8 years) or triple osteotomy	Shelf procedure or Chiari osteotomy	Ganz osteotomy or triple osteotomy	Chiari osteotomy

lateral coverage, improving the AI and CEA by about 15° at the expense of posterior coverage. This is useful in children with DDH where the dysplasia is anterolateral. They are not advised in neuromuscular dysplasia in which the posterior wall is usually deficient.

Similarly, **San Diego and Dega osteotomies** are almost equivalent and can be used interchangeably, with a few advantages of San Diego osteotomy over Dega osteotomy (see Chapter 18a). These two osteotomies provide more lateral and posterior coverage and a limited anterior coverage by folding the outer table of the ilium outward and downward. As the cut is not complete, they do not change the direction of the acetabulum, but rather the shape of the acetabulum. That is why they are useful when the socket size is large.

Triple osteotomies are powerful redirectional osteotomies because they detach the acetabulum completely from the ilium and allow complete freedom of rotation (unlike Pemberton or Salter osteotomy). Triple osteotomy involves cuts through the ilium, pubis, and ischium. Several modifications have been described, based on the sites of these cuts and the approaches to cut the bones. The commonest modifications are Steel (1973) and Tonnis (1990) triple pelvic osteotomies (Figure 4c.24). In Tonnis osteotomy, the ischial cut is extended to above the ischial spine (and its attached strong sacrospinous ligament), allowing more freedom to rotate the acetabulum. Triple osteotomy usually interferes with the birth canal in females, an important consideration in decision-making.

Ganz (or Bernese) osteotomy is an innovative advancement of the triple osteotomy. The ischial and iliac cuts join in front of the ischial spine, leaving the posterior column in continuity. The pubic cut is made closer to the acetabulum (Figure 4c.25). All these cuts are made through a single incision (anterior hip approach). This osteotomy is more stable than triple osteotomy, and patients can start partial weight-bearing shortly after surgery. It does not interfere with the birth canal. However, it is contraindicated if the triradiate cartilage is still open because the cuts go through the growth plate, which can get damaged.

Chiari osteotomy and **shelf acetabuloplasty** are salvage procedures. Although they provide mechanical support to prevent the femoral head from sliding out of the shallow socket, they do not provide hyaline cartilage coverage. Chiari osteotomy uses a cut across the ilium just above the acetabulum and moves the upper piece laterally to provide lateral coverage (Figure 4c.26). Therefore, it creates pelvic discontinuity and the patient has to wait until healing before weight-bearing.

Steel osteotomy

Tonnis osteotomy

Figure 4c.24 Triple pelvic osteotomy: Steel and Tonnis types.

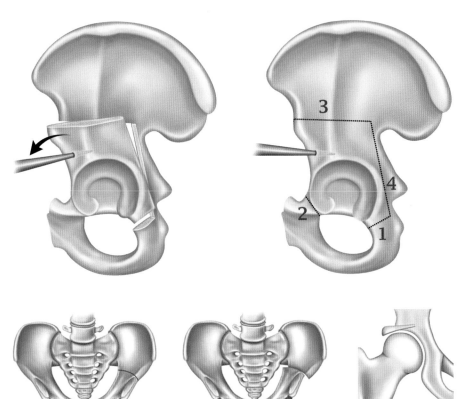

Figure 4c.25 Ganz osteotomy. The numbers represent the sequence in which pelvic bones are cut.

Figure 4c.26 Chiari osteotomy and shelf acetabuloplasty.

Chiari osteotomy

Shelf acetabuloplasty

As the name implies, shelf acetabuloplasty involves creating a bony shelf over the subluxed femoral head. It is often inserted into a trough created around the upper rim of the acetabulum.

Chiari osteotomy provides a mechanically stronger lateral coverage of the femoral head, but it is technically challenging to place in the perfect spot. Most surgeons use a bone graft below the osteotomy for perfection, which is what is often called Chiari–shelf acetabuloplasty (Figure 4c.27).

Avascular necrosis of the femoral head

AVN of the femoral head can cause long-term disability and is directly related to treatment. AVN does not occur in untreated DDH. Kalamchi and MacEwen [27] classified AVN following DDH treatment into four types. Figure 4c.28 summarizes these types and their features and treatments.

Controversies

Several controversial issues are associated with DDH treatment. We alluded to some of these earlier, including:

1. Universal versus selective hip ultrasound screening (see above)
2. The value of a medial approach to reduce dislocated hips (see above)
3. A preliminary period of traction before hip reduction

4. The timing of reduction in relation to the appearance of the ossific nucleus of the femoral head.

Proponents of a preliminary period of traction claim that traction reduces the AVN rate and the need for open reduction. To reduce costs they recommend a commercially available portable home traction device, whereas opponents claim that it is costly, and the above advantages have been challenged by various studies.

In a retrospective study [28] of 49 children aged younger than 12 months, with 57 hip dislocations, 18 hips developed partial or complete AVN and 39 hips did not develop AVN. There was no significant difference in the occurrence of AVN with respect to variables such as preliminary traction, closed versus open reduction, Pavlik harness use and age at the time of operative intervention. However, the presence of the ossific nucleus before reduction, detected either on radiographs ($P < 0.001$) or ultrasonography ($P = 0.033$), was statistically significant in predicting AVN; one (4%) of 25 hips with an ossific nucleus developed AVN, whereas 17 (53%) of 32 hips without an ossific nucleus before reduction developed AVN.

Another study of 48 patients who underwent successful closed reduction showed similar findings. At 2-year follow-up, AVN was noted post-reduction in 17 hips: 4 of 23 hips that had an ossific nucleus at reduction, compared to 13 of 25 hips reduced before ossification of the nucleus [29].

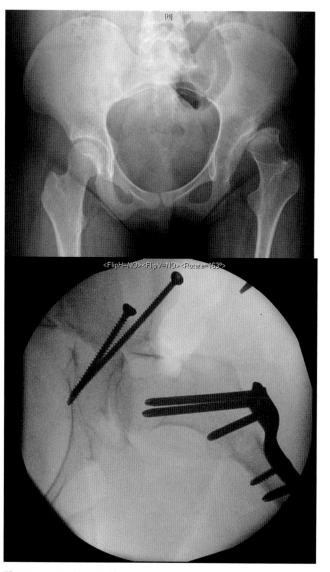

Figure 4c.27 Chiari–shelf acetabuloplasty.

Other studies disagreed with the above findings. In a study of 32 patients who underwent medial open reduction, with 40 hips and an average follow-up period of 10.3 years, AVN developed in 11 hips (27.5%) [30]. Bilateral dislocations and age older than 1 year at surgery correlated with a greater likelihood of AVN (<0.05), whereas absence of an ossific nucleus did not. AVN developed in 4 of 13 hips (30.8%) that had an ossific nucleus visible on radiographs at the time of reduction, and in 7 of 27 hips (25.9%) that did not have a visible ossific nucleus. Use of preoperative traction was not protective against AVN, because 7 of the 11 hips with AVN had undergone preoperative traction.

Analysis of other factors, such as side of dislocation, treatment with a Pavlik harness, preoperative traction, unilateral compared with bilateral involvement, closed compared with open reduction, the approach of open reduction, and failed primary reduction, demonstrated no differences with respect to the frequency of reconstructive procedures.

We believe that one should not wait to treat a hip until the ossific nucleus appears. The growth potential of the acetabulum declines with age, and hips reduced later will not remodel as well as those reduced earlier.

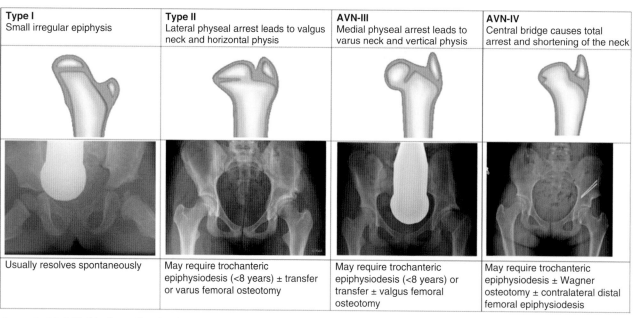

Type I Small irregular epiphysis	Type II Lateral physeal arrest leads to valgus neck and horizontal physis	AVN-III Medial physeal arrest leads to varus neck and vertical physis	AVN-IV Central bridge causes total arrest and shortening of the neck
Usually resolves spontaneously	May require trochanteric epiphysiodesis (<8 years) ± transfer or varus femoral osteotomy	May require trochanteric epiphysiodesis (<8 years) or transfer ± valgus femoral osteotomy	May require trochanteric epiphysiodesis ± Wagner osteotomy ± contralateral distal femoral epiphysiodesis

Figure 4c.28 AVN of the femoral head (Kalamchi and MacEwen classification).

References

1. de Hundt M, *et al.* Risk factors for developmental dysplasia of the hip: a meta-analysis. *Eur J Obstet Gynecol Reprod Biol.* 2012;165(1):8–17.

2. Ortiz-Neira CL, Paolucci EO, Donnon T. A meta-analysis of common risk factors associated with the diagnosis of developmental dysplasia of the hip in newborns. *Eur J Radiol.* 2011;81(3):e344–51.

3. Herring JA. *Tachdjians' Pediatric Orthopaedics*, 4th ed, Vol. 1. Philadelphia, PA: Saunders Elsevier; 2008.

4. Scheuer L, Black SM. *Developmental Juvenile Osteology*. Oxford: Elsevier Academic Press; 2000.

5. Jari S, Paton RW, Srinivasan MS. Unilateral limitation of abduction of the hip. A valuable clinical sign for DDH? *J Bone Joint Surg Br.* 2002;84(1):104–7.

6. Jones D. Neonatal detection of developmental dysplasia of the hip (DDH). *J Bone Joint Surg Br.* 1998;80(6):943–5.

7. Czubak J, *et al.* Ultrasound measurements of the newborn hip. Comparison of two methods in 657 newborns. *Acta Orthop Scand.* 1998;69(1):21–4.

8. Diaz A, Cuervo M, Epeldegui T. Simultaneous ultrasound studies of developmental dysplasia of the hip using the Graf, Harcke, and Suzuki approaches. *J Pediatr Orthop B.* 1994;3(2):185–9.

9. Sakkers R, Pollet V. The natural history of abnormal ultrasound findings in hips of infants under six months of age. *J Child Orthop.* 2018;12(4):302–7.

10. Bialik V, Bialik GM, Wiener F. Prevention of overtreatment of neonatal hip dysplasia by the use of ultrasonography. *J Pediatr Orthop B.* 1998;7(1):39–42.

11. Ashoor M, *et al.* Evidence based treatment for developmental dysplasia of the hip in children under 6 months of age. Systematic review and exploratory analysis. *Surgeon.* 2021;19(2):77–86.

12. O'Beirne JG, *et al.* International Interdisciplinary Consensus Meeting on the evaluation of developmental dysplasia of the hip. *Ultraschall Med.* 2019;40(4):454–64.

13. Thallinger C, *et al.* Long-term results of a nationwide general ultrasound screening system for developmental disorders of the hip: the Austrian hip screening program. *J Child Orthop.* 2014;8(1):3–10.

14. Ulziibat M, *et al.* Implementation of a nationwide universal ultrasound screening programme for developmental dysplasia of the neonatal hip in Mongolia. *J Child Orthop.* 2020;14(4):273–80.

15. Biedermann R, *et al.* Results of universal ultrasound screening for developmental dysplasia of the hip: a prospective follow-up of 28 092 consecutive infants. *Bone Joint J.* 2018;100-b(10):1399–404.

16. Thaler M, *et al.* Cost-effectiveness of universal ultrasound screening compared with clinical examination alone in the diagnosis and treatment of neonatal hip dysplasia in Austria. *J Bone Joint Surg Br.* 2011;93(8):1126–30.

17. Mahan ST, Katz JN, Kim YJ. To screen or not to screen? A decision analysis of the utility of screening for developmental dysplasia of the hip. *J Bone Joint Surg Am.* 2009;91(7):1705–19.

18. Shorter D, Hong T, Osborn DA. Cochrane review: screening programmes for developmental dysplasia of the hip in newborn infants. *Evid Based Child Health.* 2013;8(1):11–54.

19. Shipman SA, *et al.* Screening for developmental dysplasia of the hip: a systematic literature review for the US Preventive Services Task Force. *Pediatrics.* 2006;117(3):e557–76.

20. Patel H. Preventive health care, 2001 update: screening and management of developmental dysplasia of the hip in newborns. *CMAJ.* 2001;164(12):1669–77.

21. Murnaghan ML, *et al.* Femoral nerve palsy in Pavlik harness treatment for developmental dysplasia of the hip. *J Bone Joint Surg Am.* 2011;93(5):493–9.

22. Ramsey PL, Lasser S, MacEwen GD. Congenital dislocation of the hip: use of the Pavlik harness in the child during the first six months of life. 1976. *J Bone Joint Surg Am.* 2002;84-A(8):1478; discussion 1478.

23. Gardner RO, *et al.* The incidence of avascular necrosis and the radiographic outcome following medial open reduction in children with developmental dysplasia of the hip: a systematic review. *Bone Joint J.* 2014;96-B(2):279–86.

24. Gardner ROE, *et al.* Evidence-based management of developmental dysplasia of the hip. In: Alshryda S, Huntley JS, Banaszkiewicz PA, eds. *Paediatric Orthopaedics: An Evidence-Based Approach to Clinical Questions.* Cham: Springer; 2016. pp. 27–42.

25. Salter RB, Dubos JP. The first fifteen year's personal experience with innominate osteotomy in the treatment of congenital dislocation and subluxation of the hip. *Clin Orthop Relat Res.* 1974;98:72–103.

26. Jospeh B, *et al. Paediatric Orthopaedics. A System of Decision Making.* London: Harold Arnold; 2009.

27. Kalamchi A, MacEwen GD. Avascular necrosis following treatment of congenital dislocation of the hip. *J Bone Joint Surg Am.* 1980;62(6):876–88.

28. Segal LS, *et al.* Avascular necrosis after treatment of DDH: the protective influence of the ossific nucleus. *J Pediatr Orthop.* 1999;19(2):177–84.

29. Cooke SJ, *et al.* Ossification of the femoral head at closed reduction for developmental dysplasia of the hip and its influence on the long-term outcome. *J Pediatr Orthop B.* 2010;19(1):22–6.

30. Konigsberg DE, *et al.* Results of medial open reduction of the hip in infants with developmental dislocation of the hip. *J Pediatr Orthop.* 2003;23(1):1–9.

31. Luhmann SJ, *et al.* The prognostic importance of the ossific nucleus in the treatment of congenital dysplasia of the hip. *J Bone Joint Surg Am.* 1998;80(12):1719–27.

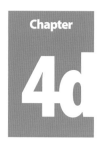
Miscellaneous Hip Disorders

Sattar Alshryda and Paul A. Banaszkiewicz

Introduction

This section covers several hip problems that are not covered earlier and are relevant to the exam (and practice). More hip disorders, including hip disorders in neuromuscular conditions, trisomy 21 and skeletal dysplasia, will be covered in their relevant sections.

Coxa Vara

Coxa vara (CV) is a term referring to the proximal femoral varus deformity in which there is a decrease in the neck shaft angle (NSA <110°) (Figure 4d.1). CV is not a single entity, but rather a wide spectrum of different types, pathologies, aetiologies, and natural history. Confusion and controversy exist in the literature as to the terminology and classification of this disorder, which can be grouped as follows.

Congenital Coxa Vara

Congenital coxa vara (CCV) is more accurately described as congenital femoral deficiency (CFD) with CV. It is caused by a primary cartilaginous defect in the femoral neck. By definition, CCV presents at birth but sometimes manifests clinically during early childhood and commonly follows a clinical course that is progressive with growth. It is commonly associated with a significant leg length discrepancy (LLD), congenital short femur (CSF), proximal femoral focal deficiency (PFFD) and congenital bowed femur (Figure 4d.1A).

Developmental Coxa Vara

Developmental coxa vara (DCV) is a term reserved for CV in early childhood, with classical radiographic features (inferior and posterior bony metaphyseal fragment) and no other skeletal manifestations. In the past, it was also referred to as infantile or cervical CV (Figure 4d.1B).

Acquired Coxa Vara

Acquired coxa vara (ACA) is caused by several conditions, including:

1. Slipped upper femoral epiphysis
2. Sequelae of avascular necrosis of the femoral epiphysis:
   a. Legg–Calvé–Perthes disease
   b. Traumatic
   c. Femoral neck fracture
   d. Traumatic hip dislocation

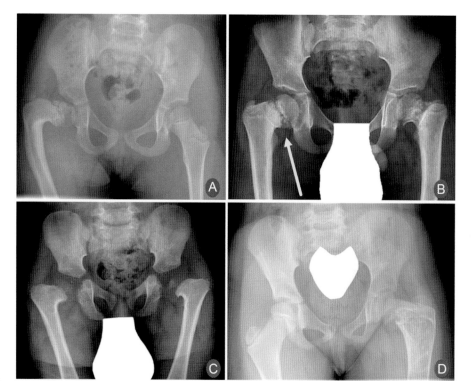

Figure 4d.1 Plain pelvic X-rays showing various types of coxa vara. (A) Congenital. (B) Developmental (notice the inverted Y appearance, which is more marked on the right hip, yellow arrow). (C) and (D) are two examples of acquired coxa vara, with (C) showing a child with chondrodysplasia punctata (see the punctated femoral head) and (D) showing a child with fibrous dysplasia.

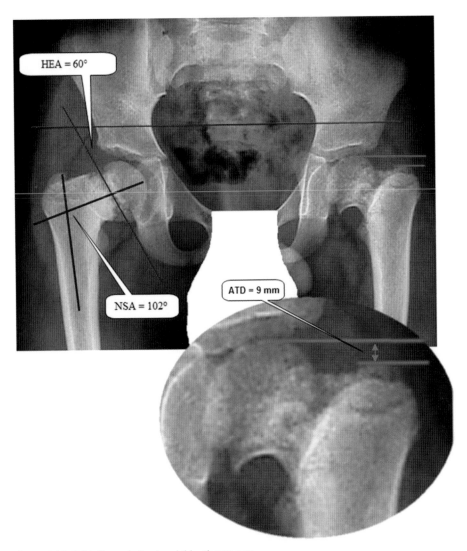

HEA = 60°

NSA = 102°

ATD = 9 mm

Figure 4d.2 Pelvic X-ray of a limping child with coxa vara.

e. Post-reduction for developmental dysplasia of the hip
f. Septic necrosis
g. Other causes of avascular necrosis of the immature femoral head
3. CV associated with pathological bone disorders:
   a. Osteogenesis imperfecta
   b. Fibrous dysplasia
   c. Renal osteodystrophy
   d. Osteopetrosis
4. Associated with skeletal dysplasia (this is often referred to as dysplastic CV. Some authors classified this group under developmental CV):
   a. Cleidocranial dysostosis
   b. Metaphyseal dysostosis
   c. Other skeletal dysplasias.

Confusion and controversy exist in the literature as to the terminology and classification of this disorder. Table 4d.1 summarizes the differences among the different types.

Presentations

DCV usually presents with a painless limp and progressive LLD. It may become painful towards the end of the day or after significant activity. There may be a family history and it can be bilateral (30–50%). Age of presentation is usually in the first 5 years of life, but older patients may be encountered. Patients may show prominent greater trochanters. There may be a pelvic tilt secondary to LLD, and there is usually a positive, or delayed positive, Trendelenburg test.

There are three important radiological measures to quantify the CV (Figure 4d.2): NSA, Hilgenreiner epiphyseal angle (HEA), and articulotrochanteric distance (ATD). A decreased ATD indicates that the location of the pathology is in the physeal or intertrochanteric area, whereas a normal ATD indicates it is in the subtrochanteric region.

Treatment

Treatment of CCV is dealt with in the following section (see Congenital Femoral Deficiency). Acquired CV treatment is

Table 4d.1 Summary of different types of coxa vara

Features	Congenital coxa vara	Developmental coxa vara	Acquired coxa vara[a]
Site	Subtrochanteric	Physis	Any (epiphysis, physis, metaphysis, subtrochanteric)
Pathology	Embryonic limb bud abnormality	Primary ossification defect in the inferior femoral neck, predisposing the local dystrophic bone to fatigue and bend by shear stress of weight	Depending on the cause; usually vascular insult (sepsis, AVN) or traumatic (fracture)
Age of onset	Birth	Walking age – 6 years	Usually older than CCV and DCV
Presenting feature	Unilateral short and deformed leg	Limping; Trendelenburg gait (unilateral) or waddling (bilateral) LLD rarely >3 cm	Presenting features of the cause
Radiological features	Features of CFD (see below)	Very typical: decreased NSA, vertical physis, a triangular metaphyseal fragment in the inferior femoral neck (Fairbank's trainable), inverted radiolucent Y pattern, decreased anteversion (may be retroversion)	Features of coxa vara and causative pathology
Natural history	Progression	Progression if HEA >60°	Progression if the physis or epiphysis is involved Fractures may remodel, resolving the varus deformity

[a] Features are closely related to the underlying pathology.
AVN, avascular necrosis; CCV, congenital coxa vara; DCV, developmental coxa vara; LLD, leg length discrepancy; CFD, congenital femoral deficiency; NSA, neck shaft angle; HEA, Hilgenreiner epiphyseal angle.

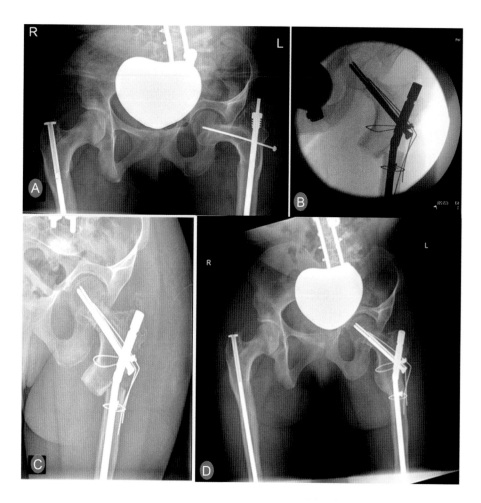

Figure 4d.3 Acquired coxa vara in a child with osteogenesis imperfecta of almost 90°. This caused subsequent impingement and stress fracture of the femoral neck. The child underwent surgical correction using a pedi-nail and wires. (A) Preoperative image. (B) Intraoperative image. (C, D) Post-operative images at 6 weeks and 1 year, respectively.

directed towards the cause; however, anatomical correction is often required to improve function and symptoms (Figure 4d.3).

As for DCV, Weinstein *et al.* [1] reviewed 42 patients with CV and introduced the HEA to aid in deciding their candidacy for surgery (average normal value is 20°):

- HEA of <45° – usually improves without intervention
- HEA of >60° – usually worsens if left untreated and is an indication for surgery
- HEA of 45–60° – requires observation for either healing or progression, the latter of which requires surgical intervention.

Surgical treatment involves corrective osteotomy to achieve the following goals:

1. NSA ≥140° and HEA to <35–40°
2. Correction of the femoral version to normal values (usually there is a retroversion)
3. Ossification and healing of the defective inferomedial femoral neck fragment
4. Restoring the ATD and abductor mechanism length–tension relationship
5. Adductor tenotomy to remove the deforming force.

Several techniques and variations to achieve the above have been described such as Pauwels Y-shaped osteotomy, Langenskiöld intertrochanteric osteotomy, and Borden subtrochanteric osteotomy. Knowing the details of these techniques is not expected for the exam. Associated abnormalities such as LLD, femoral retroversion, or trochanteric overgrowth can be corrected simultaneously or at a second stage.

Congenital Femoral Deficiency

CFD (Figure 4d.4) is a spectrum of disorder(s), rather than a single disease entity. There are two distinct forms:

1. PFFD describes a deformity in which the femur is shorter than normal and there is discontinuity (with loss of various lengths of the femur) between the femoral neck and the shaft

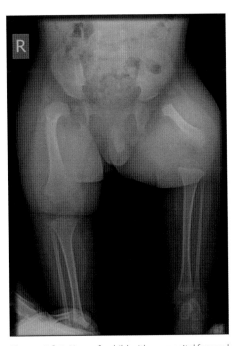

Figure 4d.4 X-ray of a child with congenital femoral deficiency showing a short and dysplastic femur. The proximal parts (head and trochanter) are not visible (may be absent or have not ossified yet); features are consistent with proximal femoral focal deficiency (PFFD). There is coxa vara of the right side, indicating the right side may be affected as well (bilateral involvement in 15%). The left fibula seems to be shorter than the right side, raising the possibility of fibular hemimelia (two-thirds of patients). It is difficult to comment on the hip and knee joint states from a single plain film, and further assessment is required.

2. CSF describes a short, but present, femur, with no bony loss or discontinuity. In most cases, the cause of the femoral deficiency is unknown; however, it can be part of genetically transmitted syndromes.

Several classifications have been advised to aid assessment and treatment.

Aitken's Classification

This classification is based on four features: presence of the femoral head, quality of the acetabulum, size of the femur and connection between the head and shaft. Composite Table 4d.2 and Figure 4d.5 illustrate the classification [2].

Paley's Classification

Aitken's classification does not consider the importance of the knee in treating CFD. Several situations do not fit neatly into the classification. Paley proposed a comprehensive classification based around lengthening reconstructive surgery that is gaining wider acceptance [4] (Figure 4d.6).

Type 1: Intact femur with mobile hip and knee

a. Normal ossification of the proximal femur
b. Delayed ossification of the proximal femur – subtrochanteric type
c. Delayed ossification of the proximal femur – neck type.

Type 2: Mobile pseudarthrosis (Hip not fully formed, a false joint) with mobile knee

a. Femoral head mobile in the acetabulum
b. Femoral head absent or stiff in the acetabulum.

Type 3: Diaphyseal deficiency of femur (Femur does not reach the acetabulum)

a. Knee motion >45°
b. Knee motion <45°
c. Complete absence of the femur.

Type 4: Distal deficiency of the femur

Type 1 is further subclassified into:
- 0 – ready for surgery; no factors to correct before lengthening
- 1 – one factor to correct before lengthening
- 2 – two factors to correct before lengthening
- 3 – three factors to correct before lengthening
- 4+, etc.

Examples of factors requiring correction prior to lengthening of the femur are NSA <90°, delayed ossification of the proximal femur, centre edge angle (CEA) <20°, subluxing patella, and/or dislocating knee.

The strategy of management is staged corrections of the abnormalities to reach stage I0, which is amenable to lengthening. For example, type 1a-3 is converted to 1a-2, then 1a-1, and then 1a-0, followed by lengthening. Pre-existing knee stiffness is the most functionally limiting factor and should be considered a relative

Table 4d.2 Aitken's classification

Type	Diagram	Femoral head	Acetabulum	Femoral segment	Relationship between components of the femur and acetabulum
A		Present	Normal	Short	Bony connections exist among all components. The cartilaginous neck ossifies later on, although this is often associated with pseudarthrosis. X-rays show severe coxa vara, with significant shortening of the femur Amstutz and Wilson subdivided class A into types 1 and 2. Type 1 is reserved for the milder form with simple femoral shortening and coxa vara (Figure 4d.4, right hip). In type 2, subtrochanteric pseudarthrosis is present. The remaining types correspond to those of Aitken's classification [3]
B		Present	Adequate or moderately plastic	Short with a proximal bony tuft	No osseous connection between the head and shaft, but the head is in the acetabulum
C		Absent or tiny ossicle	Severely dysplastic	Short and usually tapered	The hip is very unstable
D		Absent	Absent Obturator foramen enlarged Pelvis is square in bilateral cases	Short and deformed	No connection, rudimentary distal part of the femur

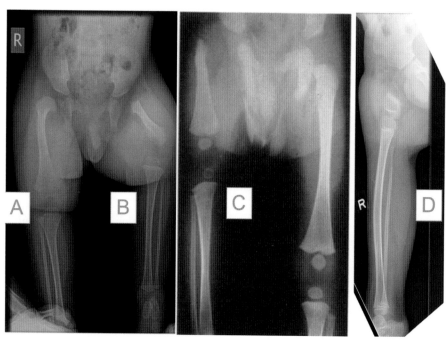

Figure 4d.5 Aitken's classification of congenital short femur. Type A-D

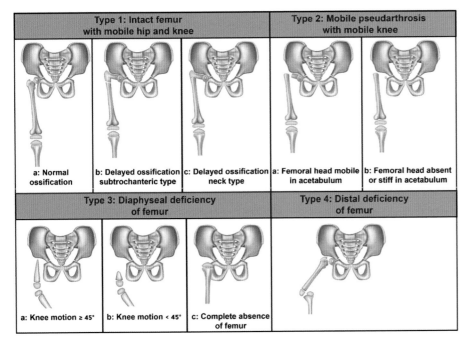

Figure 4d.6 Paley's classification of congenital femoral deficiency.

indication for amputation versus reconstruction. Hip dysplasia or deficiency is reconstructable and is not a limiting factor. Hip reconstruction should be performed prior to lengthening.

Treatment

Treatment of this condition is a challenge and it should be undertaken in specialized centres with interest and experience in its treatment. The National Institute for Health and Care Excellence (NICE) has issued guidance to National Health Service (NHS) hospitals on combined bony and soft tissue reconstruction for PFFD [5]. Treatment must be tailored to individual patients, based on LLD, hip and knee stability, femoral rotation, proximal musculature, foot condition, availability of expertise, and patient and family motivation. The two broad options are reconstructive surgery or amputation and prosthetic replacement.

References

1. Weinstein JN, Kuo KN, Millar EA. Congenital coxa vara. A retrospective review. *J Pediatr Orthop.* 1984;4(1):70–7.

2. Aitken GT. Proximal femoral focal deficiency: definition, classification and management. In: GT Aitken, ed. *Proximal Femoral Focal Deficiency – a Congenital Anomaly: A Symposium* *Held in Washington, DC, 13 June 1968.* Washington, DC: National Academy of Sciences; 1969. pp. 1–22.

3. Amstutz HC, Wilson PD. Dysgenesis of the proximal femur (coxa vara) and its surgical management. *J Bone Joint Surg.* 1962;44(1):1–24.

4. Rozbruch SR, Hamdy R. *Limb Lengthening and Reconstruction Surgery* *Case Atlas.* Cham: Springer International Publishing; 2015.

5. National Institute for Health and Care Excellence. Combined bony and soft tissue reconstruction for hip joint stabilisation in proximal focal femoral deficiency (PFFD). 2009. Interventional procedures guidance [IPG297]. Available from: www.nice.org.uk/guidance/ipg297.

Chapter 5

Traumatic Hip Disorders

Sean Duffy and Fergal Monsell

Pelvis

Pelvic injuries are uncommon in children and account for approximately 1–2% of all paediatric fractures [1–3], with high-energy motor vehicle accidents being the commonest cause [4]. Efficient primary assessment using Adult Trauma Life Support (ATLS) and Paediatric Life Support (PLS) principles, with subsequent secondary/tertiary surveys, will guide immediate management and identify associated injuries. The head, chest, and limbs are the commonest associated injuries [4], with up to 50% of paediatric pelvic fractures occurring with an associated head injury, over 40% of which are severe/critical [4]. Mortality rates between 3.6% and 5% are reported [5–8], with death rarely due to haemorrhage (0.3%) [5]

The immature skeleton differs from that of an adult, with increased elasticity in the bone, joints, and ligaments. As a result, the paediatric pelvis has a greater capacity for energy absorption in the bone, sacroiliac joints, triradiate cartilage, and pubic symphysis before bone failure. Surrounding structures will have been subject to the same force and there should be a high index of suspicion for associated injuries and a low threshold for investigation. In contrast to the adult pelvis, the immature pelvis may fail in one place, with plastic deformation or, more commonly, joint flexibility accounting for the change in pelvic ring shape.

Shaath *et al.* identified a significant difference in fracture pattern, management, and mortality rate in patients with open, compared to closed, triradiate cartilage [4]. This was considered to be related to immaturity of the pelvis, in addition to a likely difference in mechanism between these age groups. The authors suggested children with a closed triradiate cartilage have similar fracture patterns and mechanisms of injury to adults and should therefore be treated using adult algorithms.

Classification System: Modified Torode and Zeig

The original Torode and Zeig classification, with modification by Shore, is illustrated in Figure 5.1 [9, 10] and summarized in Table 5.1.

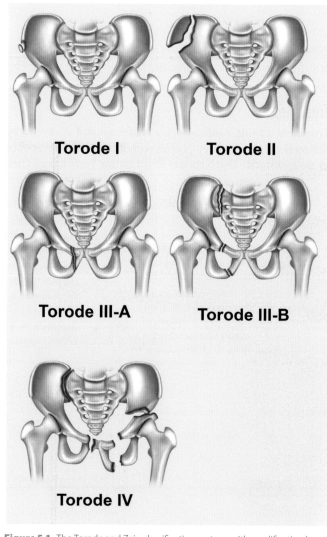

Figure 5.1 The Torode and Zeig classification system, with modification by Shore (2012) for pelvic fractures in children. Type I: avulsion; type II: iliac wing fracture; type IIIA: anterior pelvic ring fracture (stable); type IIIB: anterior and posterior pelvic fracture (stable); and type IV: ring disruption (unstable).

Table 5.1 Torode and Zeig pelvic classification system

Type I	Avulsion fractures	Consist of avulsion injuries or 'pull-off' fractures, typically of the anterior superior iliac spine
Type II	Iliac wing fractures	Include iliac wing fractures
Type III	Simple ring fractures	Simple ring fractures (stable) (e.g. rami fractures)
Type IV	Ring disruption fractures	• Bilateral fractures of the pubic rami (straddle fractures) • Fractures involving the pubic rami or disruption of the pubic symphysis, with associated posterior pelvic ring fracture or disruption of the sacroiliac joint • Fractures involving the anterior pelvic ring and acetabular segment

Shore *et al.* modified the Torode classification in 2012, and subdivided group III to delineate between lower- (IIIA) and higher- (IIIB) energy fractures. Fractures involving the anterior and posterior pelvis (group IIIB) were associated with significantly increased rates of intensive care admission, blood product resuscitation, and length of stay [10]. Increased use of CT scanning identified fractures of the posterior pelvis, which were unreliably detected with plain radiographs.

Children can tolerate longer periods of immobilization and have a greater capacity for remodelling, and the mainstay of paediatric pelvic fracture management remains supportive. Rates of operative management vary between 6% [8] and 18.5% [4], and is significantly less common in patients with an open triradiate cartilage [4]. Table 5.2 summarizes the treatment of pelvic fractures.

Table 5.2 Summary of pelvic fracture treatment

Types	Examples	Treatment recommendation
I: avulsion fractures	Avulsion (ASIS, AIIS, IT)	Bed rest for 2 weeks, then protected WB for 4 weeks. Hip should be flexed during rest in ASIS and AIIS avulsions, and extended in IT avulsion (Figure 5.2)
II: iliac wing fractures	Iliac wing fractures (Duverney)	Bed rest with abducted leg for 1 week, then WB as tolerated
III: simple ring fractures	1. Ipsilateral rami 2. symphysis pubis 3. SI joint (rare)	Bed rest for 2–4 weeks, then progress to WB
IV: ring disruption fractures	1. Bilateral pubic rami (straddle)	Bed rest for 2–4 weeks, then progress to WB
	2. Anterior and posterior ring with migration (Malgaigne)	Skeletal traction or external fixator for 3–6 weeks
Acetabular fractures	1. Small fragment with dislocation	Reduce dislocation and ambulate as able. If fragment is large, stabilize. Ensure no fragments inside the joint after reduction
	2. Linear: non-displaced	Treat associated pelvic fracture
	3. Linear: hip unstable	Skeletal traction, ORIF if incongruous
	4. Central	Lateral traction for reduction, ORIF if severe

AIIS, anterior inferior iliac spine; ASIS, anterior superior iliac spine; IT, ischial tuberosity; ORIF, open reduction and internal fixation; SI, sacroiliac; WB, weight-bearing.

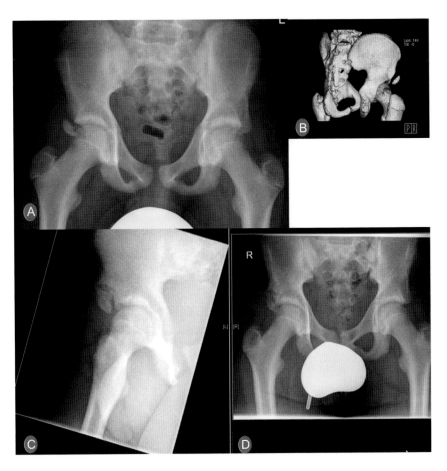

Figure 5.2 (A) Radiograph of ASIS avulsion fracture whilst playing football. CT scan demonstrating avulsion fracture (B). Radiographs demonstrating that the fracture has healed with non-operative treatment (C) and (D). Based on the displacement, this fracture may cause impingement symptoms, which should be differentiated from non-union or tendinitis. Diagnostic injection is unlikely to distinguish between these differentials, but MRI and CT may be useful.

Proximal Femur

Injuries to the femoral head and neck are rare in children, accounting for <1% of all paediatric fractures [11, 12]. They are often caused by high-energy trauma, including motor vehicle accidents and falls from height. The aim of treatment is to achieve rapid anatomic reduction of these fractures with stable internal fixation, and a hip spica may also be required to protect the fixation in younger patients.

Vascular Supply

A detailed understanding of the vascular anatomy and vascular transitions during different stages of hip development is required to treat proximal femoral fractures in children [13, 14].

Dial *et al.* described three key stages relevant to the vascular supply of the femoral head.

From birth to subcapital physeal formation at 4–6 months, the epiphysis is supplied by the medial femoral circumflex artery (MFCA), the lateral femoral circumflex artery (LFCA), and, to some degree, the artery of the ligamentum teres. After ossification of the femoral head, the physis inhibits the metaphyseal vessels from crossing the growth plate. This blocks the branches from the LFCA reaching the epiphysis. The superior and inferior retinacular branches of the MFCA pass around the growth plate and supply the epiphysis. The importance of the ligamentum teres artery has been regularly reported as minor in all age groups [14, 15].

After skeletal maturity, branches of the MFCA and LFCA form an extracapsular ring around the intertrochanteric line, from which arteries branch to supply the metaphysis and epiphysis. The physis closes, allowing the metaphyseal system to supply the femoral head, and the MFCA remains the dominant supply [15].

Classification System: Delbet

Delbet described a classification of fractures of the femoral neck in adults in 1928 (Figure 5.3). This was modified by Collona in 1929 for use in children, dividing fractures into four groups [16, 17]. Despite this amendment, the classification continues to be referred to under the original author's name. This classification is useful in predicting avascular necrosis (AVN) rates and is commonly used in contemporary paediatric practice.

Moon and Mehlman reported the results of a meta-analysis that identified the AVN rates associated with each fracture type. Type I fractures involve the physis, similar to a Salter–Harris I injury (AVN rate 38%); type II fractures are transcervical (AVN rate 28%); type III fractures are basicervical (AVN rate 18%), and type IV fractures are intertrochanteric (AVN rate 5%) [18].

Timing of Intervention

There has been a long-standing and continuing debate regarding the timing of reduction and surgical stabilization [19]. Recent studies have supported early reduction, reporting significantly lower rates of AVN [20–23]. It is axiomatic that earlier correction of distorted vessels caused by fracture displacement has the potential to re-establish circulation and therefore reduce the risk of AVN. This approach, however, has not been universal and a recent review of 239 patients did not demonstrate a temporal association [24].

Open Reduction

Whilst an anterior (Smith–Peterson) approach provides excellent direct visualization for capsular decompression, an anterolateral (Watson–Jones) approach to the hip is more useful to identify the fracture site and assists with visual reduction. In addition, this approach can be extended distally to provide access to the lateral femur for application of the fixation device through the same incision. The technique depends on surgeon preference and experience, fracture configuration, and fixation type.

An important general principle is that stable fixation has primacy over potential iatrogenic injury to the physis [25], and

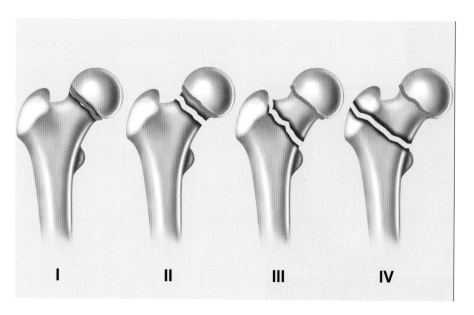

Figure 5.3 Delbet classification. Type I is a transepiphyseal separation with (type IA) or without (type IB) dislocation of the femoral head from the acetabulum. Type II is a transcervical fracture. Type III is a base cervical fracture. Type IV is an intertrochanteric fracture.

I   II   III   IV

when crossing the physis is unavoidable, to provide adequate stability, threadless fixation should be used where possible.

As the incidence for these injuries is low, there is no consensus for the optimum technique and the AO Surgery Reference (paediatrics) provides detailed information on the available options for each fracture type [26].

Undisplaced fractures may be treated with percutaneous fixation, whereas displaced fractures mandate urgent anatomical reduction and stable fixation. Intracapsular haematoma is thought to tamponade the retinacular vessels that supply the femoral head, and open reduction with capsular decompression is considered an important step in reducing the rate of AVN and also provides direct visualization of the fracture to aid reduction. Some authors advocate decompression in all paediatric hip fractures [27–29]. The procedure is safe and associated with few adverse effects, but the beneficial effects have not been unanimously reported [22].

Complications

AVN is the main factor that determines outcome after hip fracture in children, and complete, unstable fracture patterns carry the greatest risk. The majority of outcome studies contain low numbers and the true rate of AVN, particularly in the less common type (Delbet type I), is unknown. Rates of 40–75% [30] have been reported for this subtype, with an overall incidence of 24–30% [24, 31]. An observational study of 239 fractures identified the severity of the initial displacement and age over 12 years as significant independent risk factors for AVN [24] (Figure 5.4). Reduced rates of AVN were observed in patients treated with open reduction and a proximal femoral locking plate, compared to other forms of fixation, including cannulated screws or Kirschner wires, and highlights the need for stable fixation (Figure 5.5).

Radiological signs and clinical symptoms of AVN often present within 1 year of injury, but a small proportion develop late deterioration and patients require long-term follow-up. Other complications include coxa vara secondary to malunion (20–30%), non-union (8%) (as illustrated in Figure 5.6), and premature growth arrest (28%), or a combination [25].

The proximal femoral physis contributes 13% of the longitudinal growth of the entire limb, and shortening due to premature growth arrest is not usually a clinical issue, except in very young

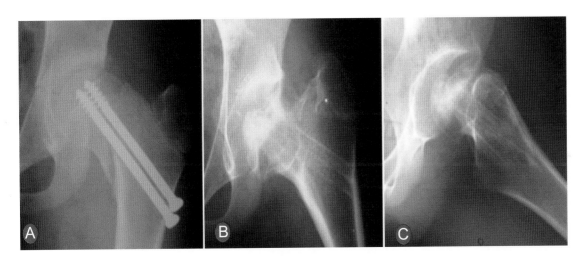

Figure 5.4 Avascular necrosis of the femoral head. (A) Partially threaded screw fixation of a displaced Delbet type II fracture with unsatisfactory reduction. (B, C) Avascular necrosis of the femoral head.

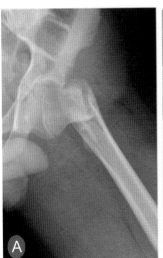 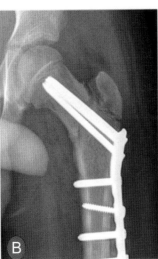 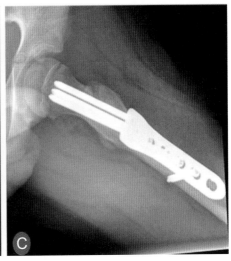

Figure 5.5 Proximal femoral fixed-angle locking plate fixation of a Delbet type III hip fracture in a 13-year-old child. (A) Pre-op radiograph (B, C) Post op radiographs

children. Non-union is generally seen after mid- and basal cervical fractures and is often due to failure to obtain, or maintain, an anatomic reduction, in addition to an unfavourable fracture configuration. CT may be helpful to identify non-union, which should be treated operatively, with either rigid internal fixation or subtrochanteric valgus osteotomy, with bone grafting reserved for persistent non-union [25].

Femoral Shaft

The American anthropologist Margaret Mead observed that femoral fractures in the animal kingdom were invariably fatal and the first sign of civilization in an ancient culture was a healed femoral fracture. This was evidence that someone had tended to the injured person, from the time of injury to eventual recovery.

Femoral fractures in children have a bimodal distribution, with an early peak incidence at 2 years and a late peak at 17 years (Figure 5.7), and with a male-to-female ratio of 2.75:1 [1, 32].

Femoral fractures in children aged under 5 years unite rapidly, and significant malunion or functional impairment is unusual. Traditional techniques, including traction and spica casting, continue to play a role in modern orthopaedic management.

Surgical intervention is recommended in the older child, with flexible and rigid intramedullary nailing recommended according to age and body weight. Conventional and minimal access plating has an expanding role in the management of these fractures, with external fixation reserved for open fractures, or rapid temporary stabilization in a polytrauma situation.

Femoral fracture in a child should prompt a detailed physical examination and careful appraisal of the circumstances of injury, and deliberate injury should be considered in all childhood femoral fractures, irrespective of the age or ambulatory status. Non-walking is the single best predictor for non-accidental injury (NAI) in paediatric femoral fracture [33]. A large epidemiological series ($n = 1358$) performed in the UK reported 3.8% of diaphyseal fractures were secondary to NAI, of which 91% were under 2 years old [32], highlighting an increased incidence of deliberate harm as the cause of femoral fracture in infants.

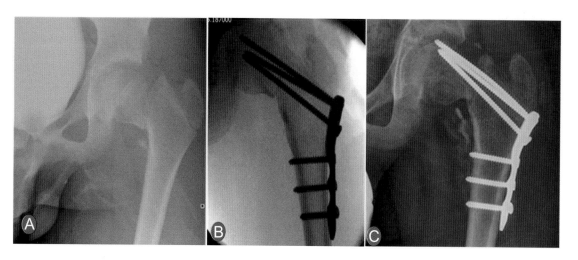

Figure 5.6 Hip fracture in a paediatric patient. (A) Anteroposterior left hip radiograph showing a displaced Delbet type II fracture. (B) Intraoperative image post-fixation. (C) Failure to unite, with subsequent coxa vara deformity and screw cut out.

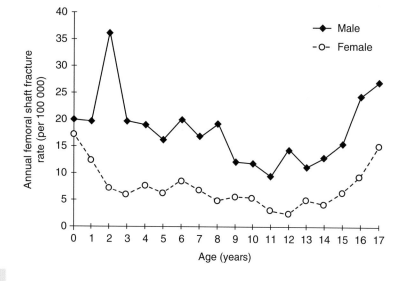

Figure 5.7 Graph showing bimodal distribution of femoral fractures in children [1].

Whilst fracture configuration is relevant, management is dependent primarily on the age/size of the child and other important considerations include the experience of the treating surgeon, disruption to education, and family circumstances.

0–6 Months

Femoral fractures in this age group heal rapidly and a 2-week period of immobilization is sufficient for the majority. Non-invasive treatment is the recommended treatment for this age group, and gallows traction is suitable for patients weighing <10–15 kg. This can be used as definitive management or with elective substitution for a hip spica. A Pavlik harness is also commonly used in this age group, particularly in the neonate with a birth fracture (Figure 5.8). Video 5.1 demonstrates how to apply a hip spica cast.

 Video 5.1 Application of a hip spica for a femoral fracture.

6 Months to 5 Years

Non-invasive treatment is also the recommended treatment for femoral fractures in this age group. Immediate traction provides fracture stability and analgesia that facilitates comfortable transport. The type of traction is age- and size-dependent, with inline skin traction, Thomas' splint, and balanced traction systems in common use. This is generally converted to a hip spica, on the next available operating list or after an interval, which may reduce the extent of malunion [34]. Malunion is rarely an issue due to the remodelling potential of these fractures in the young child. Shortening is inevitable in most fracture patterns, but overgrowth is common and clinically relevant limb length discrepancy is unusual (Figure 5.9).

5–16 Years

Non-operative management is possible in this age group, with prolonged inpatient or domiciliary traction. However, due to the associated social and financial imperatives, operative management is the treatment of choice.

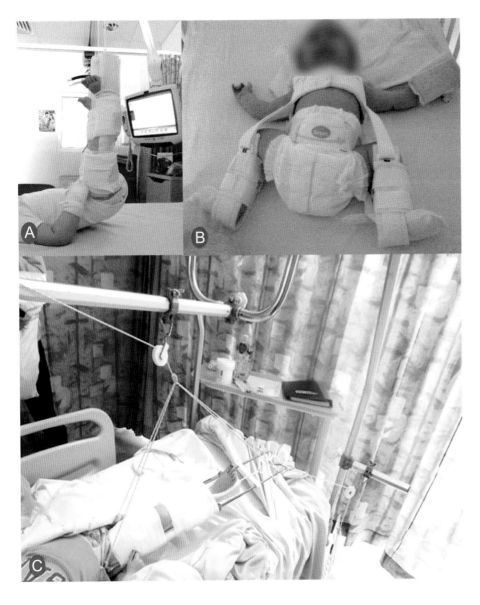

Figure 5.8 Three common methods for treating femoral shaft fractures. (A) Gallows traction (B) Pavlik harness (C) Thomas splint

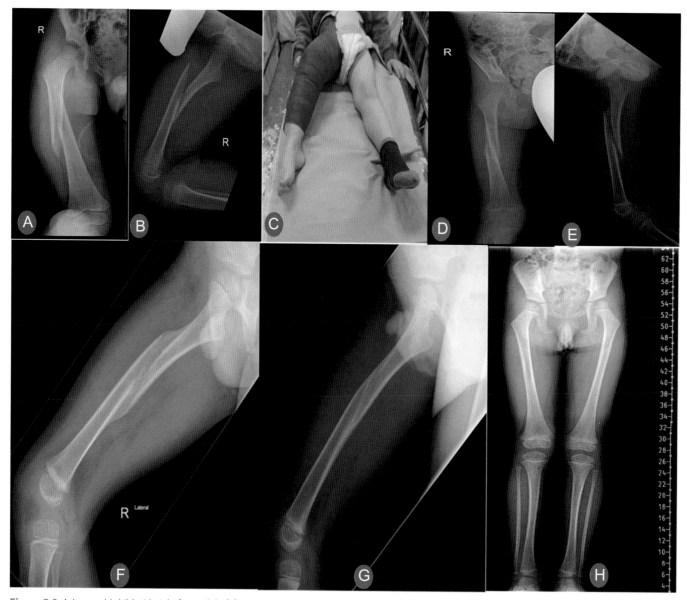

Figure 5.9 A 4-year-old child with right femoral shaft fracture who was treated with a single leg hip spica (A, B, C). (D) and (E) show healthy callus formation; the spica was removed. (F), (G), and (H) show the remodelling capacity in children.

There is no consensus opinion regarding optimal operative management, and techniques include elastic stable intramedullary nails (ESINs) and open or minimally invasive plating.

The ESIN technique is commonly used in Europe and North America for fractures in this age group. This provides excellent results in patients under 50 kg, independent of the fracture pattern, and is associated with a low complication profile [35].

Some authors discriminate on the basis of age and operatively manage femoral fractures after the age of 4 [36]. Others consider that weight is more important in determining treatment and use flexible intramedullary nails in children weighing <49 kg, and rigid nailing or plating in heavier children, with the choice of implant dependent on the fracture pattern [34, 37].

Moroz *et al.* reported that, irrespective of the fracture configuration, locked rigid nail systems were associated with a reduced rate of malunion, compared to ESINs, in children weighing over 49 kg [37].

Memeo *et al.* categorized patients by weight and fracture type, and did not identify a meaningful difference in malunion and limb length discrepancy between the rigid and flexible nail groups for length-stable fractures in heavier children (average weight 60 kg) [38].

The main consideration with the use of rigid intramedullary nails in this age group is potential injury to the femoral head blood supply with nails that enter through the piriformis fossa [39]. Trochanteric (lateral) entry nails are designed to avoid the femoral head blood supply and therefore reduce or remove the risk of AVN.

Nail entry through the piriformis fossa is associated with an AVN rate of 1–5% [39–41]. Lateral entry nails were associated with 0% AVN in two series of 246 and 78 patients, and a systematic review of 19 reports confirmed this observation [39, 42].

Proximal femoral growth disturbance is also a potential issue as the nail crosses the trochanteric apophysis. In a retrospective study (*n* = 246) with an average follow-up of 16 months, asymptomatic coxa valga was seen in two patients (2.2%) [42]. Raney *et al.* identified five cases of radiographic coxa valga following intramedullary nail fixation, none with associated functional disability [43]; it is therefore unlikely that this complication is clinically important.

After Skeletal Maturity

Operative management is common in this age group due to factors including increased time to union, difficulty in obtaining and maintaining an adequate reduction with non-operative techniques, and earlier mobilization with operative management.

Displaced femoral shaft fractures in skeletally mature patients with closed proximal femoral growth plates are usually treated with rigid locked intramedullary nails, identical to the adult population.

Elastic Stable Intramedullary Nails

Flexible nailing may be performed using steel or titanium implants. Titanium is more flexible, and the elasticity is fundamentally important to maintenance of reduction and enhancement of fracture healing. Depending on the fracture location, the nails can be inserted proximally (antegrade) or distally (retrograde). Fractures of the proximal and middle third favour a retrograde technique, and distal third fractures usually require antegrade nailing as the distal nail entry points are too close to the fracture site and the nail configuration is not sufficiently stable [26].

Key technical considerations include the following:

- Each nail should be between 0.3 and 0.4 times the diameter of the femoral canal at the narrowest point
- Both nails should have an equal diameter, so that opposing bending forces are matched
- The nails should be contoured to form a broad, symmetrical arch with the apex at the fracture site
- The maximum bend in the nails should be three times the diameter of the bone.

A simple transverse mid-diaphyseal fracture is the ideal indication. However, flexible nailing can be used for long oblique and spiral fractures (Figure 5.10), and the addition of end caps improves axial stability in suitable fractures. Anatomical reduction is not necessary, and Wallace *et al.* demonstrated remodelling with up to 25° angulation in any plane was possible [44]. Video 5.2 demonstrates how to perform elastic femoral nailing.

Femoral malrotation is common following ESIN fixation, with a reported incidence of up to 41.6% [45]. Careful

---

 Video 5.2 Flexible nailing for femoral shaft fracture.

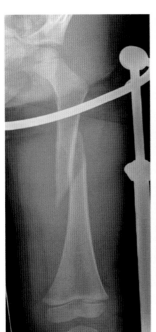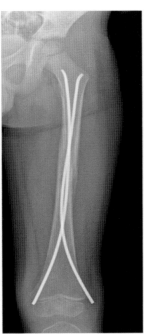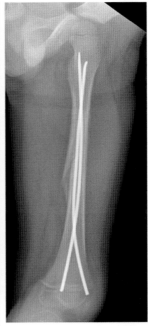

Figure 5.10 Diaphyseal spiral fracture of the femur in a 5-year-old child weighing 25 kg, treated with titanium elastic nails.

intraoperative assessment is required to avoid rotational asymmetry, which has poor remodelling potential [46].

There is controversy about removing asymptomatic flexible intramedullary nails, and potential advantages include elimination of stress risers at the tip and the complexity of treating fractures around a bent nail. Implants, however, should be left in place for a year, as premature nail removal is associated with refracture.

Rigid Intramedullary Nails

The primary indication for rigid intramedullary nailing is in the management of adolescents after skeletal maturity. Contemporary locked rigid nails stabilize the femur proximally and distally, and control rotation and alignment. This permits early rehabilitation in multifragmentary and length-unstable fracture patterns. Indications for rigid nailing in younger patients are limited by the potential for iatrogenic damage to the femoral head blood supply in the presence of an open physis, and lateral greater trochanter entry effectively eliminates this risk (Figure 5.11). Video 5.3 demonstrates how to perform rigid intramedullary femoral nailing.

 Video 5.3 Adolescent femoral fracture nailing.

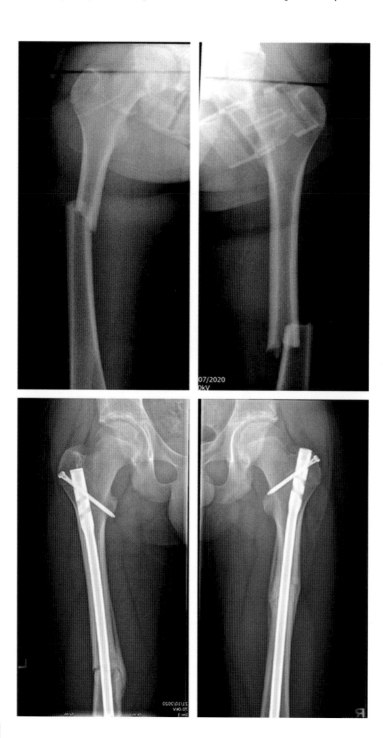

Figure 5.11 Lateral-entry rigid intramedullary nails to treat bilateral femoral shaft fractures in a 15-year-old child.

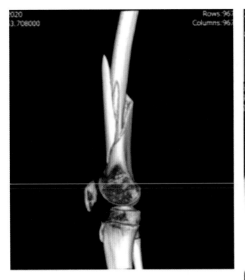

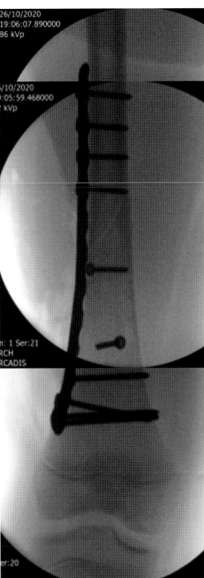

Figure 5.12 Multifragmentary spiral distal diaphyseal fracture, treated with minimally invasive submuscular plating and percutaneous lag screws.

Plating

Open or submuscular plating is an option for high-energy, multi-fragmentary injuries (Figure 5.12) and in skeletally immature patients with fractures that are unsuitable for flexible nailing, due to the anatomical location, fracture pattern, or patient's weight (Figure 5.13). The development of minimally invasive plating systems has popularized this technique in the management of paediatric femoral fractures. A retrospective review of 344 children treated with submuscular plating, rigid nailing, or flexible nailing reported an earlier return to full weight-bearing and union in the plating group [47]. Spiral fractures were more frequent in the plating group and this may have contributed to the faster time to union in this study. There is a paucity of high-level studies on submuscular plating in the paediatric population. However, favourable outcomes have been reported in multiple retrospective series [48, 49].

External Fixation

External fixation a useful technique in patients with open fractures, high-energy and multifragmentary injuries, polytrauma, or injuries requiring transfer to another centre.

Ease of application is an advantage and provides effective reduction in the short term (Figures 5.14 and 5.15), with minimal additional blood loss and the ability to avoid the zone of injury.

Bar-On *et al.* conducted a randomized trial comparing flexible nails with external fixators for definitive fixation ($n = 19$) and reported significantly improved clinical and radiographic outcomes in the flexible nail group. The authors recommended that external fixators should be reserved for open and multifragmentary injuries [50].

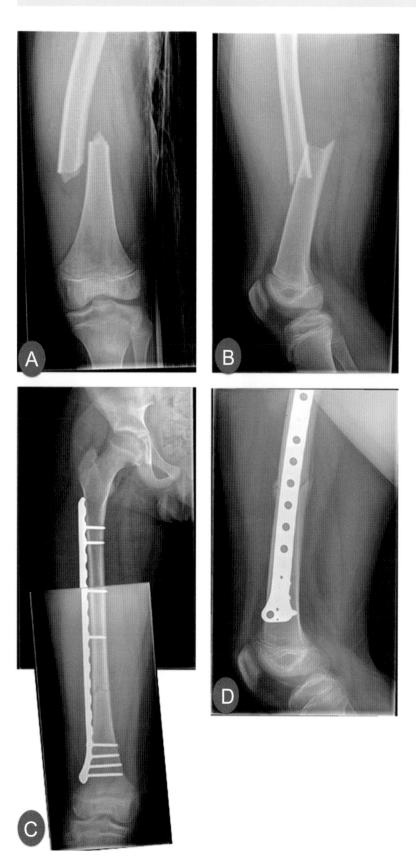

Figure 5.13 A simple transverse diaphyseal femoral fracture in a 13-year-old patient weighing 55 kg (A, B), treated with submuscular plating (C, D). Notice the screws' intensity; too many screws can make the construct too rigid which can cause non-union.

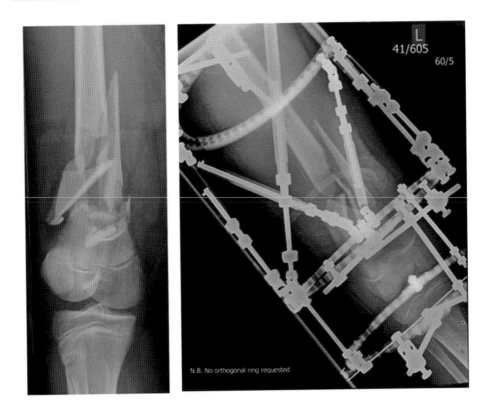

Figure 5.14 High-energy, multifragmentary open fracture of the distal femoral metaphysis, treated initially with a joint spanning Taylor spatial circular frame, restoring alignment, length, and rotation.

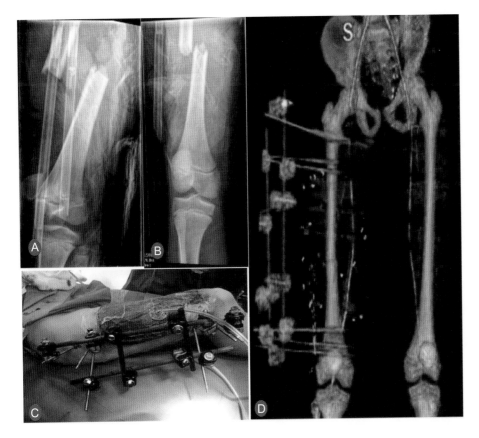

Figure 5.15 Crush injury to the thigh with an open femoral fracture and significant soft tissue injury (A, B), treated with temporizing external fixation and soft tissue debridement (C). Alignment, length, and rotation are adequately restored with the external fixation device (D).

Editors Note: A Case Study Example

An 8-year-old boy presented with hip pain after a fall. His X-ray did not show a convincing fracture, and he was reassured and discharged from the emergency room. He continued limping for 2 weeks and came back with more pain. A repeat X-ray showed sclerosis at the middle of the femoral neck. A CT scan showed a healing neck of femur fracture (Figure 5.16). He was treated with a hip spica for 6 weeks, followed by unrestricted mobilization on spica removal. When the spica was removed, he was allowed to weight-bear as tolerated.

A week later, he started limping and developed more pain. The plain radiograph and CT scan (Figure 5.17) showed a displaced, non-united femoral neck fracture. He was then subsequently referred to the regional children's hospital.

How would you treat this child now? Try to make a few notes on how to treat this fracture before you proceed.

In any non-union, infection must be excluded, which we did. Then we examined the potential biological and mechanical factors that contributed to the non-union. In this fracture, we believe that they were both contributory and needed addressing.

Non-union may be related to one, or a combination, of the following factors:

1. Infection
2. Mechanical malalignment
3. Inappropriate stabilization/fixation
4. Biological bone health problem, for example, vitamin D deficiency
5. Devascularized soft tissue envelope.

How Would You Treat This Child Now?

This patient underwent surgery, with the aim to explore the non-union site, debride the fracture ends, biopsy for infection, reduce the non-union, and decompress the capsule. Bone autograft can be considered to promote healing. Caution should be taken if infection is likely. This aspect improves the biological environment for fracture healing.

A valgus osteotomy was also performed, converting shear forces associated with a varus proximal femur into compression forces. A fixed-angle device was used to provide stable fixation (Figure 5.18).

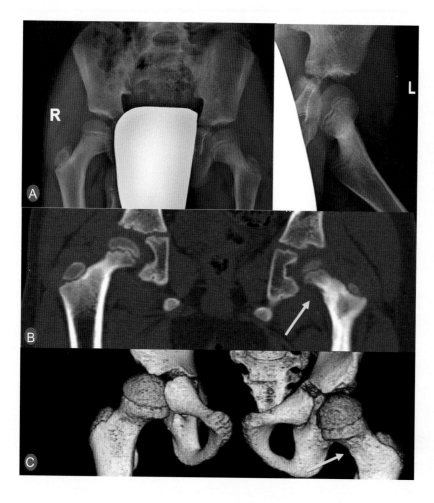

Figure 5.16 An 8-year-old boy with a subtle neck of femur fracture. He presented with left hip pain after a fall. Initial X-ray was unremarkable. He came back after 2 weeks. (A) Plain X-ray showing some neck sclerosis. CT confirmed a healing neck of femur fracture. (B, C)

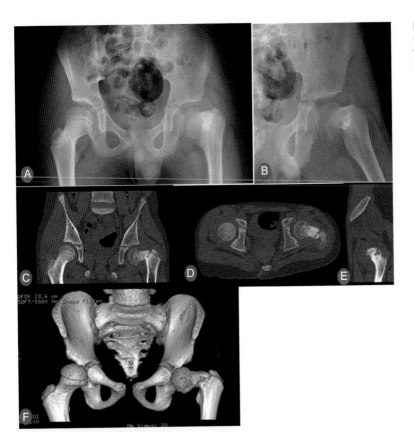

Figure 5.17 Radiological imaging showing loss of reduction. The CT scan shows cystic changes and sclerosis consistent with non-union. Although no surgery was performed, blood tests to rule out infective non-union were requested and came back normal.

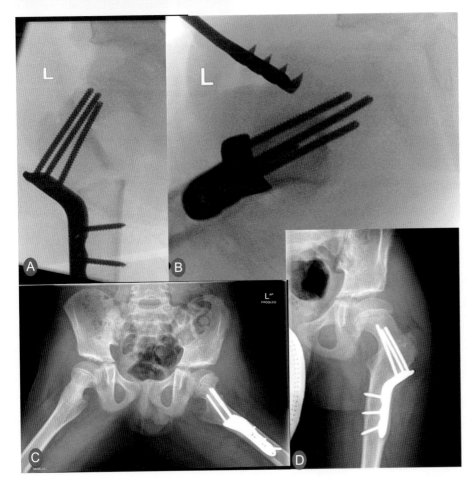

Figure 5.18 Operative fixation for a nonunited neck of femur fracture. The child had an open reduction of the fracture, a bone graft, and a valgus osteotomy (A, B). The fracture healed successfully (C, D).

Would You Remove the Metalware?

Metalware in the proximal femur may complicate subsequent future surgery, for example, total hip replacement. Removal at a later date may be challenging following bone overgrowth.

In younger patients with open physeal plates, metalwork may limit remodelling potential, for example, the valgus deformity created in this case. Therefore, metalware in the hip area is usually removed.

One exception is partially threaded cannulated screws that are used to stabilize slipped capital femoral epiphysis. These can be removed easily when the neck is cut during hip replacement.

References

1. Hinton RY, *et al*. Fractures of the femoral shaft in children. Incidence, mechanisms, and sociodemographic risk factors. *J Bone Joint Surg Am*. 1999;81(4):500–9.

2. Amorosa L. High-energy pediatric pelvic and acetabular fractures. *Orthop Clin North Am*, 2014;45(4):483–500.

3. Holden CP, Holman J, Herman MJ. Pediatric pelvic fractures. *J Am Acad Orthop Surg*. 2007;15(3):172–7.

4. Shaath MK, *et al*. Analysis of pelvic fracture pattern and overall orthopaedic injury burden in children sustaining pelvic fractures based on skeletal maturity. *J Child Orthop*. 2017;11(3):195–200.

5. Ismail N, *et al*. Death from pelvic fracture: children are different. *J Pediatr Surg*. 1996;31(1):82–5.

6. Silber JS, Flynn JM. Changing patterns of pediatric pelvic fractures with skeletal maturation: implications for classification and management. *J Pediatr Orthop*. 2002;22(1):22–6.

7. Silber JS, *et al*. Analysis of the cause, classification, and associated injuries of 166 consecutive pediatric pelvic fractures. *J Pediatr Orthop*. 2001;21(4):446–50.

8. Chia JPY, *et al*. Pelvic fractures and associated injuries in children. *J Trauma*. 2004;56(1):83–8.

9. Torode I, Zieg D. Pelvic fractures in children. *J Pediatr Orthop*. 1985;5(1):76–84.

10. Shore BJ, *et al*. Pediatric pelvic fracture. *J Pediatr Orthop*. 2012;32(2):162–8.

11. Bimmel R, *et al*. Paediatric hip fractures: a systematic review of incidence, treatment options and complications. *Acta Orthop Belg*. 2010;76(1):7–13.

12. Davison BL, Weinstein SL. Hip fractures in children: a long-term follow-up study. *J Pediatr Orthop*. 1992;12(3):355–8.

13. Joseph T. The normal vascular anatomy of the human femoral head during growth. *J Bone Joint Surg Br*. 1957;39-B(2):358–94.

14. Ogden JA. Changing patterns of proximal femoral vascularity. *J Bone Joint Surg Am*. 1974;56(5):941–50.

15. Dial BL, Lark RK. Pediatric proximal femur fractures. *J Orthop*. 2018;15(2):529–35.

16. Bartonicek J. Proximal femur fractures: the pioneer era of 1818 to 1925. *Clin Orthop Relat Res*. 2004;419:306–10.

17. Collona PC. Fracture of the neck of femur in children. *Am J Surg*. 1929;6:793–7.

18. Moon E, Mehlman C. Risk factors for avascular necrosis after femoral neck fractures in children: 25 Cincinnati cases and meta-analysis of 360 cases. *J Orthop Trauma*. 2006;20:323–9.

19. Slongo T, Audige L. AO Pediatric Classification Group. *AO Pediatric Comprehensive Classification of Long-Bone Fractures (PCCF)*. Switzerland: AO Foundation; 2007.

20. Shrader MW, *et al*. Femoral neck fractures in pediatric patients: 30 years experience at a level 1 trauma center. *Clin Orthop Relat Res*. 2007;454: 169–73.

21. Dendane MA, *et al*. Displaced femoral neck fractures in children: are complications predictable? *Orthop Traumatol Surg Res*. 2010;96(2):161–5.

22. Yeranosian M, *et al*. Factors affecting the outcome of fractures of the femoral neck in children and adolescents: a systematic review. *Bone Joint J*. 2013;95-b(1):135–42.

23. Varshney MK, *et al*. Functional and radiological outcome after delayed fixation of femoral neck fractures in pediatric patients. *J Orthop Traumatol*. 2009;10(4):211–16.

24. Wang WT, *et al*. Risk factors for the development of avascular necrosis after femoral neck fractures in children. *Bone Joint J*. 2019;101-B(9):1160–7.

25. Beaty JH. Fractures of the hip in children. *Orthop Clin North Am*. 2006;37(2):223–32, vii.

26. AO Surgery Reference. Proximal femur. Available from: https://surgeryreference.aofoundation.org/orthopedic-trauma/pediatric-trauma/proximal-femur.

27. Panigrahi R, *et al*. Treatment analysis of paediatric femoral neck fractures: a prospective multicenter theraupetic study in Indian scenario. *Int Orthop*. 2015;39(6):1121–7.

28. Bukva B, *et al*. Femoral neck fractures in children and the role of early hip decompression in final outcome. *Injury*. 2015;46(Suppl 6):S44–7.

29. Ng GPK, Cole WG. Effect of early hip decompression on the frequency of avascular necrosis in children with fractures of the neck of the femur. *Injury*. 1996;27(6):419–21.

30. Akahane T, Fujioka F, Shiozawa R. A transepiphyseal fracture of the proximal femur combined with a fracture of the mid-shaft of ipsilateral femur in a child: a case report and literature review. *Arch Orthop Trauma Surg*. 2006;126(5):330–4.

31. Omeroglu H, Inan U, Kose N. Fracture type primarily influences the final outcome in pediatric hip fractures. *Orthop Proc*. 2010;92-B(Supp V):598.

32. Talbot C, *et al*. Fractures of the femoral shaft in children. *Bone Joint J*. 2018;100-B(1): 109–18.

33. Brown D, Fisher E. Femur fractures in infants and young children. *Am J Public Health*. 2004;94(4):558–60.

34. Khoriati A-A, *et al*. The management of paediatric diaphyseal femoral fractures: a modern approach. *Strategies Trauma Limb Reconstr*. 2016;11(2):87–97.

35. Memeo A, *et al*. Retrospective, multicenter evaluation of complications

in the treatment of diaphyseal femur fractures in pediatric patients. *Injury.* 2019;50(Suppl 4):S60–3.

36. Brousil J, Hunter JB. Femoral fractures in children. *Curr Opin Pediatr.* 2013;25(1):52–7.

37. Moroz LA. Titanium elastic nailing of fractures of the femur in children: predictors of complication and poor outcome. *J Bone Joint Surg Br.* 2006;88-B(10):1361–6.

38. Garner MR, *et al.* Fixation of length-stable femoral shaft fractures in heavier children: flexible nails vs rigid locked nails. *J Pediatr Orthop.* 2011;31(1):11–16.

39. MacNeil JAM, Francis A, El-Hawary R. A systematic review of rigid, locked, intramedullary nail insertion sites and avascular necrosis of the femoral head in the skeletally immature. *J Pediatr Orthop.* 2011;31(4):377–80.

40. Letts M, *et al.* Complications of rigid intramedullary rodding of femoral shaft fractures in children. *J Trauma.* 2002;52(3):504–16.

41. Beaty JH, *et al.* Interlocking intramedullary nailing of femoral-shaft fractures in adolescents: preliminary results and complications. *J Pediatr Orthop.* 1994;4(2):178–83.

42. Crosby SN, Jr, *et al.* Twenty-year experience with rigid intramedullary nailing of femoral shaft fractures in skeletally immature patients. *J Bone Joint Surg Am.* 2014;96(13):1080–9.

43. Raney EM, Ogden JA, Grogan DP. Premature greater trochanteric epiphysiodesis secondary to intramedullary femoral rodding. *J Pediatr Orthop.* 1993;13(4):516–20.

44. ME W, EB H. Remodelling of angular deformity after femoral shaft fractures in children. *J Bone Joint Surg Br.* 1992;74-B(5):765–9.

45. Zeckey C, *et al.* Femoral malrotation after surgical treatment of femoral shaft fractures in children: a retrospective CT-based analysis. *Eur J Orthop Surg Traumatol.* 2017;27(8):1157–62.

46. Davids JR. Rotational deformity and remodeling after fracture of the femur in children. *Clin Orthop Relat Res.* 1994;302:27–35.

47. Sutphen SA, *et al.* Pediatric diaphyseal femur fractures: submuscular plating compared with intramedullary nailing. *Orthopedics.* 2016;39(6):353–8.

48. Samora WP, *et al.* Submuscular bridge plating for length-unstable, pediatric femur fractures. *J Pediatr Orthop.* 2013;33(8):797–802.

49. Sink EL, *et al.* Results and technique of unstable pediatric femoral fractures treated with submuscular bridge plating. *J Pediatr Orthop.* 2006;26(2):177–81.

50. Bar-On E, Sagiv S, Porat S. External fixation or flexible intramedullary nailing for femoral shaft fractures in children. *J Bone Joint Surg Br.* 1997;79-B(6):975–8.

Orthopaedic Knee Disorders

Sattar Alshryda and Fazal Ali

Congenital Conditions

Congenital Dislocation of the Knee

Congenital dislocation of the knee (CDK) is a relatively rare congenital condition where one or both knees are either hyperextended, subluxed, or dislocated. The reasons are not very well understood. Positional and neuromuscular conditions have been implicated. The quadriceps muscles and iliotibial (IT) band are short and fibrotic. The anterior cruciate ligament (ACL) is sometimes absent or stretched and attenuated. The condition is graded into three grades (Figure 6.1):

- Grade I (congenital hyperextension): the knee can be flexed and reduced, beyond neutral (0°) with gentle stretching of the quadriceps
- Grade II (congenital subluxation): the knee cannot be flexed beyond neutral, but the femoral and tibial epiphyses remain in contact and do not sublux with attempted flexion
- Grade III (true congenital dislocation): knee flexion is not possible, and the tibia, which is anteriorly translated in the resting position, displaces laterally on the femur when more vigorous flexion is attempted.

Bilateral CDK is commonly associated with other anomalies such as Larsen, Beals, Ehlers–Danlos syndromes, arthrogryposis and spinal dysraphism (Figure 6.2).

Anomalies of the upper extremities, face and gastrointestinal and genitourinary systems are not uncommon, but important to identify and treat timely.

Ipsilateral hip dislocation and club foot are common associations (70% and 50%, respectively). CDK should be treated first, as it is important to be able to bend the knee to 90° to treat hip dislocation and club foot effectively.

Regardless of the cause or associated conditions, treatment should be started as early as possible, with gentle manipulation and serial casting until 90° of flexion is obtained (Figure 6.3). Botox injection, femoral nerve block, and percutaneous rectus release have been practised to increase the success rates of serial casting. The evidence to support these additions is not strong.

A removable splint is then used during the night and at nap times for several months. The knee is splinted in flexion and extension on alternate nights. Aggressive manipulation can be dangerous and causes fractures, epiphyseal injuries, or rotatory subluxation of the knee (Figure 6.4).

Operative treatment is indicated if serial casting fails. This can be done between 6 months to 1 year of age. Several techniques have been advised, including the following.

Classically, surgical treatment for CDK was a distal V–Y quadricepsplasty (Thompson's procedure). Post-operatively, the knee can develop extension lag [1].

Proximal sequential quadricepsplasty in association with release of intra-articular adhesions and mobilization of the suprapatellar pouch (Judet's technique) has shown better clinical results and become more popular [2].

In recent years, femoral shortening osteotomy has been added to minimize extensive quadriceps release, whereas ACL reconstruction using the IT band has been performed to address coexisting ligament deficiency [3, 4].

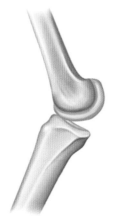 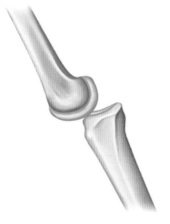 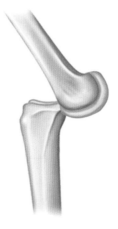

Grade I **Grade II** **Grade III**

Figure 6.1 The three grades of congenital dislocation of the knee. Grade I: congenital hyperextension; grade II: congenital subluxation; and grade III: true congenital dislocation.

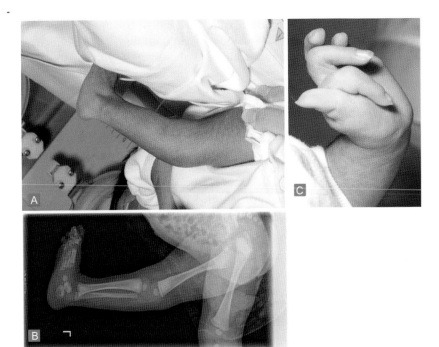

Figure 6.2 (A, B) Clinical photograph and X-ray showing a left congenital knee subluxation. Note the anterior translation of the tibial epiphysis relative to the femoral epiphysis. (C) A patient's hand with finger contractures and lack of normal skin creases. The patient was subsequently diagnosed with arthrogryposis.

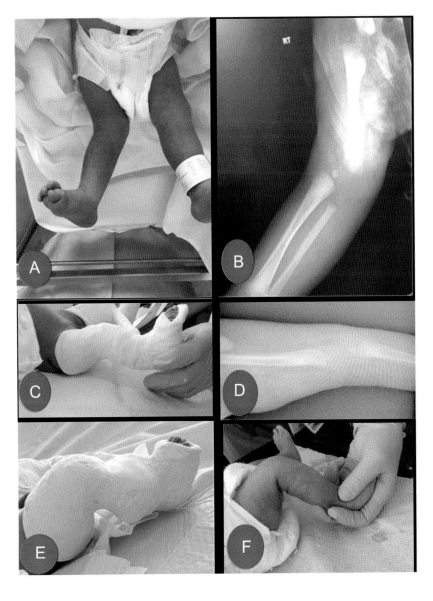

Figure 6.3 Serial casting of a congenital knee subluxation. (A, B) Before serial casting. (C, D) After the second set of serial casting. (E, F) At the end of six sets. No Botox or tenotomy was required. Unlike club foot serial casting, X-ray is usually required to ensure that there is no fracture or metaphyseal deformity. This is easier to do by fluoroscopy, rather than by plain X-ray, to ensure a perfect image.

Congenital Dislocation of the Patella

Congenital dislocation of the patella is a rare condition. The patella is usually hypoplastic and dislocates laterally with knee flexion, an important differentiation from other types of patellar dislocations which occur in extension and reduce in flexion (Figure 6.5). In congenital patellar dislocation, the quadriceps

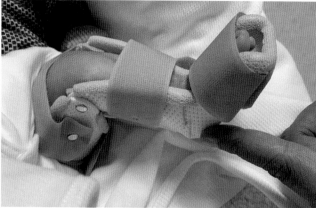

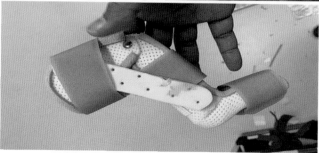

Figure 6.4 Bracing of the knee after serial casting. In bilateral cases, two options are in common use – either using two solid knee–ankle–foot orthoses (KAFOs), one in flexion and one in extension and switching between the legs on alternate nights, or using a hinged KAFO as in the images shown.

muscles are short and contracted, and with increasing knee flexion, the patella (and the attached short muscle) dislocates over the lateral femoral condyle to allow for more flexion.

Mild forms of dislocation may not present until school age, with weak knee extension, inability to extend the knee fully, slight valgus deformity of the knee and external tibial torsion. In some cases, parents often notice a knee click. X-ray is often not helpful because the patella is not ossified until about 3 years of age. MRI requires sedation or general anaesthesia in small children. Ultrasound can be diagnostic in expert hands.

The severe form needs to be differentiated from other causes of congenital flexion contractures, such as:

1. Limb dysplasia such as congenital femoral deficiency or tibial hemimelia
2. Syndromes with soft tissue contracture such as arthrogryposis, pterygium syndromes and Beals syndrome (congenital contractural arachnodactyly)
3. Neurological syndromes such as sacral agenesis and myelodysplasia
4. Skeletal dysplasia with bony flexion deformity such as diastrophic dysplasia.

Treatment is surgical and involves a stepwise approach until the patella stops dislocating. This involves extensive soft tissue releases, including:

1. Extensive lateral patellar release and advancing the vastus medialis obliquus (VMO) distally and medially
2. Lengthening of the quadriceps tendon (V–Y) ± distal patellar tendon realignment using the Goldthwait technique (or tibial tuberosity transfer in older children)
3. Immobilization of the knee at 20° for 6–8 weeks, followed by intensive physiotherapy.

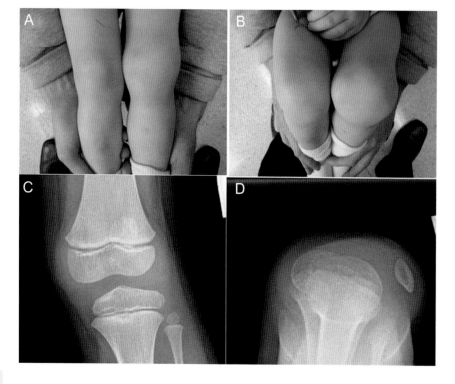

Figure 6.5 Congenital dislocation of the patella. (A, B) The left patella is dislocated in flexion and partially reduced in extension. This was also shown on X-ray(C,D). The patella does not normally ossify until about 3 years of age, and this may be delayed even further in the presence of congenital dislocation.

Discoid Meniscus

This is an abnormally thick meniscus that covers a large proportion of the tibial surface and is thought to be of congenital origin. It is almost always located on the lateral side. Incidence varies from 1.5% to 15%, and the condition occurs mostly in girls.

It presents in various ways, from an incidental finding on MRI or arthroscopy to a frank tear. Children frequently describe 'popping', 'locking', or 'snapping'. Diagnosis can be confirmed by MRI. The most accurate criterion for the diagnosis of discoid meniscus on MRI is a ratio of the minimal meniscal width to the maximal tibial width on the coronal slice of >20% (Figure 6.6). Another less precise criterion is continuity between the anterior and posterior meniscal horns on three consecutive sagittal images. If a plain X-ray is taken, it may characteristically show a widened lateral joint space and squaring of the lateral femoral condyle.

Watanabe classified the discoid meniscus into three types: complete, incomplete, and Wrisberg. Both the complete and incomplete types have a stable posterior attachment via the meniscotibial ligaments. The difference is that the complete type covers the whole of the tibial surface, whereas the incomplete type does not. The Wrisberg type is the most mobile, as it is bounded posteriorly only by the meniscofemoral ligament of Wrisberg (Figure 6.7).

If asymptomatic, the discoid meniscus is left alone. Tears are excised to a stable margin (saucerization) if the meniscus

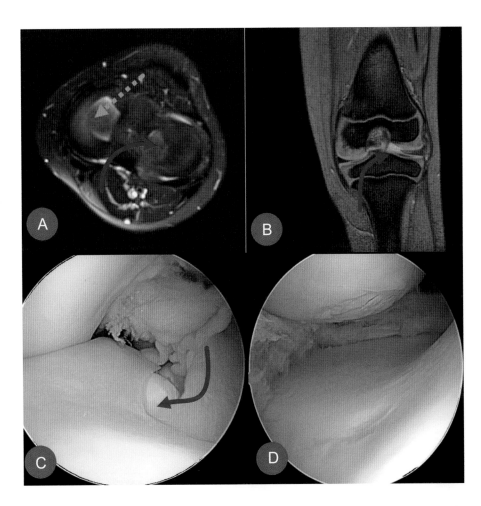

Figure 6.6 Discoid meniscus. (A, B) MRI scans of the knee showing an almost complete discoid meniscus, with the edge reaching the midline (curved red arrow), in comparison with the normal side (dashed green arrow). (C0 Pre-operative arthroscopic picture (D) Post-operative saucerization.

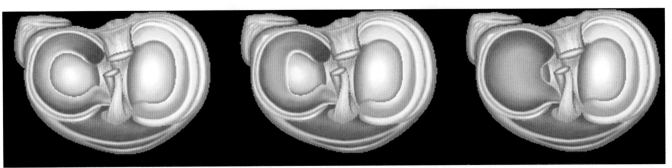

Figure 6.7 Types of meniscus based on their size.

has adequate peripheral attachment. A hypermobile meniscus (Wrisberg type) may be repaired onto the capsule, or in some cases, a complete meniscectomy may be necessary.

Blount's Disease

Blount's disease (BD) is a type of idiopathic tibia varus. It is uncommon and characterized by disordered ossification of the medial aspect of the proximal tibial physis, epiphysis, and metaphysis, causing unilateral or bilateral genu varum (Figure 6.8). Though the cause is unknown, it is thought to be a combination of excessive compressive forces on the proximal medial metaphysis of the tibia and altered endochondral bone formation. There are two recognized types of BD: infantile (<4 years) and adolescent (>10 years) (Table 6.3). A third type, juvenile tibia vara, shares features of both types and has been described for BD in children aged 4–10 years.

Table 6.1 Differences between Blount's disease and physiological genu varum

Measurements	Favouring Blount's disease	Favouring physiological genu varum	Notes
Mechanical axis deviation (MAD)[a]	NA	NA	See also mechanical axis zones
Tibiofemoral angle (TFA)[b]	28 ± 11°	22 ± 8°	Correlate with the Salenius curve
Epiphyseal–metaphyseal angle (EMA)[c]	>20°	<20°	
Metaphyseal–diaphyseal angle (MDA)[d] (also called TMDA where T stands for tibial)	17 ± 4°	8 ± 4°	A few modifications on how to measure these exist to accommodate for natural bowing of bones
Femoral–metaphyseal–diaphyseal angle (FMDA)	7.4 ± 5°	14 ± 5°	
Femoral:tibial ratio of McCarthy (FTR)[e]	0.48 ± 0.4	2.6 ± 3	TMDA greater than FMDA is associated with persistent varus

[a] The MAD is the distance between the mechanical axis and the centre of the knee. The ideal adult MAD is zero (±3 mm). In children, this varies based on age. Therefore, MAD is useful in monitoring progress, rather than supporting the diagnosis. Some authors prefer to use the mechanical axis zones, instead of the actual value of MAD (Figures 6.10 and 6.11), to remove the magnification effect.
[b] The TFA is the angle between the femur and the tibial diaphysis. The diaphyseal line is usually drawn in the middle of the diaphysis.
[c] The EMA is the angle formed by the epiphyseal line (a line through the proximal tibial physis parallel to the base of the epiphyseal ossification centre) and a line connecting the midpoint of the epiphyseal line to the most distal point on the medial beak of the proximal tibia.
[d] The MDA is the angle formed by a line connecting the most distal point on the medial and lateral beaks of the metaphysis (the distal femur in the FMDA and the proximal tibia in the TMDA) and a line perpendicular to the anatomical axis (or the lateral cortex) of the bone.
[e] The FTR is defined as the FMDA divided by the TMDA.

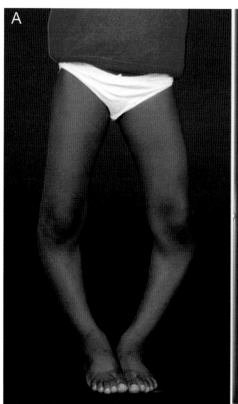
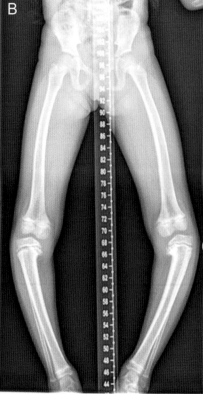

Figure 6.8 A clinical photograph (A) and a plain X-ray (B) of a child with bilateral infantile Blount's disease. There is an obvious bilateral tibia varus deformity. Both feet point inwards, although the patellae point outwards, indicating bilateral internal tibial torsion which is commonly associated with Blount's disease.

Infantile Blount's Disease

This is bilateral in 80% of cases and more prevalent in girls, blacks and children with marked obesity (Figure 6.8). These children generally start walking early (before 10 months of age). Associated clinical findings include a lateral thrust of the knee when walking, internal tibial torsion, and limb length discrepancy (LLD). It is important to differentiate infantile BD from physiological genu varum (see Chapter 3). Physiological genu varum is rare in children over 3 years old. The cover-up test is a useful screening test to differentiate the two in children aged between 1 and 3 years (Figure 6.9). A negative test (slight valgus at the upper tibia) indicates physiological bowing. A positive test (bowing in the upper tibia) or neutral test (a straight thigh–upper leg axis) is an indication for radiographic evaluation [5].

Plain long leg alignment views are usually characteristic in children with BD. These usually show:

1. Genu varum (unilateral or bilateral)
2. Sharp varus angulation in the proximal tibial metaphysis, with prominent beaking
3. Widened and irregular physeal line medially
4. Medially sloped and irregularly ossified epiphysis

None of the above features are exclusively diagnostic of infantile BD, and several radiological measurements have been proposed to predict the risk of progression. Table 6.1 and Figure 6.10 show common measurements that are in current use. None of these measurements guarantee a correct prediction, but they do aid clinical judgement. In general, when the epiphyseal–metaphyseal angle (EMA) is <20°, tibial–metaphyseal–diaphyseal angle (TMDA) <10°, tibiofemoral angle (TFA) <10° and femoral:tibial ratio (FTR) >1.4, BD is very unlikely, whereas when the EMA is >20°, TMDA ≥16° and FTR <0.7, BD is likely. The grey zone is when values lies between these range.

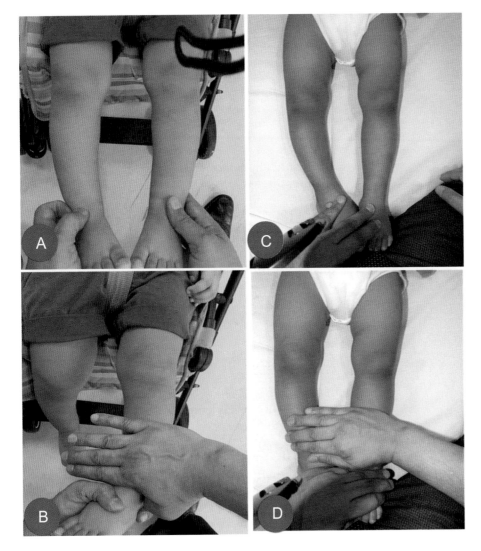

Figure 6.9 (A, B) A negative cover-up test; slight valgus of the upper tibia in relationship to the femur. (C, D) A positive test with the knee in varus (right knee) or neutral (left knee). A positive test is an indication for an X-ray.

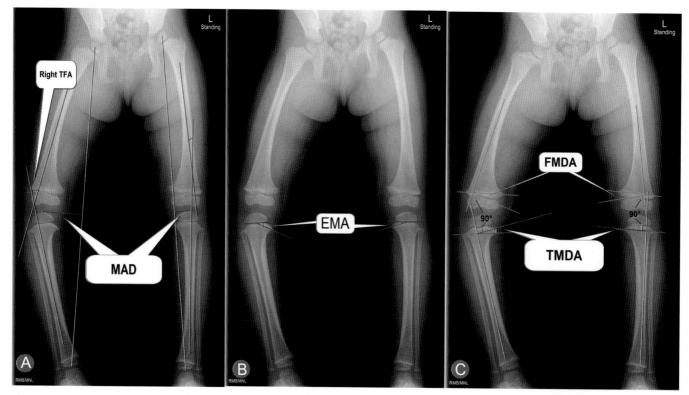

Figure 6.10 Radiological measurements to diagnose and monitor genu varum. The MAD is the distance between the mechanical axis and the centre of the knee(A). The TFA is the angle between the femur and the tibial diaphysis. The diaphyseal line is usually drawn in the middle of the diaphysis proper. The EMA is the angle formed by the epiphyseal line (a line through the proximal tibial physis parallel to the base of the epiphyseal ossification centre) and a line connecting the midpoint of the epiphyseal line to the most distal point on the medial beak of the proximal tibia(B). The MDA is the angle formed by a line connecting the most distal point on the medial and lateral beaks of the metaphysis (the distal femur in the FMDA, and the proximal tibia in the TMDA) and a line perpendicular to the anatomical axis (or the lateral cortex) of the bone. The femoral:tibial ratio (FTR) is defined as the FMDA divided by the TMDA(C).

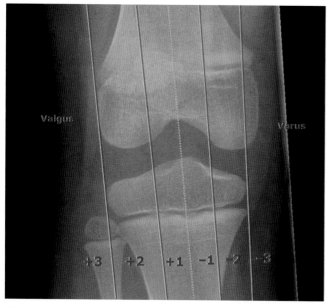

Figure 6.11 Mechanical axis zones. In children aged above 6 years, the knee is divided into quadrants. The ideal mechanical axis would bisect the knee (0), with the medial zone (−1) and lateral zone (−1) being within the physiological range. Symptomatic zone 2 and asymptomatic zone 3 require correction.

Langenskiold described six stages of the disease, based on radiological findings (Figure 6.12; Table 6.2) [6]. Although several shortfalls of the classification have been identified,

Key Points: Physiological Genu Varum or Infantile Blount's Disease

Several radiological measurements have been proposed to differentiate between these two conditions. None guarantees a correct diagnosis. See Table 6.1.

In general, when the EMA is <20°, TMDA <10°, TFA <10°, and FTR >1.4, BD is very unlikely, whereas when the EMA is >20°, TMDA ≥16°, and FTR <0.7, BD is likely. The grey zone is when values fall between these ranges.

including inter- and intra-observer reproducibility and prognostic values, it remains a useful descriptive tool and a rough guidance for treatment.

Adolescent Blount's Disease

This is unilateral in 80% of cases. Patients are usually overweight and complain of pain at the medial aspect of the knee. A leg length discrepancy is generally observed, and femoral alignment is often abnormal (Figure 6.13). Table 6.3 summarizes the main differences between infantile and adolescent BD.

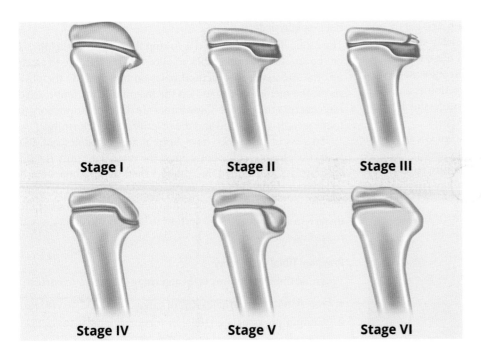

Figure 6.12 Langenskiold classification of Blount's disease. Stage I: medial beaking, irregular medial ossification with protrusion of the metaphysis. Stage II: cartilage fills the depression. Progressive depression of the medial epiphysis with the epiphysis sloping medially as the disease progresses. Stage III: ossification of the inferomedial corner of the epiphysis. Stage IV: epiphyseal ossification filling the metaphyseal depression. Stage V: double epiphyseal plate (cleft separating the two epiphyses). Stage VI: medial physeal closure.

Table 6.2 Langenskiold staging

Stages	Descriptions
I	Medial beaking, irregular medial ossification with protrusion of the metaphysis
II	Cartilage fills the depression. Progressive depression of the medial epiphysis with the epiphysis slopes medially as the disease progresses
III	Ossification of the inferomedial corner of the epiphysis
IV	Epiphyseal ossification filling the metaphyseal depression
V	Double epiphyseal plate (cleft separating the two epiphyses)
VI	Medial physeal closure

Treatment

Bracing

It is indicated in children younger than 3 years of age and at stages I and II, with a reported success rate of 50% using a three-point BD brace (Figure 6.14). Risk factors for failure are instability, obesity, delayed bracing and non-compliance.

Raney reported their experience in 38 patients (60 tibia vara) with an MDA of >16° or between 9° and 16°, with a clinical risk factor for progression such as ligamentous instability, patient weight above the 90th percentile, bilateral involvement and late initiation of bracing. The success rate was 90% (54 tibae); 27 were

Table 6.3 Summary of differences between infantile and adolescent tibia vara

	Infantile type	Adolescent type
Clinical	The typical patient is an obese female <4 years with lateral knee thrust. She/he is usually followed up for physiological genu varum	The typical patient is a male teenager, often black, whose body weight greatly exceeds 2 SDs above the mean
Radiological	Medially sloped and irregularly ossified epiphysis, sometimes triangular Prominent beaking of the medial metaphysis, with lucent cartilage islands within the beak Widened and irregular physeal line medially Lateral subluxation of the proximal end of the tibia Varus angulation at the epiphyseal–metaphyseal junction	Shape of the epiphysis relatively normal Lack of beaking of the medial tibial metaphysis Widening of the proximal medial physeal plate, sometimes extending across to the lateral side of the physis Widening of the lateral distal femoral physis, in comparison to either the medial femoral physis of the same knee or the distal femoral physis of the normal knee
Treatment	Treatment is based on the stage of the disease. Orthosis is indicated in the early stages The goal of surgical treatment is to overcorrect the mechanical axis Hemi-epiphysiodesis (alone) is not usually effective or adequate	Treatment is usually surgical as orthosis is usually ineffective The goal of surgical treatment is to correct the mechanical axis to normal (avoiding overcorrection), so that physeal growth is restored and degenerative arthritis of the medial compartment of the knee can be avoided Lateral hemi-epiphysiodesis (alone) can be successful treatment in 50–70% of cases

See reference [7].

treated by full-time bracing, 23 by night-time bracing only, and 4 by daytime use. Three of the six tibias requiring surgery had been treated with full-time orthotic use, and three with night-time use only [8]. Valgus correction should be increased every 2 months to promote correction; if no correction is achieved within a year, the brace has probably not been successful. Bracing is not recommended for children older than 3 years.

Some children present with mild BD (stage I) early, with most radiological measurements in the grey areas. There is merit in observing these children for 6–12 months, particularly if they are much younger than 3 years old, without jeopardizing the bracing treatment potential (Figure 6.15).

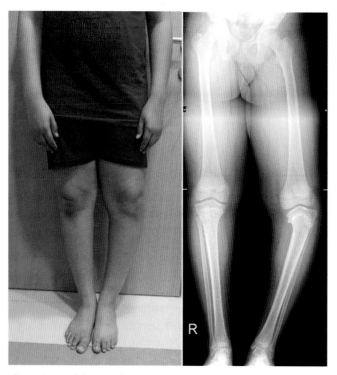

Figure 6.13 Adolescent Blount's disease in an overweight teenager boy. Notice the shape of the epiphysis that is relatively normal and the lack of beaking of the medial tibial metaphysis.

Hemi-epiphysiodesis

The rationale of this method is to stop the growth of the physis on the lateral side of the tibia, to allow the medial side to catch up. The success of this method relies on how healthy the physis on the medial side is and on the magnitude of compressive forces across the physis. These forces are directly proportionate to the weight of the child and the severity of the deformity.

Successful outcomes have been noted in adolescent BD when the physis is sufficiently open, the varus deformity is mild to moderate, and patients are younger than 10 [9]. About a third of children with adolescent BD have a distal femoral deformity also, which responds very well to hemi-epiphysiodesis of the distal femur. Chapter 23 covers how to identify the site, side, and magnitude of deformity.

Proximal Tibial Osteotomy

Proximal tibial osteotomy is the mainstay of surgery to correct:

1. Mechanical axis to at least 5° of valgus
2. Commonly associated tibial in-torsion (Figure 6.16)
3. Physeal bar and any associated shortening
4. Tibial joint surface depression.

The following are important factors to be considered:

1. Age of the child as a reflection of remaining growth. The more growth that is left, the more effort to save the physis
2. The Silverskiöld stage. Complete growth plate recovery has been reported in stages I, II and III. Growth restoration could occur in type IV, but not in types V and VI. Therefore, protection of the growth plate is essential in types I, II and III, and, to a lesser extent, in type IV
3. The severity of medial joint depression. This can be corrected through intra-epiphyseal osteotomy and hemi-elevation whilst protecting the growth plate, or by transphyseal osteotomy and hemi-elevation, sacrificing the growth plate based on the remaining growth and the Silverskiöld stage (Figure 6.17)

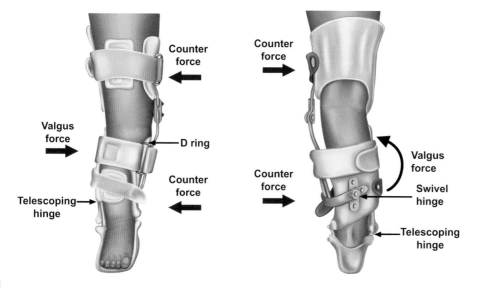

Figure 6.14 Three-point Blount's disease brace, showing the mechanism by which it reduces the compressive forces through the medial physis.

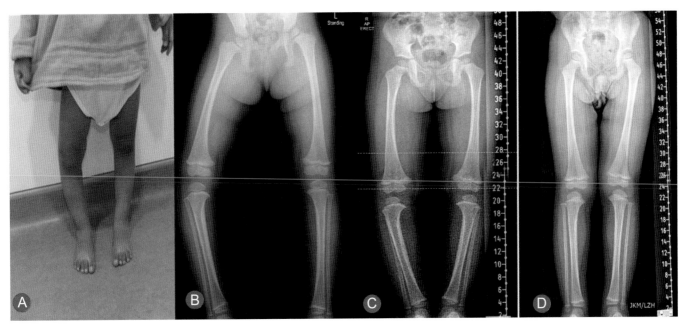

Figure 6.15 Mild borderline cases of Blount's disease can correct spontaneously. This child presented with unilateral genu varum. Most radiological measurements indicated that it is more physiological, rather than pathological. A decision was made to observe the child for 6 months (C) and when she was improving, for another 6 months (D) when her leg alignments became normal.

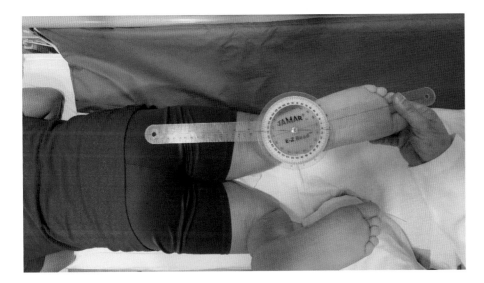

Figure 6.16 Left tibial in-torsion associated with Blount's disease (same patient shown in Figure 6.13).

4. The estimated height at maturity to decide whether to lengthen the leg using the same osteotomy or to perform epiphysiodesis of the contralateral side. It is quicker and safer to do epiphysiodesis of the other side, but this means the overall height will be shorter than the natural height.

All the above factors represent a spectrum. On the extreme ends of the spectrum, the decision can be obvious. However, in the middle of the spectrum, the decision requires clinical judgement and experience.

A very young child of 6 with BD stage III will benefit from proximal tibial corrective osteotomy. Overcorrection (more valgus than the normal) is desirable to give the best chance for the growth plate to function again. If there is a small physeal bar, it can be excised and an interposition graft, such as fat or bone wax, is used to prevent re-formation. If there is medial joint depression, intra-epiphyseal osteotomy can be utilized to level the joint surface whilst protecting the growth plate.

By contrast, a 12-year-old child with BD stage V will benefit from proximal tibial osteotomy to correct the mechanical axis to normal. There is no potential benefit from overcorrection (given the child's age and stage of the disease). It is more practical to perform epiphysiodesis to prevent recurrence, rather than trying to save the physis. If there is medial joint depression, transphyseal osteotomy and hemi-elevation of the tibial plateau can be

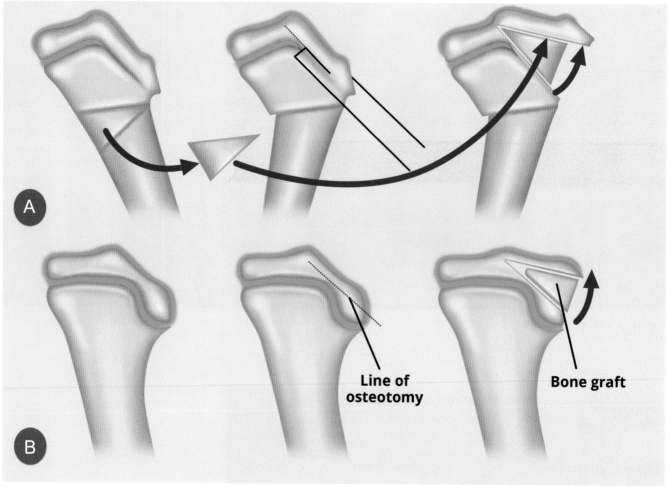

Figure 6.17 Transphyseal (A) versus intra-epiphyseal (B) osteotomies to correct joint surface depression in Blount's disease.

performed (Figure 6.17). There are two options to keep the leg length equal: epiphysiodesis of the proximal tibia on the other side (particularly if the child is likely to be naturally tall at maturity) or lengthening at the osteotomy site using an external fixator (particularly if the child is likely to be naturally short at maturity).

The methods of stabilizing osteotomy depends on the age of the child, the bone stock, the desire to fine-tune the correction, and the child's and parents' preference. Figure 6.18 shows various methods that have been used for stabilization. Prophylactic minimal invasive anterior compartment fasciotomy is advisable to prevent compartment syndrome during osteotomy. Careful assessment of the whole lower limb is important to identify and address all associated deformities in other bones.

Focal Fibrocartilaginous Dysplasia

Focal fibrocartilaginous dysplasia (FFCD) is a rare, benign disorder that has been reported as a cause of unilateral deformity of the tibia in young children, and sometimes gets confused with BD (Figure 6.19). It was first described in 1985 in three cases of proximal tibia varus deformity that was caused by a metaphyseal defect created by fibrocartilaginous tissue.

FFCD has also been reported in the femur, humerus, and ulna, as well as causing tibia valga. Clinically, there is significant hyperextension of the knee in FFCD. Radiologically, there is an abrupt varus at the metaphyseal–diaphyseal junction of the tibia, with surrounding cortical sclerosis; usually a radiolucent area just proximal to the area of cortical sclerosis and the physis appears normal. FFCD is a benign condition and often does not need treatment, unless the deformity is very severe, worsening, or causing significant symptoms [10].

Bowing of the Tibia

There are three classical types of tibial bowing, depending on the direction of the bow (Table 6.4).

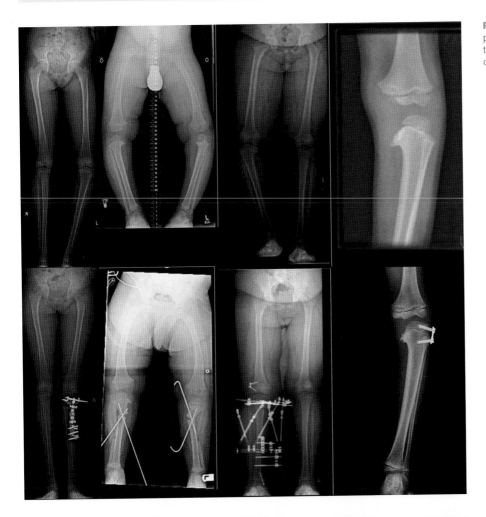

Figure 6.18 Various methods of stabilizing proximal tibial osteotomy. It is essential to assess the whole limb for associated deformities, which can be corrected at the same time.

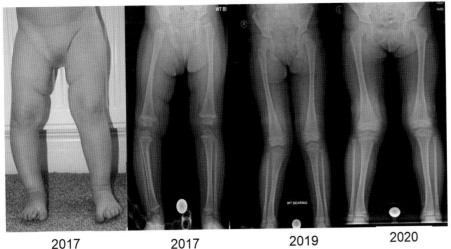

2017   2017   2019   2020

Figure 6.19 Focal fibrocartilaginous dysplasia of the proximal tibia, a rare, often self-limiting condition that may get confused with Blount's disease.

Table 6.4 Tibial bowing

Type	Cause	Treatment
Posteromedial	**P**hysiological	Observation, rarely causes limb length discrepancy
Antero**m**edial	Fibular he**m**imelia	See fibular hemimelia treatment
Anterolateral	Congenital pseudoarthrosis	Bracing, intramedullary fixation, vascularized bone graft, or amputation

Posteromedial Tibial Bowing

Posteromedial tibial bowing is seen shortly after birth and is often associated with calcaneovalgus deformity of the foot (Figure 6.20). It is considered to be physiological due to intrauterine malposition and resolves spontaneously. The foot deformity is generally resolved by 9 months. Tibial bowing usually resolves over 3–5 years, with rapid resolution in the first year, moderate resolution in the second year, slow resolution over the third year, following by plateauing after that.

Gentle stretching of the calcaneovalgus foot contracture may speed recovery and keep the parents satisfied. In severe cases, serial casting into plantar flexion and use of splints or bracing to maintain the position until weight-bearing may be necessary. Parents should be counselled about the probable need for limb lengthening in the future (Figure 6.21).

Anterolateral Tibial Bowing

This is commonly associated with tibial pseudoarthrosis (also called tibial dysplasia; see Figure 6.22) which is a rare and not very well-understood condition. Many cases have been linked to neurofibromatosis (50%, but only 10% of patients with neurofibromatosis have this disorder), fibrous dysplasia and amniotic band syndrome. Callus does not form at the fracture site, resulting in pseudoarthrosis. The site universally has fibrous tissue.

Depending on the severity of the condition, the diagnosis can be made at birth when the deformity is evident. If there is already pseudoarthrosis, there is abnormal movement at the fracture site. Milder forms may present later in childhood with bowing, limping, and actual fracture.

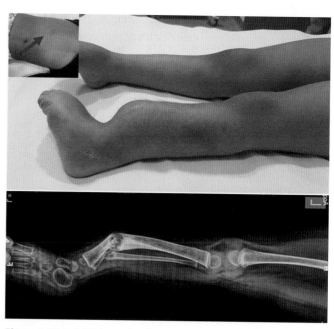

Figure 6.22 Left tibial pseudoarthrosis in a 4-year-old child. The child has a single large café-au-lait spot (inset picture), but genetic tests ruled out neurofibromatosis.

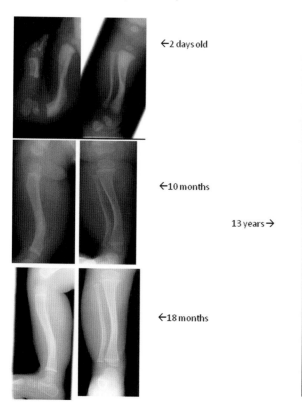

Figure 6.20 Calcaneovalgus deformity of the foot.

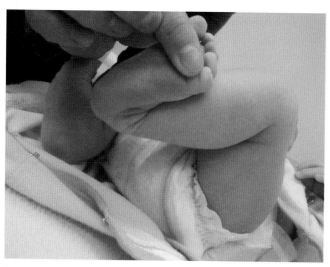

← 2 days old

← 10 months

← 18 months

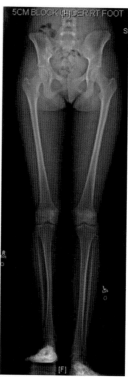

13 years →

Figure 6.21 Posteromedial bowing of the right tibia. These X-rays show how the posteromedial bowing almost fully resolved over 19 months (can take up to 3 years). However, the patient had a 5-cm limb length discrepancy at 13 years of age.

A few classifications, such as Boyd's, Crawford's, and Paley's, have been advocated, but none provide guidance to management or eventual outcome.

Crawford's Four Radiographic Types

- Type I: anterolateral bowing. The medullary canal is preserved and dense. Cortical thickening might be observed. Best prognosis may never fracture.
- Type II: anterolateral bowing with thinned medullary canal, cortical thickening, and tabulation defect. This should be protected with a brace and surgery should be considered.
- Type III: anterolateral bowing with a cystic lesion. There is a high risk of fracture and this should be treated with fixation and bone graft.
- Type IV: anterolateral bowing with fracture (as in the patient shown in Figure 6.22) or pseudoarthrosis, which has the worst prognosis.

Paley's Four Classification Types

- Type 1: no fracture
- Type 2: no tibial fracture, but fibular fracture:
  - Type 2a: fibula at station
  - Type 2b: fibula migrated proximally

- Type 3: tibial fracture, but no fibular fracture
- Type 4: fractures of both bones:
  - Type 4a: fibula at station
  - Type 4b: fibula migrated proximally
  - Type 4c: bone defect, with fibula migrated proximally.

Treatment

Treating anterolateral bowing with pseudoarthrosis and fracture is very challenging. Parent education is an essential part of treatment. Type I and, to a lesser extent, type II can be observed or protected with a brace (Figure 6.23).

In higher-grade, recurring fractures or unhealed fractures, alignment should be corrected and the fracture stabilized. Several forms of surgical interventions have been tried, with low success rates of around 50% (range 12–80%). However, the tibia and fibula cross-union technique showed a much higher success rate of 100% [11]. This technique involves (Figure 6.24):

1. Excision of the pseudoarthrosis
2. Stabilization of the tibia with intramedullary telescopic nailing
3. Stabilization of the fibula with intramedullary nail or thick wire

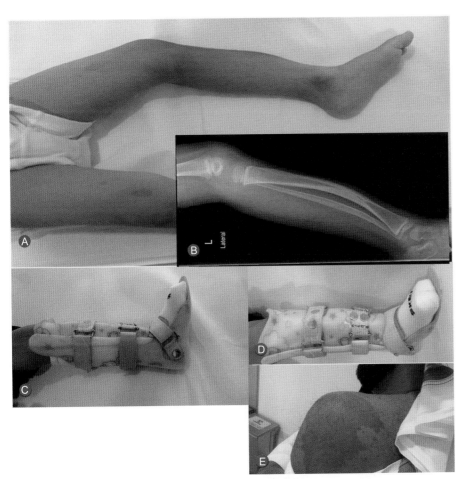

Figure 6.23 Clinical picture of a child with neurofibromatosis (see the multiple café -au-lait spots (A). Radiograph demonstrating tibial pseudoarthrosis type II (B). Clam shell brace for tibial pseudoarthrosis (C, D) In exam situations, show your knowledge and ask parents whether they have neurofibromatosis as well, as in the case with the dad of this child (E).

4. Tibia and fibula cross-union using autologous bone graft, meshed periosteum, bone morphogenetic protein 2 (BMP 2), and bisphosphonate infusion
5. External fixator (or internal locking plate) to control rotation and distraction which cannot be controlled by the above telescoping nail alone
6. Temporary cast followed by a brace, until solid union achieved

Other options that have been used include:

1. Excision of the pseudoarthrosis and bone transport using a circular frame
2. Ipsilateral or contralateral vascularized fibular graft
3. Amputation which may be considered if reconstructive surgery fails

Reported poor prognostic signs include:

1. Neurofibromatosis
2. Fracture or treatment in <3 years
3. Previous failed surgery
4. Narrow sectional area of healed segment
5. Persistent fibular pseudoarthrosis
6. Persistence of deformity
7. Removal of intramedullary rod
8. Non-compliance

Anteromedial Tibial Bowing

Anteromedial tibial bowing is usually caused by fibular hemimelia (Figure 6.25) and treatment is directed towards the hemimelia. Fibular hemimelia is the commonest long bone deficiency (1 in 600). It is usually associated with ankle instability, equinovarus foot, congenital absence of lateral foot rays, tarsal coalition, ball-and-socket ankle joint, proximal femoral focal deficiency (PFFD), and significant LLD. The fibular deficiency can be intercalary or terminal. The aetiology is unknown.

Several classifications have been proposed to describe the condition and plan management.

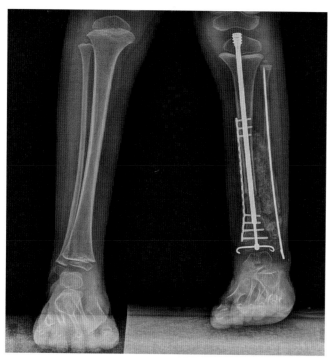

Figure 6.24 Cross-union of the tibia and fibula (the Paley technique).

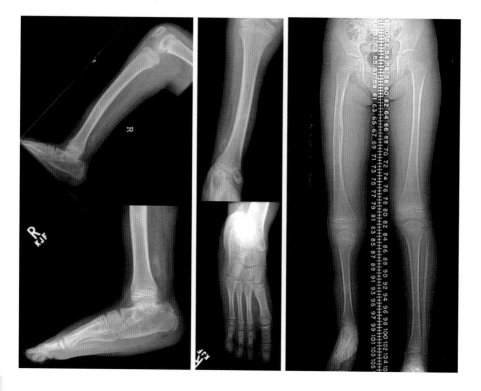

Figure 6.25 Anteromedial tibial bowing associated with fibular hemimelia. There is an almost complete absence of the fibula (apart from a high-riding lateral malleolus), with slight anteromedial bowing and a short right limb. There are four foot rays, with an absent lateral ray. There are some sclerosis and bony changes in the right femur, which may reflect an associated congenital short femur.

Birch's Functional Classification

The classification was developed to overcome problems with previous classifications which did not provide satisfactory guidelines for managing fibular hemimelia. Table 6.5 summarizes Birch's functional classification. The foot condition was the major factor in persevering the limb or not. Limb salvage was possible in 95% of patients with five-ray feet, 81% of those with four-ray feet, 49% of those with three-ray feet, and about 10% of those with fewer-than-three-ray feet.

Table 6.5 Birch's functional classification and treatment guidelines for fibular hemimelia

	Classification	Treatment
Type I: functional foot (can be made plantigrade and have three or more rays)		
IA	0–5% inequality	No treatment, orthosis or epiphysiodesis
IB	6–10% inequality	Epiphysiodesis ± limb lengthening
IC	11–30% inequality	One to two limb lengthening procedures ± epiphysiodesis or extension orthosis
ID	>30% inequality	More than two limb lengthening procedures or amputation
Type II: non-functional foot		
IIA	Functional upper limb	Early amputation (Figure 6.26)
IIB	Non-functional upper limb	Consider limb salvage procedure

Paley's Classification

Paley appreciated the importance of the foot in salvaging the limb and so he developed his classification with reconstruction only in mind [12] (Table 6.6; Figure 6.27).

Table 6.6 Paley's classification of fibular hemimelia

Types	Description and subtypes		Treatment	Note
1	Stable ankle		Tibia and fibula lengthening	
2	Dynamic valgus ankle		SHORDT,[a] then lengthening	
3	Fixed equinovalgus	3A: ankle type 3B: subtalar type	SUPERankle,[b] combined with lengthening	Calcaneo–talus coalition fixed in valgus
		3C: combined ankle and subtalar		
4	Fixed equinovarus			Calcaneo–talus coalition fixed in varus

[a] SHORDT stands for shortening osteotomy realignment distal tibia, to correct the valgus and stabilize the ankle. After SHORDT, or in combination with it, the tibia can be lengthened.
[b] SUPERankle stands for systematic utilitarian procedure for extremity reconstruction. It involves supramalleolar and/or subtalar osteotomies, combined with soft tissue release, to stabilize the foot and ankle. It is often combined with tibia and fibula lengthening.

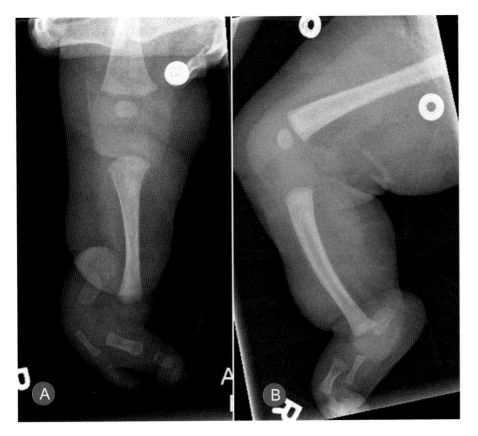

Figure 6.26 Birch's type IIA fibular hemimelia that was treated with Syme's amputation.

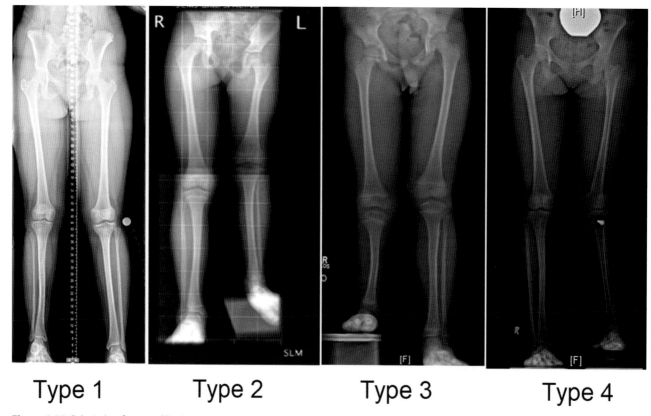

Figure 6.27 Paley's classification of fibular hemimelia. Lateral views (not shown) are important in assessing the deformity.

Key Points: Fibular Hemimelia Management

Although Birch's and Paley's classifications seem complicated, the general principle that underpins the treatment is simple: lengthening (±contralateral epiphysiodesis) in patients with a discrepancy of <10%; or amputation and prosthetic replacement in those with a discrepancy of >30%, particularly with a badly affected foot. Management of patients with a discrepancy of 10–30% should be individually tailored.

Tibial Hemimelia

Tibial hemimelia has an autosomal dominant mode of inheritance and is less common than fibular hemimelia. However, it is more commonly associated with other bony anomalies (preaxial polydactyly, cleft hand) or syndromes (75% of patients) (Figure 6.28). Clinical features include a short tibia that is bowed anterolaterally, with a prominent proximal fibula and an equinovarus foot. There are four recognized classifications. Weber and Paley classifications are very comprehensive and complicated and they are not expected to feature in the exam; however, the below two classifications are relatively easy and provide enough material to tackle potential exam questions.

Kalamachi Classification

- Type I: complete absence; the knee and ankle are grossly unstable
- Type II: absence of distal half; the ankle is unstable

- Type III: hypoplastic; tibial shortening, proximal migration of the fibula, and diastasis of the distal tibia–fibular joint.

Jones' Classification

Table 6.7 and Figure 6.29 show Jones' classification of tibial hemimelia and treatment guidelines [13].

Osteochondritis Dissecans

This is a condition which most commonly affects the knee, although it can occur in other joints such as the ankle (talus) and elbow (trochlea). The cause of osteochondritis dissecans is unknown. However, it is thought that articular trauma and subchondral ischaemia may be contributing factors.

In the knee, it occurs on the lateral aspect of the medial femoral condyle in 70% of cases (the lateral condyle 20%, and the patella in 10%). Males are affected more commonly, and the condition is bilateral in 1 in 4 patients.

The patient may present with a general limp or with pain in the knee joint, with or without swelling. There is often a history of injury. Sometimes there are mechanical symptoms such as locking.

Diagnosis is confirmed by plain radiographs (Figure 6.30), including tunnel views where it is best seen. MRI is useful for evaluating the status of the overlying cartilage and the amount of subchondral oedema. It helps with the staging of the lesion, and hence predicting the outcome [14].

In Guhl's MRI classification:

- Type I lesions have a signal change on MRI and the cartilage is intact

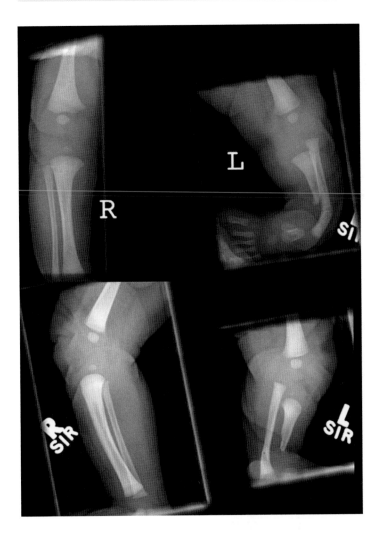

Figure 6.28 X-rays of a child with tibial hemimelia, showing the left and right lower limbs. There is partial absence of the tibia (type II) and a hypertrophied fibula, and the ankle is in severe varus. The foot has five rays and a well-developed calcaneum, talus and cuboid. Before recommending any treatment, a thorough history should be obtained and thorough examination and investigation should be performed. Treatment should be provided by a multidisciplinary team. It is surgically possible to fuse the proximal tibia and fibula at this stage and perform lengthening in the future. The ankle should be stabilized in plantigrade or a Syme's amputation should be performed.

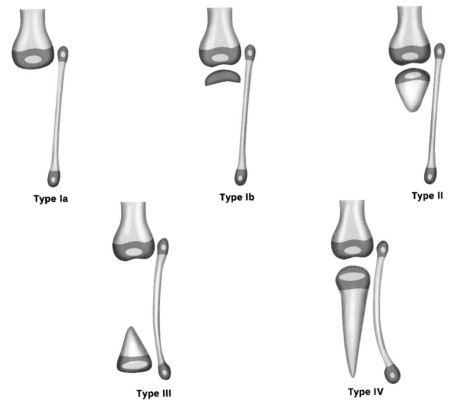

Figure 6.29 Jones' classification of tibial hemimelia.

Table 6.7 Jones' classification and treatment guidelines

Type	Radiological description	Clinical description and treament
Ia	Tibia not seen, with hypoplastic lower femoral epiphysis	The child has a knee flexion contracture and hamstring function, but not quadriceps function; the patella is typically absent, and the foot, which is fixed in severe varus, has minimal functional movement. Treatment options include knee disarticulation or centralization of the fibula (Brown's procedure)
Ib	Tibia not seen, but normal lower femoral epiphysis	Hamstring and quadriceps function is normal, and the knee moves normally. The fibular head is displaced proximally and laterally, and the limb is in a varus position, with significant varus instability. At the ankle joint, the foot is displaced medially relative to the fibula and is also in varus.
II	Distal tibia not seen	Good functional results can be obtained by fusing the proximal fibula to the upper part of the tibia (fusion cannot be obtained until there is sufficient ossification of the upper tibia to allow for successful synostosis with the fibula). A Syme's amputation, with subsequent prosthetic management, is the best treatment for the distal part of the limb because of severe foot and ankle instability
III	Proximal tibia not seen	The knee is unstable, and there are extra digits distally. The tibial shaft is palpable, and there is a severe varus deformity of the leg. Some of these patients may benefit from tibial lengthening, with or without Syme's or Chopart amputation, depending on the anatomy of the ankle joint
IV	Diastasis of tibia and fibula	There is diastasis of the distal tibia and fibula; the limb is short, and the foot is in a severe, rigid varus, positioned between the tibia and the fibula. This can be treated by Syme's ankle disarticulation performed at walking age. Tibial lengthening and foot repositioning may make it possible to retain a plantigrade foot. The functional outcome may not be better than amputation

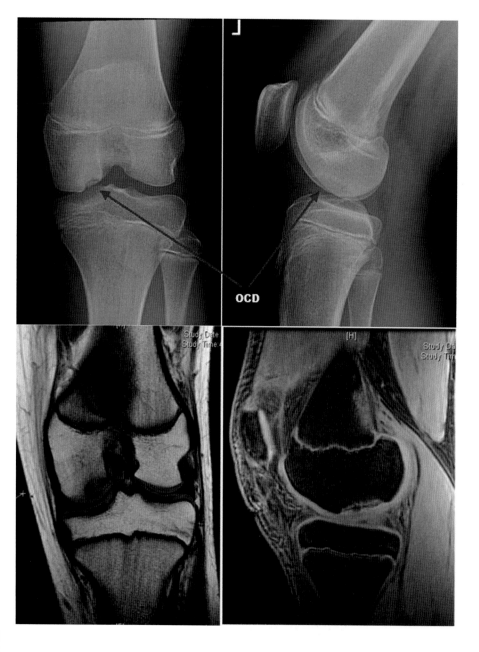

Figure 6.30 Osteochondritis dissecans.

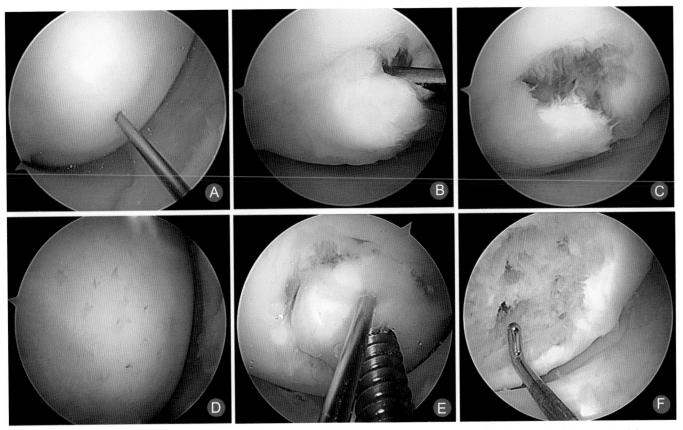

Figure 6.31 Three sets of arthroscopic pictures showing three different modality interventions to treat osteochondritis dissecans. (A, B) Transarticular drilling (notice the classical baseball-on-basketball appearance of osteochondritis dissecans). (C, D) Fixation using headless screw. (E, F) Debridement and microfractures.

- Type II lesions show a bright signal surrounding the bone portion, indicating detachment, but the cartilage is not breached
- Type III lesions show detachment of the bone and the cartilage is breached
- Type IV lesions involve displacement of the osteochondral fragment.

Good prognostic factors include early stage of disease, small lesion (<20 mm), typical location on the medial femoral condyle, younger age at presentation, and the physis being still open.

Treatment of osteochondritis dissecans is controversial. Patients with stable lesions are first treated with activity modification, rest, and sometimes area-specific offloading splints. If after a prolonged period of treatment (3–6 months), pain is still significant, then surgical drilling may be considered. This may be done transarticularly using arthroscopy or retroarticularly under image intensifier guidance. Although none of these approaches have been shown to have superiority, the retroarticular approach is recommended if the lesion appears healed arthroscopically.

The aim of drilling is to stimulate new bone formation. Unstable or loose lesions are treated by debridement of the bed, followed by fixation with bioabsorbable pins or screws. Cancellous bone graft harvested from the tibia may be needed to restore the joint line. Non-viable fragments should be removed, and the bed debrided and microfractured (Figure 6.31).

If the above interventions fail, techniques to fill the defect can be utilized such as osteochondral grafting, mosaicplasty, and chondrocyte transplantation. Evidence for these techniques in skeletally immature patients is not available. About 25% of patients with osteochondritis dissecans have long-term problems.

Popliteal Cyst in Children

Popliteal cysts are a relatively common condition in children and present as a variable-sized cystic swelling at the back of the knee. Anatomically, it is located between the semimembranosus muscle and the medial head of the gastrocnemius. It can be seen or felt medial to the midline at the back of the knee joint. It does not usually communicate with the joint, and therefore, the swelling does not vary in size. It is best palpated with the knee extended. It is self-limiting and surgical treatment is not necessary.

Sometimes popliteal cysts (called a Baker's cyst in adults) are a result of bulging of the posterior capsule and synovial herniation. They are in the midline and at the level of the joint or just below. They communicate with the joint, and therefore, their size can be variable. No direct treatment is necessary for the

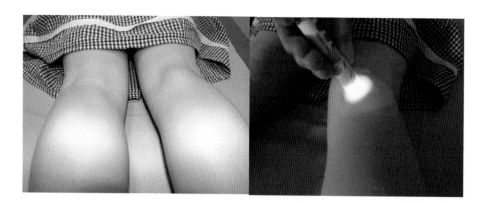

Figure 6.32 Popliteal cyst showing classical transillumination.

swelling. As the cyst is full of fluid, it usually transilluminates (Figure 6.32).

Plain X-ray is usually normal; ultrasound findings are consistent with a cystic lesion, and MRI shows a fluid-filled cyst. In children (unlike in adults), there is often no intra-articular pathology.

The natural history of popliteal cysts is spontaneous resolution, often within 30 months [15–17]. Surgery is reserved for very large symptomatic cysts that do not resolve spontaneously after a reasonable period of observation. The risk of recurrence after surgery is around 40%.

References

1. Thompson TC. Quadricepsplasty to improve knee function. *J Bone Joint Surg.* 1944;26(2):366–79.

2. Judet T. L'arthrolyse dans les raideurs post-traumatiques du coude. In: Bureau de La Société Française de Chirurgie Orthopédique et Traumatologique (SOFCOT 2010). *Conférences d'Enseignement 2010, No. 99.* Elsevier; 2010. pp. 333–49.

3. Johnston CE. Simultaneous open reduction of ipsilateral congenital dislocation of the hip and knee assisted by femoral diaphyseal shortening. *J Pediatr Orthop.* 2011;31(7):732–40.

4. Klingele KE, Stephens S. Management of ACL elongation in the surgical treatment of congenital knee dislocation. *Orthopedics.* 2012;35(7):e1094–8.

5. Davids JR, Blackhurst DW, Allen BL, Jr. Clinical evaluation of bowed legs in children. *J Pediatr Orthop B.* 2000;9(4):278–84.

6. Langenskiold A. Tibia vara (osteochondrosis deformans tibiae): a survey of 23 cases. *Acta Chir Scand.* 1952;103(1):1–22.

7. Herring JA. *Tachdjians' Pediatric Orthopaedics*, 4th ed, Vol. 1. Philadelphia, PA: Saunders Elsevier; 2008.

8. Raney EM, Topoleski TA, Yaghoubian R, Guidera KJ, Marshall JG. Orthotic treatment of infantile tibia vara. *J Pediatr Orthop.* 1998;18(5):670–4.

9. Park SS, Gordon JE, Luhmann SJ, Dobbs MB, Schoenecker PL. Outcome of hemiepiphyseal stapling for late-onset tibia vara. *J Bone Joint Surg Am.* 2005;87(10):2259–66.

10. Pavone V, Testa G, Riccioli M, Sessa A, Evola FR, Avondo S. The natural history of focal fibrocartilaginous dysplasia in the young child with tibia vara. *Eur J Orthop Surg Traumatol.* 2014;24(4):579–86.

11. Paley D. Congenital pseudarthrosis of the tibia: biological and biomechanical considerations to achieve union and prevent refracture. *J Child Orthop.* 2019;13(2):120–33.

12. Paley D. Surgical reconstruction for fibular hemimelia. *J Child Orthop.* 2016;10(6):557–83.

13. Jones D, Barnes J, Lloyd-Roberts GC. Congenital aplasia and dysplasia of the tibia with intact fibula. Classification and management. *J Bone Joint Surg Br.* 1978;60(1):31–9.

14. Pill SG, Ganley TJ, Milam RA, Lou JE, Meyer JS, Flynn JM. Role of magnetic resonance imaging and clinical criteria in predicting successful nonoperative treatment of osteochondritis dissecans in children. *J Pediatr Orthop.* 2003;23(1):102–8.

15. Dinham JM. Popliteal cysts in children. The case against surgery. *J Bone Joint Surg Br.* 1975;57(1):69–71.

16. Akagi R, Saisu T, Segawa Y, *et al.* Natural history of popliteal cysts in the pediatric population. *J Pediatr Orthop.* 2013;33(3):262–8.

17. O'Connor D, Clarke NMP, Hegarty SE, Fairhurst JJ. The natural history of popliteal cysts in children: an ultrasound study. *Knee.* 1998;5(4): 249–51.

Traumatic Knee Disorders

Nick Nicolaou and Joanna Thomas

Distal Femur Fractures

The distal femoral physis grows at 10 mm per year and contributes to 70% of the femoral growth and to 40% of the growth of the lower limb [1]. Distal femur fractures account for 1% of all physeal injuries and are often caused by motor vehicle accidents [2] and sporting activities [3].

Distal femur fractures are usually classified according to the Salter–Harris (SH) injury classification system [4]. They are associated with a high incidence of complications, the most serious of which include neurovascular injury [5] and growth disturbance, which can be as high as 70% [6].

Type I and undisplaced type II injuries are usually treated conservatively. Other injuries may require closed or open reduction followed by internal fixation. With internal fixation, care should be taken to avoid the physis. If the physis needs to be crossed, then smooth wires should be used, and these removed after 3–4 weeks (Figures 7.1 and 7.2).

Compartment syndrome and neurovascular injuries are rare but may be seen with displaced fractures, especially if the displacement is anterior.

Growth arrest is seen in 30–50% of physeal injuries. Limb length discrepancy and angular deformity may be obvious in these fractures because of the rapid growth that takes place at the distal femur.

Patellar Dislocation, Instability, and Maltracking

Traumatic patellar dislocation or subluxation is relatively common in children; it is the commonest cause of haemarthrosis in children. The incidence of recurrent dislocations following an initial episode of dislocation is as high as 60% in patients aged 11–14 years, and 30% in patients aged 15–18 years [7].

Our understanding of patellofemoral pathology in general and dislocation in particular is advancing. It is recognized that

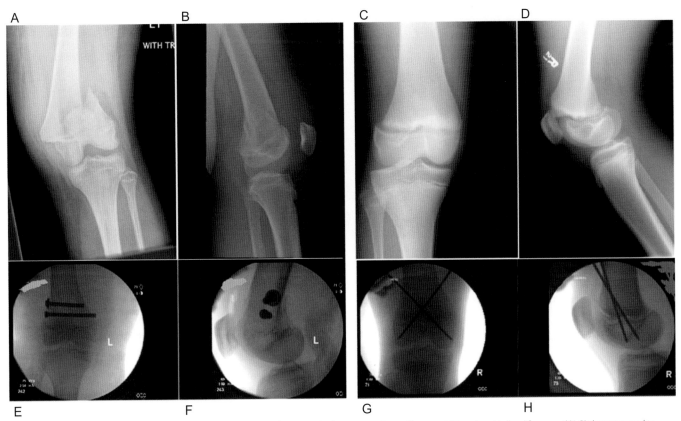

Figure 7.1 Distal femoral fractures. Salter-Harris type II on the left side, with a large metaphyseal fragment (Thurstan-Holland fragment)(A,B) that was used to stabilize the fracture with two cannulated screws(C,D). Salter-Harris type I distal femoral fracture(C,D) which was treated with smooth K-wires(G,H).

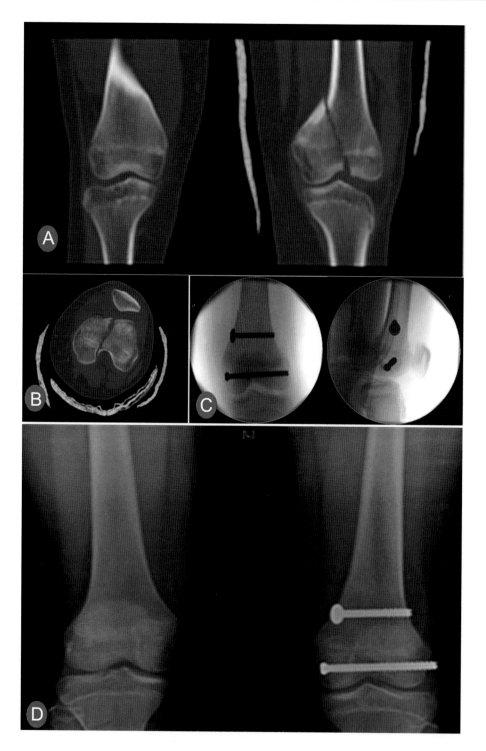

Figure 7.2 Salter -Harris type IV distal femoral fracture(A,B) that was reduced and stabilized using two cannulated screws, one through the epiphysis and another through the metaphysis(C,D). It is essential to ensure the joint surface is reduced anatomically by direct visualization using a small opening or arthroscopy.

these conditions are underdiagnosed and undertreated. Similar to hip dysplasia, these conditions represent a spectrum of pathologies [8]:

1. Patellofemoral pain without clinical or radiological findings
2. Patellofemoral maltracking, in which patellar motion during the gait cycle does not match its femoral track but remains within the track. This can cause abnormal tilting, deviation, or excessive localized pressure at the patellofemoral joint (PFJ) surfaces

3. Patellofemoral instability when the patella actually comes out of its femoral track but spontaneously reduces during motion
4. Patellar dislocation when the patella comes out of its track and requires reduction.

There are several reasons why a patella may dislocate. These can be grouped into:

1. Bony abnormalities such as:
   a. Femoral torsion (usually internal)

b. Tibial torsion (usually external). Where both (a) and (b) are present, it is termed miserable malalignment syndrome (Figure 7.3)

c. Valgus knee alignment

d. Trochlear dysplasia. A shallow patellofemoral sulcus angle (ABC >144° is abnormal) (Figure 7.3) – more relevant to adult practice, as traditional trochleoplasty is contraindicated in skeletally immature children

e. Abnormal congruence angle of Merchant (OBX is normally 6–8°). This angle is abnormal if it is more than +16°. Positive (+) means lateral, whilst negative (–) means medial (Figure 7.3)

f. Patellar dysplasia (as in nail patella syndrome)

g. Patella alta (high-riding patella)

h. High Q-angle (normal is 10° in males and 15° in females) (Figure 7.4)

i. High tibial tuberosity trochlear groove (TTTG) distance. This is the distance between the deepest trochlear groove and the summit of the tibial tuberosity on axial views of a CT or MRI scan (Figure 7.6). Normal value is about 13 mm. It is considered abnormal when above >20 mm

2. Muscular abnormalities:

a. Vastus medialis obliquus (VMO) weakness

b. Vastus lateralis contracture

c. Rectus contractures

d. Hypotonia as in trisomy 21

3. Ligament abnormalities:

a. Medial patellofemoral ligament complex

b. Laxity

4. Trauma.

In most cases, several of the above factors coexist in varying degrees of severity, making decision on what to correct and what to leave less clear.

In Figure 7.4, panel B shows the sulcus angle ABC of 150°. The line BO is the bisector of the sulcus angle ABC. The line BX passes through the lowest point of the patella. The angle OXB is the congruence angle of Merchant, which is abnormally high (+20°) in this X-ray. Also, notice the avulsion fracture of the mPFL. Panel C shows the lateral patellofemoral angle, which should open laterally, as in this example.

Management

Two distinctive clinical entities are encountered in clinical practice:

1. Acute traumatic patellar dislocation

2. Chronic instability – this group of patients can present with an acute episode of patellar dislocation, fuzzing the clinical picture and treatment further.

Most acute patellar dislocations are reduced spontaneously by simply extending the knee with or without gentle force directed anteromedially on the lateral patellar edge to lift the patella over the femoral condyle. Immobilization of the knee in full

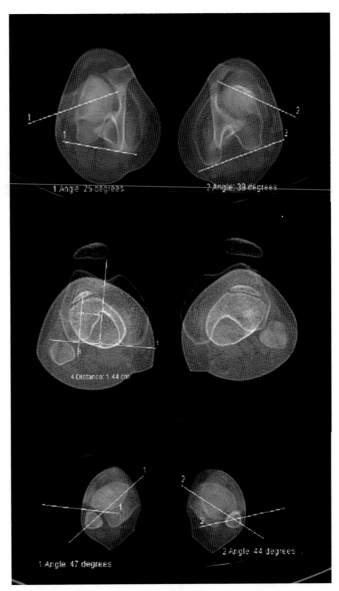

Figure 7.3 Miserable malalignment syndrome. Femoral in-torsion of 25° on the right and 39° on the left, and tibial ex-torsion of about 45°. Left patellar dislocation and right patellar subluxation. Notice the bony changes of the left patellofemoral joint, with loss of patellar height and sclerosis of the lateral femoral condyle. There is also narrowing of the joint space (articular cartilage). The TTTG distance is 1.44 cm, which is normal.

extension for comfort for a short duration with early mobilization is indicated. However, there is increasing evidence that not all patients do well with conservative treatment, and risk stratification can identify individuals at high risk of recurrence who would benefit from early surgical intervention. Risk factors that have been identified include younger age, skeletal immaturity, contralateral instability, trochlear dysplasia, patella alta, increased tibial tubercle–trochlear groove distance, and increased patellar tilt (see the list above). The PAPI (Pediatric and Adolescent Patellar Instability) randomized controlled trial and JUPITER (Justifying Patellar Instability Treatment by Early Results) prospective cohort study are under way and will provide further guidance [9].

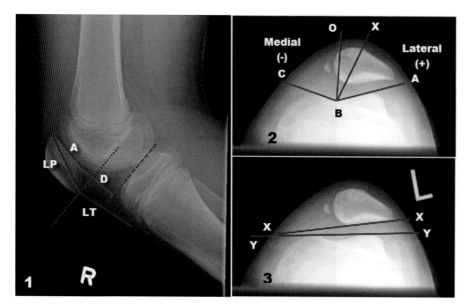

Figure 7.4 Radiological markers for patellar instability. (1) With the knee flexed to 30°, the Blumensaat's line (fine dashed) touches the lower border of the patella. The Insall -Salvati index is the ratio of the patellar tendon length (LT) to the patella length (LP) and should be 1.0. An index of 1.2 is alta, and 0.8 is baja. The Blackburne -Peel index is the ratio of the distance from the tibial plateau to the inferior articular surface of the patella, D, to the length of the articular surface of the patella, A, and should be 0.8. An index of 1.0 is alta.Sulcus angle (B). Patella tilting angle.(C)

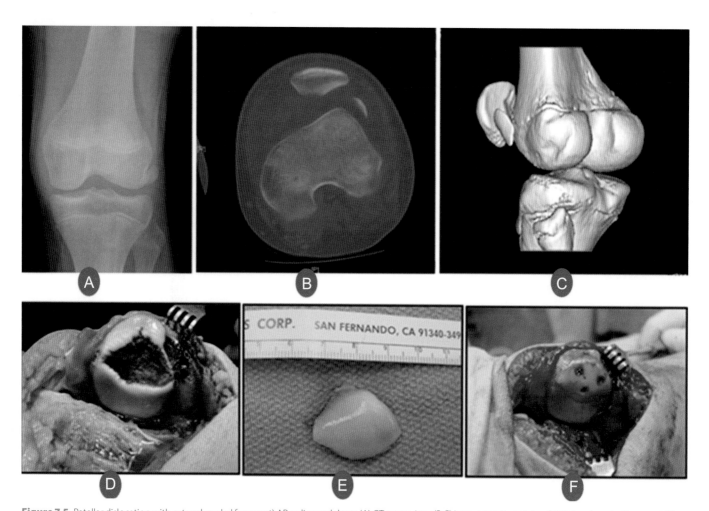

Figure 7.5 Patellar dislocation with osteochondral fragment).AP radiograph knee (A) CT scans views(B,C).Intra-operative picture(D).Osteochondral fragment (E) with reattachment of fragment(F)

Immediate surgery for first-time dislocations is widely recommended in situations where there is an osteochondral fracture of the patella or femoral condyle (Figure 7.5). Small fragments are excised, whilst large fragments are fixed. The presence of a haemarthrosis with dislocation should raise suspicion of osteochondral injury.

In patients with chronic patellar instability or those who fail to respond to physiotherapy, the consensus is to undertake surgery. There are over 100 procedures that have been described to stabilize the patella, implying none of them is 100% successful. Surgical interventions can be summarized as:

- Proximal:
  - mPFL reconstruction (extraosseous in skeletally immature, or transosseous in mature, children)
  - Lateral retinaculum release
  - Medial (VMO) advancement and reefing
- Distal (recommended with high TTTG distance or high Q-angle):
  - Roux–Goldthwait (half of the patellar tendon transferred to the Sartorius insertion). Grammont transfer of the whole patella tendon medially
  - Elmslie–Trillat procedure (osteotomy of the tibial tuberosity, preserving the distal attachment of the patellar tendon; the tuberosity is then moved medially and fixed with a single screw)
  - Fulkerson technique (similar to Elmslie–Trillat procedure, but longer osteotomy). The direction of the cut should allow anteromedialization of the tibial tuberosity; usually fixed with 2–3 screws (Figure 7.6)
  - Galeazzi (for immature skeleton). The semitendinosus is released proximally and passed through the patella, and resutured on itself
- Combined:
  - Hughston (involves lateral retinaculum release, medial (VMO) advancement and reefing (proximally), and Fulkerson technique distally; 70% reported excellent result
- Others:
  - Hemi-epiphysiodesis or corrective osteotomy in patients with genu valgum
  - Derotation osteotomy if there are significant torsional abnormalities
  - Patellectomy (last resort).

Selecting which operations to perform in individual patients is challenging. We recommend the use of a problem matrix to list and quantify the potential problems that have led to recurrence of dislocations (Table 7.1). Video 7.1 demonstrates how to use the matrix approach to treat patellar instability.

Table 7.1 Problem matrix in chronic patellar dislocation

Bony	Ligaments	Muscles	Trauma
Femoral torsion	mPFL	Weakness	Accidental
Tibial torsion	Laxity	Hypotonia	Habitual
Valgus knee alignment		Spasticity	
Trochlear dysplasia		Contractures	
Patellar dysplasia			
Patella alta			
High Q-angle			
High TTTG distance			

Red problems benefit from surgery, whereas blue problems benefit from physiotherapy. The more severe the problem is, the more likely surgery is required. Indications for correction are clearer with some problems such as TTTG distance >20 mm; however, this is not the case for tibial torsion or a valgus knee.

MRI scanning of the knee is helpful. Damage to the patellar or femoral cartilage should prompt a proactive approach to stabilize the patella (Figure 7.7).

 Video 7.1 The Matrix Approach to PF instability.

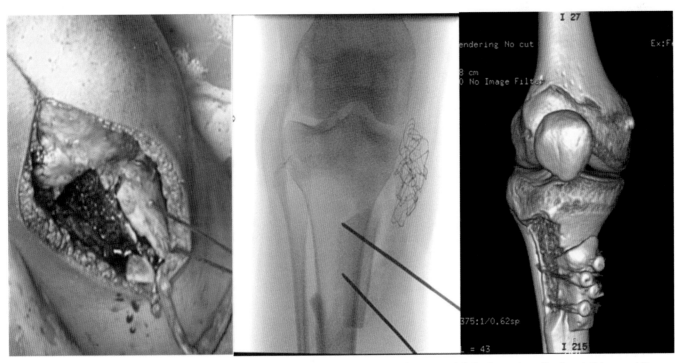

Figure 7.6 Fulkerson technique in which a long osteotomy of the tibial tuberosity is then moved anteromedially (and sometimes distally, as in this example) to allow realignment of the patella and reduce pressure at the patellofemoral joint.

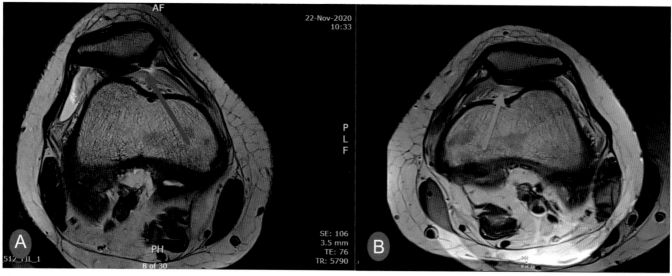

Figure 7.7 MRI scan of both knees in an adolescent with bilateral recurrent patellar dislocations. (A) shows substantive damage to the cartilage, with fissuring and delamination. (B) shows a high signal within the articular cartilage of the patella (blue arrow), but no cartilage breakdown yet.

Patellar Fractures

These usually result from a direct blow or a forced flexion injury to the knee. If the fracture is through the bony part of the patella, the diagnosis is usually obvious from the radiographs. This must be differentiated from a bipartite patella. In a bipartite patella, the edges are typically rounded and are characteristically located in one of the recognized places of the patella (Figure 7.8).

A patella sleeve fracture is a variation seen in children (Figure 7.9). The bony component is usually small, but there is a large chondral segment that is attached to the bone. This chondral part is not seen on the radiographs, and the only clue on the images may be a small bony fragment or a patella alta (or baja with proximal pole injuries). Hence, these injuries are frequently missed in the initial assessment.

Fractures through the bone may be treated as in adults with plaster immobilization for undisplaced fractures and tension band or cerclage wires for displaced fractures.

Tibial Spine Fractures

These fractures typically occur in children 8–14 years of age. They are the result of forced hyperextension of the knee or a direct blow to the distal femur with the knee flexed. These mechanisms create excessive tension on the bone and, because of the decreased resistance to tensile stress, the bone fractures whilst the anterior cruciate ligament (ACL) is spared.

Meyers and McKeever classified these injuries into types I–III (and type IV as a later addition) (Figure 7.10):

- Type I: the fracture is undisplaced
- Type II: the fracture is hinged posteriorly, but lifted anteriorly
- Type III: the spine is completely displaced (Figure 7.11)
- Type IV: this is a displaced and comminuted fracture.

Type I and some type II injuries can be treated conservatively in a plaster cylinder. There is some debate on the position of the knee in plaster. Hyperextension is recommended but causes

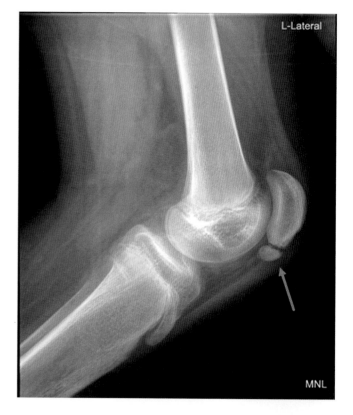

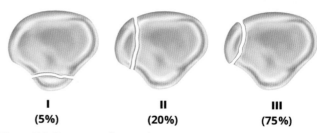

Figure 7.8 Bipartite patella type I showing typical site and the edges which are rounded, with no signs of healing. The Saupe classification describes the bipartite patella according to the location of the secondary ossification centre: type I, inferior pole (5%); type II, lateral margin (20–25%); type III, superolateral portion (75%).

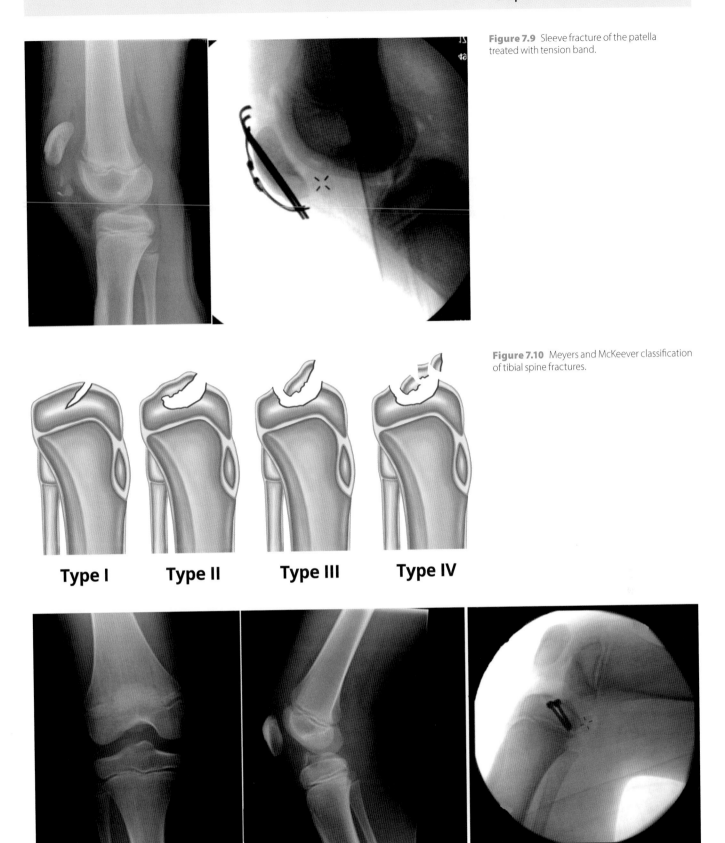

Figure 7.9 Sleeve fracture of the patella treated with tension band.

Figure 7.10 Meyers and McKeever classification of tibial spine fractures.

Type I   **Type II**   **Type III**   **Type IV**

Figure 7.11 Type III tibial spine fracture treated with arthroscopic assisted fixation.

extreme stiffness. If flexion of 20–30° holds the fracture reduced, then it is preferable. Immobilization for around 4 weeks is then followed by gentle rehabilitation.

Surgery is for type III fractures and type II fractures that cannot be reduced. It is not uncommon for the anterior horn of the meniscus to block the reduction. Reduction and fixation can be achieved via open or arthroscopic techniques. Fixation can be by sutures, wires, or a screw. Care must be taken not to cross the proximal tibial physis. Complications of this injury include ACL laxity and sometimes loss of full extension if there is malunion of the tibial spine fragment resulting in notch impingement on extension of the knee.

Proximal Tibial Physeal Fractures

Proximal tibial physeal fractures (Figure 7.12) are classified by the SH method. Treatment is dictated by the degree of displacement.

- Undisplaced fractures can be treated by cast immobilization.
- Displaced type I and II fractures are reduced and held with smooth wires which need to be removed after 3–4 weeks.
- Displaced type III and IV fractures and type II fractures with a large metaphyseal fragment are treated by reduction and screw fixation. These screws are placed parallel to the physis.

Neurovascular complications occur in 10–15% of injuries and include compartment syndrome, peroneal nerve injury, and popliteal artery damage. Popliteal artery damage is commonest after hyperextension injuries where the distal fragment is displaced posteriorly. Growth arrest occurs in 25% of patients with physeal injuries.

Tibial Tubercle Fractures

Tibial tubercle fractures usually result from the pull of the patella tendon. There is a spectrum of injuries, ranging from an undisplaced fracture involving only the tibial tubercle to injuries where the fracture line extends into the knee joint (Ogden modification of the Watson–Jones classification; Figures 7.13 and 7.14). An avulsion of the patella tendon with a periosteal sleeve can also be seen.

These injuries are usually treated surgically. An exception is an undisplaced fracture with no extensor lag, which can be treated in a plaster cast.

Although complications from this injury are uncommon, growth disturbance is seen, leading to genu recurvatum.

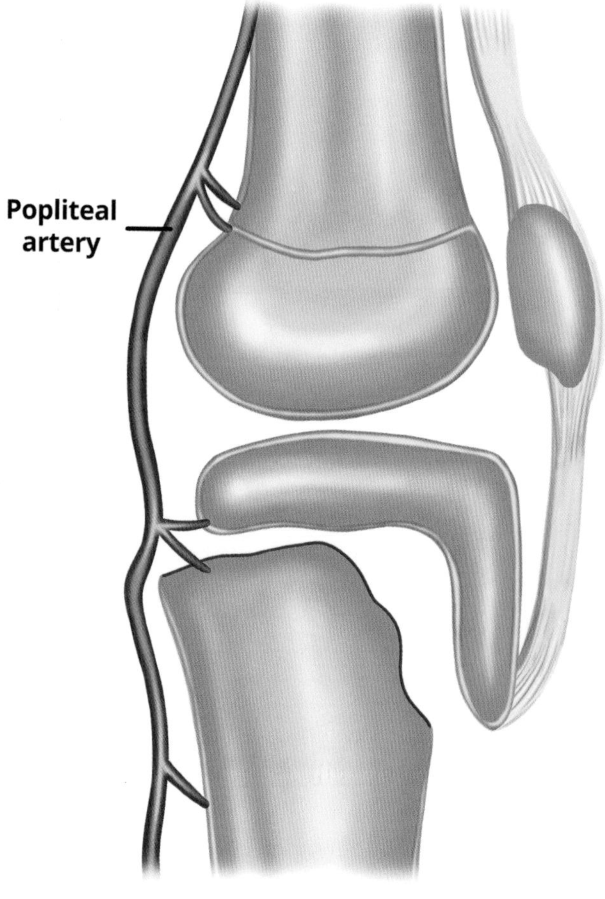

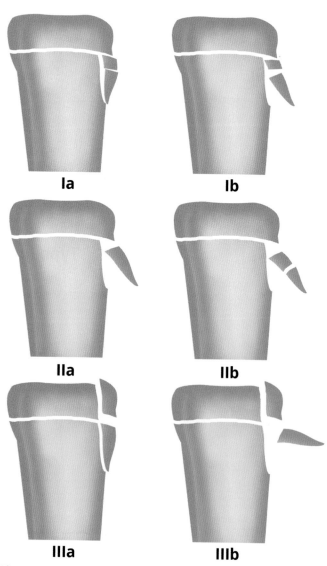

Figure 7.13 Ogden classification of the tibial tuberosity. Type I tuberosity fracture is distal to the physis; type Ia is undisplaced, and type Ib displaced. Type II fractures are through the physis; type IIa is not comminuted, and type IIb is comminuted. Type III fractures cross the physis; type IIIa is not comminuted, and type IIIb is comminuted.

Figure 7.12 Proximal tibial physeal fracture and the anatomical proximity of the vascular structure to the fracture.

Popliteal artery

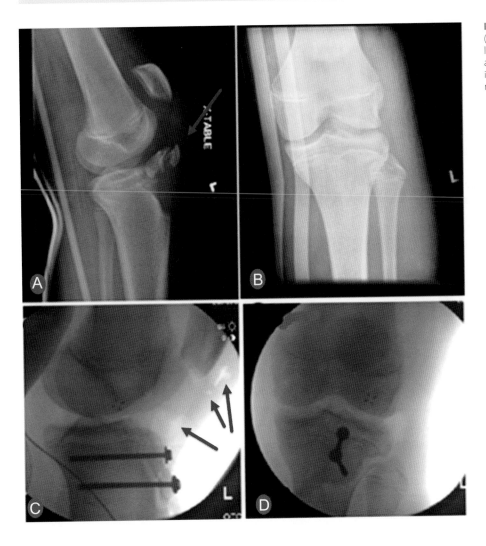

Figure 7.14 Type IIIb tibial tuberosity fracture (red arrow) that was stabilized with two cannulated screws on either side of the physis. There are a few air bubbles in the joint (blue arrows), indicating the joint was opened to check for meniscal entrapment or ensure good reduction.

Proximal Tibia Metaphyseal Fracture and Cozen Fracture

A characteristic pattern of injury occurs with some metaphyseal fractures (Cozen fracture) (Figure 7.15). Here the proximal tibial fracture results in the leg going into valgus, possibly due to medial overgrowth, lateral growth suppression, or periosteal incarceration. The child's parents need to be warned that this may happen and that usually no treatment is needed, as it would remodel with time, although this may take up to 3 years. The deformity progresses rapidly in the first year and can continue to progress over 20 months after the injury.

Surgery in the form of corrective osteotomies within the first 2–3 years after the injury has not yielded better results than non-operative treatment. The valgus deformity is thought to recur because corrective surgery recreates the conditions of the initial fracture [10]. Persistence of deformity after 3 years may warrant surgery such as medial hemi-epiphysiodesis (Figure 7.16).

Knee Ligament Injuries

Knee ligament injuries are rare in the skeletally immature patient. This is because the mechanisms that cause these injuries in the adult will result in a physeal or an avulsion-type fracture in children.

A medial collateral ligament (MCL) rupture is the commonest knee ligament injury, followed by an ACL rupture. Injuries to the posterior cruciate ligament (PCL) and lateral collateral ligament (LCL) are very uncommon.

Most controversies surround the management of ACL injuries, as these injuries are more likely to require surgical treatment.

- Isolated MCL and LCL tears are usually treated non-operatively in a locked brace for 2 weeks, followed by a hinged brace for 2 weeks.
- MCL or LCL tears, in combination with other injuries, such as ACL injuries, usually require surgery.
- MCL and LCL tears, combined with other injuries, such as ACL injuries and some isolated grade III injuries, may need direct repair.

Posterior Cruciate Ligament Injuries

These are rare. When they occur, they are frequently combined with other ligament injuries and require surgery. Isolated PCL injuries can be effectively treated by non-operative means. Quadriceps strengthening exercises are the mainstay of treatment.

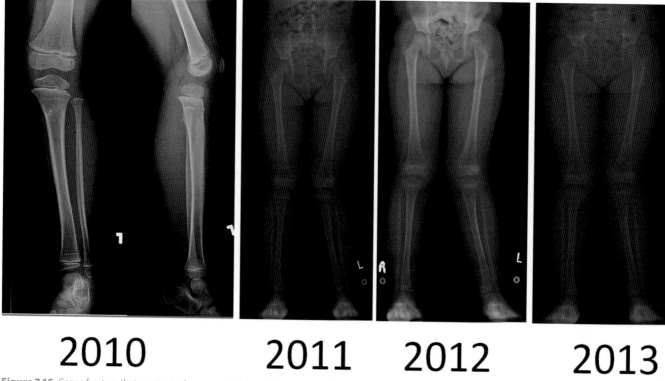

2010 2011 2012 2013

Figure 7.15 Cozen fracture that was treated non-operatively and almost completely normalized naturally.

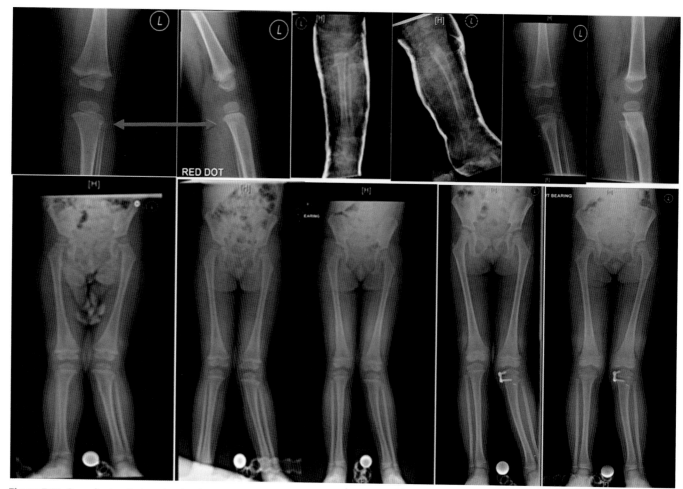

Figure 7.16 Cozen fracture that persisted and consequently treated with proximal tibia medial hemi-epiphysiodesis.

Anterior Cruciate Ligament Injuries

The mechanism of injury is the same as in the adult. The younger patient is more likely to sustain a tibial spine fracture, whereas the older child will suffer an ACL rupture. A haemarthrosis is usually present and the diagnosis is confirmed by a positive Lachman test and with MRI. Plain radiographs may show a lateral capsule avulsion fracture (Segond fracture; Figure 7.17) or the arcuate sign. The latter represents an avulsion fracture of the proximal fibula at the site of insertion of the arcuate ligament complex, and is usually associated with a cruciate ligament injury (~90% of cases).

Although MRI in the skeletally immature child is less sensitive than in the adult, it is the gold standard for confirming the diagnosis and detecting associated injuries. FRCS candidates are expected to describe knee joint MRI confidently and be able to identify ACL tears on MRI. Several features can be identified (Figure 7.18):

1. Joint swelling and effusion
2. ACL fibre discontinuity or bruises. ACL tears typically occur in the middle portion of the ligament (mid-substance tears) and appear as discontinuity of the ligament or an abnormal contour
3. Abnormal ACL orientation relative to the intercondylar (Blumensaat's) line (less steep than Blumensaat's line)
4. Empty notch sign: a fluid signal at the site of femoral attachment at the intercondylar notch – denotes avulsion at the femoral attachment. These types of tears are more amenable to ACL repair rather than to reconstruction

5. Footprint sign: incomplete coverage of the lateral aspect of the tibial spine by the distal ACL attachment, seen only on coronal MRI images
6. Bone contusion in the lateral femoral condyle and posterolateral tibial plateau
7. Deep sulcus (terminalis) sign (depression on the lateral femoral condyle at the terminal sulcus, a junction between the weight-bearing tibial articular surface and the patellar articular surface of the femoral condyle)
8. >7 mm of anterior tibial translation, also known as the anterior tibial translocation sign or anterior drawer sign
9. Uncovered posterior horn of the lateral meniscus
10. Buckling of the PCL
11. Associated meniscal and ligament tear.

Because of the potential damage to the physis associated with reconstructive surgery and the resulting growth disturbance, the following factors must be considered before undertaking reconstructive surgery:

- Age of the patient
- Time to skeletal maturity
- Level of planned activity
- Parental influence.

Non-operative treatment is a viable option if there is no other intra-articular pathology, and involves hamstring rehabilitation, ACL brace, and activity modification. If instability continues after return to sport, surgery should be undertaken to prevent subsequent damage to the knee [11].

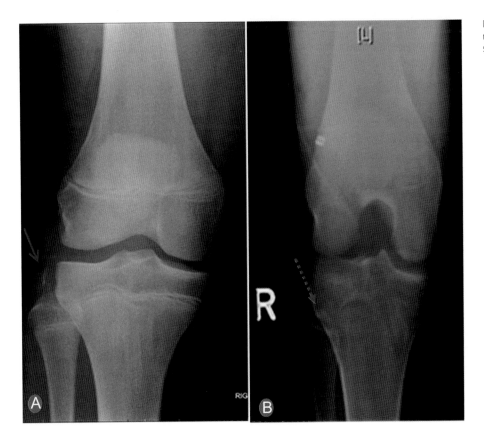

Figure 7.17 (A) shows a Segond fracture (solid red arrow) – a lateral capsule avulsion fracture. (B) shows the arcuate sign.

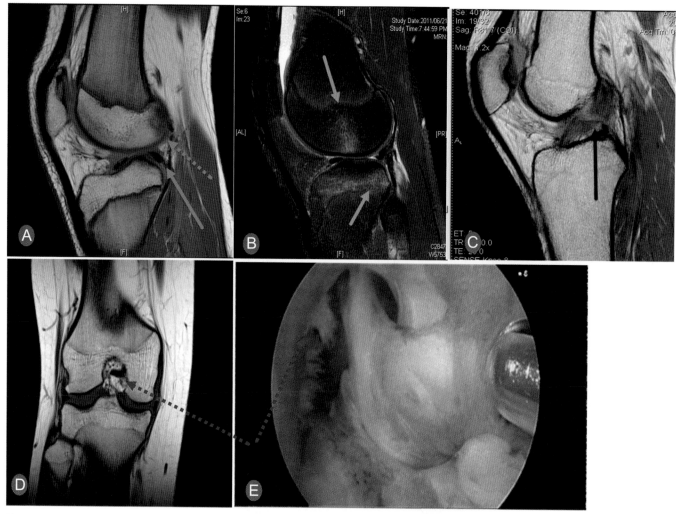

Figure 7.18 Magnetic resonance findings in ACL rupture. Anterior tibial translation (dashed blue arrow), uncovering of the meniscus (solid blue line)(A), bruises in the middle of the femoral and posterior tibial condyles (green arrows)(B), fibre discontinuity (black arrow)(C), empty notch sign (equivalent to the arthroscopic empty wall sign; dashed red arrow)(D,E).

The following points should be considered when undertaking an ACL reconstruction in a skeletally immature patient:

- The skeletal age should be assessed using clinical (menarche in girls) and radiological methods (Greulich and Pyle). It is relatively safe to proceed to an ACL reconstruction within 2 years of skeletal maturity using transphyseal techniques, with low risk of growth disturbance (girls aged over 13 years and boys aged over 14 years).
- If surgery is to be performed in the younger patient, physeal-sparing techniques should be considered such as all-epiphyseal, partial transphyseal, and extraphyseal reconstructions (Figures 7.19 and 7.20).
- With transphyseal techniques, a more vertical tunnel position in the femur will reduce the volume of physeal damage.
- Hamstring grafts are more commonly used, although use of the quadriceps tendon is increasing in popularity and bone–patella tendon–bone in those with closed growth plates may be a better option for reducing re-rupture. Bioabsorbable screws or cortical fixation devices are

preferred. Avoid using metal screws or any fixation device across the physis.

The results of most studies show that the incidence of growth disturbance following ACL reconstruction is low, although most do not quantify this with standardized imaging post-treatment.

- Patients undergoing surgery should be monitored for coronal or sagittal plane growth disturbance by performing leg alignment views preoperatively once full extension has been achieved and at 1 year post-operatively.
- Rehabilitation is vitally important to reduce the re-rupture rate. Consider delaying return to cutting sports activities for a year post-operatively. Rehabilitating the injured and uninjured leg is done simultaneously to reduce the re-rupture rate. Ensure return-to-sport testing has occurred, or make sure the limb is adequately rehabilitated.
- Consider discussing these injuries in a multidisciplinary setting with adult knee surgeons, paediatric surgeons, and physiotherapists.

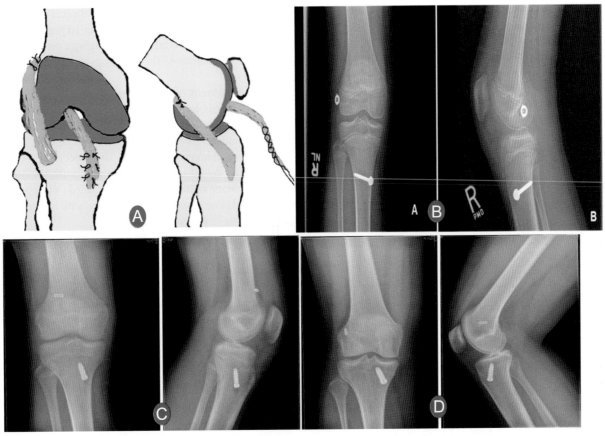

Figure 7.19 ACL reconstructions using various techniques. (A) Over-the-top technique using the iliotibial band. (B) All-epiphyseal (physeal-sparing). (C) Transphyseal (vertical tunnels to minimize damage to the physis). (D) Adult-type with a more lateral femoral tunnel.

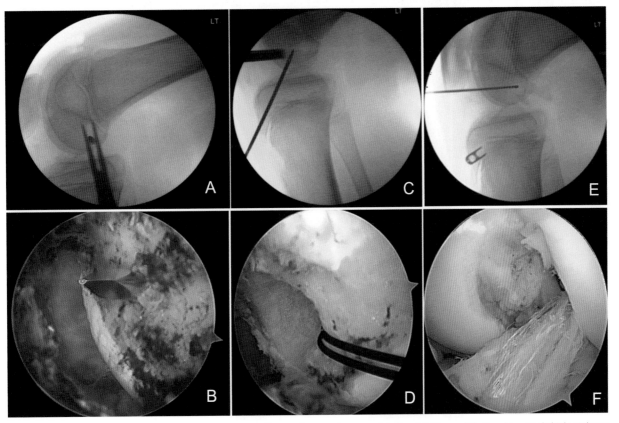

Figure 7.20 All-epiphyseal technique of ACL reconstruction. This involves creating tunnels in the distal femoral (A, B) and proximal tibial epiphyses (C) using an image intensifier and an arthroscope. Direct endobutton (E) was used to secure the graft distally first, then was pulled through the femoral tunnel (D, F) and secured using a bioabsorbable interference screw.

ACL repair was the first treatment for ACL rupture that has been superseded by ACL reconstruction; however, there is increasing interest in repairing ACL rupture in selective cases. The potential benefits are:

1. Less invasive
2. No graft morbidity
3. Maintenance of native ligament function, including proprioception
4. Faster healing
5. Faster rehabilitation.

Patient selection is vital. The ideal patient is a non-high athlete older than 25 years and who has an acute proximal one-bundle ACL rupture. Risk factors for failure are young age, high pre-injury sports activity level, mid-substance ruptures, and impaired integrity of the ACL bundles and synovial sheath [12].

Meniscal Injuries

Meniscal tears in children are much less common than in adults. The mechanism of injury is usually a twisting force on a planted knee. Diagnosis can usually be made by the history and the presence of joint line tenderness on clinical examination (Figure 7.21). Especially in children under 10 years, MRI is usually not as accurate as in adults in diagnosing a tear because of the increased vascularity of the meniscus resulting in false positive findings.

The aim of treatment of symptomatic cases should be to preserve the meniscus by repairing it where possible. If the meniscus is irreparable, a partial meniscectomy should be performed. Total meniscectomy should be avoided, as it leads to early degenerative changes in the knee. The success of meniscal repair is largely based on the blood supply, with the outer third (red zone) being better than the inner third (white zone) (Figure 7.22), and time to surgery from injury, with long delays to surgery resulting in poorer outcomes.

Meniscal repair methods include:

- Inside-out repair (used to be the gold standard using the double-lumen inside-out cannula)
- Outside-in (especially for anterior horn repair using meniscal Mender II from Smith and Nephew)
- All-inside technique which is, at present, the most popular method using modern suture equipment such as Fast-Fix 360. This technique is not ideal for anterior horn tears.

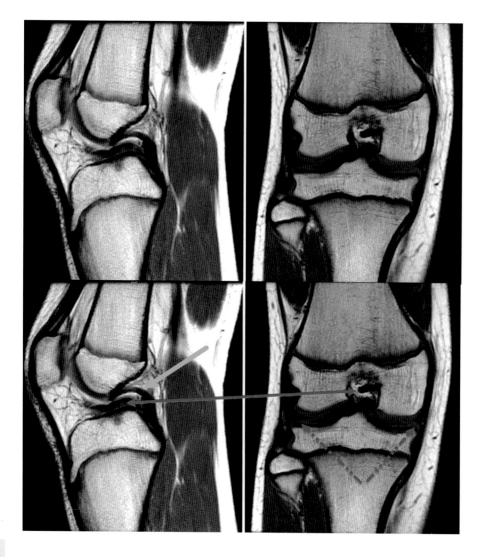

Figure 7.21 Bucket handle tear of the medial meniscus. MRI shows a large bucket handle tear of the medial meniscus, evident by a double posterior cruciate ligament (PCL) sign on the sagittal section (the green arrow points at the PCL, whereas the solid red arrow points at the meniscal tissue in the notch). Compare the shape of the normal wedge-like lateral meniscus to that of the torn medial meniscus (dashed red arrows).

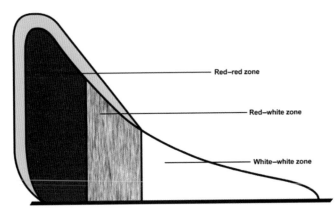

Figure 7.22 Zones of the meniscus based on vascularity and probability of healing. The red–red zone is more vascular and heals much better than the other zones.

Use of a fibrin clot has been suggested to improve the healing potential of the meniscus. Meniscal transplantation is an option for salvage.

Discoid Meniscus

This is an abnormally thick meniscus that covers a large proportion of the tibial surface and is thought to be of congenital origin. It is almost always located on the lateral side. The incidence varies from 1.5% to 15% and occurs mostly in girls. It can be bilateral.

It presents in various ways, from an incidental finding on MRI or arthroscopy to a frank tear. Children frequently describe 'popping', 'locking', or 'snapping'. Diagnosis can be confirmed by MRI scanning. The most accurate criterion for the diagnosis of discoid meniscus on MRI is a ratio of the minimal meniscal width to the maximal tibial width (on the coronal slice) of >20%. Another less precise criterion is continuity between the anterior and posterior meniscal horns on three consecutive sagittal images. If a plain X-ray is taken, it may characteristically show widened lateral joint space and squaring of the lateral femoral condyle.

Watanabe classified the discoid meniscus into three types:

- Complete
- Incomplete
- Wrisberg type.

Both the complete and incomplete types have a stable posterior attachment via the meniscotibial ligaments. The difference is that the complete type covers the whole of the tibial surface, whereas the incomplete does not. The Wrisberg type is the most mobile, as it is bounded posteriorly only by the meniscofemoral ligament of Wrisberg.

If asymptomatic, discoid menisci are left alone. Tears are excised to a stable margin (saucerization) if the meniscus has adequate peripheral attachment. Where the meniscus is hypermobile (Wrisberg type), it is attached to the capsule. Meniscectomy should be avoided.

References

1. Anderson M, Messner MB, Green WT. Distribution of lengths of the normal femur and tibia in children from one to eighteen years of age. *J Bone Joint Surg Am.* 1964;46:1197–202.

2. Czitrom AA, Pritzker KP. Simple bone cyst causing collapse of the articular surface of the femoral head and incongruity of the hip joint. A case report. *J Bone Joint Surg Am.* 1980;62(5):842–5.

3. Arkader A, Warner WC, Horn BD, Shaw RN, Wells L. Predicting the outcome of physeal fractures of the distal femur. *J Pediatr Orthop.* 2007;27(6):703–8.

4. Salter R, Harris W. Injuries involving the epiphyseal plate. *J Bone Joint Surg Am.* 1963;45A:587–622.

5. Eid AM, Hafez MA. Traumatic injuries of the distal femoral physis. Retrospective study on 151 cases. *Injury.* 2002;33(3):251–5.

6. Ilharreborde B, Raquillet C, Morel E, *et al.* Long-term prognosis of Salter–Harris type 2 injuries of the distal femoral physis. *J Pediatr Orthop B.* 2006;15(6):433–8.

7. Cash JD, Hughston JC. Treatment of acute patellar dislocation. *Am J Sports Med.* 1988;16(3):244–9.

8. Alshryda S, Tsang K, Dekiewiet G. Evidence-based treatment for slipped upper femoral epiphysis. In: Alshryda S, Huntley JS, Banaszkiewicz P, eds. *Paediatric Orthopaedics: An Evidence-Based Approach to Clinical Questions.* Cham: Springer; 2016. pp. 51–70.

9. Rund JM, Hinckel BB, Sherman SL. Acute patellofemoral dislocation: controversial decision-making. *Curr Rev Musculoskelet Med.* 2021;14(1):82–7.

10. Dormans JP. *Pediatric Orthopaedics.* Philadelphia, PA: Elsevier Mosby; 2005.

11. Kocher MS, Saxon HS, Hovis WD, Hawkins RJ. Management and complications of anterior cruciate ligament injuries in skeletally immature patients: survey of the Herodicus Society and The ACL Study Group. *J Pediatr Orthop.* 2002;22(4):452–7.

12. Heusdens CHW. ACL repair: a game changer or will history repeat itself? A critical appraisal. *J Clin Med.* 2021;10(5):912.

Orthopaedic Foot and Ankle Disorders

Anthony Cooper, Akinwande Adedapo, and Stan Jones

Introduction

The foot has 26 bones, 33 joints, and over 100 muscles and tendons; therefore, it is not a surprise that it is one of the commonest causes for parents to see a paediatric orthopaedic surgeon. At birth, the talus, calcaneus, cuboid, metatarsals, and phalanges are ossified, whereas the navicular and three cuneiforms are not (see Chapter 3, Figure 3.11). The lateral cuneiform ossifies at 1 year, the medial cuneiform at 2 years, and the intermediate cuneiform at 3 years. The navicular bone ossifies between 2 and 5 years [1].

The foot grows rapidly in the first year of life (Table 8.1).

Longitudinal arches develop with advancing age. In infants, the foot does not show arches well due to abundant fat along the medial arch, ligamentous laxity, and the fact that most tarsal bones are still not ossified (still cartilaginous). Fifty per cent of children have a visible arch by the age of 8 years, and around 90% when they are adult.

Table 8.1 Growth of children's feet

Age	Growth rate in centimetres per year	Shoe size changes
1–3	≤2	Half size every 2–3 months
3–6	1	Half size every 3–4 months
6–12	≤1	

Most feet reached adult size by the age of 12. Limited growth may still happen, but this is <10%. On average, boys' shoes are one size longer and one size wider than girls'.

Congenital Talipes Equino Varus (or Club Foot)
Overview

Club foot is a congenital and complex foot deformity (Figure 8.1), consisting of:

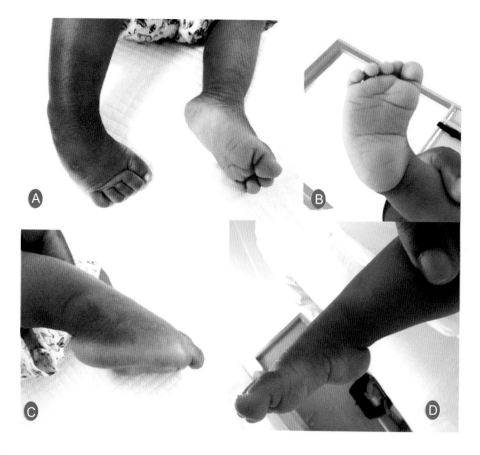

Figure 8.1 Club foot(A) is a congenital and complex foot deformity consisting of ankle equinus (C, D), heel varus (B), and (midfoot/forefoot) adductus (B). There is forefoot pronation (can be appreciated in C and D), producing a high-arched foot (cavus). The word *talipes* is derived from *talus* = ankle and *pes* = foot.

1. Equinus (ankle)
2. Varus (heel)
3. Adductus (midfoot/forefoot).

Incidence varies with race. In Europe, the incidence is 1 in 1000 live births, with boys twice as commonly affected as girls. In 50% of cases, both feet are affected. In affected families, the likelihood of club foot occurring in the offspring is 30 times greater than in the general population.

The exact cause is unknown but is thought to be multifactorial. Various aetiologies have been proposed, including primary muscle, bone, nerve, or vascular pathology, developmental arrest, and retracting fibrosis.

Anomalies are present in the bones, muscles, tendons, and ligaments. Key components of the deformities are medial and plantar subluxation of the navicular on the talar head, and a medially rotated calcaneum, such that the talus and calcaneum are parallel in all three planes (sagittal, coronal, and axial).

Diagnosis and Evaluation

Diagnosis is often made prenatally by ultrasonography (Figure 8.2). In the absence of a prenatal diagnosis, diagnosis is made at birth by clinical examination. Club foot may be positional, idiopathic, or syndromic. Syndromic club foot is associated with conditions such as arthrogryposis, myelodysplasia, amniotic band syndrome, and diastrophic dysplasia.

Common clinical findings are a small foot, a thin calf, and prominent medial and posterior skin creases. A full clinical examination is required to determine whether a child presenting with club feet has an associated syndrome.

Minimal ossification of the bones in the foot limits the usefulness of radiographs in the newborn. In addition, radiological appearances correlate poorly with clinical outcome.

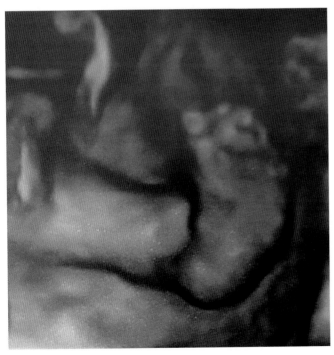

Figure 8.2 Antenatal ultrasound scan showing an infant with a left club foot.

Grading

Two grading systems are in use: the Pirani score (Table 8.2) and the Diméglio grading.

Both classifications assign points based on severity of the clinical findings.

Treatment

The aim of treatment is to achieve a mobile, pain-free, and functional foot that will fit in a shoe.

Initial treatment is non-operative, and the Ponseti method of manipulation and serial casting, followed by bracing, is the technique most commonly favoured. (A success rate of 80–90% is achieved with the Ponseti method.) The French method is another non-operative treatment but is not popular in the United Kingdom. It involves daily manipulations of the newborn's club foot by a specialized physical therapist, stimulation of the muscles around the foot, and temporary immobilization of the foot with elastic and inelastic adhesive taping. A comparative study of 176 patients treated by the Ponseti method and 80 patients treated by the French functional method showed improved results with use of the Ponseti method, although the difference was not statistically significant [2].

Ponseti Method

1. Treatment starts soon after birth but may be delayed for a few weeks in a premature baby (until the weight reaches 3.5 kg, which is the average birthweight).

2. The sequence of deformity correction is cavus, adduction, varus, and finally equinus (CAVE) (Figure 8.3; Video 8.1).

   a. Cavus correction. This can be corrected by positioning the forefoot in proper alignment with the hindfoot.

   b. Adduction and varus are corrected simultaneously around the talus head which act as a fulcrum. The forefoot is held supinated, and not pronated. Lateral pressure with the thumb is over the neck of the talus, and not the calcaneocuboid joint (Figure 8.4). On average, it takes three sets of cast to correct these two deformities.

   c. Equinus should be corrected without causing a midfoot break. It is usually possible to bring the ankle to neutral (0° of dorsiflexion) before performing tenotomy. The following signs are useful to indicate the correct time to start correcting the equinus deformity:

      i. Forefoot abduction of about 60° in relation to the frontal plane of the tibia

      ii. The heel in neutral or valgus position

      iii. The ability to feel the anterior process of the calcaneus, as it abducts out from beneath the talus.

   d. Residual equinus is corrected by a percutaneous Achilles tenotomy using a single incision (required in up to 90% of feet); this is followed by a last cast for 3 weeks.

3. Before each cast application, the foot is gently manipulated to the desired position. A thin layer of cast padding is applied. The foot is maintained in the maximum corrected

Table 8.2 Pirani score for club feet

Six clinical signs are used in the Pirani score, equally divided between the hindfoot and the midfoot.

Hindfoot Contracture Score (HFCS), 0–3: equinus (0 = dorsiflexion; 0.5 come to neutral; 1 = cannot reach neutral); posterior crease (0 = multiple fine creases – normal; 0.5 = superficial single crease which is obliterated on dorsiflexion; 1 = deep persistent crease); and empty heel (0 = easily palpable calcaneum; 0.5 = deep calcaneum; 1 = not palpable.)

Midfoot Contracture Score (MFCS), 0–3: curved lateral border (0 = straight; 0.5 = mildly curved; 1 = severely curved); medial crease (as in posterior crease); and lateral head of talus (0 = fully covered with the navicular bone; 0.5 = partially covered; 1 = not covered at all).

Total Pirani score (TPS) = 0–6.

Source: Pictures courtesy of Dr Lynn Staheli and Global Help Publication.

position by holding the toes, with counterpressure applied against the talus head, whilst the cast is applied.

4. A below-knee cast is applied and moulded well around the foot to maintain the correction. When this is set, the knee is bent to 90° and the cast is extended to above the knee.

5. Casts are changed on a weekly basis, although this can be done at 5-day intervals. Removal of the cast can be done by using a cast knife, as an electric saw can frighten children. Alternative ways include soaking the cast in water until completely soft, then unwrapping it like a bandage.

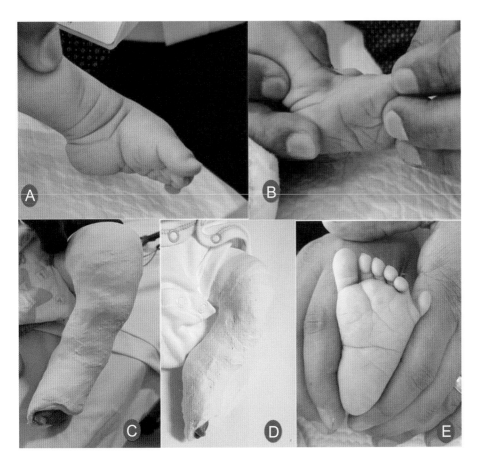

Figure 8.3 The first set of Ponseti serial casting is to correct cavus by elevating the first ray of the foot, so that the plantar aspect of the forefoot aligns well with that of the hindfoot(A,B). This causes the foot to face more inwards and the deformity looks worse in and after the first cast (C, D). However, if the limb is covered, the plantar surface should look flat after the first cast (E).

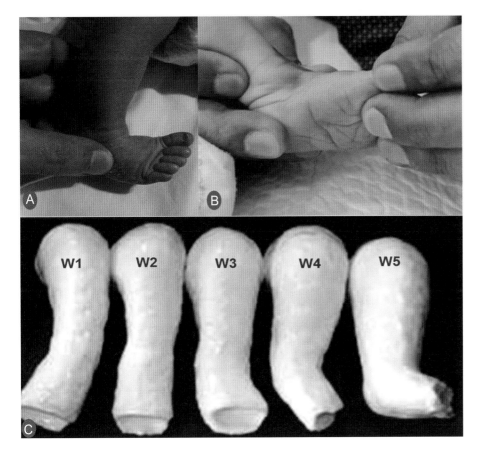

Figure 8.4 Simultaneous correction of the forefoot adductus and heel varus. The thumb is placed over the talus neck/head (which is immediately in front of the lateral malleolus) (A), with the left hand holding the supinated forefoot and gently pulling it into further valgus (B). Gradual correction of adductus and varus deformities over weeks 2, 3, and 4(C).

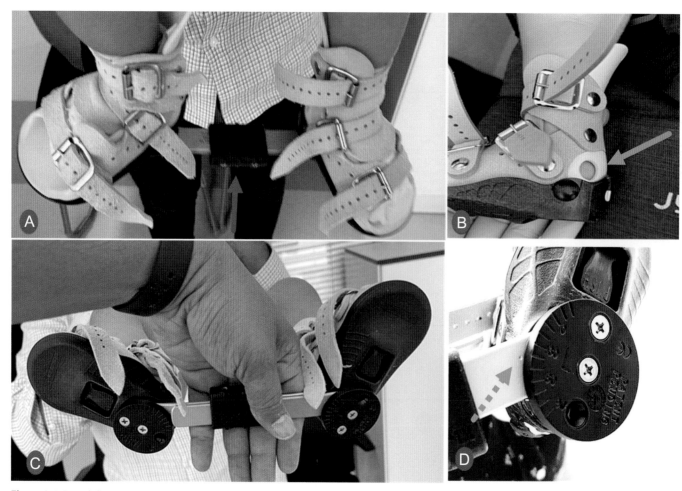

Figure 8.5 Foot abduction brace (Ponseti boots and bar). This is a Denis Browne brace; the bar should be of sufficient length, so that the heels of the shoes are at shoulder width. This can be adjusted using the sliding clamp in the middle (A, red arrow). The bar is bent around 10 -15Åã to hold the feet in dorsiflexion. For unilateral cases, the brace is set at 60 -70Åã of external rotation on the club foot side, and 30 -40Åã of external rotation (D, dashed green arrow) on the normal side (D). In bilateral cases, it is set at 70Åã of external rotation on both sides (C). It is important that the foot is well seated in the boot and the heel is visible through the heel hole (B, green arrow).

6. After removing the last cast, a foot abduction orthosis (e.g. Denis Browne boots and bar) (Figure 8.5) is applied and worn for 23 hours a day, initially for 3 months, then only at nap- and night-time (this is usually around 14 hours) for 3–4 years. This is required to facilitate remodelling of the foot and prevent relapse of the deformity.

7. The commonest cause of relapse of the deformity is poor compliance with the Denis Browne boot and bar. Relapse is treated by rescue serial casting, with or without an Achilles tenotomy.

> **Video 8.1** Ponseti treatment for club foot.

Complications and Technical Errors

Figure 8.6 shows the complications following Ponseti serial casting:

1. Pressure sores. If they are superficial, they can be dressed and treatment is continued. However, if they are deep, casting is withheld for a week or so for them to be treated, but special care must be taken to avoid recurrence

2. Crowded toes, tight cast, loose cast, and broken cast

3. Rocker-bottom deformity. This happens when the foot is dorsiflexed too early against a tight tendo Achilles

4. Residual deformity or relapses.

Surgery

Ponseti serial casting is a successful treatment for club foot. It has almost removed the need for surgical intervention. However, surgery sometimes is required in the situations outlined in Table 8.3.

Atypical Club Foot

This term is loosely applied to several types of club foot, including later-presented typical club foot, neuromuscular club foot, and those associated with arthrogryposis, spina bifida, Mobius syndrome, etc.

One type is of particular interest because of the unique features. The foot is short and stubby. It is very stiff with severe plantar flexion of all metatarsals, with a deep crease just above the heel and across the side of the midfoot, with a short big toe (Figure 8.7). Some modification of the Ponseti method is required. More sets of cast may be needed.

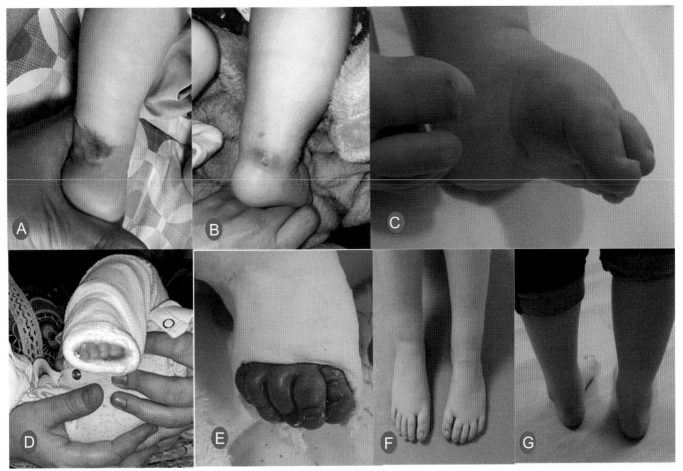

Figure 8.6 Complications following Ponseti serial casting. (A) and (B) show skin pressure sores. (C) shows a pronated foot; this is usually caused by a technical error when the foot is pronated, rather than supinated, during treatment. (D) shows a loose cast. This should be treated on an urgent basis by removing the cast to prevent any skin breakdown (Do not leave them until morning!). (E) shows a too tight cast causing swollen and crowded toes. (F) and (G) show a residual deformity (varus and adductus).

Table 8.3 Indications for surgery in club foot

Persistent supination	Whole or split tibialis anterior tendon transfer
Relapse despite repeat serial casting	Limited posteromedial release or soft tissue distraction using a circular external fixator
Severe multiplanar residual deformity in the older child	Osteotomies of the mid- and/or hindfoot with or without a circular external fixator

Key Points: Evidence-Based Note

Morecuende *et al.* reported a success rate of 98% in 256 consecutive cases of club foot over 10 years. The relapse rate was 11%. Most were treated successfully with repeat serial casting ± tenotomy; 2.5% required tibialis anterior tendon transfer. The authors investigated predictive factors for relapses. The only predictive factor was compliance with the boot and bar brace. Age, previous treatment, and number of cases were not significantly predictive factors [3].

Metatarsus Adductus

This condition is covered in Chapter 3.

Flat Foot (Pes Planus)

Flat foot is not a disease as such, but it is a clinical sign that presents in normal physiological conditions, as well as in pathological conditions. The commonest cause for flat feet is developmental flat feet present in all infants, most children, and some adults. Developmental flat feet are covered in Chapter 3.

In this section, we cover pathological flat feet, which are summarized in Table 8.4.

Congenital Vertical Talus
Overview

Congenital vertical talus (convex pes valgus) is an irreducible dorsal dislocation of the navicular bone on the talus. The foot assumes a rocker-bottom shape (Figure 8.8).

The incidence is 1 in 150 000 births, with no sex predilection, and is bilateral in 50% of cases. It may occur as an isolated foot

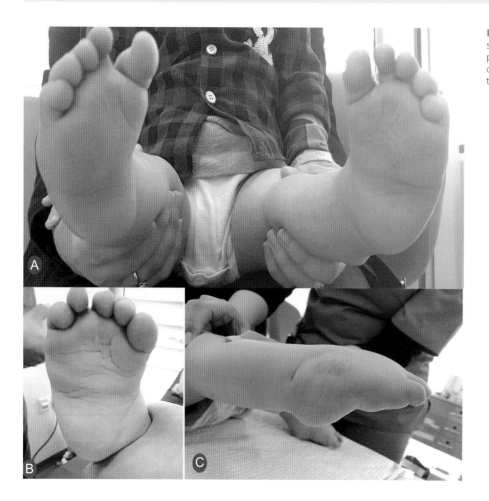

Figure 8.7 Atypical club foot (A). The foot is short and stubby (B). It is very stiff with severe plantar flexion of all metatarsals, with a deep crease just above the heel and across the side of the midfoot, with a short big toe (C).

Table 8.4 Common pathological flat feet

Causes	Notes
Congenital vertical talus	Usually apparent in the first year of life. It should be differentiated from the oblique talus, which is a common radiological finding in developmental flat feet
Tarsal coalition	Usually presents with recurrent twisting injuries or difficulty walking on uneven surfaces
Accessary navicular bone	Flat feet are commonly associated with an accessory navicular bone, but it is not a constant feature. This is not always symptomatic and not always rigid
Tibialis posterior insufficiency	This is very common in elderly women (often termed acquired adult flat feet). Rare in children unless there is trauma, including surgical transfer of the tendon
Tight gastrocnemius muscles (or tendo Achilles) with or without midfoot break	This is getting commoner with changes in lifestyle. Many children spend long periods of time being sedentary
Trauma, including surgical	
Juvenile rheumatoid arthritis	

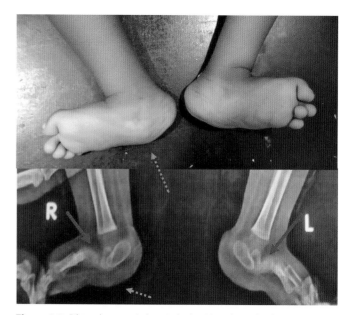

Figure 8.8 Bilateral congenital vertical talus. Note the rocker-bottom-shaped feet (dashed green arrows). Both tali are plantar subluxed (red arrows).

anomaly or in association with other neuromuscular conditions such as myelomeningocele, arthrogryposis, or chromosomal abnormalities [4].

Pathoanatomy

The cause is unknown, but muscle imbalance, intrauterine compression, and growth arrest during fetal development have been suggested. The navicular articulates with the dorsal aspect of the neck of the talus. The calcaneum is displaced posterolaterally with respect to the talus and is in equinus.

Diagnosis and Evaluation

Diagnosis is made by clinical and radiological examinations (lateral radiograph of the foot in maximum plantar flexion).

On clinical examination, the foot has a convex plantar surface; the talar head is prominent medially, and the midfoot is dorsiflexed and abducted in relation to the hindfoot. The hindfoot is in equinovalgus, giving the appearance of a Persian slipper. In addition, the Achilles, tibialis anterior, and peroneal tendons are contracted. Passive correction of this deformity is not possible.

On a lateral radiograph taken with the foot in maximum plantar flexion, the hallmark of vertical talus is that a line drawn along the long axis of the talus appears vertical (almost parallel to the tibia) and also passes plantarward to a line drawn along the first metatarsal cuneiform axes (Figures 8.9 and 8.10).

Differential Diagnosis

1. Oblique talus is a benign condition, with a good prognosis, and must be distinguished from vertical talus. In oblique talus, the valgus deformity of the hindfoot is passively correctable and this restores the medial arch. Moreover, on a lateral radiograph, the navicular is reduced on the talus, with the foot maximally plantar flexed.

2. Calcaneovalgus foot deformity. The calcaneum is in calcaneus, and not in equinus.

3. Paralytic pes valgus. Neurological features are usually present.

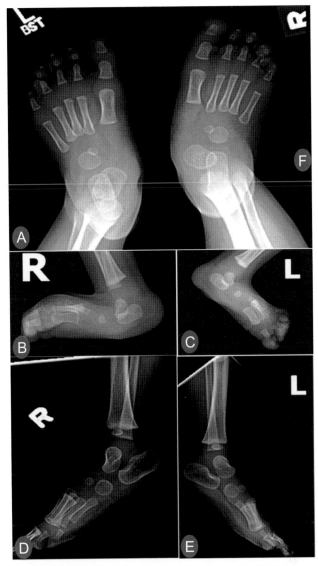

Figure 8.9 Radiological assessment of congenital vertical talus (A-E). The right talus bone is vertical and almost aligned with the tibial axis (A). The calcaneal pitch is reversed on the right side, and the calcaneum is in marked equinus. This has created a rocker-bottom soft tissue shadow (B). On forced plantar flexion views (D, E), the left talus is aligned very well with the first ray, but the right talus is still flexed.

Figure 8.10 Forced plantar flexion views demonstrating the alignment of the left and right talus bones with the first ray. On the left, they are aligned well and the soft tissue shadow of the foot arch is nicely visible, but this is not the case on the right side.

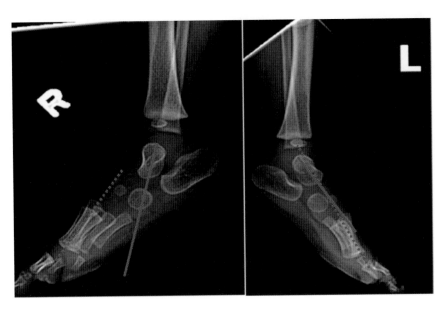

4. Severe flat foot (also called planovalgus foot). Unless there are neurological problems, this is usually flexible and easily correctable, in contrast to congenital vertical talus.

Treatment

Non-surgical

Initial treatment involves manipulation and serial casting, with the corrective forces applied opposite to those required during Ponseti casting for congenital talipes equino varus (often termed the reversed Ponseti method).

Manipulation and serial casting are usually not sufficient to correct the deformity fully and surgery is often required.

Surgical

Surgery is usually undertaken between 6 and 12 months of age and involves soft tissue releases, including tendo Achilles lengthening, reduction of the talonavicular joint, and K-wire stabilization (Figure 8.11). Additional surgery may be required such as reconstruction of the spring ligament and transfer of the tibialis anterior tendon to the dorsum of the talus.

In older children or neglected cases, it may be necessary to excise the navicular and carry out more extensive surgery. The outcome is less predictable.

Tarsal Coalition

Overview

Tarsal coalition is an abnormal connection between two or more bones in the foot. The connection may be fibrous, cartilaginous, or bony. The reported incidence varies between 1% and 6%; in 50% of affected individuals, it is bilateral.

Coalitions may be solitary or multiple. The commonest site is calcaneonavicular, followed by talocalcaneal. Talocalcaneal coalitions usually involve the middle facet. Coalitions are associated with limb abnormalities such as fibular hemimelia and proximal femoral focal deficiency.

Pathoanatomy

Tarsal coalitions are thought to be the result of failure of segmentation of mesenchymal tissue in the developing foot. Although coalitions may be present at birth, symptoms such as pain appear later in life, usually at age between 10 and 12 years for calcaneonavicular coalitions, and between 12 and 15 years for talocalcaneal coalitions [5].

Evaluation

The presenting history and physical examination are suggestive, but radiographs, CT, or MRI are required to confirm the diagnosis. (MRI is more accurate than CT in demonstrating fibrous coalitions.)

Pain is usually the initial complaint and is typically localized over the sinus tarsi, although it may be present in other parts of the foot. It is aggravated by sporting activities. Clinical evaluation reveals a planovalgus foot. On tiptoeing, the hindfoot valgus does not correct and the medial arch does not reconstitute (Figure 8.12). In addition, the range of movement to the subtalar joint is decreased.

A standing oblique radiograph provides the best view for diagnosing a calcaneonavicular coalition. A CT scan may be required to diagnose a talocalcaneal coalition and, in addition, to determine the size of the coalition, as this provides useful information regarding surgical options.

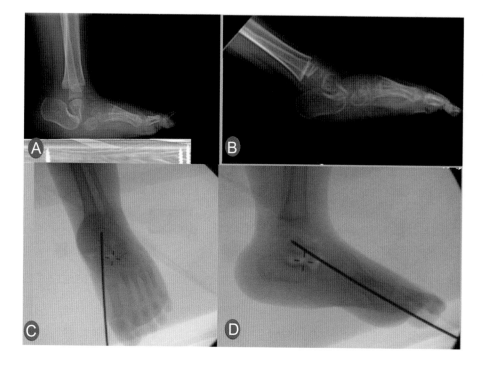

Figure 8.11 Congenital vertical talus (A)which does not correct in forced plantar flexion views. (B) The patient underwent serial casting, followed by open reduction and K-wire stabilization of the joint(C,D).

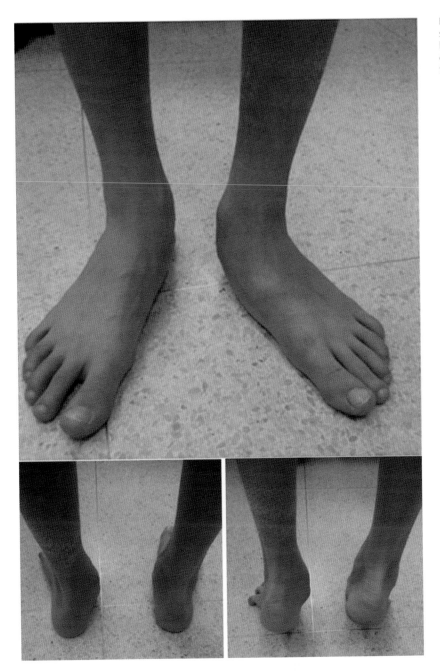

Figure 8.12 Tarsal coalition. The clinical photographs show a left flat foot, an abducted forefoot, and a valgus heel that does not correct to varus on tiptoeing, in comparison to the right foot. The underlying diagnosis is tarsal coalition.

Lateral standing radiographs will show features such as the anteater sign and C-sign that are suggestive of calcaneonavicular and talocalcaneal coalitions, respectively (Figure 8.13).

Treatment

The goal of treatment is pain relief and to improve joint motion.

Non-surgical

An initial trial of non-operative management is recommended; this involves use of non-steroidal anti-inflammatory drugs (NSAIDs), activity modification, insoles, and/or a period of immobilization in a below-knee weight-bearing cast for 4–6 weeks.

Surgery should be considered in patients who continue to have symptoms despite a period of non-operative management.

Surgery

Several studies reported excellent results in over 85% of patients with excision of calcaneonavicular coalitions and graft interposition (Figure 8.14). The reported recurrence rate ranged from 0% to 30% [6]. Several types of graft have been used, including bone wax, fat, and extensor digitorum brevis tendon. The literature is contradictory, although use of tendon grafts is falling out of favour [7].

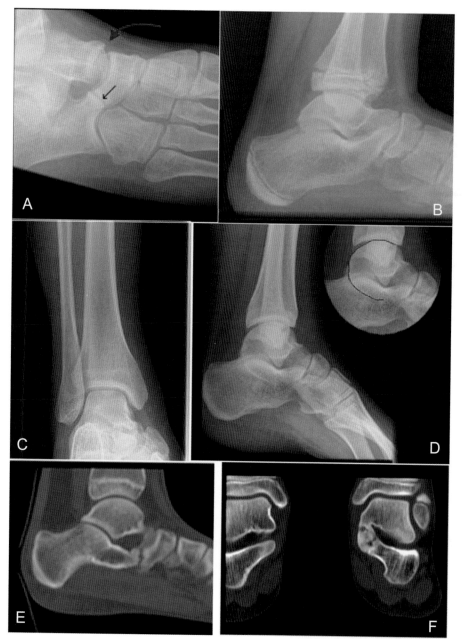

Figure 8.13 Tarsal coalition radiology. These X-rays show various recognized radiological signs of tarsal coalition seen in different patients. (A) Calcaneonavicular coalition marked by a straight black arrow. The anterior process of the calcaneum can be elongated, mimicking the anteater nose (B). Talar peaking is another sign of tarsal coalition and is marked by a curved red arrow (A). (C) Ball-and-socket ankle joint secondary to remodelling of the joint to compensate for subtalar motion loss. (D) C-sign. (E) CT scan (sagittal cut) showing a calcaneonavicular fibrous tarsal coalition. (F) CT scan (coronal cut) showing a talocalcaneal tarsal coalition on the right, in comparison to the normal left side.

Excision of talocalcaneal coalitions (Figure 8.15) is less successful, in comparison with that of calcaneonavicular coalitions. It is not recommended if it is >50% of the middle facet. A medial hindfoot approach is advised. Associated deformity (such as valgus heel of >20°) requires correction for better outcome.

A triple or subtalar arthrodesis may be required in the presence of degenerative changes or multiple coalitions, or if symptoms persist despite previous surgery to excise a coalition.

Accessory Navicular
Overview

An accessory navicular is an accessory ossification centre at the medial side of the navicular; it is considered a normal anatomical variant. It is observed in 12% of the population.

Evaluation

Most accessory naviculars are asymptomatic and are diagnosed incidentally, following radiographic examination after an

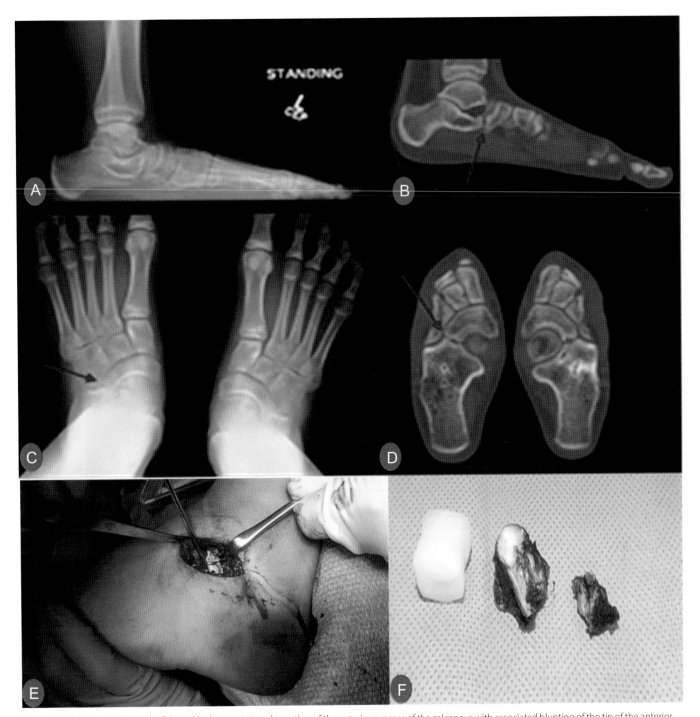

Figure 8.14 Lateral radiograph of the ankle demonstrates elongation of the anterior process of the calcaneus with associated blunting of the tip of the anterior process of the calcaneus known as the anteater sign(A). Calcaneonavicular tarsal coalition (red arrows)(B, C). (E) and (F) are photographs taken intraoperatively of the coalition before and after excision. Bone wax is made of the shape of the excised bone to fill the gap. Obvious advantages of use of bone wax include: quick procedure; no donor site morbidity; unlimited availability; and strong bone inhibition. That is why use of bone wax is our preferred option

injury to the foot (Figure 8.16). Three types have been described (Figure 8.17).

A child with a symptomatic accessory navicular bone will present with pain over the medial aspect of the midfoot that is usually aggravated by tight-fitting shoes. A tender prominence will be observed to this area of the foot, and resisted inversion may be painful.

Treatment

If asymptomatic, reassurance is usually all that is required. If symptomatic, initial management is non-operative and involves the use of soft insole, or a below-knee weight-bearing cast for a short period, to relieve pressure and symptoms.

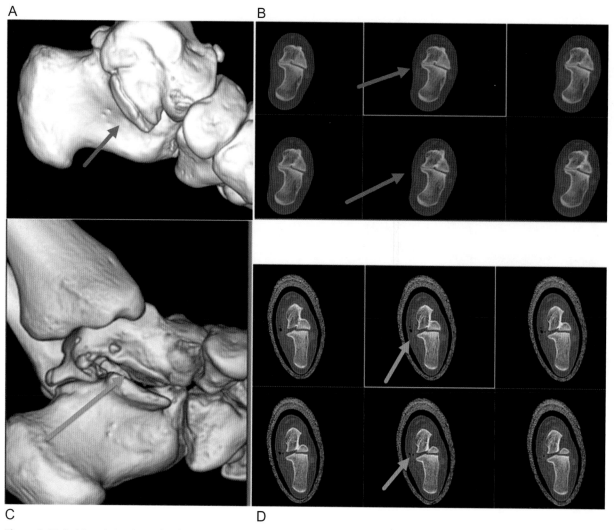

Figure 8.15 Excision of talocalcaneal coalitions. (A) and (B) show the coalition (red arrows) before excision, and (C) and (D) after excision.

If pain persists despite a trial of non-operative treatment, surgery may be required to excise the accessory navicular. The tibialis posterior tendon is peeled off subperiosteally to allow complete excision of the accessory navicular bone. However, sometimes, the tendon becomes fully detached from the bone. In this case, it must be reattached either through a bone tunnel or an anchor suture (Figure 8.18).

Tight Gastrocnemius Muscle (or Tendo Achilles) with or without Midfoot Break

There has been a significant change in lifestyle with more children spending more time on screen watching videos than playing in the playground. This causes many children to develop muscle tightness, particularly in the muscles that cross several growth plates such as the gastrocnemius and hamstrings. Bones grow longer through the growth plate; then muscles get stretched to match the adjacent bones during playing. Sedentary lifestyles do not promote muscle stretching and lead to relative shortening of the muscles.

This is initially present with a bouncy gait (children go on their toes towards the end of the terminal stance phase). Careful assessment of ankle dorsiflexion (Silfverskiöld test) reveals tightness in the gastrocnemius muscle. Normal walking requires at least 20° of ankle dorsiflexion to allow the body to move forward on planted foot during the stance phase of the gait. Gastrocnemius muscle tightness prevents the required ankle dorsiflexion and the foot is forced into equinus and abduction (manifests as out-toeing and loss of the medial arch). Eventually, with increasing body weight, the talonavicular joint subluxates (this is known as midfoot break among orthopaedic surgeons) (Figure 8.19).

Plain weight radiograph often shows talonavicular joint subluxation where the navicular bone does not cover the talus head fully. The angle between the talus bone axis and the first metatarsal is increased (normally is 10 ± 7°) (Figure 8.20).

Prevention is better than treatment. Education about the importance of healthy lifestyle is important. Muscle tightness should be treated promptly with physiotherapy to stretch the muscles, but also parents and children should be educated.

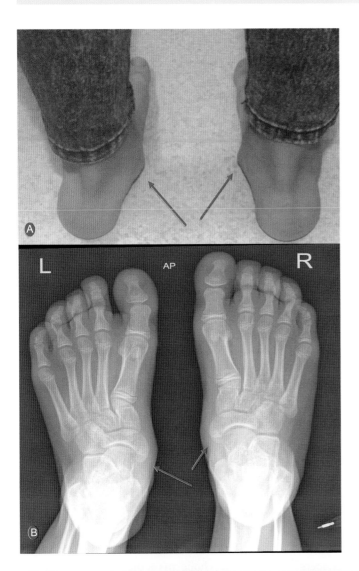

Figure 8.16 Accessory navicular bones marked with red arrows on the clinical photograph (A) and the plain radiograph of the feet (B).

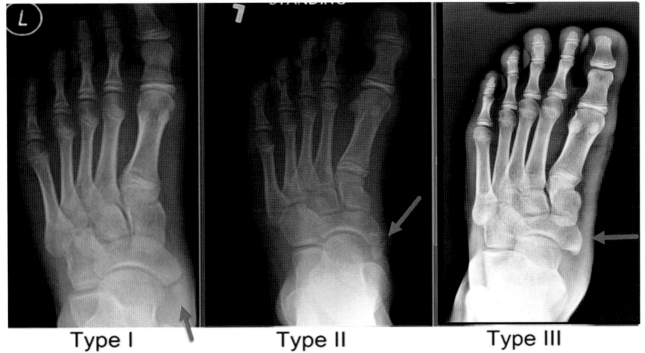

Figure 8.17 Types of accessory navicular bone. Type I is a small, round ossicle within the substance of the posterior tibialis tendon. Type II is larger and triangular-shaped, and is connected to the navicular by a cartilaginous or fibrocartilaginous synchondrosis. Type II is a cornuate-shaped navicular, following fusion between the accessory and the anatomical navicular bones. Type IV has been also described when there is a small extra bony ossicle beside type III.

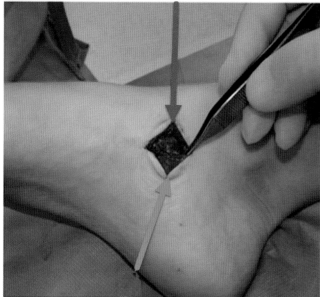

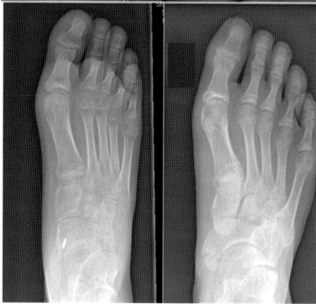

Figure 8.18 Excision of accessory navicular bone. The green arrow points to the tibialis posterior tendon, which was initially peeled off the bone subperiosteally. However, complete detachment was necessary to remove the accessory bone and reshape the main bone. The tendon was reattached using an anchor suture.

Serial casting to stretch the gastrocnemius muscle can be employed if physiotherapy is not effective. However, when talonavicular joint subluxation occurs (Figure 8.20), physiotherapy and serial casting are not usually effective and may make the joint subluxation worse. Surgery is required to correct the foot and for lengthening of either the tendon or the gastrocnemius muscle, depending on which one is involved (Video 8.2).

 Video 8.2 Gastrocnemius fractional lengthening and calcaneal lengthening.

Kohler's Disease

Overview

Kohler's disease is osteochondritis of the tarsal navicular. It is frequently bilateral and is seen more commonly in boys (4:1), usually between the ages of 2–8 years. It is a self-limiting condition and resolves over a period of 18 months to 3 years.

Pathoanatomy

Like other osteochondritides, Kohler's disease is thought to be due to avascular necrosis.

The navicular is the last tarsal bone to ossify (after 2 years), and it is thought that it is therefore more susceptible to mechanical compression injury causing avascular necrosis.

Evaluation

Patients present with midfoot pain. Tenderness and swelling may be observed over the dorsum of the midfoot; in addition, the child may have a limp.

Radiographs confirm the diagnosis. Flattening, sclerosis, or fragmentation of the navicular are observed (Figure 8.21). These radiographic changes disappear over time.

Treatment

The mainstay of treatment is activity modification. Immobilization of the affected limb in a below-knee weight-bearing cast for 4–6 weeks may be required and has been shown to reduce the duration of symptoms. Surgery is never indicated.

Freiberg's Disease

Overview

Freiberg's disease is osteochondritis of the metatarsal head. The second metatarsal is most commonly affected, although occasionally the third may be involved. It is commonly seen in girls over the age of 13 years.

The cause is unknown. However, it is thought to be due to avascular necrosis of the metatarsal head due to microfracture secondary to repetitive stresses.

Evaluation

Patients may present with pain, with or without a prominence to the dorsum of the foot overlying the second metatarsal head, although occasionally the diagnosis is made incidentally after radiographic examination of the foot following an injury.

Clinically, localized tenderness, with or without a swelling, may be observed. There may also be an associated deformity of the respective toe, and the patient may have a limp.

An MRI scan may help make the diagnosis before radiographic changes occur. Radiographs show irregularity of the articular surface, sclerosis, and fragmentation of the metatarsal head (Figure 8.22).

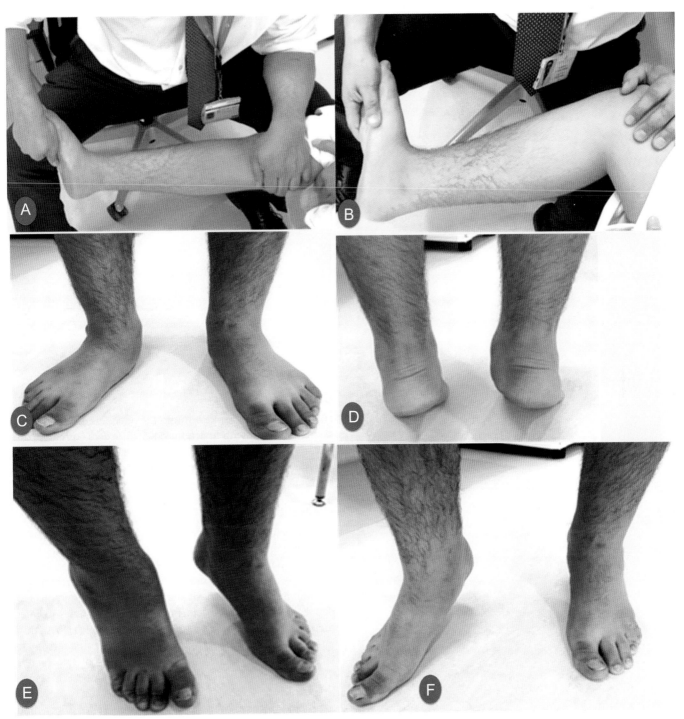

Figure 8.19 Gastrocnemius muscle tightness and midfoot break. (A) and (B) demonstrate gastrocnemius tightness mainly (around −30° of equinus, with the knee fully extended). There is some tightness of the soleus, but this is very minor (ankle dorsiflexion with the knee flexed around +15°). (C) and (D) show a fallen medial arch of the right foot, mainly causing a rigid flat foot (the heel does not move to varus and the medial longitudinal arch does not correct on tip-toeing) (C–F). The resultant flat foot is not always rigid, particularly early in the disease.

Treatment

A trial of conservative management is usually advised in symptomatic cases. Options include rest, activity modification, use of hard-soled shoes, and a below-knee weight-bearing cast.

Surgery may be required if the patient is symptomatic despite a trial of non-operative treatment. Surgical options include joint debridement or cheilectomy, or a dorsiflexion osteotomy of the metatarsal neck.

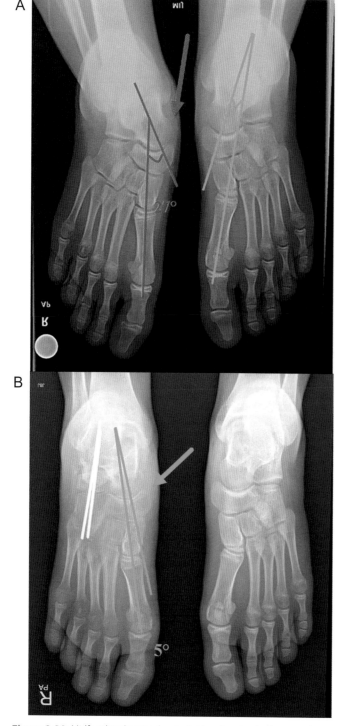

A

B

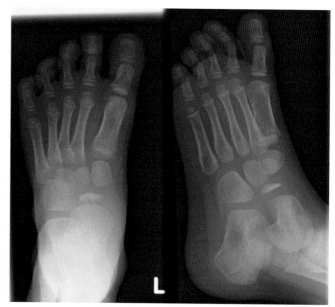

Figure 8.21 Kohler's disease. Notice flattening and sclerosis of the navicular bone.

Hallux Valgus

Overview

Hallux valgus or juvenile bunions are often familial but may be seen in children with neuromuscular disorders (cerebral palsy or connective tissue diseases such as Ehlers–Danlos syndrome).

There is often a familial preponderance (88%), and it is often bilateral.

Evaluation

Diagnosis is clinical, but radiographs are required to assess the severity of the deformity. In addition to examination of the foot, a full examination is required, to check for signs of generalized ligamentous laxity or other underlying causes such as cerebral palsy.

Standing foot (dorsal–plantar and lateral) radiographs help define the severity of the deformity. The normal angles are intermetatarsal angle (IMA ≤10°), hallux valgus angle (HVA ≤15°), distal metatarsal articular angle (DMAA ≤15°), first tarsometatarsal angle (TMA <25°), and length of the first metatarsal relative to the second are important parameters to be measured (Figure 8.23).

Hallux valgus may be classified into mild (HVA <30°), moderate (HVA 30–40°), or severe (HVA >40°).

Treatment

Some conservative treatment options may help relieve pain but do not correct the deformity. Patients should be encouraged to wear comfortable shoes and to avoid high-heeled or pointed shoes. Various hallux valgus orthoses have been used

Figure 8.20 Midfoot break secondary to tight gastrocnemius (same patient as in Figure 8.19). (A) is a preoperative plain radiograph showing the uncovering of the talus head (red arrow) with an increased talo-first metatarsal angle. The patient underwent gastrocnemius muscle lengthening and calcaneus bone lengthening (B). Notice the improved covering of the talus head and the restoration of the talo-first metatarsal angle.

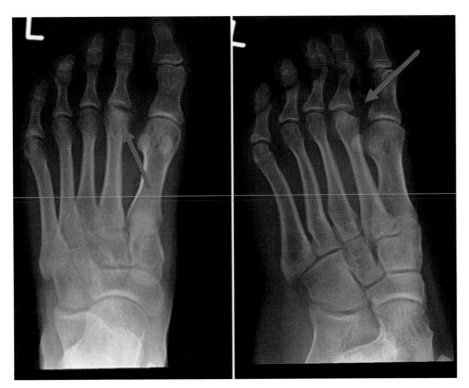

Figure 8.22 Freiberg's disease.

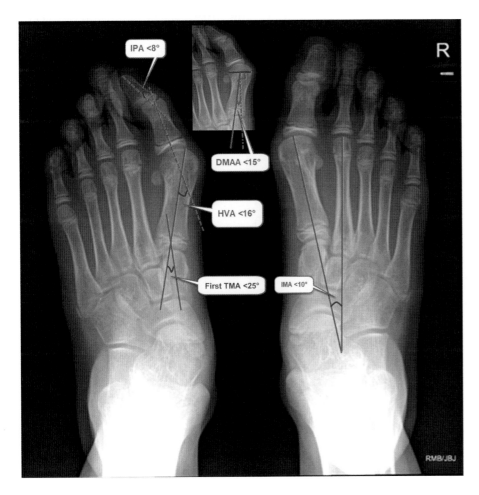

IPA <8°

DMAA <15°

HVA <16°

First TMA <25°

IMA <10°

R

Figure 8.23 Hallux valgus radiology measurements. The interphalangeal angle (IPA) uncovers any hallux interphalangeus. The hallux valgus angle (HVA) indicates the severity of the valgus deformity. Excessive intermetatarsal angle (IMA) indicates metatarsus primus varus (varus of the first metatarsal). This may be an indication for proximal corrective osteotomy either at the metatarsal base or through the medial cuneiform. The distal metatarsal articular angle (DMAA) is the angle between the first metatarsal longitudinal axis and the line perpendicular to the articular line. Some books use the angle between the articular line and the main axis, quoting 85° as a normal value. The numbers on the X-ray represent the normal values, and not the actual measurement of this patient. Notice the presence of the accessory navicular bone and bilateral midfoot breaks (talonavicular subluxations), which were caused by tight gastrocnemius muscle.

(Figure 8.24). They may help with pain and buy time, but their effectiveness in slowing the deformity or reversing it is not proven.

Surgery may be considered if symptoms are unacceptable and non-surgical measures fail. Patients and their parents must be warned of the high rate of recurrence after surgery and complications such as overcorrection, hallux varus, and joint stiffness.

Surgical intervention often involves soft tissue balance of the metatarsophalangeal joint (MTPJ) and bunionectomy. The joint is approached medially. A Y-V capsulotomy is performed to allow bunionectomy and capsular repair. The abductor halluces are released if tight. These are often not enough and an osteotomy is often required.

Osteotomy options can be distal, such as Chevron ostetomy, when the IMA is within normal. Proximal osteotomy is indicated when the IMA is high. Options include Scarf or proximal medial opening wedge osteotomy of the first metatarsal. Guided growth using the proximal physis of the first metatarsal is being explored. Given the slow growth of the bone, it is slow to show effect and it is often inadequate.

Abnormal DMAA should be considered when designing the above osteotomies. A small wedge at the end of osteotomized bone can improve the direction of the MTPJ, improving outcome and minimizing recurrence. Akin osteotomy of the proximal phalanx can be added when there is hallux interphalangeus (interphalangeal angle >8°) [8].

Hallux Varus
Overview

This is medial deviation of the big toe (also called atavistic big toe) (Figure 8.27). It is often congenital (although acquired cases happen after hallux valgus overcorrection). Three types are described:

1. Isolated hallux varus (normal first metatarsal and proximal phalanx). This is usually caused by a tight band (fibrotic abductor hallucis muscle). There is also mild metatarsal adductus
2. Associated with other malformations such as bracket epiphysis or polydactyly
3. Associated with skeletal dysplasia (such as diastrophic dwarfism).

Evaluation

Diagnosis is clinical. Complaints are usually about how they look, pain, and interference with shoe wear.

Treatment

1. Observation (they usually, however, get worse)
2. Surgical:
   a. Abductor hallucis muscle releases in type I.
   b. Excision of the central portion of the epiphyseal bracket ± corrective osteotomy for type II (Figure 8.28)

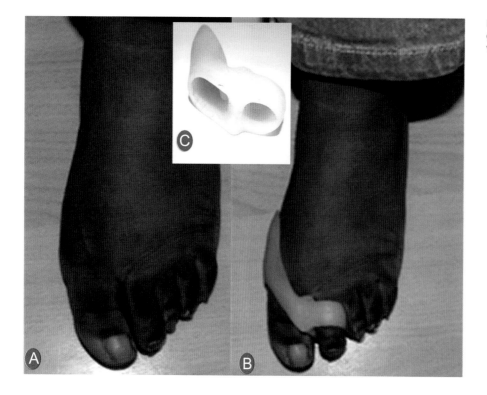

Figure 8.24 Interdigital spacer and bunion guard(B,C) to alleviate symptoms of hallux valgus.(A)

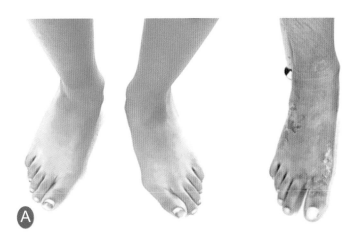

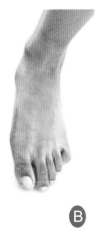

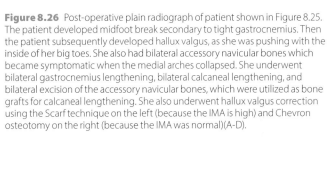

Figure 8.25 Hallux valgus. (A) shows a preoperative clinical photograph. (B) shows a post-operative radiograph. Other operations were performed (see Figure 8.26 for radiograph).

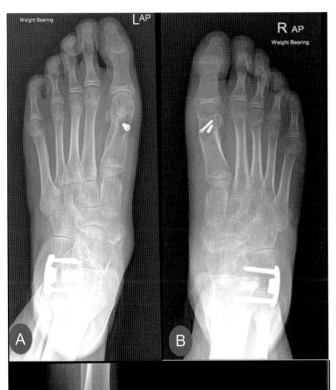

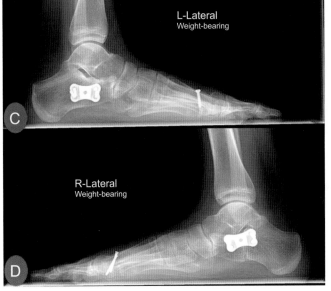

Figure 8.26 Post-operative plain radiograph of patient shown in Figure 8.25. The patient developed midfoot break secondary to tight gastrocnemius. Then the patient subsequently developed hallux valgus, as she was pushing with the inside of her big toes. She also had bilateral accessory navicular bones which became symptomatic when the medial arches collapsed. She underwent bilateral gastrocnemius lengthening, bilateral calcaneal lengthening, and bilateral excision of the accessory navicular bones, which were utilized as bone grafts for calcaneal lengthening. She also underwent hallux valgus correction using the Scarf technique on the left (because the IMA is high) and Chevron osteotomy on the right (because the IMA was normal)(A-D).

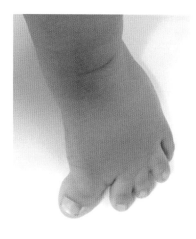

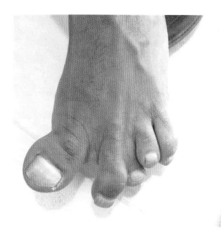

Figure 8.27 Hallux varus in a father and son. Always ask whether there are any other family members who have the same deformity. Parents do not always volunteer this information. Hallux varus usually gets worse, but not always.

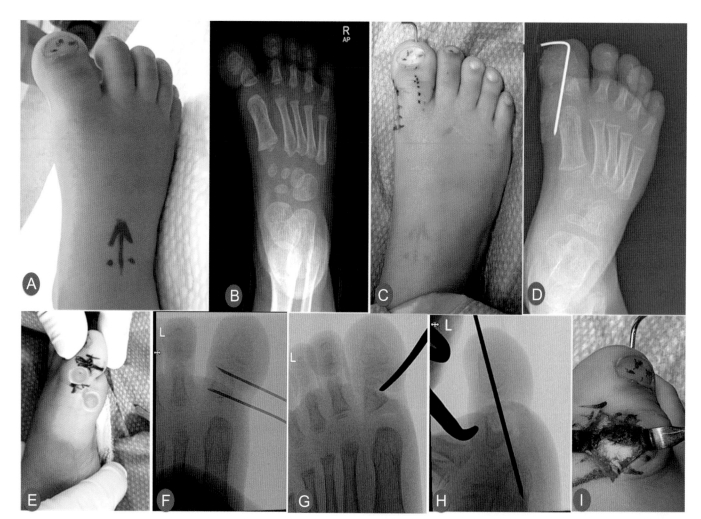

Figure 8.28 Hallux varus type II with epiphyseal bracket which underwent excision and corrective osteotomy. (A, B) Preoperative clinical photograph and radiograph, respectively. (C, D) Post-operative clinical photograph and radiograph, respectively. (E) to (I) show the steps of surgery: medial approach; the bracket is identified using a needle and an image intensifier; careful excision; osteotomy of the phalanx; and stabilization of the phalanx in the corrected position. *Source:* Images are courtesy of Dr Ibrar Majid, Al Jalila Children's Speciality Hospital, Dubai.

c. Farmer and McElvenny procedure. Soft tissue balancing procedure with syndactylization of the second toe and hallux

d. Arthrodesis reserved for recurrent hallux varus with arthritic MTPJ.

Overlying Fifth Toes
Overview

An overlying fifth toe (varus fifth toe) is a dorsal adduction deformity of the fifth toe. It is usually present at birth and is typically familial and bilateral. The extensor digitorum longus tendon is contracted.

Evaluation

Diagnosis is clinical (Figure 8.29). Pain may develop over time due to footwear irritation.

Treatment

Conservative measures, such as buddy strapping, are ineffective and surgery is usually advised. Surgery involves a double racquet skin incision around the toe, tenotomy of the extensor digitorum longus, and dorsal capsulotomy of the MTPJ, with or without temporary stabilization of the toe with a K-wire in the corrected position for 2–4 weeks (Butler's procedure). The risk of vascular injury with surgery is real and parents must be warned accordingly.

Curly Toes

This deformity is characterized by flexion and medial deviation of the proximal interphalangeal joint of the affected toe, and results in the affected toe underlying an adjacent one. Contracture of the flexor digitorum longus and brevis tendons is the commonest cause.

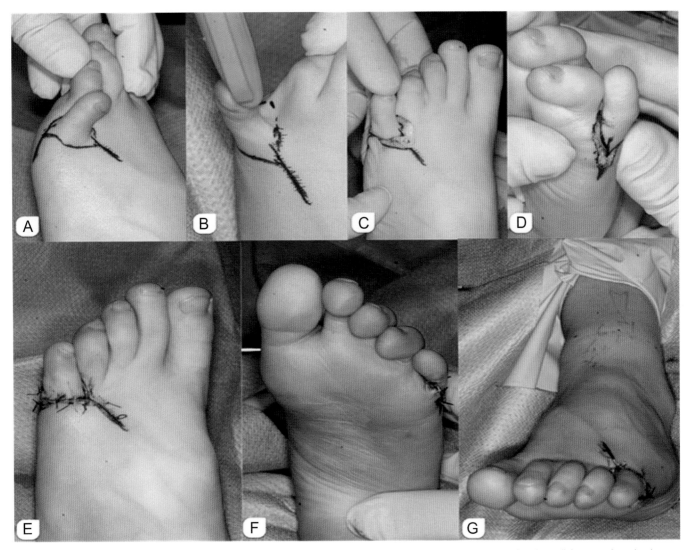

Figure 8.29 Overlapping and curly toes. The essence of Butler's procedure is to lengthen all the tight structures at the back and to pull the toe in the right place using the dermodesis principle(A,B). A double racket incision releases the extensor digitorum longus and also releases the dorsal capsule(C,D). The skin is then closed (Y in V on the plantar aspect(E), and V in Y on the dorsal aspect(F)). A K-wire may be used to keep the corrected position when there are bony changes that prevent stability(F).Post-op picture following surgical correction (G)

Curly toes are usually bilateral; the third and fourth toes are commonly affected. There is often a positive family history.

In 76% of children affected, the deformity persists and surgery may be required, as toe strapping only improves the deformity temporarily. The recommended surgical option is an open tenotomy of the flexor digitorum longus and brevis tendons (Figure 8.30). A randomized controlled trial did not show a superior result with flexor-to-extensor tendon transfer. Rarely, when there are bony changes, osteotomy may be required.

Pes Cavus
Overview

Pes cavus is a foot with a high longitudinal arch. It is often associated with clawing of the toes and a varus hindfoot. Two-thirds of patients with pes cavus have an underlying neurological condition such as hereditary sensorimotor neuropathy (HSMN), for example, Charcot–Marie–Tooth (CMT) disease, cerebral palsy, spinal dysraphism, poliomyelitis, or Friedreich's ataxia. It may also be secondary to compartment syndrome following an injury to the leg.

Morphologically, there are four types of pes cavus (Figure 8.31):

1. Cavovarus (commonest)
2. Calcaneocavus
3. Calcaneus
4. Plantaris.

Pathoanatomy

Muscle imbalance prevents the foot from positioning correctly. Strong muscles pull the foot to one direction, for example, in CMT disease, which is one of the commonest causes for pes cavus. The tibialis posterior is stronger than the peroneus brevis, pulling the hindfoot in varus. This elevates the first ray of the floor by virtue of anatomical connection. The body compensates by depressing the first ray down through the peroneus longus (the tripod theory; Figure 8.31). This creates the typical high-arched foot (cavovarus type) that is seen in CMT disease. This is initially flexible, but later it becomes fixed. The Coleman block test is used to differentiate between flexible and fixed deformity (see Chapter 2, Figure 2.11).

Furthermore, the weak tibialis anterior causes foot drop. The extensor hallucis and long toe extensors compensate for this weakness and this leads to clawing of the lesser toes (Figure 8.32).

Evaluation and Diagnosis

Diagnosis of the cavus deformity is usually made after a thorough examination of the foot/ankle.

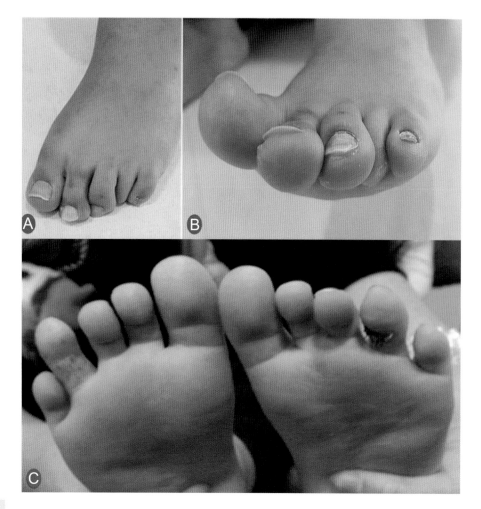

Figure 8.30 Curly fourth toes (A,B) treated with flexor tenotomies (C).

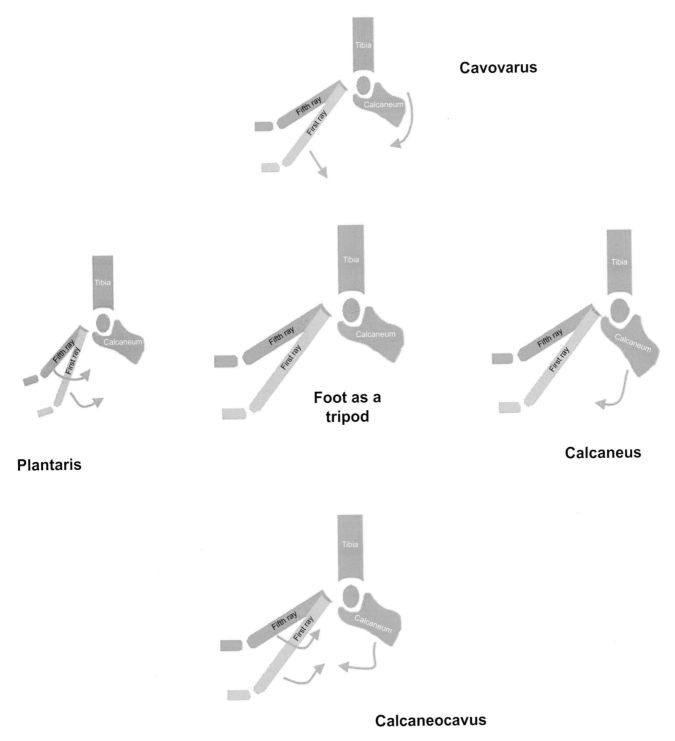

Figure 8.31 Pes cavus: morphological types.

A family history and a full neurological examination, including examination of the spine, are paramount. A hairy patch on the back is suggestive of spinal dysraphism. Unilateral limb involvement suggests a focal diagnosis, that is, spinal cord or nerve injury, whereas bilateral involvement suggests generalized neuropathy such as HSMN. In the latter, examination of the dorsum of the hand may reveal guttering due to intrinsic muscle wasting.

In a cavovarus foot, it is essential to carry out a Coleman block test to determine if the hindfoot varus is flexible or fixed (see Chapter 2, Figure 2.11). This has important implications when planning surgical treatment. In unilateral cavus feet, calf muscle atrophy may be observed and the affected foot often appears shorter.

Standing radiographs of the foot/ankle help quantify the severity of the deformity. Meary's angle (normal = 0°) is

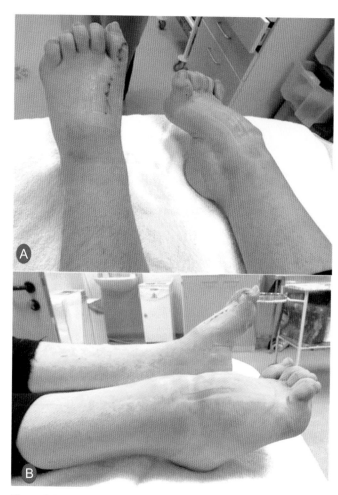

Figure 8.32 Pes cavus in a child with hereditary sensorimotor neuropathy disease. She had corrective surgery for the left side. Notice the varus heel, flexed first ray, and clawed toes.

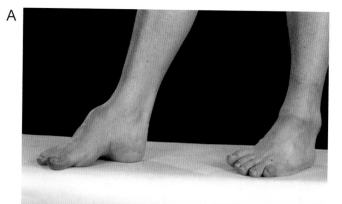

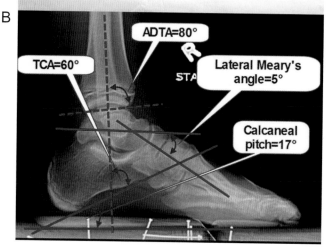

Figure 8.33 Pes cavus. (A) A clinical photograph of a child with pes cavus (high-arched foot). (B) Common radiological measures around the foot and ankle in the context of pes cavus: anterior distal tibial angle (ADTA) = 80° (78–82°); lateral Meary's angle (tibiocalcaneal axis and first metatarsal axis) = 5° (1–9°); calcaneal pitch = 17° (11–23°); tibiocalcaneal angle (TCA): longitudinal axis of the tibia and calcaneum (more useful than calcaneal pitch if there is associated equinus deformity) = 60° (60–80°). Hibbs angle (not shown) is the angle between the longitudinal axis of the calcaneum and the first metatarsal axis = 150°. Some references quote slightly different values of these angles or use the complementary angle instead, which can create some confusion.

increased in cavus feet, whereas Hibbs angle (normal >150°) is usually decreased (Figure 8.33).

Consultation with a neurologist is useful. Nerve conduction studies, MRI of the brain and/or spine, muscle biopsy, and DNA assay may be required to help establish the underlying cause.

Treatment

The aim of treatment is to relieve symptoms (pain, ankle instability), correct deformity, and minimize the risk of recurrence of the deformity.

Asymptomatic patients do not usually require treatment. Conservative treatment options, such as orthosis, muscle stretching, and strengthening exercises, play a limited role.

The mainstay of treatment is surgical. The type of surgery undertaken depends on the age of the patient, symptoms, muscle strength/weakness, and rigidity of the deformity, as well as the underlying causes. The following are commonly used to address pes cavus deformity:

1. Tendo Achilles lengthening if there is equinus deformity

2. Lateral calcaneal slide or lateral calcaneal closing wedge osteotomy to correct heel valgus. The former is preferable, as the closing wedge makes the heel shorter

3. First (±second) metatarsal base osteotomy to correct plantar flexion deformity

4. Jones transfer in which the extensor hallucis longus tendon is freed and reattached to the first or second metatarsal to act as ankle dorsiflexors. To prevent contracture of the big toe flexor caused by the unopposed flexor hallucis longus, either MTPJ tenodesis (using the remnant of the extensor hallucis longus as a checkrein) or arthrodesis is performed

5. Weak muscle powering to prevent recurrence by tendon transfers. The commonest is tibialis posterior (whole or split) transfer to the peroneus brevis OR to the tibialis anterior; peroneus longus to peroneus brevis tendon transfer.

References

1. Herring JA. *Tachdjians' Pediatric Orthopaedics*, 5th ed. Philadelphia, PA: Saunders Elsevier; 2014.

2. Steinman S, Richards BS, Faulks S, Kaipus K. A comparison of two nonoperative methods of idiopathic clubfoot correction: the Ponseti method and the French functional (physiotherapy) method. Surgical technique. *J Bone Joint Surg Am*. 2009;91 Suppl 2:299–312.

3. Morcuende JA, Dolan LA, Dietz FR, Ponseti IV. Radical reduction in the rate of extensive corrective surgery for clubfoot using the Ponseti method. *Pediatrics*. 2004;113(2):376–80.

4. Drennan JC. Congenital vertical talus. *Instr Course Lect*. 1996;45:315–22.

5. Mubarak SJ, Patel PN, Upasani VV, Moor MA, Wenger DR. Calcaneonavicular coalition: treatment by excision and fat graft. *J Pediatr Orthop*. 2009;29(5):418–26.

6. Chytas A, Chaudhry S, Alshryda S. Evidence-based treatment for tarsal coalition. In: Alshryda S, Huntley JS, Banaszkiewicz PA, eds. *Paediatric Orthopaedics: An Evidence-Based Approach to Clinical Questions*. Cham: Springer; 2016. pp. 175–82.

7. Masquijo J, Allende V, Torres-Gomez A, Dobbs MB. Fat graft and bone wax interposition provides better functional outcomes and lower reossification rates than extensor digitorum brevis after calcaneonavicular coalition resection. *J Pediatr Orthop*. 2017;37(7):e427–31.

8. Robinson AH, Limbers JP. Modern concepts in the treatment of hallux valgus. *J Bone Joint Surg Br*. 2005;87(8):1038–45.

Traumatic Foot and Ankle Disorders

Vittoria Bucknall and Mohammed Al-Maiyah

Anatomical Considerations

The ankle joint is a modified hinge joint between the tibial plafond, the medial and lateral malleoli proximally, and the talus distally. It is stabilized by several ligaments which are essential for normal function (Figure 9.1). These ligaments are:

1. The anterior talofibular (ATFL), calcaneofibular (CFL), and posterior talofibular ligaments (PTFL) on the lateral side. These are collectively called the lateral ligament complex of the ankle

2. The deltoid ligament medially

3. The anterior tibiofibular interosseous ligament (ATiFL) and the posterior tibiofibular ligament (PTiFL) which stabilize the lower ends of the tibia and fibula that articulate together to form the inferior tibiofibular joint (ITFJ) [1].

The distal tibial and fibular epiphyses (secondary ossification centres) begin to appear between the ages of 6 months and 2 years. The tibial secondary ossification centre extends into the medial malleolus at around the age of 7 years and it is usually completed

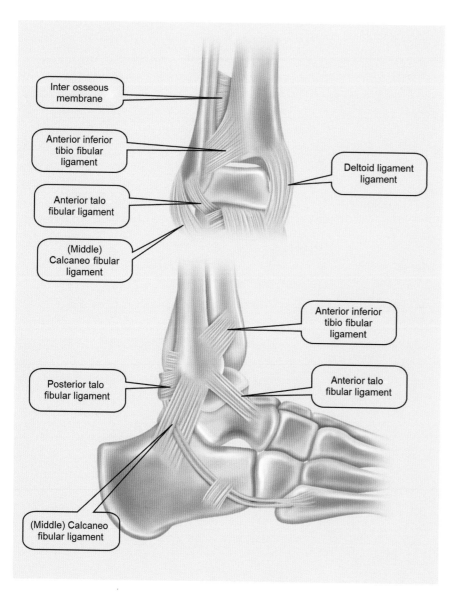

Figure 9.1 Ankle joint ligaments.

at around the age of 10 years. In 20% of cases, there is a separate ossification centre in the medial malleolus. Furthermore, an accessory bone (called os subtibiale) can be found just distal to the tibia. These are two different entities and should not be confused with a fracture. The secondary ossification centre usually appears at around the age of 7 and fuse with the rest of the medial malleolus at around the age of 10, whereas the os subtibiale usually ossifies at various ages and does not fuse with the medial malleolus. The os subtibiale and the secondary ossification centre of the medial malleolus are two different entities [2, 3].

The distal tibial physis closes between the ages of 13 and 16 years during adolescence over an 18-month period. Closure of this physis follows a unique pattern that explains the pattern of fractures seen in this age group, namely the Tillaux and triplane fractures (also called transitional ankle fractures).

The distal tibial physis begins to close centrally, continues medially, and completes laterally. The physes are the weakest spot around the ankle and they usually fail before the ligaments.

Ankle Fractures

Ankle fractures are common injuries in children, constituting approximately 5% of all paediatric fractures, and are the second commonest physeal injury after the distal radius. Although the mechanisms resulting in paediatric ankle fractures may be similar to those in adults, the forces act differently on the paediatric skeleton. Compared to the surrounding ligaments and bone, the physis is relatively weak and fracture lines often propagate through these physeal regions, resulting in unique fracture patterns.

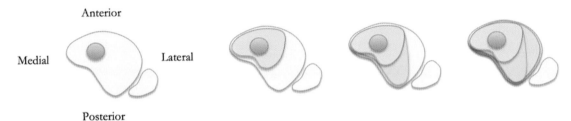

Figure 9.2 Distal tibial physis fusion pattern. The distal tibial physis begins to close centrally (blue dot), expands medially first (pink area), then continues laterally, initially posterolaterally (light green), and finishes in the anterolateral area (light brown).

Figure 9.3 Salter -Harris classification of fractures, as applied to the distal tibia.(A)Normal (B) Salter Harris I (C) Salter Harris II (D) Salter Harris III (E) Salter Harris IV (F) Salter Harris V

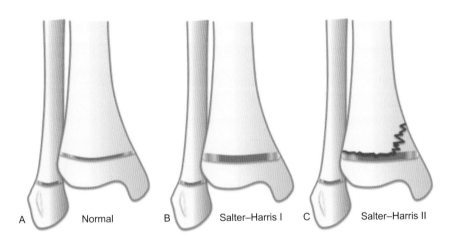

A Normal B Salter–Harris I C Salter–Harris II

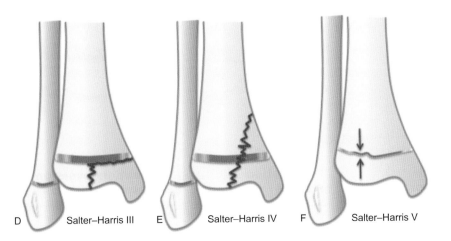

D Salter–Harris III E Salter–Harris IV F Salter–Harris V

The widened physis of a Salter–Harris (SH) type I fracture (Figure 9.3B) or the crushed physis of a SH type V fracture (Figure 9.3F) may be difficult to visualize on plain radiographs. Consequently, a high index of suspicion must be maintained. SH type II fractures account for almost half of ankle fracture patterns and can be diagnosed by the presence of a Thurstan Holland fragment (Figure 9.3C). Type III and IV fractures exit through the epiphysis into the joint line and could represent Tillaux or triplane fractures, respectively. Care must be taken when assessing joint congruity in these injuries, with the ultimate need to achieve anatomical restoration of the joint surface. Type III to V injuries (Figure 9.3D–F) have an increased risk of physeal growth arrest and will need careful follow-up with serial radiographs for up to 2 years.

A further classification of paediatric ankle fractures has been described by Dias and Tachdjian (Figure 9.4; Table 9.1) [4]. This classification takes into account the SH classification, in addition to the familiar Lauge–Hansen classification widely used in adult-pattern injuries. It is used to describe the foot position and deforming forces at the time of injury. Reversing these forces assists in achieving reduction of the fracture. However, if a fracture of the paediatric ankle fails to reduce anatomically with closed reduction, there should be a low threshold for open reduction. This is due to large amounts of thick paediatric periosteum which often incarcerates into the fracture site, causing a physical block to reduction and subsequent union.

Table 9.1 Dias and Tachdjian paediatric ankle fracture classification

Types	Sequence of structure failure with increasing force caused by an injury
Supination–inversion injury (the foot is supinated and the force is pure inversion; commonly described as 'I twisted my ankle') (Figure 9.5)	Stage I: traction by the lateral ligaments produces SH type I or II fracture of the distal fibular physis. Lateral ligamentous injury can occur but is rare, as the physis is usually weaker than the ligament Stage II: the talus impacts against the medial malleolus, causing SH type III or IV injury; occasionally SH type II and rarely type I injury of the medial malleolus
Supination–plantar flexion injury (the typical mechanism of injury is jumping off a high wall and landing on a plantar flexed foot which buckled underneath the body weight)	The resultant force fractures the posterior malleolus, causing SH type II physeal injury of the distal tibial physis, with posterior displacement of the epiphyseal–metaphyseal fragment and no fracture of the fibula. The metaphyseal fragment of the tibia is posterior and best seen on a lateral radiograph
Supination–external rotation (SER) Similar to supination–inversion ('twisted my ankle'), but there is external ankle moment as twisting whilst running, rather than just landing (see triplane fractures) (figures)	Stage I: SH type II fracture of the distal tibial epiphysis, with a posterior metaphyseal–epiphyseal fragment displaced posteriorly. The distal tibial fracture begins on the lateral distal aspect and spirals medially and proximally. The fibula remains intact. This fracture is similar to a supination–plantar flexion injury, especially when seen on a lateral radiograph; the distinction is that the distal tibial fracture line begins on the distal lateral aspect and spirals medially when viewed on the AP projection Stage II: spiral fracture of the fibula. The fracture begins medially and extends superiorly and posteriorly
Pronation–eversion–external rotation fracture (this happens during contact sports when the victim tries to avoid a collision. With the foot planted on the ground, the whole body turns away from the planted foot) (Figure 9.6)	SH type I or II fracture of the distal tibia, with a transverse or short oblique fibular fracture located 4–7 cm proximal to the tip of the lateral malleolus When SH type II fracture occurs, the metaphyseal fragment is located laterally or posterolaterally and the distal tibial fragment is displaced laterally and posteriorly

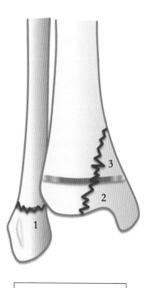
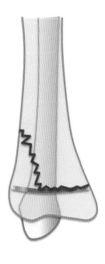
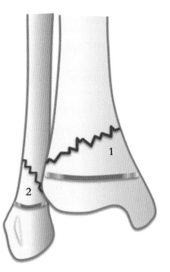
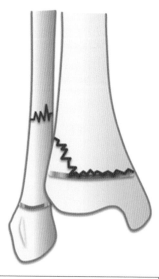

| Supination–inversion | Supination–plantar-flexion | Supination–external rotation | Pronation–eversion–external rotation |

Figure 9.4 Dias and Tachdjian paediatric ankle fracture classification.

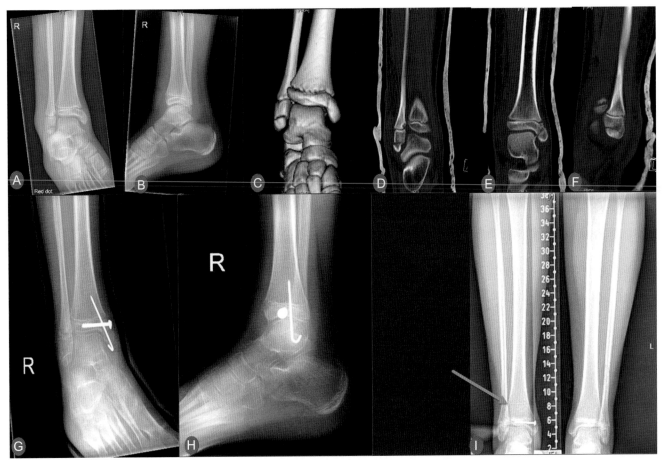

Figure 9.5 Supination–inversion injury. (A) and (B) show a transverse fracture of the lateral malleolus caused by traction of the lateral collateral ligament. This is unusual as the growth plate is usually weaker than the bone and it should give first. There is SH type III fracture of the medial malleolus. The fracture was treated by stabilizing the medial malleolus only and allowing the lateral malleolus to heal naturally (G, H). (I) shows a plain radiograph after 1 year with the fracture fully healed. Note the Harris arrest line which is parallel to the growth plate (good sign).

Medial malleolus physeal fractures (SH type III or IV) merit special attention. They are also called McFarland fractures and they can occur with any of the above-mentioned mechanisms (Figure 9.7). They have been associated with a high rate of growth disturbance (35%) [5, 6]. Early surgery (within 24 hours) and anatomical reduction have been proposed to reduce the risk of growth disturbance. However, there is controversy about stabilizing the undisplaced fractures to ensure non-displacement.

Key Points: Ankle Fracture Classification

The Salter–Harris classification of physeal fracture is important to understand for practice and exams. It is easy to remember, aids fracture description, and is closely related to the outcome of ankle fracture treatments. In a retrospective study of 376 children with distal tibial physeal injury, Schurz et al. [7] reported poor outcome in 0.5%, 5%, 12%, and 6% in SH types I, II, III, and IV, respectively.

Understanding the Dias–Tachdjian classification is helpful to predict typical patterns, prevent missing subtle fractures, and assist in planning closed reduction; however, it is not essential. Moreover, a substantive proportion of ankle fractures do not fit the described types as is the case with the Lauge–Hansen classification in adults.

Transitional Fractures

Unusual fracture patterns occur during the transitional phase into skeletal maturity when the distal tibial physis is closing. These patterns of injury include Tillaux and triplane fractures. These occur because of the way in which the distal tibial physis is formed and closes (see above).

Tillaux Fractures

A Tillaux fracture occurs when the anterolateral portion of the distal tibial epiphysis is avulsed off by the anterior inferior tibiofibular ligament during an external rotational force injury (Figure 9.8). This anterolateral region of the physis is last to fuse and therefore represents an area of relative weakness.

These injuries can often be reduce-closed by internal rotation and above-knee cast application. Patients should remain non-weight-bearing for a minimum of 6 weeks. Consideration of exchange to a below-knee cast can be made at 3 weeks. However, serial imaging is required to ensure that there is no displacement of the fracture.

As this fragment is intra-articular, any displacement exceeding 2 mm requires anatomical reduction and fixation. An anterolateral approach is used to visualize the articular surface for congruency, and the fracture stabilized using a 4.5-mm partially threaded cannulated screw (Figure 9.8). It is valuable to note the

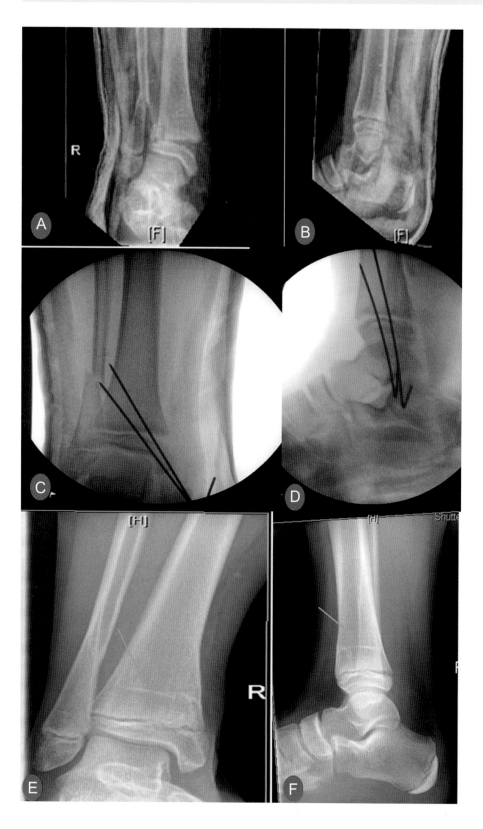

Figure 9.6 Pronation -eversion -external rotation fracture. SH type II fracture of the distal tibia, with a short oblique fibular fracture located 4 -7 cm proximal to the tip of the lateral malleolus(A,B). Good reduction and minimal stabilization using K-wires(C,D). Although fixing the fibula is possible and will add more to stability, in children, this is often not required as it heals quickly and remodelling is usually good. (E) and (F) show the fractures have fully healed. The Harris arrest lines are parallel to the growth plates of the tibia and fibula (green arrows).

trajectory of the screw in the AP plane. A non-weight-bearing below-knee cast should be applied and worn for a full 6 weeks.

Triplane Fractures

A triplane fracture, as the name suggests, is an injury that has a fracture line extending in three planes: frontal, lateral, and transverse (X, Y, and Z, respectively). On an AP radiograph, the fracture may appear as an SH type III injury. However, on a lateral radiograph, the fracture appears to be an SH type II or IV. In actual fact, a triplane fracture is an SH type IV injury, as the fracture line extends all the way from the epiphysis to the metaphysis and crosses the physis.

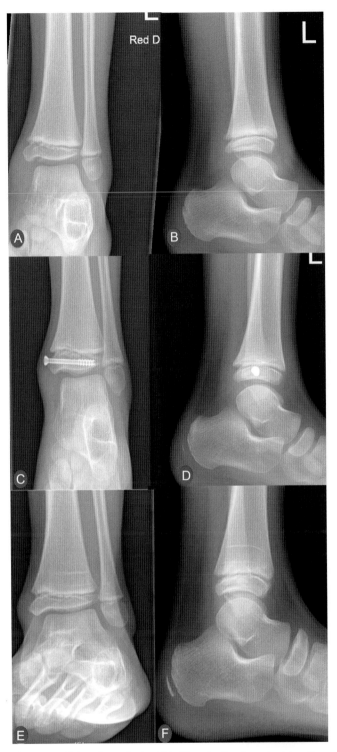

Figure 9.7 Plain radiograph of a child with supination -inversion injury. It is difficult to ascertain whether the fibula is fractured. There is a SH type III medial malleolus fracture (McFarland fracture)(A,B). These fractures have a high tendency for growth arrest, particularly displaced ones. Opened reduction and stabilization were performed using a single cannulated screw(C,D). One-year follow-up showed no growth arrest(E,F).

As the medial distal tibial physis is first to close, the lateral side is left vulnerable to injury. Triplane fractures result from an SER force, and it is believed that forces required to produce this pattern of injury are greater than those which result in a Tillaux fracture.

The simple two-part triplane fracture can be traced as follows (Figure 9.9):

- A vertical fracture through the epiphysis
- A horizontal fracture through the physis
- An oblique fracture through the metaphysis where it exits.

Triplane fractures can be more complex and consists of two, three, or four parts (Figure 9.10). Understanding the fracture's exact configuration is essential for proper surgical treatment. CT is a valuable tool to better understand the pathoanatomy of fracture patterns (Figures 9.10 and 9.11). This enables a thorough assessment and appreciation of the congruency of the articular surface, the number of fragments, and the degree of displacement, so that surgical management can be planned precisely.

Fractures with displacement of <2 mm can be treated conservatively in a non-weight-bearing above-knee cast, with early further reimaging to ensure maintenance of optimal fracture position. A non-weight-bearing below-knee cast can be applied in the third week and should be worn for a further 3 weeks. If there is joint incongruency of >2 mm, or if there has been loss of reduction after a trial of conservative treatment, operative intervention is required.

Surgical intervention may involve percutaneous fixation or open reduction and fixation with wires or screws. An anterolateral approach is best used to visualize the articular surface and ensure anatomical restoration. Where minimal comminution has occurred, a single 4.5-mm partially threaded cannulated screw may be passed from lateral to medial across the epiphysis to restore joint congruency. However, where greater comminution has occurred, a second screw may be passed from anterior to posterior to capture the posterior epiphyseal fragment. Having a CT scan is paramount in order to discern the trajectory of this anterior-to-posterior screw (Figure 9.12). A non-weight-bearing below-knee cast should be applied and worn for a full 6 weeks, and the patient should be followed up for a minimum of 2 years to assess for the occurrence of growth arrest.

Lawnmower Injuries

In 2016, Over 86 000 adults and 4500 children in the United States were treated for injuries related to lawnmowers, according to the US Consumer Product Safety Commission. Boys sustain the vast majority of lawnmower injuries, which most often occur on the arms or in the hands [8].

The SH classification has been extended to include SH type VI – injury to the perichondral ring. In the ankle, this represents a medial malleolar injury that results in disruption or loss of the medial portion of the distal tibia, physis, or zone of Ranvier (Figure 9.13). It is most commonly known for being caused by the blades of a lawnmower but can also result from severe abrasions and burns such as those resulting from gravel rash. These injuries have a high incidence of growth disturbances and often require plastic surgical input for debridement and soft tissue reconstruction.

Other Foot and Ankle Injuries

Children can sustain several foot and ankle injuries, just like adults. In most of these injuries, treatments are based on adult types of treatment. Intra-articular fractures require anatomical reduction. Joint dislocation requires reduction and stabilization. Remodelling of foot bone fracture is impaired after the age of 8.

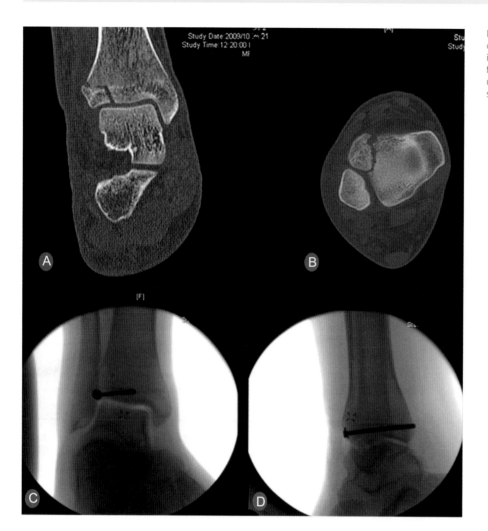

Figure 9.8 Tillaux fracture. (A, B) CT scan in the coronal and axial planes showing a displaced intra-articular Tillaux fracture. (C, D) Intraoperative fluoroscopic images of a Tillaux fracture fixation using a singular partially threaded cannulated screw.

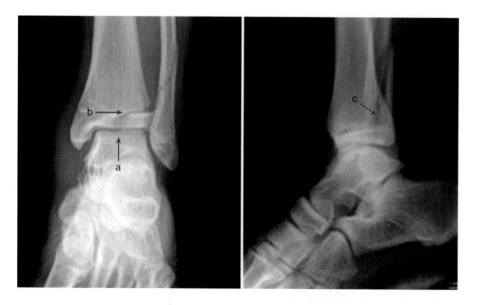

Figure 9.9 AP and lateral plain radiographs showing the fracture lines of a simple two-part triplane fracture: (a) a vertical fracture through the epiphysis; (b) a horizontal fracture through the physis; and (c) an oblique fracture through the metaphysis.

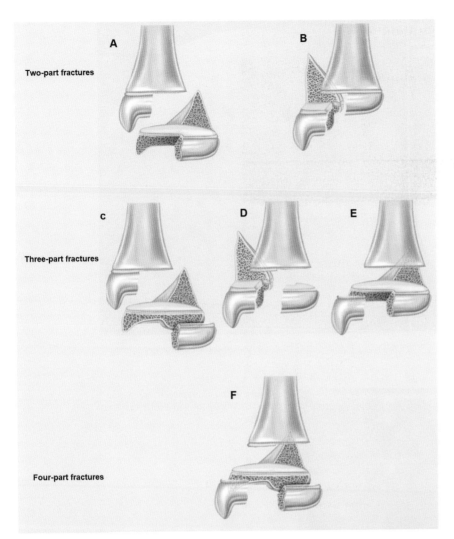

Two-part fractures

Three-part fractures

Four-part fractures

Figure 9.10 Types of triplane fractures. (A) and (B) represent a two-part fracture, with the medial malleolus attached to a large metaphyseal spike. (A) The medial malleolus is attached to the shaft fragment; (B) the medial malleolus is not attached to the shaft fragment. (C), (D), and (E) represent three-part fractures. (C) A three-part fracture with the medial malleolus attached to the shaft fragment and a separate anterolateral epiphyseal free fragment. (D) A three-part fracture with the epiphysis completely detached from the shaft, and the medial malleolus on the large metaphyseal spike. (E) A three-part fracture with a completely detached medial malleolus. (F) A rare four-part fracture (also called quadriplane variant) with free medial malleolus and anterolateral epiphyseal fragments.

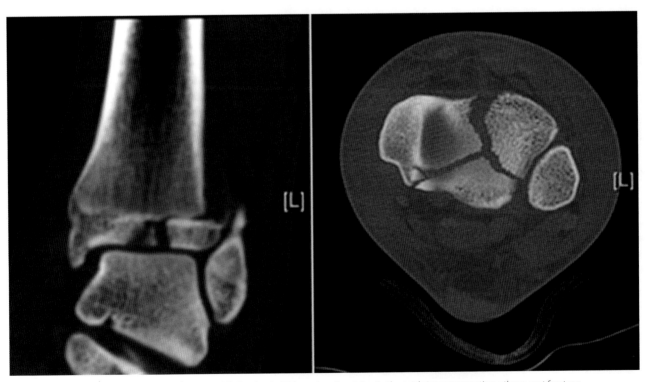

Figure 9.11 CT scan showing a triplane fracture, with the classical 'Mercedes–Benz' sign in the axial view representing a three-part fracture.

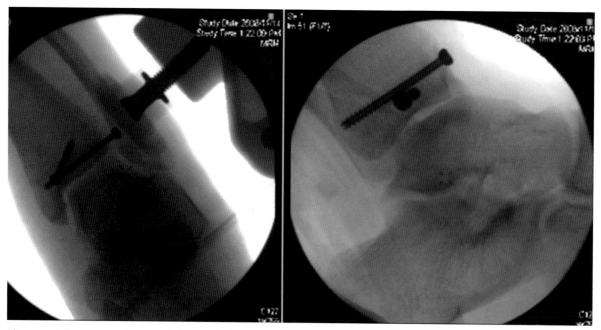

Figure 9.12 Intraoperative fluoroscopic images of a three-part triplane fracture fixation showing lateral-to-medial and anterior-to-posterior cannulated screw fixation.

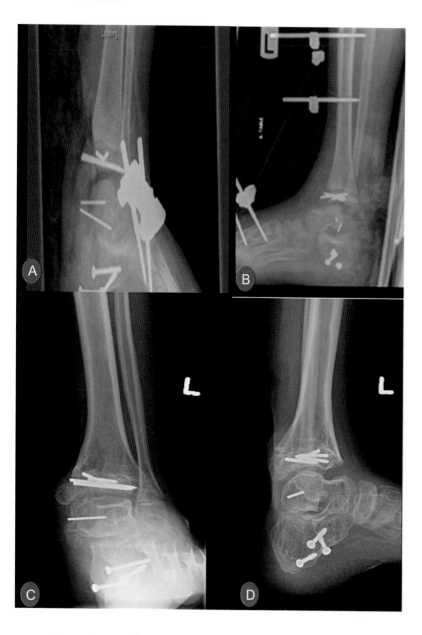

Figure 9.13 Lawnmower injury causing substantive damage to the soft tissue and bones(A-D).

References

1. Barrie J, Hope R, Lishman J. Ankle instability. 2014. Available from: www.foothyperbook.com/elective/ankleInstability/ankleInstabBasic.htm.

2. Topal M, Köse A, Dinçer R, Baran T, Köse M, Çağatay Engin M. Os subtibiale: mimicking medial malleolar fracture. *Am J Emerg Med.* 2017;35(6):940.e1–3.

3. Turan A, Kilicaslan OF, Kose O. Os subtibiale and secondary ossification center of medial malleolus are two different entities. *Am J Emerg Med.* 2017;35(6):929.

4. Dias LS, Tachdjian MO. Physeal injuries of the ankle in children: classification. *Clin Orthop Relat Res.* 1978(136):230–3.

5. Petratos DV, Kokkinakis M, Ballas EG, Anastasopoulos JN. Prognostic factors for premature growth plate arrest as a complication of the surgical treatment of fractures of the medial malleolus in children. *Bone Joint J.* 95B(3):419–23.

6. Cooperman DR, Spiegel PG, Laros GS. Tibial fractures involving the ankle in children. The so-called triplane epiphyseal fracture. *J Bone Joint Surg Am.* 1978;60(8):1040–6.

7. Schurz M, Binder H, Platzer P, Schulz M, Hajdu S, Vecsei V. Physeal injuries of the distal tibia: long-term results in 376 patients. *Int Orthop.* 2010;34(4):547–52.

8. American Academy of Orthopaedic Surgeons. Lawn mower injuries in children. 2022. Available from: https://orthoinfo.aaos.org/en/diseases--conditions/lawn-mower-injuries-in-children/.

Orthopaedic Spine Disorders

Ashley A. Cole and Lee M. Breakwell

Spinal Deformity

Spinal deformities are probably the most complex deformities to understand, analyse, and treat in orthopaedic practice. This is because of the many small vertebrae in the spine, inherent instability of facet joints, reliance on muscle strength to maintain stability, various compensatory mechanisms to accommodate for a deformity, and strong bending forces that the spine endures.

Spine deformities are often described in one of three planes: scoliosis – in deviation or rotation in the coronal plane; kyphosis and lordosis – rotation or bending the sagittal plane; spondylolisthesis and retrolistheisis – translation in the sagittal plane; and rotatory subluxation and unilateral facet dislocation – rotation in the axial plane. The reality is that these deformities often involve more than one plane.

Scoliosis

Scoliosis is defined as a frontal or coronal plane curvature of the spine with a Cobb angle of >10°. The Cobb angle is defined as the maximal angle subtended by the end plates of the vertebrae within the curve.

Classification includes:

1. Congenital
2. Idiopathic
3. Syndromic
4. Neuromuscular
5. Degenerative
6. Paralytic.

Congenital

Congenital scoliosis, which may not present with a curve at birth, is due to a developmental defect in the formation of the mesenchymal anlage. The resulting abnormal vertebra conveys uneven growth, creating angulation of the end plates, which leads to unbalanced growth in adjacent vertebrae.

The defects could be (Figure 10.1):

- Failure of formation: the commonest abnormality in this group is a hemivertebra, which can be fully or partially segmented, or unsegmented
- Failure of segmentation: common abnormalities in this group are block vertebrae and unsegmented bars
- A combination of the above.

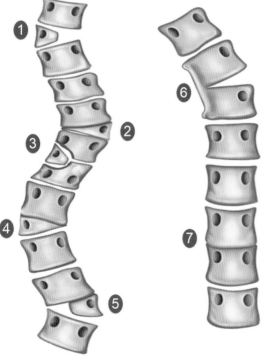
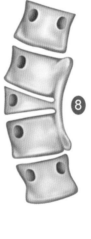

Figure 10.1 Congenital scoliosis. Failure of formation: (1) fully segmented hemivertebra; (2) unsegmented hemivertebra; (3) incarcerated hemivertebra; (4) wedge vertebrae; (5) partially (semi-) segmented hemivertebra. Failure of segmentation: (6) unilateral unsegmented bar; (7) block vertebra. Mixed: (8) unilateral unsegmented bar with contralateral hemivertebra.

Failure of formation   **Failure of segmentation**   **Mixed**

Association

Once a diagnosis of congenital scoliosis is identified, the following associated anomalies must be sought and excluded:

- Spinal abnormalities – dysraphism (21–37%: MRI)
  o Myelomeningocele
  o Diastematomyelia
  o Tethered cord
  o Chiari malformation ± syringomyelia
- Cardiac anomalies (12–26%: echocardiography)
- Renal anomalies (20%: ultrasound)
- VACTERL association (vertebral defects, anal atresia, cardiac defects, tracheo-oesophageal fistula, renal anomalies, and limb abnormalities). The cause of such association has not been identified.

Risk of Progression

On assessing a patient, several factors will help to indicate the risk of progression, and hence the indications for treatment:

1. Age of patient (remaining growth)
2. Site of the anomaly (worse at junctional regions such as thoracolumbar and lumbosacral)
3. Type of anomaly (from worst to best)
   a. Unilateral unsegmented bar with contralateral fully segmented hemivertebra
   b. Unilateral unsegmented bar
   c. Fully segmented hemivertebra
   d. Partially segmented hemivertebra and wedge vertebra
   e. Incarcerated hemivertebra
   f. Non-segmented hemivertebra
4. Size of curve at presentation.

Treatment

The mainstay of treatment is observation, as the large majority of congenital curves result in minor deformity. Bracing is of little value in this type of abnormality. Surgery is indicated once progression has been confirmed. Surgical management has three broad principles:

- Convex growth arrest to allow corrective growth
- Correction and fusion of an abnormal section to arrest abnormal growth and correct malalignment
- Excision of abnormal bone and correction of surrounding vertebrae.

It is prudent to delay surgery in young children if possible. Growing rods have been used to buy time and protect internal organs in complex congenital scoliosis (Figure 10.2).

Idiopathic

Idiopathic scoliosis is by far the commonest form of the condition and affects approximately 3% of girls. Although the aetiology is unknown, there is growing evidence of a genetic causation, especially in adolescent scoliosis.

Right thoracic curves are the commonest, followed by double major (right thoracic and left lumbar), then thoracolumbar, curves.

Idiopathic scoliosis is subdivided into three types, based on age of onset:

- Infantile (IIS; 0–3 years)
- Juvenile (JIS; 4–10 years)
- Adolescent (AIS; 10–18 years).

Infantile Idiopathic Scoliosis

This represents <1% of all idiopathic curves, and is commoner in boys and more commonly left-sided.

It is the only true scoliosis that can resolve spontaneously: this can be predicted by measuring the rib–vertebra angle difference (RVAD) of Mehta on an AP radiograph. This is derived by measuring the angle between a line along the rib 'neck' and a perpendicular line from the apical vertebra, and subtracting the convex from the concave angles (Figure 10.3).

Eighty-three per cent of the curves that resolved had an initial RVAD measuring <20°, whereas 84% of the curves that progressively worsened had a RVAD exceeding 20° [1].

Early treatment can, in this group, reverse the deformity, leading to normal growth of the spine. Elongation, derotation, and flexion (EDF) casting has been shown to successfully treat IIS if managed in the first year of life (Figure 10.4). Casting in even severe curves can significantly delay progression and prevent serious cardiorespiratory harm from developing [2].

Surgery may be required if repeated casts fail to control the curve. This involves the use of growing rods (Luque trolley, surgically lengthened rods, or magnetically lengthened rods) without spinal fusion. The concept is for the rods to maintain an applied correction whilst the spine grows.

Juvenile Idiopathic Scoliosis

Juvenile curves have a relatively high risk of progression due to the remaining growth potential. Children's growth velocity, however, progresses relatively slowly over these years. Approximately 70% will progress, and many will require treatment. As many as 1 in 10 JIS patients have a neural axis abnormality on MRI.

This group attracts the most interest in terms of varied treatments. Various forms of braces exist, the evidence for which is weak. The aim of bracing is to prevent curve progression, or at least delay surgery long enough to allow for lung development.

It is advisable to delay surgery until the adolescent growth period, as spinal fusion before the age of 10 years reduces the final lung volume and chest expansion, thus compromising respiratory function. Apparent trunk shortening can also be a cosmetic issue in some patients, as can the crankshaft phenomenon [3] which occurs in posterior-only fusions in immature spines due to the significant remaining anterior growth.

Various 'growing' constructs exist for surgical treatment of the immature spine. The basic concept is for an implant to hold an applied correction whilst the spine continues to grow, allowing lung volume increase and maintenance of the trunk-to-lower limb ratio.

Types of growing implants include:

- Luque trolley [4]
- Single or dual surgically lengthened growing rod (traditional growing rods) (Figure 10.5)

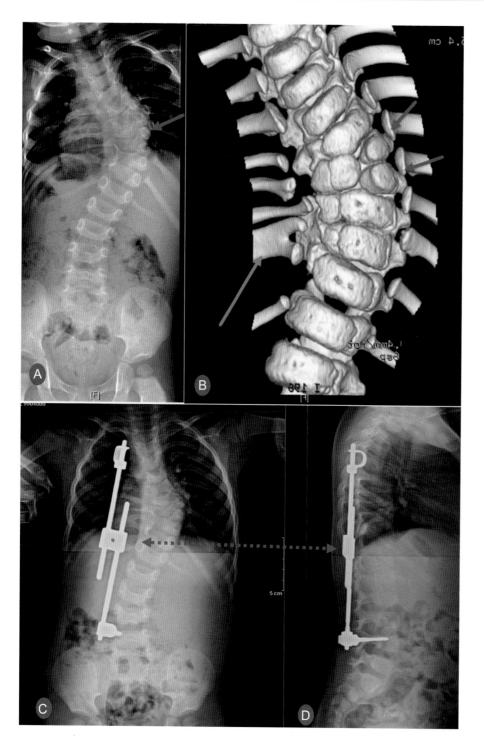

Figure 10.2 Congenital scoliosis with hemivertebra on the left (A, red arrow) and fused rib and a bar on the right (B, blue arrow). This was treated with a hybrid (spine to rib) growing rod (C, D). The growing rod was elongated every 6 months using a small incision over the domino connector (dashed red arrow).

- Magnetically driven expandable rods
- Shilla technique.

A recently developed new non-fusion procedure has offered the prospect of controlling growth whilst maintaining motion of the spine. Vertebral body tethering is an anterior construct with screws in the vertebral bodies over the whole curve, connected (tethered) on the convex side of the curve with a cord. This allows some compression between the screws to correct the curve but retains movement and does not impede growth on the concave side of the spine, which improves the correction over time. This has shown early potential promise, but there are no long-term studies available to support routine implementation of the technique [5].

Adolescent Idiopathic Scoliosis

This is the commonest form of scoliosis; it is more commonly seen in girls.

Factors that aid in identifying risk of progression:
- Curve size (>20°)
- Remaining growth (curves worsen with growth). This is usually assessed:

RIB VERTEBRAL ANGLE DIFFERENCE (RVAD)

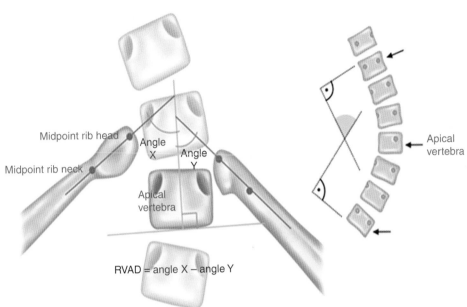

Figure 10.3 Rib–vertebra angle difference of Mehta. This is the difference between the scoliosis convex side rib vertebra angle and the concave one.

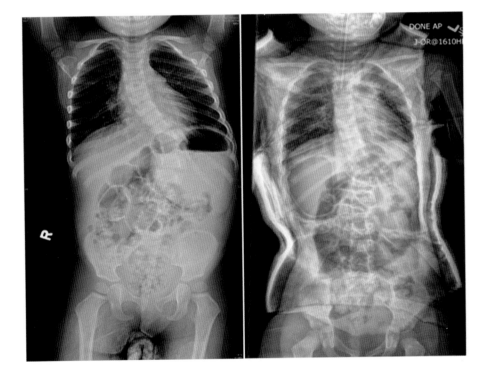

Figure 10.4 Infantile idiopathic scoliosis treated with serial casting. Notice the improvement in the magnitude of the curve.

- Clinically (age, menarche, Tanner system (sexual maturity) staging, and peak height velocity (PHV))
- Radiologically (Risser stage, triradiate cartilage closure, Sanders' stage assessed using a left hand and wrist radiograph, distal radius and ulna classification)
- Curve type (progression more likely in thoracic and thoracolumbar curves than in double curves).

In clinical practice, the PHV (i.e. the adolescent growth spurt) is documented serially by measuring the patient's height over time. This is about 8.0 cm per year for girls and 9.5 cm per year for boys. The average age of the PHV occurs at 11.5 years in girls. Triradiate cartilage closure occurs after PHV and before both Risser stage 1 and menarche (Figure 10.6).

Factors of no predictive value for curve progression before skeletal maturity include:

- Family history
- Patient's body mass index
- Lumbosacral transitional anomalies

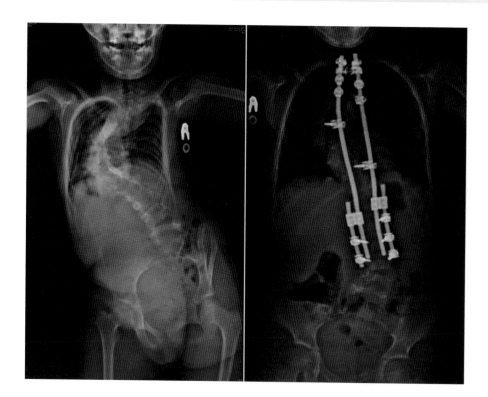

Figure 10.5 A child with juvenile idiopathic scoliosis treated with growing rods, which were elongated every 6 months, using a small incision over the domino connector and subsequent elongation of the rods.

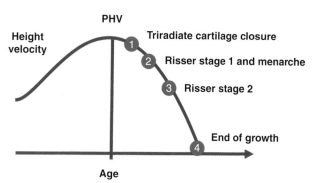

Figure 10.6 Estimation of remaining growth.

- Thoracic kyphosis
- Lumbar lordosis
- Spinal balance.

Treatment

Reassurance is the most commonly required treatment in this group, as the majority of curves will not progress, and if they do, they will not exceed cosmetic or health-challenging size. Long-term studies have shown minimal, if any, impact on the health of patients with curves below 80°.

Curves below 30° at skeletal maturity do not progress during adult life; curves of 30–50° very rarely progress, whilst curves above 50° will usually progress slowly (1° per year) over many years [6]. Treatment focuses on maintaining curve size below 50°, and this can involve bracing.

Options include braces and surgery.

Braces

Braces are used for curves with a Cobb angle of 20–40° and significant remaining growth (Risser stages 0, 1, and 2). A large prospective trial has shown rigid bracing to be effective at reducing the risk of progression to surgery; 72% of braced patients were successfully treated (did not reach the primary end point of 50°, taken as a surrogate marker of surgery), with only 48% of non-braced patients successfully treated [7]. The main types of braces include the Boston-style thermoplastic brace and CAD/CAM designed braces to optimize in-brace correction (Figure 10.7).

Predictive features for brace treatment failure include:

1. Curves >40°
2. Correction of <50% in brace (comparing X-ray with and without the brace) (Figure 10.10)
3. Brace worn for <16 hours per day.

A positive family history has not been shown to be related to curve progression or chance of control.

Surgery

Surgery aims to reduce the Cobb angle of the curve and involves spinal fusion with instrumentation. A safe, partial correction, achieving good frontal and sagittal plane spinal balance, is the goal. Modern pedicle screw-based instrumentation has dramatically improved the ability of the surgeon to derotate the spine and translate the apex towards the midline. Most systems are built around the use of two contoured rods, with segmental fixation of the spine with hooks and screws. These implants are sequentially connected to the rods, allowing gradual deformity correction prior to bony fusion. The vast majority of procedures are now performed posteriorly as a result of these techniques (Figure 10.8).

Spinal cord monitoring is used to monitor the sensory and motor tracts within the spinal cord during surgery. This reduces the risk of post-operative neurological deficit by warning of problems and allowing, where possible, a reversal of the cause. Sometimes elevation of blood pressure is all that is required;

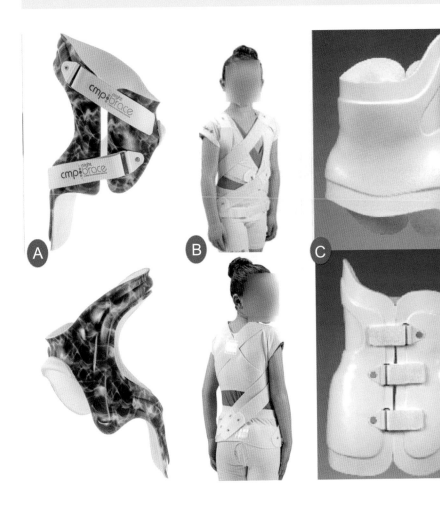

Figure 10.7 Three different brace designs used in scoliosis treatment. The top row represents the front view, and the bottom row shows the back view. (A) Night brace to be worn when lying or sleeping. (B) SpineCore dynamic brace. (C) Boston brace.

sometimes screw malposition may be the cause, and sometimes it is the correction manoeuvre as the rod is connected.

Anterior surgery is generally reserved for thoracolumbar scoliosis, with the apex at or below T12, whereby preservation of mobile levels at L3/4 and L4/5 can sometimes be maintained preferentially over posterior surgery. This is usually achieved via a thoraco-abdominal approach, which requires temporary detachment of the diaphragm.

Surgery enables a significant reduction in the size of the curve and commensurate improvement in the cosmetic appearance of the trunk. On average, the Cobb angle improves by 60–70%, and the apical trunk rotational angle by 40–50%. Long-term studies have found no advantage of surgery in improving back pain.

Complication rates for posterior surgery are 5–10%, with infection and pain being the commonest. With modern implant designs, loss of correction is rare and the incidence of revision surgery is low. The risk of paralysis following surgery in an adolescent idiopathic scoliosis (AIS) patient with a normal MRI scan is 1 in 800.

Syndromic

Scoliosis is a common feature of many well-known syndromes. In addition, it is present in many rare syndromes that are regularly seen in spinal clinics. Common syndromes with scoliosis include:

- Neurofibromatosis
- Marfan syndrome
- Ehlers–Danlos syndrome.

Rarer syndromes with scoliosis include:

- Rett syndrome
- Prader–Willi syndrome
- Osteogenesis imperfecta
- Multiple pterygium
- Noonan syndrome
- Angelman syndrome
- Sotos syndrome.

The majority of these patients already have a diagnosis prior to identification of the scoliosis. However, in some, the spinal deformity is the index problem.

Neurofibromatosis scoliosis is the commonest skeletal manifestation of neurofibromatosis. The cause is unknown, but various theories have been proposed such as primary mesodermal dysplasia, erosion or infiltration of the bone by localized neurofibromatosis tumours, and endocrine disturbances. Neurofibromatosis scoliosis can be either:

- Non-dystrophic or
- Dystrophic.

Differentiation between the two types is important because prognosis and management differ significantly.

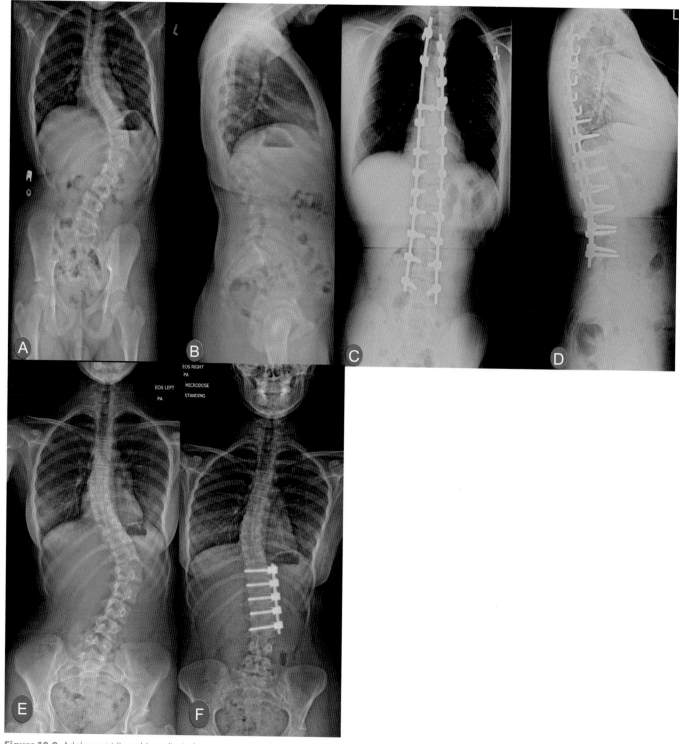

Figure 10.8 Adolescent idiopathic scoliosis that was treated with posterior spinal fusion using pedicles screws, hooks, and rods (A-D). Similar thoracolumbar scoliosis that was treated with anterior spinal fusion (E,F). Notice the apex is below the T12 vertebra. The length of spine fusion is shorter in an anterior approach, which is an advantage.

Dystrophic scoliosis is commoner, is usually located in the thoracic region, and has a short (4–6 vertebrae), sharply angled curve, often associated with kyphosis. It has a greater tendency to progress and is at risk of developing neurological deficits. Bony abnormalities are common, with thin pedicles and dural ectasia (Figure 10.9). Non-dystrophic scoliosis more closely resembles idiopathic scoliosis in both curve patterns and behaviour.

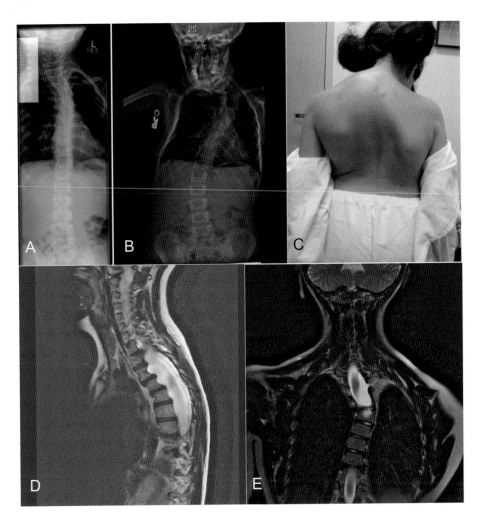

Figure 10.9 Dystrophic scoliosis in a child with neurofibromatosis (C). There was rapid progression in severity over 2 years (A, B). The clinical photographs show café-au-lait spots and a sharply angled kyphoscoliosis. The kyphosis is more pronounced than the scoliosis. The MRI scan shows large dural ectasia and scalloping of the posterior vertebrae (D, E). A large plexiform neurofibroma in continuity with a nerve root is seen (E).

Neuromuscular

These curves are usually long and less likely to have compensatory curves, and may progress after maturity. Pulmonary problems, such as decreased lung function, are observed.

This form of scoliosis is divided into two subgroups:

- Cerebral palsy
- True neuromuscular diseases, in which there is a primary nerve or muscle disorder.

Cerebral Palsy

The incidence of spinal deformity increases with severity of cerebral palsy. It is around 20%; however, in the quadriplegic group, the incidence is in excess of 70%.

The ability to walk is relatively protective, and therefore, wheelchair dependence is a risk factor for development and progression of scoliosis.

Duchenne Muscular Dystrophy

This X-linked recessive condition, affecting the production of dystrophin, almost exclusively affects boys, with their mothers as the carrier. Historically, wheelchair dependence happened at about 10–11 years of age, following which the patient developed scoliosis. Curves beyond 20° were seen to progress inexorably and surgery was advised at an early stage, to prevent further respiratory embarrassment.

Since the advent of steroid treatment, the progression of weakness has significantly slowed, and many continue with some form of ambulation into their teens. This, coupled with the effect that untreated curves do not always progress, means that the indication for surgery has changed, and not all patients require surgery. The decision to proceed to corrective surgery can now often be left until the curve has progressed to ≥40°, as the child is often older and lung function better than in the historical cohort.

Spinal Muscular Atrophy

This autosomal recessive muscle wasting disease commonly causes scoliosis, which is often progressive. A defect in the *SMN1* gene leads to loss of the SMN protein, which is vital for nerve function. There are three types of spinal muscular atrophy (SMA) in children, with function and life expectancy increasing from type I through to type III. Respiratory function can be severely restricted; hence, scoliosis is a major concern.

The median survival in type I SMA is 7 months, with a mortality rate of 95% by the age of 18 months. In type II SMA, the age of onset is between 6 and 18 months and the age of death varies. The decision to undertake surgery for spinal deformity must be made in close collaboration with respiratory physicians, ideally considering life expectancy and function, as well as the risk of curve progression.

Key Points: Gene Therapy

The natural history of SMA (and some other neuromuscular diseases) has been influenced substantially with the introduction of gene therapy, bringing new challenges for orthopedic surgeons.

Two genes are involved in the pathogenesis of SMA: *SMN1* and *SMN2*. The SMN protein is made from the two genes. Patients with SMA lack the *SMN1* gene but have the *SMN2* gene, which mostly produces a short SMN protein that does not work as well as the full-length protein. Mutations in the *SMN1* gene cause all types of SMA. The number of copies of the *SMN2* gene (from one to eight copies) modifies the severity – the more copies, the better function.

Traditionally SMA treatments have been supportive: physiotherapy, occupational therapy, and assistive devices such as braces, crutches, walkers, and wheelchairs. However, two forms of treatments have been introduced recently:

1. Disease-modifying therapy (2016): these drugs stimulate production of the SMN protein by enabling the *SMN2* gene to produce the full-length protein, which is able to work normally. Nusinersen (Spinraza®) is for children aged 2–12 years, given intrathecally every 3 months. Risdiplam (Evrysdi®) is given orally and is for adults and children older than 2 months.
2. Gene replacement therapy (2019). Zolgensma® contains a functional copy of the *SMN1* gene. It passes into the nerves, from where it provides the correct gene to make enough of the protein, thereby restoring nerve function. It is given once by intravenous infusion.

In a study, 20 out of the 22 babies given Zolgensma® were alive and breathing without a permanent ventilator after 14 months, when normally only a quarter of untreated patients would survive without needing a ventilator. The study also showed that 14 out of the 22 babies were able to sit for 30 seconds after 18 months, a milestone that is never achieved in untreated babies with severe forms of the disease [8].

Degenerative

This form of curve typically develops in the fifth, or later, decade in life, often in a previously normal spine. This is therefore beyond the scope of this book.

Paralytic

Spinal cord injury with resultant paralysis before the onset of the adolescent growth spurt leads to development of scoliosis in 97% of patients [9].

Treatment of Syndromic and Neuromuscular Scoliosis

Treatment in these patients is variable, dependent upon the underlying diagnosis and ambulatory status. The principles, however, are the same for both groups.

In ambulant patients, pelvic obliquity is rare and treatment is aimed at maintaining ambulation and preventing curve progression. Treatment is similar as for those with idiopathic scoliosis; hence, it depends on remaining growth, curve size, progression rate, and comorbidities.

In non-ambulant patients, the aim is to maintain sitting function. The long C-shaped curves that are commonly seen can lead to pelvic obliquity and associated postural difficulties. Smaller curves are often tolerated very well, and agreement with carers for observation and seating modification are sufficient. Braces have no scientific evidence and are poorly tolerated in this group, but may be considered in very flexible 'collapsing' curves (Figure 10.10).

In some cases, however, the degree of curvature and pelvic obliquity and imbalance lead to pain and poor quality of life. In this scenario, posterior fusion usually from T2 or T3 to the pelvis is possible (Figure 10.11). Major improvements in comfort, eating, sleeping, and sitting can be achieved, but at the risk of major complications such as infection, wound problems, implant failure, and prolonged paralytic ileus. Mortality is about 2%.

Combined anterior and posterior surgery is reserved for the worst cases with a stiff, deformed spine. This can be undertaken as either a single or a staged procedure, and involves some form of release anteriorly by removing either discs or a whole vertebra, prior to posterior fixation.

Assessment

The main areas of concern for the doctor and the patient are:
- Risk to long-term health
- Risk to neurological structures
- Cosmesis
- Pain
- Function.

Clinical examination aims to assess first the likely type of scoliosis and then the nature of the curve itself.

Observation of the child for skin markers, such as hairy patches, café-au-lait spots, axillary freckling, and sacral dimples, may indicate underlying disorders (see Chapter 2). Scars indicating previous spinal surgery or even thoracotomy are likely to be relevant.

Assessment of the overall standing or sitting balance is next, with a plumb line from the vertebra prominence which should pass through the natal cleft. Leg length discrepancy, real or apparent, must be calculated.

Curve geometry gives the most basic form of classification, such as right thoracic, when the apex of the curve is in the thoracic spine convex aspect to the patient's right.

Flexibility of the curve can be estimated by bending the spine left and right or by prone traction, or if the child is small enough, by suspension.

Rotation of the spine, a fundamental aspect of the deformity in scoliosis, can be estimated by the Adam's forward bend test. On flexing forward, such that the spine is horizontal in the sagittal plane, the true rotation of the curve apex can be measured with a scoliometer (Figure 10.12).

Neurological examination, including abdominal reflexes, will help identify a neural axis abnormality, whereas inspection of the feet may show cavus deformities due to hereditary motor and sensory neuropathy.

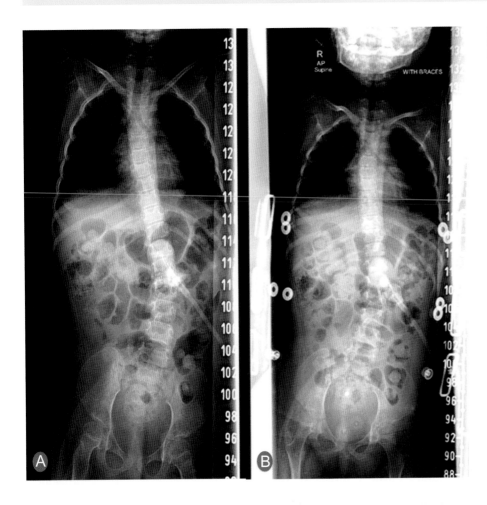

Figure 10.10 A child with Rett syndrome and a flexible curve (A) that has been treated with a brace (B).

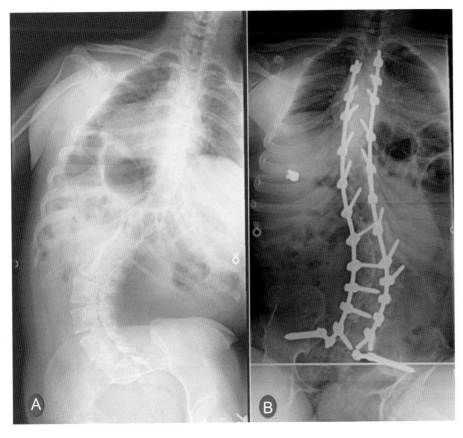

Figure 10.11 Typical long curve neuromuscular scoliosis with pelvic obliquity (A) that has been treated with spinal fusion down to the pelvis (B).

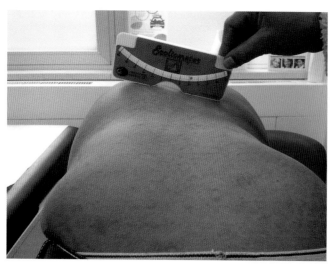

Figure 10.12 Measurement of the angle of trunk rotation (ATR) using a scoliometer. The ATR is a term for the paraspinal rib hump that is accentuated by forward bending in structural scoliosis. This accentuation does not occur in non-structural scoliosis like the ones that are caused by leg length discrepancy. An ATR of 5–7° is associated with a Cobb angle of 15–20°.

Investigations

A full posteroanterior (PA) film, as well as a lateral spine view, standing where possible, will allow the diagnosis of a congenital anomaly and estimation of the Cobb angle. Plain radiographs are used for assessing progression over time using the Cobb angle, as we understand the natural history of this measurement over time both before and after skeletal maturity. **Most studies suggest an increase in Cobb angle of >5° (measurement error) as indicative of definite curve progression.**

Supine bending views may be requested to confirm flexibility of the curve and aid classification. Classification systems, such as King and Lenke, are also largely based on findings from plain radiographs [4, 5].

The following radiological terms are useful to assess radiographs:

- **Cobb angle**: the angle subtended by the upper end plate of the most tilted vertebra above the curve apex and the lower end plate of the most tilted vertebra below the curve apex
- **Harrington's stable zone**: this is defined by two vertical lines drawn up from the lumbosacral facets
- **Plumb line**: a vertical line drawn vertically from the mid body of C7 towards the floor
- **Central sacral vertical line (CSVL)**: this is drawn as a vertical line extended cephalad from the spinous process of S1
- **Apical vertebra**: the most laterally displaced vertebra or disc space in the curve
- **Apical vertebral translation**: the distance of the centre of the apical vertebra on the thoracic curve from the plumb line and the lumbar curve from the CSVL
- **Apical vertebral rotation**: this indicates the magnitude of the apical vertebral rotation. There are two methods to measure the vertebral rotation: the Perdriolle and Nash–

Moe methods. The former uses a transparent torsionometer that is overlaid on the radiograph. In the Nash–Moe method, the relationship of the pedicle to the centre of the vertebral body is observed on AP radiographs (Figure 10.13)

- **Stable vertebra**: the vertebra at the caudal end of the curve which is most closely bisected by the CSVL
- **Neutral vertebra**: the vertebra at the caudal end of the curve which has the most neutrally rotated pedicles
- **Major curve**: the largest curve and the one with the greatest degree of rotation. The direction of the curve is determined by its convex side
- **RVAD**: this is derived by taking the angle of the concave and convex ribs to the apical vertebra bisector, and subtracting the convex from the concave angles.

The following signs of skeletal maturity are used to assess the remaining growth:

- Risser's sign: the iliac crest apophysis is divided into four quarters (Risser 0 = no ossification; Risser 1–4 = increasing number of ossified quarters; Risser 5 = when the apophysis is fused with the iliac wing)
- Triradiate closure
- Vertebral apophysis fusion on the lateral X-ray – a good indicator of skeletal maturity of the vertebra
- Sander's stage (1–8) – based on epiphyseal development and closure on the left hand and wrist radiograph [6].

MRI is excellent at identifying cord (tethered cord, diastematomyelia, syringomyelia) and hindbrain (Chiari malformations) anomalies present in spinal deformities. It can also be used to demonstrate the stretched or compressed cord sometimes seen in severe kyphosis.

As noted, early-onset scoliosis (<10 years old) has a relatively high incidence of neural axis abnormality; hence, routine MRI scans are performed as part of the assessment of these patients.

Adolescent scoliosis patients very rarely exhibit positive findings on MRI (1 in 1 000), so in practice, the scan is reserved only for those undergoing surgery or those who have a neurological abnormality on clinical examination. All ambulant patients undergoing corrective spinal surgery require an MRI scan as part of the preoperative workup.

In spinal deformity, MRI is used in:

- All ambulant patients undergoing surgery
- Severe kyphosis
- Early-onset scoliosis
- Congenital deformity
- Significant pain
- Neurological abnormality on clinical examination.

CT scanning, in particular three-dimensional reconstruction imaging, is helpful in understanding and planning treatment of complex deformities such as congenital scoliosis and dystrophic curves. This is especially the case for identifying the posterior element anatomy. Three-dimensional models can be made to better appreciate the anatomy and aid surgical planning in more complex spinal deformities with severe curves and combined scoliosis and kyphosis.

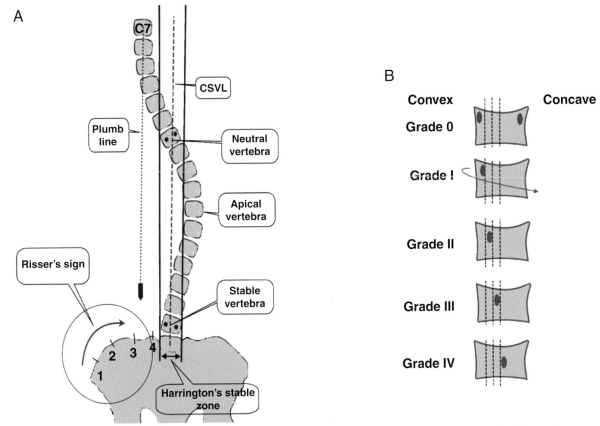

Figure 10.13 Scoliosis radiology. (A) A diagram showing various radiological terms of scoliosis. (B) The Nash–Moe method for assessing vertebral rotation. Grade 0: both pedicles are symmetrical; grade I: the convex pedicle has moved away from the side of the vertebral body; grade II: the rotation is between grades I and III; grade III: the convex pedicle is in the centre of the vertebral body; and grade IV: the convex pedicle has moved past the midline. The curved arrow denotes the direction of the rotation.

EOS imaging is becoming a more popular alternative to plain radiographs and CT scanning in scoliosis. It uses very low-dose radiation to capture two- and three-dimensional images of the patient's entire body in natural, load-bearing positions whilst standing or sitting.

Natural History and Treatment

Scoliosis is not always progressive, and as we have seen in the infantile group, it can actually resolve spontaneously. Many curves, however, will progress and it is important to understand the long-term effect of this in order to plan management.

In normal, healthy subjects, lung alveolar budding is not complete until the age of 4 years, and the full lung structure is not complete until the age of 8 years. Following this, the lungs expand significantly due to thoracic spine and ribcage growth.

It can be seen therefore that any effect on thoracic spine growth prior to the age of 8 years can be catastrophic and, beyond this, can affect cardiorespiratory function in the long term.

Congenital deformity is often associated with complex rib anomalies and, in up to 20%, cardiac problems. This infers a risk to the long-term health of the subject, and quantification of this risk aids in treatment planning.

IIS and JIS (onset prior to the age of 10 years) can therefore be seen to convey significant mortality risk.

AIS rarely causes major health concern and only affects respiratory function when the curve progresses beyond 90°.

A major problem in the more severe syndromic and neuromuscular cases is the ability to sit, as many are non-ambulant. Respiratory embarrassment can be a feature particularly in those with muscular weakness or thoracic cage restriction.

Treatments for individual scoliosis types were discussed above to emphasize the difference among the various types.

Kyphosis

Kyphosis is a forward curvature of the spine in the sagittal plane. A certain degree of thoracic kyphosis (20–50°) is normal and indeed desirable for spinal balance. Thoracic kyphosis does not strictly have a normal value, as it exhibits a range throughout different body shapes in the different sagittal spinal shapes described.

Classification

- Congenital
- Idiopathic
- Neuromuscular
- Syndromic
- Traumatic
- Degenerative.

Congenital

As in scoliosis, this deformity develops due to an underlying structural disorder. The same basic types exist as in the coronal plane scenario.

A hemivertebra positioned posteriorly will gradually deform the spine in a kyphotic direction (Figure 10.14). This causes a localized angular deformity called a gibbus.

As the angulation progresses with growth, the centre of gravity of the body moves forward, increasing the load on the anterior aspect of the vertebral ring apophysis. This impedes anterior growth, in compliance with the Hueter–Volkmann Law, unbalancing in favour of posterior height increase and leading to worsening of the kyphosis. By this process, kyphosis progresses throughout growth, and even during adulthood if beyond 90° or very localized.

Whereas scoliotic deformity causes neurological deficit extremely rarely, congenital kyphosis has a relatively high risk of curve progression and neurological deficit when the angle is localized and beyond 90°.

Idiopathic

Scheuermann's kyphosis (Figure 10.15) is seen in children older than 10 years and is commoner in boys. The incidence ranges from 1% to 8%. The accepted pathoaetiology is that slight kyphosis in the growing spine causes an anterior shift in the body weight centre, unevenly loading the anterior apophysis. This then leads to fragmentation and poor growth, as seen in the anterior vertebral body. It is characterized by vertebral wedging, disc space narrowing, end plate irregularities, including Schmorl's nodes, and kyphosis.

Long-term natural history studies have shown that pain and function levels are not affected until the kyphosis progresses beyond 75° [10].

Neuromuscular

This is often noted in the wheelchair-dependent patient, as it is related to seating position and a preference to leaning forward when sitting. It is typically passively correctable.

Syndromic

Sagittal plane deformity is a common feature of some syndromes, in particular the mucopolysaccharidoses (MPS), with Hurler (type I), Hunter (type II), and Morquio (type IV) being the commonest. Severe localized kyphosis can occur in the presence of abnormal bone, as in neurofibromatosis, making surgical treatment very complex (Figure 10.16).

Severe localized kyphosis can occur in the presence of abnormal bone, making surgical treatment very complex.

Kyphosis beyond 90° will progress beyond maturity and carries a significant neurological risk in adult life. The cord becomes progressively draped and stretched over the apex, leading to myelopathic change. In general, angular kyphosis is more problematic than global kyphosis for neural structures.

Treatment

Rigid braces are often used to try and prevent progression in adolescents with Scheuermann's kyphosis who have remaining growth potential. Posterior corrective surgery can be undertaken either for cosmesis, as in Scheuermann's kyphosis, or

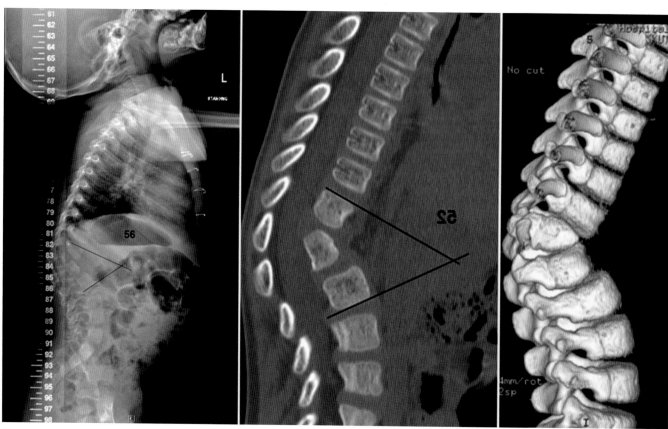

Figure 10.14 Congenital kyphosis caused by a hemivertebra.

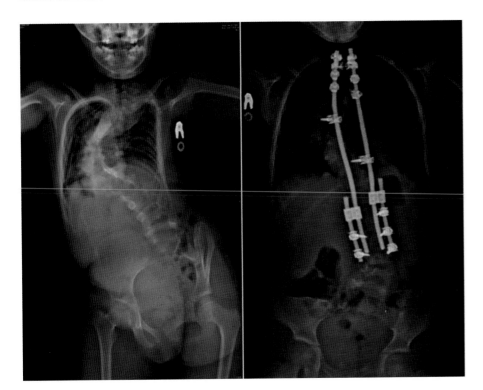

Figure 10.15 Scheuermann's kyphosis or disease. It is traditionally defined by anterior wedging of at least 5° of three or more adjacent thoracic vertebral bodies.

to prevent future neurological problems when a significant kyphotic deformity is present.

Long posterior constructs are required to give stable fixation and balance, without the risk of implant failure. Careful attention must be paid to the overall sagittal balance, and posterior-based osteotomies are often performed. The risks are similar to scoliosis in most cases and depend predominantly on the size of the curve and patient comorbidities.

Some patients present with early symptoms of spinal cord compression: ataxia, lower limb sensory abnormality or motor weakness, and bladder and bowel dysfunction. The spinal cord is usually being stretched by the deformity. Surgery involves posterior spinal osteotomy removing the lamina and the vertebral body stabilized with posterior instrumentation, which has a 10–20% chance of neurological deficit.

Key Points: Exam Tips

When presented with a question regarding spinal deformity at the FRCS (Tr & Orth) exam, the main aim is to show a logical approach to a complex and largely specialist area.

A clear description of the presenting problems from the patient's perspective and an understanding of the types of deformity will suffice.

An ordered exposition of the classification of scoliosis, with a logical order of either congenital or acquired, with some recognition of prevalence, is helpful.

With regard to the presentation, appearance is the commonest problem in idiopathic forms of spinal deformity, although with increasing severity of the risk of cardiopulmonary restriction with earlier onset.

Untreated, the neurological risk is generally low for scoliotic deformities, with an increased incidence seen in angular kyphosis, in particular congenital kyphosis.

In non-idiopathic curves, the cardiorespiratory risk may be higher and function becomes more important with regard to pelvic obliquity and sitting.

Clinical assessment is aimed at excluding underlying causes such as syndromes, in particular neurofibromatosis and spinal dysraphism. A description of alignment and balance when standing and of the forward bend test demonstrates the deformity. Neurological examination must include abdominal reflexes.

Investigations begin with plain full-length weight-bearing radiographs, with CT generally reserved for complex deformities. MRI is performed on all ambulant patients undergoing surgery and in any cases with abnormal neurological signs or a higher incidence of anomaly such as congenital or juvenile curves.

Treatment, as with all conditions, is based around an understanding of the natural history of the deformity in question, including the present and future functional or cosmetic issues.

Bracing has an important role, reducing the incidence of progression to a significant sized curve in AIS, and in younger patients, it may be helpful in delaying progression sufficiently to prevent early growth-restrictive surgery. Surgery is limited to the more severe curves with a risk of future progression or functional limitation. Most surgery is currently performed via a posterior approach, with pedicle screw instrumentation.

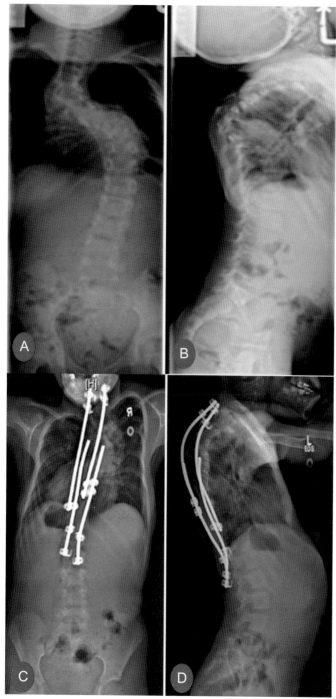

Figure 10.16 Typical long curve neuromuscular scoliosis with pelvic obliquity (A) that has been treated with spinal fusion down to the pelvis (B).

Infection

Aetiology/Definition

Usually younger children aged 2–8 years are affected. The aetiology is usually haematogenous spread and is thought to be due to good blood supply to the vertebral bodies and cartilaginous vertebral end plates. Direct invasion from a local infection may also occur. The lumbar spine is the commonest site. Some suspected spinal infections in children may be just inflammatory or low-virulence organisms.

There are four general groups:

- Pyrogenic: the commonest (>90%) is *Staphylococcus aureus*, especially at age >4 years. *Kingella Kingae* is commonest among those aged 6 months to 4 years
- Tuberculosis (TB)
- Iatrogenic: usually after instrumented spinal deformity corrections. Idiopathic scoliosis, 1%; neuromuscular scoliosis, 4%
- Fungal: *Aspergillus*, *Cryptococcus*, *Candida*.

Classification

There is no accepted classification, but, in children, the vertebra and/or disc can be involved, resulting in:

- Discitis
- Vertebral osteomyelitis (rare in children and usually involves *S. aureus*)
- Paraspinal abscess (e.g. psoas)
- Epidural or subdural abscess.

Natural History

Low-virulence infections in non-immunocompromised patients may resolve spontaneously. However, in general, progression is expected with vertebral body destruction or abscess formation.

Clinical Presentation

The lumbar spine is the commonest place, and symptoms include:

- Axial pain (50%)
- General malaise
- Fever
- Limp
- Abdominal pain.

Always consider this diagnosis in a young child who is limping or unable to weight-bear. Examination may reveal spinal tenderness or evidence of paraspinal muscle spasm. Neurological deficit is very rare and is due to:

- Epidural abscess
- Vertebral destruction with kyphosis.

Thorough history taking is essential, as suspicion of TB or any immunosuppression (HIV, chemotherapy, long-term steroids) may raise the possibility of a non-staphylococcal cause.

Investigations

Blood Tests

White cell count (WCC), erythrocyte sedimentation rate (ESR), and C-reactive protein (CRP) are raised in about 50% of patients [11] but could also be raised with infection elsewhere or malignancy. There is no information on procalcitonin in paediatric spinal infection.

Blood Cultures

These are positive in only 10% of cases (much less than in adults) and should be repeated with temperature spikes.

Plain Radiographs

This may be normal in early infection, although 75% show disc height loss, irregular end plates, or bone destruction or collapse.

Isotope Bone Scan

This is a useful screening investigation in a child who presents with diffuse back pain, to try to localize further imaging investigations, although the radiation dose is high. A chronic, low-grade post-operative infection presenting with back pain can be detected with a bone scan once normal post-operative inflammation has settled.

Magnetic Resonance Imaging

This is the investigation of choice, as it shows oedema from inflammation, pus, and granulation tissue. If required, contrast MRI can distinguish between granulation tissue (enhancing) and pus (non-enhancing) (Figure 10.17). With disc involvement, this is usually diagnostic, although low-virulence infections may be difficult to distinguish from Sheuermann's changes. Vertebral

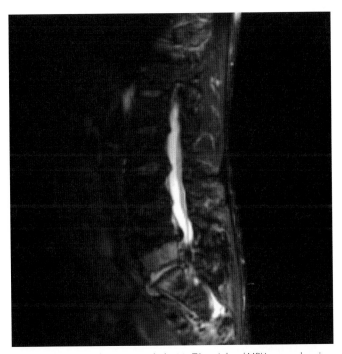

Figure 10.17 MRI of a patient with discitis. T2-weighted MRI images showing a high signal in the L5/S1 disc and pus collecting anterior to the disc.

involvement may raise the possibility of tumour, including leukaemia or lymphoma (Figure 10.18). Vertebral collapse, especially vertebra plana, may raise the possibility of histiocytosis or eosinophilic granuloma. Vertebral body changes may suggest SAPHO (synovitis, acne, pustulosis, hyperostosis, and osteitis). MRI changes always lag behind the clinical picture, making this a poor modality for monitoring response to treatment. Consider including the sacroiliac joints if clinically indicated, as infection or inflammation (ankylosing spondylitis) may occur.

Biopsy

There is less need for biopsy in children than in adults, except in older teenagers. Biopsies should be sent for microbiological and histological analyses. Prolonged culture should be requested, and the possibility of fungal infections considered.

Indications for biopsy include:

- Vertebral osteomyelitis where other diagnoses need to be excluded
- Failure of clinical and blood test improvement on flucloxacillin. The antibiotic should ideally be stopped for 1 week
- Suspicion that the infection may not be caused by *S. aureus* – immunosuppression, possible TB, sickle cell disease, long and indolent course suggestive of possible fungal infection
- QuantiFERON: if TB is suspected. Beware false positives in other *Mycobacterium* infections. Limited data for this test in children.

Management

Treatment aims are to eradicate infection and prevent or minimize spinal deformity. This is achieved by:

1. A short period of bed rest, usually a few days
2. Peripherally inserted central catheter for antibiotics
3. Intravenous flucloxacillin initially for 7–14 days; depending on clinical and blood test improvement, this can be changed to oral antibiotics for a further 4–6 weeks
4. Weekly monitoring of WCC, ESR, and CRP level. The CRP level settles faster than ESR
5. The requirement for bracing is controversial. Brace immobilization may help with 'instability'-type pain to assist mobilization. Thoracolumbar braces are unlikely to prevent deformity. Hard cervical collars may prevent kyphosis

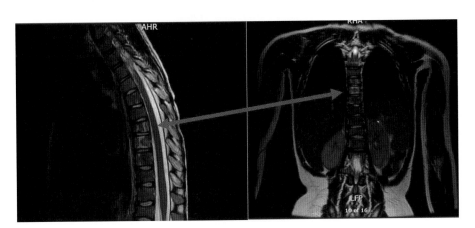

Figure 10.18 A child presented with back pain, fatigue, and high levels of inflammatory markers. MRI scan showed abnormal signals in T7–9 and partial collapse and anterior wedging of the T7 vertebra. Although infection was suspected, biopsy demonstrated that this child has acute lymphoblastic leukaemia.

6. If persistent or worsening pain, or failure of inflammatory marker improvement, consider stopping antibiotics for 1 week and biopsy
7. Plain radiograph at 12 months to document restoration of disc height, loss of disc height, or fusion.

Tuberculosis Infections

These infections can affect multiple vertebral bodies, leading to anterior abscess formation, and cause anterior collapse, resulting in deformity or neurological deficit.

Anterior abscesses in the cervical or upper thoracic spine can cause respiratory compromise in children. Ideally, a biopsy is required for diagnosis and antibiotic sensitivity, as resistant strains are becoming commoner. In the absence of an abscess, bony destruction, or collapse, treatment is non-surgical using appropriate antibiotics.

The aims of surgical treatment are to eradicate infection and stabilize the spine to achieve fusion and prevent late progressive deformity that may result in paraplegia.

An abscess with minimal bone involvement should be surgically drained (often by a costotransverse approach in the thoracic spine) to prevent it from spreading and involving more vertebrae.

An anterior abscess with significant bony involvement and no neurological deficit should be drained, and the bone debrided from an anterior or posterolateral approach. The cavity should be supported with a rib strut graft, which can be oversized to improve any deformity.

Where there is a neurological deficit, the spinal cord should be decompressed and the spinal column reconstructed and stabilized.

If the cord compression is due to acute bony collapse or pus, the neurological outlook is good. However, if the compression is caused by chronic deformity with organized fibrosis, the neurological outlook is poor. In the lumbar spine and lumbosacral junction, it is important to prevent localized kyphosis to reduce the risk of late back pain.

Indications for Surgery

A neurological deficit from an epidural abscess, especially at the spinal cord level, is treated by laminectomy or multiple laminectomies, using a small catheter to wash out the abscess. Preoperative MRI with contrast is good for distinguishing pus (enhancing rim with contrast) from infected granulation tissue (generalized enhancement with contrast) that cannot be washed out. A costotransverse approach can be used to drain a thoracic epidural abscess, especially in TB infection.

Occasionally, bone loss may cause severe deformity requiring surgical reconstruction. The aims of surgery are:

1. Decompression of compressed neurological elements
2. Biopsy (if required)
3. Thorough debridement
4. Stabilization
5. Fusion (usually spontaneous, no requirement for bone graft).

Iatrogenic spinal infections are usually treated with a thorough washout and debridement, as the infection often involves posterior instrumentation. Multiple tissue samples should be taken before any antibiotics have been given. These should be sent to the microbiology department for immediate processing and prolonged culture.

Mildly infected wounds can be closed primarily, and broad-spectrum antibiotics started initially; this should be narrowed once culture results are available. Unless the metalwork is loose, it should be left in situ. Bone graft should probably be removed and discarded. There should be a low threshold for further washouts if the wound is leaking or inflammatory markers do not settle.

Heavily infected wounds may be treated with vacuum therapy after initial washout and debridement, with a planned second return to theatre for redebridement and closure. Intravenous antibiotics should be given for at least 2 weeks, followed by oral antibiotics for 3 months. If infection persists or presents very late after surgery and is low grade, it can be suppressed with antibiotics until the spine has fused, so long as the instrumentation is not loose. The instrumentation can then be removed.

Removal of instrumentation for suspected low-grade or chronic infection will usually settle the infection. Samples should be taken at the time of surgery. The link between postoperative pain and low-grade infection is not well established, although *Propionibacterium*, a low-virulence skin organism, is a common cause.

Tumour

Aetiology/Definition

This section provides an overview of spinal tumours. A detailed description of individual tumours is covered in Chapter 20, but intradural spinal tumours or spinal dysraphism are not considered. In children, 70% of primary bone tumours are benign. Generally, most tumours of cervical vertebrae are benign, whereas thoracic and lumbar tumours are more commonly malignant.

The following tumours are known to affect the spine (Figure 10.19):

1. Benign:
   a. Osteoid osteoma
   b. Osteoblastoma
   c. Aneurysmal bone cyst (ABC)
   d. Giant cell tumour
   e. Eosinophilic granuloma
   f. Osteochondroma
   g. Neurofibroma
   h. Haemangioma
   i. Fibrous dysplasia
2. Malignant:

   a. Ewing's sarcoma
   b. Osteosarcoma
   c. Chondrosarcoma
   d. Lymphoma
   e. Leukaemia
   f. Metastasis.

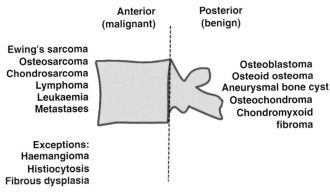

Figure 10.19 A summary of the predilection of spinal tumours.

Clinical Presentation

Worrying symptoms include:

- Severe pain requiring regular analgesia
- Waking up at night in pain
- Pain that prevents engagement in enjoyable activities
- Fever (pyrexia)
- Neurological symptoms, including bladder or bowel dysfunction
- Rapid, new-onset deformity, especially if associated with pain.

Investigations

Blood Tests

Full blood count (including film), ESR, and CRP levels are useful screening investigations, as the child will probably present with back pain and other causes, such as infection, must be considered.

Plain Radiograph

These may show bone destruction or collapse. An absent pedicle is a classic sign (winking owl sign).

Bone Scan

As with spinal infection, this can be useful in localizing tumours and is a good screening tool in children who would require general anaesthesia or sedation for an MRI scan where the level of clinical suspicion is low. However, the radiation dose is quite high and MRI is becoming the preferred investigation.

Magnetic Resonance Imaging

This is excellent for diagnosis and looking at neurological involvement. It is also useful for defining location:

- Intradural, intramedullary
- Intradural, extramedullary
- Extradural
- Bone.

Computed Tomography

This is useful for evaluating bony involvement and can be used to diagnose osteoid osteoma where MRI only shows inflammation (central nidus with surrounding lytic area). It is essential to stage malignant tumours with CT of the chest, abdomen, and pelvis.

Biopsy

Biopsy may be excisional or incisional. An incisional biopsy track must be excisable if en bloc (potential curative) resection is planned.

Management

In the spine, surgical treatment consists of:

1. Decompression, with some intralesional tumour removal aimed at decompressing neurological elements, obtaining a biopsy, and achieving some local control. Stabilization may be required if spinal instability exists or results from surgical decompression. This is often an emergency treatment, when there is spinal cord compression and tumours are usually high grade. Surgery is supplemented with chemotherapy or radiotherapy (or both). Outcome is not always poor (e.g. lymphoma).

2. Intralesional excision aimed at removing all macroscopic tumours. This is often performed for benign tumours and has a low recurrence rate. Stabilization is rarely required.

3. Marginal en bloc resection. This is rarely possible in the spine and involves removal of the whole vertebra (vertebrectomy), attempting to remove the tumour with a wide margin of resection. Preoperative chemotherapy may be used to reduce the size of the tumour. Neurological structures may need to be sacrificed in the en bloc resection.

Bone Tumours of the Spine

This section provides an overview of spinal tumours. Detailed description of individual tumours is covered in Chapter 20. It will not consider intradural spinal tumours or spinal dysraphism. Seventy per cent of primary bone tumours in children are benign. The following tumours are known to affect the spine.

Osteoid Osteoma and Osteoblastoma

They tend to occur mainly in the posterior elements of the spine, and 20% of osteoid osteomas occur in the spine. Osteoid osteomas present with back pain which is worse at night and is relieved with aspirin. Associated muscle spasm can cause scoliosis or torticollis, and osteoid osteoma is the commonest cause of painful scoliosis. Neurological compromise is rare and commoner in osteoblastoma where radicular pain is commonest. CT will show a well-circumscribed bony lesion with a central nidus. MRI shows surrounding oedema, which can be dramatic and suggest a more sinister process.

Treatment can be conservative, with pain resolving in approximately 3 years. Radiofrequency ablation for osteoid osteoma of the spine should be considered if technically possible and not too close to the spinal cord. Otherwise, excision is performed, as recurrence rates are low and pain relief is reliable. Treatment is best if there is spinal deformity, as this often resolves, whereas fixed deformities develop with conservative treatment. Total en bloc excision with curettage and grafting has a recurrence rate of up to 10%.

Aneurysmal Bone Cyst

These are thin-walled, blood-filled cystic cavities that expand, causing bony destruction mostly in the posterior elements. They tend to involve adjacent vertebrae and can cause vertebral collapse (vertebra plana). Patients present with back pain and may develop neurological deficit. X-ray shows an expansile, well-demarcated lesion with a 'bubbly' appearance. CT and MRI often show a fluid level and trabecular struts within the lesion, confirming the diagnosis. Treatment is with excision and curettage after preoperative embolization. Sometimes, neurological decompression and stabilization may be required. Recurrence rates are approximately 15%.

Giant Cell Tumour

These are rare before the adolescent growth spurt, and although benign, they are locally aggressive and rarely 'metastasize' to the lungs. Presentation can be with paralysis. En bloc excision is curative, whereas embolization, curettage, and radiotherapy result in a high recurrence rate and 10% chance of sarcoma development.

Eosinophilic Granuloma

This is the most benign form of histiocytosis and usually occurs in children aged <10 years. It is a self-limiting destruction of bone by lipid-containing histiocytes. Presentation is with pain and occasionally with neurological deficit, especially if adjacent vertebrae are involved. There is usually vertebral body collapse (often vertebra plana), with preserved disc spaces. Biopsy may be required to distinguish from other benign tumours or Ewing's sarcoma. Vertebral reconstitution often occurs and is more noticeable in younger patients. Radiotherapy or chemotherapy (or both) is used, especially for multifocal disease.

Osteochondroma

These cartilaginous capped, benign bony lesions are an abnormality of the perichondral ring. They are rare in the spine as solitary tumours (3%), and only slightly commoner in hereditary multiple osteochondromas (autosomal dominant). They are commoner in the cervical spine. They usually present as a bony swelling, often painless, but can cause nerve root or spinal cord compression. There is a small risk of malignant transformation of the cartilaginous cap, especially in hereditary multiple osteochondromas. Plain spinal radiographs are usually normal. MRI is used to define the cartilaginous cap and the degree of cord or nerve root compression. CT scan is used to define the bony anatomy and the origin of the osteochondroma. They can be removed piecemeal, with low recurrence rates and good neurological recovery. Patients with multiple hereditary osteochondromas should be screened with a full-spine MRI at least once during the adolescent growth spurt.

Neurofibromas

These are attached to the peripheral nerves and can be solitary, with a low risk of malignant transformation. They only require treatment for persistent pain, as weakness is unlikely to recover with excision and may be made worse. They also commonly occur in neurofibromatosis type I (von Recklinghausen, autosomal dominant, chromosome 17) where the risk of malignant transformation is higher. Diagnosis is on MRI, with T2-weighted imaging showing a hyperintense rim and a hypointense centre (target lesion) and heterogenous enhancement with contrast. Resection can involve nerve sacrifice in the thoracic region, but for more important nerve roots, the tumour can be microscopically resected off the nerve.

Ewing's Sarcoma

Ewing's sarcoma is commonest between the ages of 5 and 15 years, and most locate in the sacrum. Patients present with back and often radicular pain or weakness. Fever occurs in 25%, and 50% have raised ESR. Plain X-ray may show vertebra plana. MRI shows a large soft tissue mass. Biopsy confirms the diagnosis. Treatment usually involves chemotherapy to shrink the tumour to enable an en bloc resection. Metastases can occur in the spine, lungs, abdominal viscera, lymph nodes, and brain.

Osteosarcoma

The commonest age is 10–20 years, and osteosarcoma can occur post-irradiation and in some benign bone tumours. Although commoner than Ewing's sarcoma and chondrosarcoma, it is rare in the spine. Radiographs show a mixed osteosclerotic and lytic lesion, with MRI showing a soft tissue mass and helping to distinguish from benign lesions, although biopsy is usually required. CT evaluation is required to rule out metastatic lesions. Treatment involves initial chemotherapy to treat micrometastases and reduce the size of the primary tumour, and hopefully enable an en bloc resection.

Chondrosarcoma

Chondrosarcomas are very rare in children and have a poor prognosis. They sometimes arise in existing osteochondromas. Treatment is surgical wide excision, if possible. Radiotherapy and chemotherapy are usually for metastases or local recurrence.

Lymphoma

Lymphoma presents with pain or neurological symptoms (or both). Lymphoma can invade bone, causing collapse, or can present with neurological symptoms from invasion of the epidural space. There is usually a history of progressive symptoms over a few weeks, with paralysis or cauda equina being common presentations. Biopsy gives the diagnosis, and chemotherapy results in a rapid reduction in tumour size. Surgery is not required, unless biopsy can only be achieved at the time of emergency spinal cord decompression and stabilization is required.

Leukaemia

In children, 6% of cases of leukaemia present with back pain and vertebral collapse. They usually have an elevated ESR and can be mistaken for infection. Anaemia and leucopenia may be present to help with diagnosis.

Metastases

These are rare in children and are usually secondary to Ewing's sarcoma or neuroblastoma.

Back and Radicular pain

Back pain is a common presentation in childhood, with an incidence of approximately 40% in teenagers. In general, back pain in patients younger than 10 years is likely to be pathological, whereas the opposite is true for those older than 10 years. The various causes of back pain have been considered already. Sinister causes of back pain tend to have a relatively short history and the pain will be continuous and worsening. In addition, the pain interferes with activities that the child likes and is present at night, preventing sleep. A history of pyrexia is suspicious. Neurological symptoms or signs are obviously significant.

Investigations

Blood tests (full blood count, ESR, and CRP) should be performed in all children with persistent back pain. Plain radiographs may be considered if there is suspicion of tumour, deformity, spondylolysis, or spondylolisthesis.

Bone scan or MRI should always be performed in children younger than 10 years with back pain, and should be considered in older children with sinister features or who fail to resolve with physiotherapy.

Lumbar disc protrusions are rare in children and will often present with only back pain, although some will present with radicular pain. Straight leg raise is usually restricted. MRI is diagnostic. Initial treatment is physiotherapy, and nerve root injections may be considered for radicular pain, although the success rate is only about 50%. Chemonucleolysis with chymopapain, although a successful treatment, is no longer available. Lumbar discectomy will usually improve back and leg pain, but there is a high incidence of recurrence and many patients have chronic low back pain and require further surgery.

Surgical Complications

Reported complications of spinal surgery in children include:

- Neurological – spinal cord injury, nerve root injury, dural tear
- Infection – early and late
- Vascular injury
- Failure of fusion (pseudarthrosis), failure of instrumentation
- Paralytic ileus
- Bleeding requiring transfusion.

References

1. Mehta MH. The rib-vertebra angle in the early diagnosis between resolving and progressive infantile scoliosis. *J Bone Joint Surg Br.* 1972;54(2):230–43.

2. Mehta MH. Growth as a corrective force in the early treatment of progressive infantile scoliosis. *J Bone Joint Surg Br.* 2005;87(9):1237–47.

3. Dubousset J, Herring JA, Shufflebarger H. The crankshaft phenomenon. *J Pediatr Orthop.* 1989;9(5):541–50.

4. Luque ER. Paralytic scoliosis in growing children. *Clin Orthop Relat Res.* 1982;163:202–9.

5. Samdani AF, *et al.* Anterior vertebral body tethering for idiopathic scoliosis: two-year results. *Spine (Phila Pa 1976).* 2014;39(20):1688–93.

6. Weinstein SL, *et al.* Health and function of patients with untreated idiopathic scoliosis: a 50-year natural history study. *JAMA.* 2003;289(5):559–67.

7. Weinstein SL, *et al.* Effects of bracing in adolescents with idiopathic scoliosis. *N Engl J Med.* 2013;369 (16):1512–21.

8. European Medicines Agency. Zolgensma. 2021. Available from: www.ema.europa.eu/en/medicines/human/EPAR/zolgensma.

9. Dearolf WW, 3rd, *et al.* Scoliosis in pediatric spinal cord-injured patients. *J Pediatr Orthop.* 1990;10(2):214–18.

10. Sachs B, *et al.* Scheuermann kyphosis. Follow-up of Milwaukee-brace treatment. *J Bone Joint Surg Am.* 1987;69(1):50–7.

11. Dayer R, *et al.* Spinal infections in children: a multicentre retrospective study. *Bone Joint J.* 2018;100-b(4):542–8.

Traumatic Spine Disorders

Ashley A. Cole and Lee M. Breakwell

General Considerations

The initial management of a child with a suspected spine injury is the same as for an adult. Advanced Trauma Life Support (ATLS) protocols of primary and secondary survey must be followed. Cervical spine protection is linked to airway management, which is the first step in managing an injured person. A paediatric spinal board should be used in children aged <8 years to avoid neck flexion due to their relatively large heads. In younger children, injury is commoner in the upper cervical spine, whereas after the age of 8, the mid-cervical spine is more commonly injured.

The National Institute for Health and Care Excellence (NICE) guidelines (NG41) for spinal injury assessment and initial management recommend using the Canadian C-spine rule [1]. This considers:

- High-risk factors: a dangerous mechanism of injury, neurological symptoms, including numbness or tingling in the extremities
- Low-risk factors: cervical spine pain or tenderness.

If there are no risk factors and the patient can actively rotate the neck 45° each way, regardless of pain, then no imaging is required. If there is a low suspicion, then a cervical spine X-ray is indicated. MRI is indicated if there is a high level of suspicion, which includes neurological signs.

Spinal Cord Injury

Spinal cord injury without radiological abnormality (SCIWORA) is rare. Physeal injuries (separation of the vertebral end plate from the vertebral body) which are not easily visible radiologically can result in spinal cord injury. SCIWORA is commoner in the cervical spine and in younger children. Complete cord injury has a poor prognosis, whereas incomplete cord injury often results in good functional recovery. The onset of SCIWORA can be delayed, with most patients recalling transient neurological symptoms at the time of injury.

The American Spinal Injury Association (ASIA) classification is used to determine the severity of neurological involvement and any recovery:

- ASIA A: complete paralysis
- ASIA B: sensory function only below the injury level
- ASIA C: incomplete motor function (grades 1–2/5 in more than half of the key muscles below the injury)

- ASIA D: incomplete motor function (grades 3–4/5 in more than half of the key muscles below the injury)
- ASIA E: normal motor function (grade 5/5).

Radio-anatomy

Proper assessment of spine X-rays is well covered in the ATLS manual and courses, and it is beyond the scope of this chapter. However, certain specialized areas would be covered to enhance understanding. Ossification centres and synchondrosis of cervical spine vertebrae can pose serious challenges when interpreting X-rays.

The atlas has three ossification centres: one for the anterior arch and two for the posterior arches. These are separated by synchondroses, which usually fuse by 7 years of age. The posterior synchondrosis, which separates the two posterior ossification centres, closes earlier by 3 years of age. However, sometimes it remains unfused, giving the appearance of a fracture [2].

The axis has five primary ossification centres: one for each neural arch, one for the body, and two for the odontoid process. The odontoid is separated from the body of the axis by a cartilaginous physis that fuses between 3 and 6 years of age. It can be mistaken for a fracture up to 11 years of age. The posterior arches fuse in the midline by 2–3 years and fuse to the body by 3–6 years of age.

The radiological appearance of the cranio-cervical junction is complex. Clear understanding is important to identify some serious disorders. Figure 11.1 summarizes some important features.

Anterior subluxation of C2 on C3 of up to 4 mm is considered normal in children up to 8 years of age. Occasionally, C3/4 may be involved. Radiographs may also reveal the absence of soft tissue swelling and normal alignment of the posterior spinolaminar line (Figure 11.2).

The rest of the cervical, thoracic, and lumbar vertebrae are typical; they have three primary ossification centres: one for the body and one for each neural arch. These fuse in the midline between 2 and 4 years, and the neural arch central synchondroses close at 3–6 years. As children grow, the ossification centres enlarge and replace all cartilaginous parts.

Apophyseal rings on the upper and lower surfaces of the vertebral bodies begin to ossify late in childhood and complete their fusion to the vertebral body by 25 years of age. Fractures of the apophyseal ring (Salter–Harris type I) have been reported and are commoner in the inferior end plates [3].

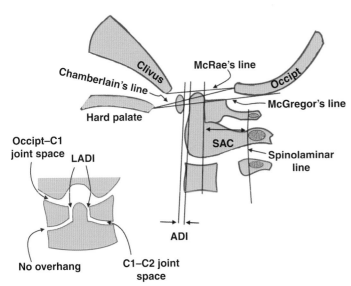

Figure 11.1 Cranio-spinal junction radio-anatomy. This diagram shows extremely important radiological measurements. Anterior atlanto-dens index (ADI): <3–5 mm; space available to the cord (SAC), also called posterior atlanto-dens index (PADI): >13; lateral atlanto-dens index (LADI) 2–3 mm (symmetrical on both sides); OC1 and C1–C2 = 1–2 mm. McRae's line defines the opening of the foramen magnum. The tip of the dens may protrude slightly above this line, but if the dens is below this line, then impaction is not present. McGregor's line is a line drawn from the posterior edge of the hard palate to the caudal posterior occipital curve; cranial settling is present when the tip of dens is >4.5 mm above this line. Chamberlain's line (an Englishman between two Scots) is a line from the dorsal margin of the hard palate to the posterior edge of the foramen magnum; this line is often hard to visualize on standard radiographs, and if the dens is >6 mm above this line, this is consistent with impaction.

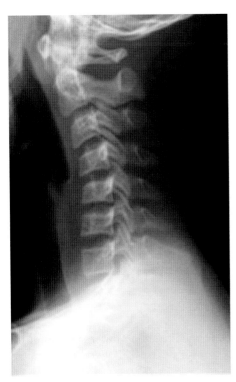

Figure 11.2 Pseudo-subluxation of the cervical spine in children.

Occipito-atlantal Dislocation

This is a rare injury but is commoner in younger children because of the tendency for upper cervical spine injuries. The relatively large head and weak nuchal muscles cause a shift in the fulcrum of movement in the upper cervical spine, with maximum movement at C2–C3. These injuries are usually fatal.

Atlantoaxial Rotatory Subluxation

Although this can be traumatic, it is usually secondary to an upper respiratory tract infection (Grisel's syndrome). Patients usually present with a torticollis and often have pain. Diagnosis is made with dynamic CT, with the head rotated to the left and right.

The Fielding and Hawkins classification is used:

- Type I – rotation without anterior displacement of C1 (transverse ligament intact)
- Type II – rotation with 3–5 mm anterior translation (transverse ligament deficient)
- Type III – rotation with >5 mm anterior translation
- Type IV – rotation with posterior translation due to deficient odontoid.

If detected early, 1–2 weeks in a soft cervical collar, with analgesia, usually results in resolution. If this fails or detection is delayed, halter or halo traction (depending on the age of the patient) for 1–2 weeks may resolve the torticollis. If this occurs quickly and completely, 6 weeks in a rigid cervical collar should be sufficient. If traction only achieves partial resolution over 2 weeks, then a halo vest for 8–12 weeks is indicated. Posterior instrumented C1/2 fusion is indicated if conservative treatment fails.

C1/2 Instability

A normal atlanto-dens interval is up to 4.5 mm. Causes of instability include:

1. Previous or acute trauma
2. Down syndrome
3. Juvenile rheumatoid arthritis
4. Spondyloepiphyseal dysplasia
5. Kniest syndrome
6. Mucopolysaccharidoses
7. Other skeletal dysplasias.

Surgery in the form of a C1/2 fusion is required in the presence of neurological symptoms or if the space available for the spinal cord is <14 mm. Ideally, lateral mass screws are inserted in C1, and pedicle screws in C2 (Figure 11.4).

Basilar Impression

Basilar impression is an acquired cephalad migration of the odontoid peg into the foramen magnum due to abnormal bone quality. Basilar invagination is rarer and is a congenital displacement of the odontoid peg into the foramen magnum with normal

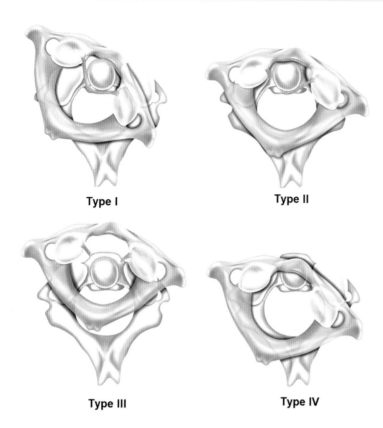

Figure 11.3 Fielding and Hawkins classification. Type I: rotation without anterior displacement of C1 (transverse ligament intact); type II: rotation with 3–5 mm anterior translation (transverse ligament deficient); type III: rotation with >5 mm anterior translation; type IV: rotation with posterior translation due to deficient odontoid.

Type I

Type II

Type III

Type IV

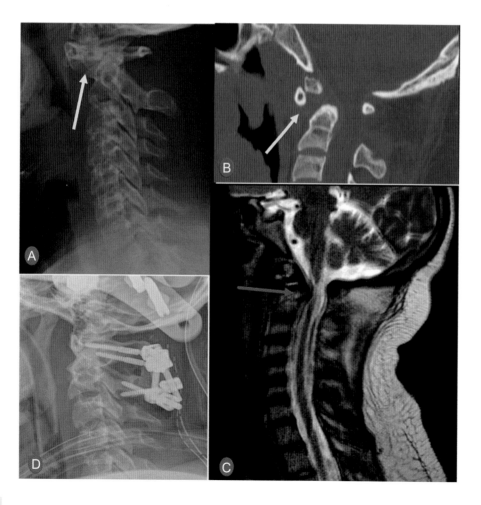

Figure 11.4 C1/2 instability in a child with Down syndrome. Notice the long anterior atlanto-dens index (ADI) distance (yellow arrow) and the pressure on the spinal cord, with effacement of synovial fluid (A,B). The child had neck flexion and extension views in the preoperative assessment clinic. The ADI is normal on MRI (<3 mm). The patient was stabilized with C1/C2 stabilization (D).

bone quality. These conditions narrow the space available for the spinal cord at the cranio-cervical junction. Patients will usually present with headaches, lower cranial nerve abnormalities, nystagmus, and cervical myelopathy. On X-ray or MRI, the tip of the odontoid peg should not be above the line joining the clivus with the posterior rim of the foramen magnum (McRae's line).

Treatment decisions are complex, but treatment usually requires cranio-cervical decompression and instrumented fusion from the occiput (C0) to the mid-cervical spine.

Atlas Fractures (Jefferson Fractures)

This fracture is caused by axial compression such as falling directly on the head (diving in shallow water). The ring of C1 is commonly broken at more than one site. Over 6.9 mm of combined lateral overhang of the lateral masses on an AP radiograph is diagnostic of potential instablity. These fractures require immobilization in a cervical orthosis or halo device for up to 6 months. Halo traction, followed by halo immobilization, may be necessary if there is >6.9 mm or widening of lateral masses.

Axis Fractures

The odontoid peg may not fuse with the rest of the axis completely until the age of 7. This can be a weak spot where fractures can happen (odontoid synchondrolysis). Lateral C-spine radiographs will reveal the odontoid process to be angulated anteriorly and, rarely, posteriorly.

Treatment involves closed reduction and external immobilization with a Minerva jacket or a halo ring for approximately 10 weeks (80% fusion rate). If not fused, then surgical stabilization is performed.

Traumatic spondylolisthesis of C2 (hangman's fracture) can happen in younger patients. Hyperextension and axial loading of a relatively large head size can cause this fracture. Non-accidental injury (NAI) must be ruled out.

Closed reduction in extension and immobilization in a Minerva jacket or a halo ring are performed. If there is non-union or continual instability, posterior C1–3 arthrodesis or anterior C2–3 arthrodesis is undertaken.

Torticollis

Torticollis is lateral flexion of the head to the affected side and rotation towards the unaffected side – that is, in a right-sided torticollis, the head will tilt to the right and rotate anticlockwise to the left. Patients can present at any age. Torticollis can be classified as follows:

- Congenital:
  - Congenital muscular torticollis (commonest cause)
  - Vertebral anomalies:
    - Failure of segmentation – occipitalization of C1
    - Failure of formation – congenital hemi-vertebra (Figure 11.5)
    - Combined
  - Ocular (have a low threshold to refer to an ophthalmologist)
- Acquired: painful:
  - Traumatic – C1 fracture

  - Inflammatory – atlantoaxial rotatory subluxation, juvenile rheumatoid arthritis, infection
  - Tumour – osteoid osteoma, eosinophilic granuloma
- Acquired – non-painful:
  - Central nervous system tumour – posterior fossa, acoustic neuroma, cervical cord
  - Syringomyelia
  - Ligamentous laxity – Down's syndrome, spondyloepiphyseal dysplasia.

Congenital muscular torticollis is the commonest type (see Figure 2.2 in Chapter 2). The cause is unknown, although it is thought to be due to an abnormality of the sternomastoid muscle. If the history dates back to birth, there is a palpable 'tumour' in the sternomastoid muscle (disappears by 4 months of age), and the sternomastoid feels tight (often difficult to be sure in a baby), a diagnosis of congenital muscular torticollis can be made. This is treated with stretches and postural encouragement, with the baby encouraged to rotate their head to the tight side.

If stretching fails to improve the condition (<10%), or the presentation is abnormal, other causes should be considered. In practice, this means an ophthalmic examination, CT of the cervical spine, and MRI of the cervical spine and head (Figure 11.5).

Congenital muscular torticollis should be treated at around 6 years of age, if still significant. This involves muscle release, which can be unipolar (distal release of the clavicular head and z-lengthening of the sternal head) or bipolar (as for unipolar, and proximal release just below the mastoid attachment). Bipolar release produces better results, whereas proximal release has a risk of accessory nerve injury. Other causes should be treated based on the aetiology.

Chance Fracture

Chance fractures are common following road traffic accidents, with the commonest mechanism being a lap-belt injury (hyperflexion), and are often associated with intra-abdominal injury (Figure 11.6). Spinal cord injury is common and bony chance fractures are commoner in children than in adults (weaker bone, ligaments laxer).

Spondylolysis/Spondylolisthesis

There is no diagnosis for back pain in 78% of patients. Spondylolysis and spondylolisthesis are the commonest diagnosis in the remaining 22%. Below, spondylolysis will be considered to be at L5, and spondylolisthesis at L5/S1, which are the commonest sites.

Definition and Aetiology

Spondylolysis is a stress fracture of the pars intra-articularis. It is commonest at L5 but does occur at other lumbar levels. It is caused by repetitive trauma to the pars from the inferior L4 facet in extension; sporting activities involving lumbar spine extension are known risk factors. Approximately 6% of athletic children have a spondylolysis, which is the same percentage observed in adults. Athletic children with low back pain have a higher incidence, with this being up to 43% in those

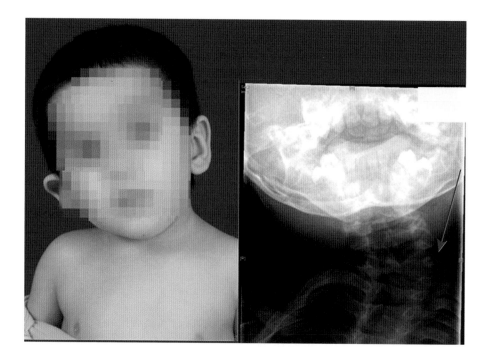

Figure 11.5 A child with congenital torticollis. X-ray shows a congenital hemi-vertebra (red arrow).

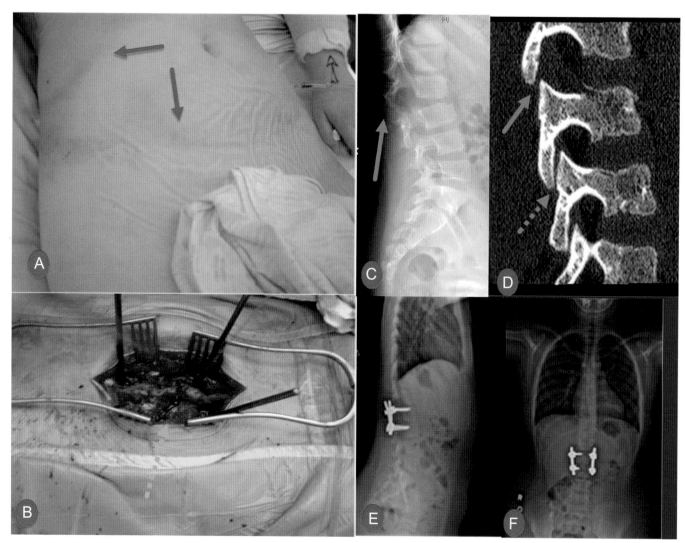

Figure 11.6 Chance facture. This is a seat-belted passenger involved in a front-impaction car collision. There are seat belt bruises (A, red arrows). The operative picture shows the torn supraspinous and interspinous ligaments caused by flexion distraction injury (B, dashed green arrow). (C) and (D) are the preoperative plan radiograph and CT scan, respectively, showing the typical appearance with subluxation of the facet joint (blue arrow, in comparison to the normal facet joint indicated by the dashed blue arrow). (E) and (F) are the post-operative images.

participating in some high-risk sports such as dancers, divers, and bowlers. The incidence may be higher if CT is used.

Spondylolisthesis is where the cranial vertebra slips anteriorly on the caudal vertebra. The opposite of this is called retrolisthesis.

Classification

Spondylolisthesis can be classified by the cause, using the Wiltse classification (Table 11.1) [4].

The degree of slip is graded by dividing the superior end plate of S1 into quarters and observing how far the postero-inferior corner of the L5 vertebral body slips forward on S1 [5], such that:

- Grade 1 = 0–25% slip
- Grade 2 = 25–50% slip
- Grade 3 = 50–75% slip
- Grade 4 = 75–100% slip
- Grade 5 >100% slip = spondyloptosis (not in the original description).

Natural History

Many patients remain asymptomatic and management depends on symptoms. Reported risk factors for spondylolisthesis progression include:

- Age (10–15 years)
- Female
- Dysplastic spondylolisthesis:
  - Sacral doming
  - Trapezoidal shape to L5
  - Short L5 transverse processes
  - Spina bifida occulta
  - Pars elongation
- High grade >50%
- Lumbosacral angle <100° (Figure 11.7) [6].

Clinical Presentation

In childhood, spondylolysis usually presents with low back pain, gait abnormalities, and occasionally leg pain secondary to L5 root irritation, which lies just below the pars in the L5/S1 foramen.

Spondylolisthesis is usually secondary to spondylolysis (isthmic or lytic spondylolisthesis), although occasional cases of dysplastic spondylolisthesis are seen. Both will present with back pain and L5 radicular leg pain, with the L5 nerve root compressed in the foramen at L5/S1. In dysplastic spondylolisthesis, the S1 roots are also commonly compressed in the lateral recess at L5/S1.

On examination, straight leg raise is usually decreased due to bilateral hamstring tightness. Neurological findings are usually normal, and any weakness or other neurological abnormality should raise questions as to whether the spondylolysis or spondylolisthesis is just an incidental finding and whether there is another cause for the patient's symptoms.

Investigation

Plain radiographs show the spondylolysis in 40–60% of cases (Figure 11.7). The radiation doses of oblique radiograph imaging of the lumbosacral junction are as high as those of localized CT scanning, so this should no longer be performed. A lateral standing radiograph will show the degree of slip and comparison with supine investigations (CT or MRI) will demonstrate whether the spondylolisthesis is mobile. The sagittal plane alignment of the spine is thought to be important. Full spine standing lateral radiographs, including the hips, will allow an overall assessment of sagittal balance and measurement of pelvic incidence and sacral slope, which may be clinically significant when managing high-grade (grades 3 and 4) spondylolisthesis.

CT is diagnostic, showing the spondylolysis and any spondylolisthesis in the supine position. Sagittal reconstructions are the best images to view. CT also shows the gap width in a spondylolysis, which, if <2 mm with small fragments in the fracture (progressive phase), has a 39% chance of healing. Sclerosis on CT at the fracture margins indicates the terminal phase, with no chance of healing [7].

MRI in spondylolysis has 81% sensitivity and 99% specificity, so it can miss a spondylolysis. However, it does show oedema on T2 imaging, which is present in a stress reaction without fracture or early acute or hairline fractures which have at least 73% chance of healing. MRI will also show any nerve root compression and any degenerative change in the discs.

Management

Spondylolysis

- Reassurance and analgesia
- Stop any sporting activity for 3 months
- Physiotherapy, but avoiding extension exercises
- Reintroduce activities at 3 months if the pain has settled, mobility is unrestricted, and there is no hamstring spasm. There is an 85% success rate at 1 year, with return to previous levels of sporting activity; however, 26% of cases recur
- No evidence for brace or steroid injection, although a pars injection (steroid + local anaesthetic) may allow further physiotherapy, with reduction in pain
- For the 15% of patients who fail conservative treatment:
  - Pars repair (Buck's fusion with a 3.5-mm lagged cortical screw and bone grafting) [8] (Figure 11.8).

Table 11.1 Spondylolisthesis classification

Type	Age	Pathology
I: dysplastic	Child	Congenital dysplasia of S1 superior facet
II: isthmic	5–60 years	Predisposition leading to elongation or fracture of the pars
III: degenerative	>40 years	Facet arthrosis leading to subluxation
IV: traumatic	Any age	Acute fracture
V: pathological	Any age	Destruction of posterior bony elements
VI: post-surgical	Adult	Excessive resection of the pars or facets during decompression

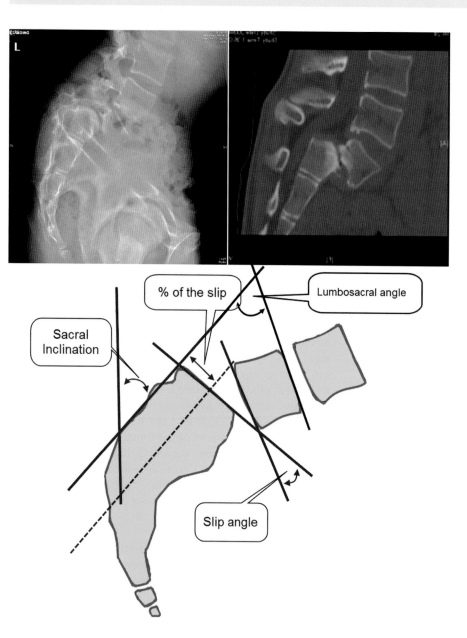

Figure 11.7 Spondylolisthesis and useful radiological features.

This is useful for unilateral spondylolysis; however, it can be considered for bilateral lysis, but an uninstrumented fusion may be better
- Uninstrumented fusion. Bilateral Wiltse approach, iliac crest graft, and 2–3 months in a lumbosacral orthosis. This would be at L5/S1 for an L5 spondylolysis.

Spondylolisthesis (Low Grade = Grades 1 and 2)
The initial treatment is the same as for spondylolysis. Pars injections are rarely beneficial but may have a role in diagnosing the source of back pain. If non-operative measures fail to relieve back pain, an uninstrumented fusion is advised. This has a 70% chance of improving the back pain.

If the main problem is radicular leg pain and there is nerve compression in the foramen, instrumented fusion and L5 decompression through a midline approach and using an iliac crest graft are the best option. The L5 root decompression is in the foramen at L5/S1, rather than in the lateral recess at L4/5.

Spondylolisthesis (High Grade = Grades 3, 4, and 5)
High-grade spondylolisthesis is more likely to progress. Non-operative management should be considered, as there is evidence of good outcome, equivalent to outcome from surgery, at 5–15 years. If the presentation is back pain only, an in situ L5/S1 instrumented fusion with an iliac crest graft through a bilateral Wiltse approach is advised.

If there is significant radicular leg pain, with or without back pain, a midline approach with L5/S1 instrumented fusion and L5 decompression should be performed.

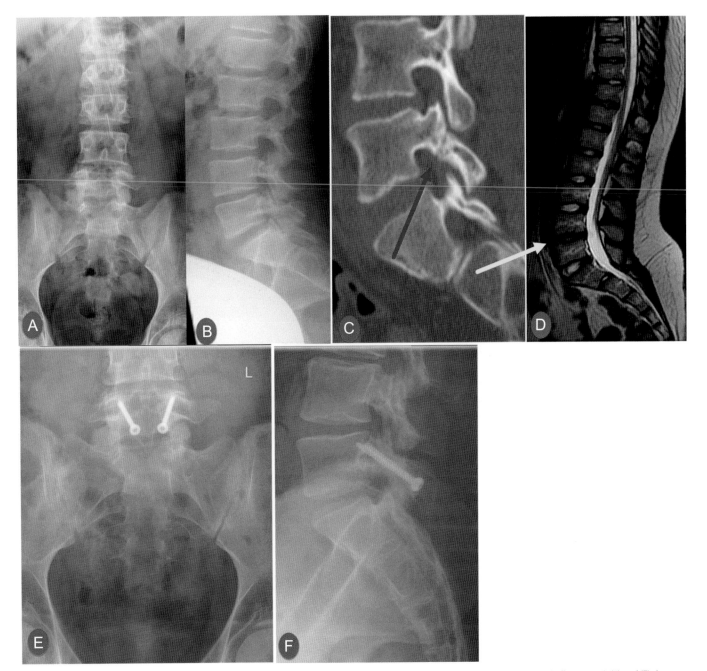

Figure 11.8 Spondylolysis of L5/S1(A,B).Pars defect (C, red arrow). (D) is an MRI scan showing a degenerative disc between L4/L5 (yellow arrow). (E) and (F) show Buck's fusion.

Reduction of high-grade spondylolisthesis is sometimes performed in children and involves a posterior instrumented fusion from L4 to S1 and total removal of the L5/S1 disc usually from a posterior approach with interbody fusion (Figure 11.9). This procedure has the advantage of improved cosmesis and a high fusion rate, but it is a much more complex procedure and has a 10% chance of neurological injury (L5 = foot drop). There is no evidence that reduction of spondylolisthesis improves outcome.

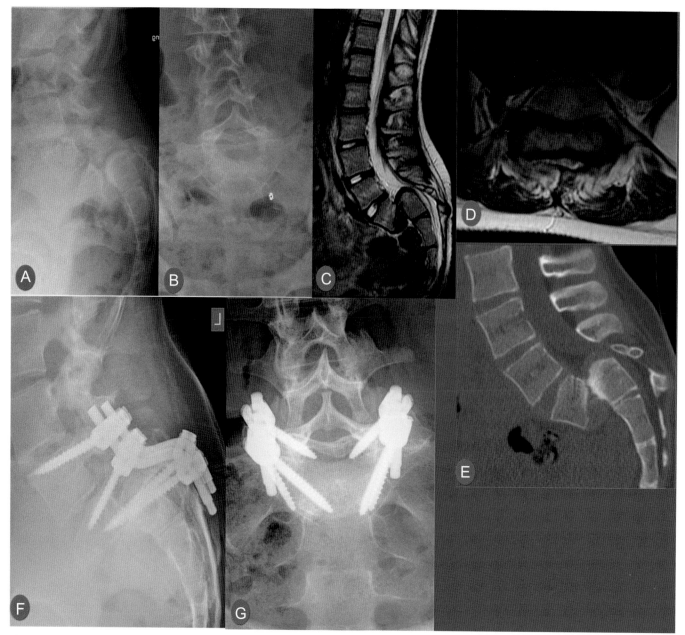

Figure 11.9 Lateral and AP radiographs demonstrating severe spondylosis L5/S1(A,B). T2 weighted sagittal and axial MRI scans (C,D)and CT scan (E.)demonstrating slip. Instrumented fusion of the L4/L5/S1 (F,G).

References

1. National Institute for Health and Care Excellence. Spinal injury: assessment and initial management. NICE guideline [NG41]. 2016. Available from: www.nice.org.uk/guidance/ng41/resources/spinal-injury-assessment-and-initial-management-pdf-1837447790533.

2. Mortazavi M, *et al.* Pediatric cervical spine injuries: a comprehensive review. *Childs Nerv Syst.* 2011;27(5):705–17.

3. Alshryda S, Huntley JS, Banaszkiewicz PA, eds. *Paediatric Orthopaedics: An Evidence-Based Approach to Clinical Questions.* Cham: Springer; 2018.

4. Wiltse LL; Newman PH, Macnab I. Classification of spondylolisis and spondylolisthesis. *Clin Orthop Relat Res.* 1976;Jun(117):23–9.

5. Meyerding HW. Spondyloptosis. *Surg Gynecol Obstet.* 1932;54:371–7.

6. Boxall D, *et al.* Management of severe spondylolisthesis in children and adolescents. *J Bone Joint Surg Am.* 1979;61(4):479–95.

7. Morita T, *et al.* Lumbar spondylolysis in children and adolescents. *J Bone Joint Surg Br.* 1995;77(4):620–5.

8. Schlenzka D, *et al.* Direct repair for treatment of symptomatic spondylolysis and low-grade isthmic spondylolisthesis in young patients: no benefit in comparison to segmental fusion after a mean follow-up of 14.8 years. *Eur Spine J.* 2006;15(10):1437–47.

Orthopaedic Shoulder Disorders

Obstetric Brachial Plexus Injury

Aetiology

The incidence of obstetric brachial plexus injury (OBPI) is approximately 1 per 1 000 live births. Without intervention, around 25% of patients are left with permanent disability [1]. The shoulder is the most commonly affected joint and, owing to the subsequent imbalance of musculature, the abnormal deforming forces cause dysplasia of the glenohumeral joint [2]. In the growing child, this presents with a changing pattern of pathology, which requires a multidisciplinary approach and a broad range of treatment modalities to optimize function.

A common cause is traction injury to the brachial plexus during the later stages of vaginal delivery when the head is pulled away from the shoulder. The mechanism of injury is a forced lateral flexion of the cervical spine, resulting in injury initially to the upper cervical roots (C5–C7), causing Erb's palsy, and, in more severe cases, to the entire brachial plexus (C5–T1). With this mechanism, isolated lower root injuries (C8–T1; Klumpke's palsy) do not tend to occur in OBPI. Other rare causes are abnormal forces on the shoulder over the sacral promontory or abnormal forces in an abnormal uterus such as a bicornuate or fibroid uterus.

The followings are recognized risk factors:

1. Large babies (>4 kg)
2. Difficult labour. Prolonged labour and difficult delivery, and fetal distress with relative hypotonia allow stretching of nerves
3. Abnormal fetal presentation such as breech delivery or shoulder dystocia
4. Multiple pregnancies
5. A previous child with OBPI.

Typical scenarios are large babies (birthweight >4 kg) with a cephalic presentation and shoulder dystocia, requiring excessive traction force to deliver the shoulder, and resulting in traction to C5 and C6 roots. In small babies – weighing under 3 kg – with a breech presentation, manipulation of the neck to deliver the arms and head results in traction on the upper and lower roots. This mechanism may be associated with nerve root tearing or avulsion of nerve roots.

Classifications

OBPI has been variously classified, based on the location of the lesion, clinical picture, and neuronal injury.

Anatomical (Narakas)

The severity of injury has been classified by Narakas into four prognostic grades:

- Grade 1: this involves only C5/6 roots and presents with weakness of shoulder abduction and elbow flexion
- Grade 2: the C7 nerve root is also involved with associated wrist drop. This group has a higher rate of spontaneous recovery
- Grade 3: complete paralysis
- Grade 4: this is also associated with Horner's syndrome.

Narakas grade 3 and 4 patients have a significantly worse prognosis.

Erb's Palsy

OBPI lesions involving the upper roots in isolation (Narakas grades 1 and 2) cause weakness to the supra- and infraspinatus muscles (due to involvement of the suprascapular nerve) and the rhomboids (dorsal scapular nerve palsy), leading to weakness of external rotation and abduction of the shoulder joint. Unopposed action of the subscapularis (supplied by the upper and lower subscapular nerves) leads to an internal rotation contracture of the shoulder.

Deltoid function is often abnormal in these patients. However, the axillary nerve is supplied from multiple levels and the deltoid muscle belly often appears healthy at the time of surgery, and it is more likely deltoid dysfunction is a result of lack of synergistic function of the supraspinatus. The teres minor (also supplied by the axillary nerve) may have some function in Narakas grade 1 or 2 injuries, but it is too weak to oppose the action of the subscapularis. The pectoralis muscles may also be weak, but their supply from both the medial and lateral pectoral nerves ensures that some function remains in isolated upper root injuries.

The internal rotation muscle imbalance leads to progressive flattening and retroversion of the humeral head. The glenoid becomes biconcave, with a false postero-inferior facet, which is lined by hyaline cartilage. With time, the humerus dislocates posteriorly, creating a pseudoglenoid, in which the humeral head articulates with the joint capsule overlying cortical bone (Figure 12.1).

Secondary adaptive changes occur with overgrowth of the acromion and lateral clavicle. The coracohumeral and coracoacromial ligaments become elongated and tight, further restricting external rotation.

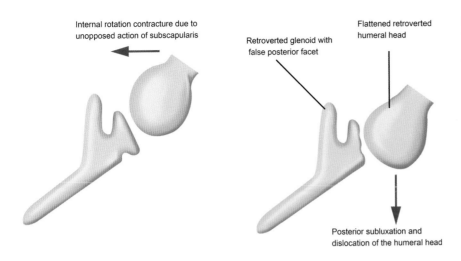

Internal rotation contracture due to unopposed action of subscapularis

Retroverted glenoid with false posterior facet

Flattened retroverted humeral head

Posterior subluxation and dislocation of the humeral head

Figure 12.1 Secondary pathological changes of the glenohumeral joint. The unopposed subscapularis muscle internally rotates the joint, and with time, pressure on the posterior part of the glenoid causes glenoid dysplasia and subsequent dislocation.

THE BRACHIAL PLEXUS

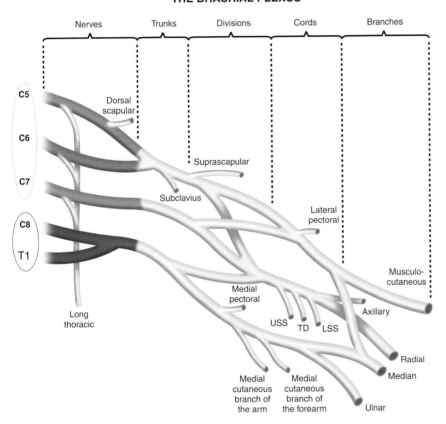

Figure 12.2 The pattern of pre- and post-ganglionic injury depends on the nerve root level. Roots for C5, C6, and C7 are more likely to have post-ganglionic root rupture in obstetric brachial plexus injury, whereas C8 and C9 roots are more likely to have a pre-ganglionic root avulsion. USS, upper subscapular; LSS, lower subscapular; TD, thoracodorsal; MBC, medial brachial cutaneous nerve; MABC, medial antebrachial cutaneous nerve.

Distally, the commonest secondary changes are:

1. Elbow weak flexion and subsequent contracture
2. Forearm pronation contracture with weak supination
3. Wrist drop (lack of extension) and sometimes wrist instability
4. Lack of finger extension.

Total Plexus Injuries

In total plexus injuries (Narakas grades 3 and 4), lower root involvement leads mainly to hand weakness, but also to increased weakness of the deltoid, subscapularis, and pectoralis muscles. This results in a flail shoulder, but with less internal rotation contracture.

Types of Neuronal Injury

Seddon's classification (neurapraxia, axonotmesis, and neurotmesis) is important in determining the type of injury, and hence recovery. However, it can be difficult to determine which type of injury has occurred, and by the time it is known, it may be too late to perform primary reconstructive surgery to the damaged nerve roots.

Binding of the nerve roots to the axial skeleton by connective tissue is important. This is greater in the upper roots, resulting in a more distal post-ganglionic nerve rupture, compared to the pre-ganglionic avulsion directly from the spine seen in lower roots. Surgically, this is important as the presence of a root stump can be used in the neonatal period for nerve grafting, which has connotations on surgical options and prognosis (Figures 12.2 and 12.3).

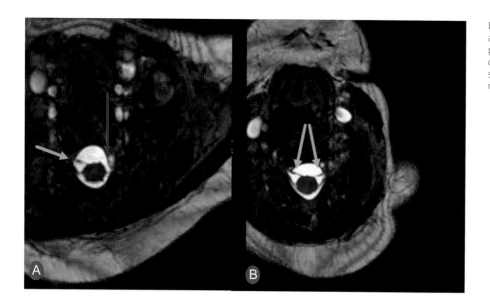

Figure 12.3 MRI scan of the neck showing a root avulsion with the formation of a pseudomeningocele (A, red arrow), in comparison to the normal roots on the other side (A and B, green arrows) and lower-level roots (B).

Key Points: Level of Lesion – Pre-ganglionic or Post-ganglionic

- Pre-ganglionic: avulsions from the spinal cord, so spontaneous recovery is not possible. The presence of Horner's syndrome (sympathetic innervation), an elevated hemi-diaphragm, or a winged scapula indicate a pre-ganglionic lesion.
- Post-ganglionic: full or partial spontaneous recovery is possible.
- Prognostic value of biceps recovery in the first 3 months.

Assessment

The child should be relaxed, warm, and recently fed. A head-to-toe examination should include all four extremities to confirm that the lower limbs are not involved – involvement of all four limbs or one upper and one lower limb involvement suggests other neurological causes such as cerebral palsy. Typical positions of the upper limb in Erb's palsy are the shoulder in internal rotation, the elbow in extension, and the fingers in flexion (waiter's tip position) (Figure 12.4).

Horner's syndrome is a consequence of sympathetic neuronal involvement at the level of T1. It signifies a severe, total plexus injury and presents with dry skin, miosis, ptosis, and enophthalmos. Being a consequence of more severe injuries, it may also be associated with phrenic nerve involvement (a chest X-ray is indicated), which is important as this poses a higher anaesthetic risk and also limits the use of the intercostal nerves as potential nerve donors.

Differential Diagnosis

In the infant, the differential diagnosis of a flail (not moving) limb includes clavicular or humeral fracture and septic arthritis. An isolated clavicular or humeral fracture without concomitant brachial plexus injury causes pseudoparalysis of the arm, but the arm does not adopt the typical posture of a brachial plexus

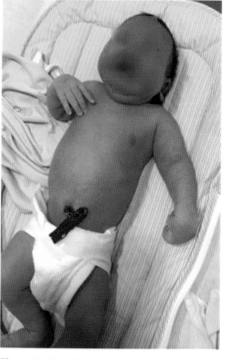

Figure 12.4 A clinical photograph of a 5-month-old baby with a left brachial plexus injury. The left arm is internally rotated; the elbow is extended and the fingers are flexed.

injury, and spontaneous contraction in the deltoid and biceps is observed after 24–48 hours. Localized swelling and bruises give a clue to the diagnosis. X-ray usually confirms the diagnosis. In septic arthritis or osteomyelitis, temperature and raised inflammatory markers raise suspicion. Ultrasound or MRI confirm the diagnosis.

Scoring Systems

Several scoring systems have been used across the world. Knowing these scores and how they are applied in decision-making is beyond the exam scope. However, some basic understanding is useful to appreciate some key principles in treating OBPI.

The Global Function Score is one of the most widely used and scores shoulder abduction, elbow flexion, and wrist, digit, and thumb extensions, with normal function scoring 2, reduced function scoring 1, and no function scoring zero (Table 12.1). A score of zero is the lowest possible score, and 10 is the highest possible score.

In older children (>2 years), the Mallet score (Figure 12.5) is a more comprehensive clinical assessment of shoulder function (abduction, external rotation, hand to neck, hand to back, and hand to mouth), with normal function scoring grade V and no function scoring grade I.

The 'trumpet sign' is named after the way of holding a trumpet, that is, 90° of shoulder abduction. Some children with OBPI assume this position when asked to bring the affected arm to

Table 12.1 Global Function Score

Tests	Score 2 (normal function)	Score 1 (partial function)	Score 0 (no function)
Shoulder abduction			
Elbow flexion			
Wrist extension			
Finger extension			
Thumb extension			
Total			

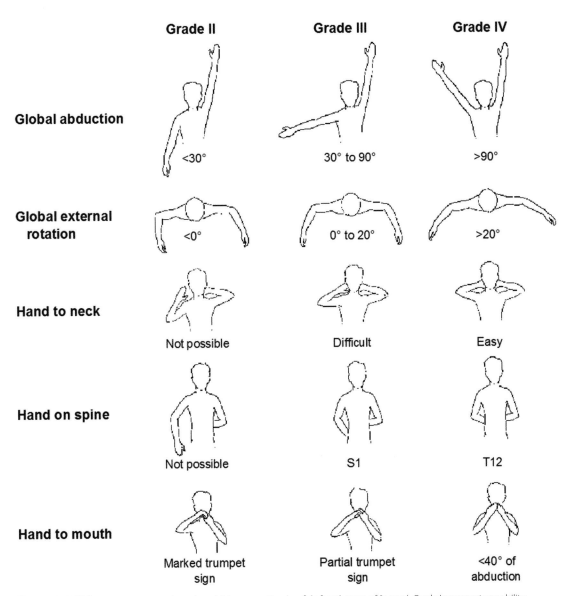

Figure 12.5 Mallet score assessment requires child cooperation (useful after the age of 2 years). Grade I represents no ability, whereas grade V is normal. The 'trumpet sign' is named after the way of holding the trumpet (almost 90° abduction of the affected arm when bringing the hand to the mouth).

213

the mouth (Figure 12.6). This is to compensate for weak elbow flexion (to get gravity assistance) and shoulder internal rotation contracture.

The 'cookie test' is used to assess biceps function at 9 months of age. A cookie is placed in the child's hand on the affected side and the examiner holds the child's elbow adducted at the side to prevent shoulder abduction (the 'trumpet sign'). If the child can bring the cookie to the mouth without bending the neck forward >45°, she or he passes the 'cookie test'.

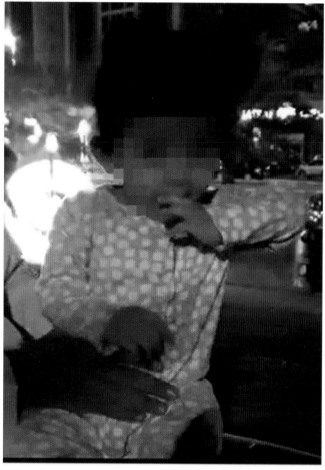

Figure 12.6 The trumpet sign in a child with a left brachial plexus injury.

Investigation

Diagnosis of OBPI is generally clear on clinical examination, so diagnostic tests are generally not needed. However, distinguishing between root avulsions and extraforaminal injury is important to plan surgical interventions. Most clinicians rely on clinical examination to assess severity and the level of injury.

Horner's syndrome indicates severe injury. The rate of recovery of biceps function, shoulder abduction, and wrist extension in the first 3–6 months is generally used to predict recovery [3], although this remains controversial. Myelography, CT, and MRI have all been shown to distinguish between root avulsions and extraforaminal injuries (Figure 12.3).

MRI has the added advantage of showing detailed imaging of the plexus in the neck, as well as of the shoulder joint. Using axial slices, the glenoid version can be measured, relative to the spine of the scapula, and is normally 10–20° retroverted. Joint reduction may be assessed using the posterior humeral head articulation (PHHA) – a measure of the percentage of the humeral head anterior to the middle of the glenoid fossa (Figure 12.7). Unfortunately, MRI requires general anaesthesia in this age group, which carries some risk that parents (and physicians) should consider. CT and ultrasound scanning are alternatives; the former has a risk of radiation, whereas the latter is operator-dependent (Figure 12.8).

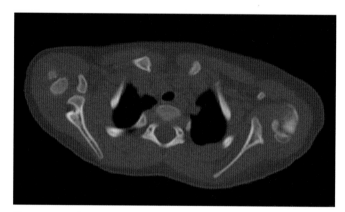

Figure 12.8 Glenohumeral dysplasia of the shoulder in a child with obstetric brachial plexus injury. Cross-sectional CT scan showing a posterior subluxation of the humeral head with substantive dysplasia of the glenoid.

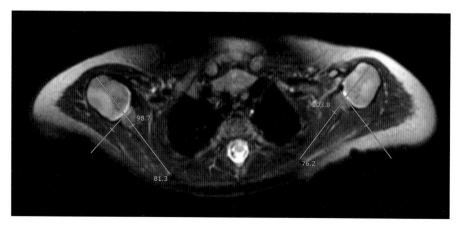

Figure 12.7 MRI scan of the shoulder showing a subtle subluxation of the left glenohumeral joint, as depicted by the percentage of the humeral head anterior to the middle of the glenoid fossa (posterior humeral head articulation, PHHA). Both glenoid versions are within 5° of each other (left side 76.2° versus right side 81.3°), which is acceptable.

Electrophysiological studies are not helpful in assessing severity because electrical motor activity does not always predict acceptable levels of motor function. Dynamic chest fluoroscopy can be used to assess phrenic nerve function.

Surgical Planning

The management of OBPI has been evolving with advancing knowledge and surgical skills; therefore, there is controversy about the timing of, and indications for, primary surgical repair (Figure 12.9). Surgical exploration enables direct assessment of the injury and nerve stimulation, and is often combined with neurolysis and primary nerve reconstruction. Total plexus involvement, pre-ganglionic injury, Horner's syndrome, or a Global Function Score of <4 at 3 months are all indications for surgical exploration. Exploration is usually performed by plastic surgeons or neurosurgeons with interest in brachial plexus repair. Orthopaedic surgeons may be involved in performing clavicle osteotomy to ease access to the surgical field or if there is any concomitant orthopaedic surgery.

Management

Non-surgical Treatment

It is important to maintain passive range of movement in all joints of the affected upper limb whilst waiting for the pattern and extent of recovery in 3–6 months. A specialist physiotherapist should be involved as soon as possible in caring for these children. Shoulder contracture prevention by passive gentle stretching, whilst stabilizing the scapula, is commenced early on.

Surgical Treatment
Primary Interventions

Current recommendations are excision of neuroma and sural nerve grafting for extraforaminal injuries. In the case of root avulsions, nerve transfers are performed using thoracic intercostal nerves and/or branches of the spinal accessory nerve beyond trapezius innervation. A typical nerve transfer in Erb's palsy involves using a branch of the spinal accessory nerve to reconstruct the suprascapular nerve with nerve grafting of the upper and posterior trunks to the C5/6 stumps. After the age of 2 years, the results of nerve transfer procedures are poor and a different approach to management is required.

Interventions to Treat Secondary Pathological Changes

The aims are to reduce the glenohumeral joint and rebalance the shoulder to promote remodelling and restore function. The fundamental principles are to release tight anterior structures, ensure concentric reduction, and restore external rotational power.

The primary structure causing anterior tightness is the subscapularis muscle. Although physiotherapy and Botox injection are used, they are not always effective and surgical release is warranted. This is often done proximally by releasing the subscapularis off the scapula through a small incision over the lateral border of the scapula.

Release alone does not last long. Therefore, powering shoulder external rotation is important.

The most commonly transferred muscle is the latissimus dorsi ± teres major (both are internal rotators of the shoulder), which is transferred to the infraspinatus attachment at the back of the greater tuberosity.

If the glenohumeral joint is subluxed or dislocated, it needs reduction. This is usually done via a posterior approach. Any glenoid dysplasia is corrected through glenoid osteotomy and bone graft (Video 12.1). However, if the joint is badly damaged and the cartilage is worn out, humeral external rotation osteotomy to optimize the upper limb position is preferred.

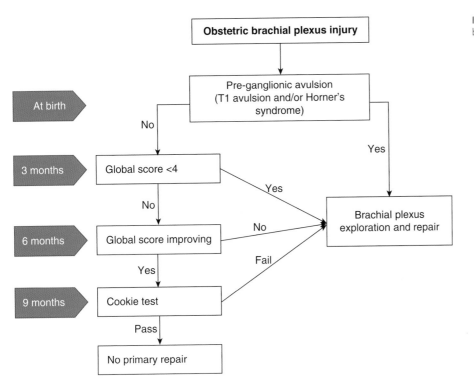

Figure 12.9 Clinical pathway to repair the brachial plexus.

Sometimes, if the joint is good, but there is substantive retroversion (>40°), osteotomy is combined with joint reduction.

 Video 12.1 The glenoid osteotomy and latissmus dorsi transfer.

Elbow flexion paralysis or weakness is disabling. If there is no recovery, it must be powered. Options are:

1. Nerve transfer; the following are popular:
   a. Modified Oberlin's nerve transfer. A fascicle of the ulnar nerve is transferred to the musculocutaneous nerve branch to the biceps
   b. Intercostal nerves
   c. Nerve to the pectoralis major
2. Steindler flexorplasty – transfer of the common flexor tendon to the front of the humerus to act as an elbow flexor. It needs strong wrist extension (or wrist fusion) to work!
3. Free muscle and nerve transfer (the gracilis muscle is the commonest).

Forearm pronation is rarely problematic in these children (unlike cerebral palsy), as it puts the hand in a more functional position. Severe cases can be treated by pronator muscle release or transfer to the supinator (when there is no active supination) and/or radius osteotomy.

Wrist extension weakness can be treated by flexor carpi ulnaris or radialis transfer to the extensor carpi radialis. Severe wrist instability merits bony fusion.

Key Points: Brachial Plexus Injury

Unfortunately, treatment of orthopaedic problems of the upper limbs in neuromuscular conditions in general, and OBPI in particular, is lagging behind lower limb treatment. However, the situation has improved significantly over the last 10 years. We have started seeing a change in practice and teaching modules, but not in the exam yet!

Sprengel's Shoulder

This is a rare congenital anomaly known as Sprengel's deformity and is the result of failure of descent of the scapula from the fetal position in the neck. The scapula remains hypoplastic and elevated (Figure 12.10).

It is associated with other abnormalities in 70% of cases. Muscles that attach the scapula to the spine and chest wall, such as the rhomboids, trapezius, and levator scapulae, show varying degrees of hypoplasia or aplasia. Bony abnormalities include cervical hemivertebra, with or without scoliosis, hypoplasia of the clavicle, and the presence of omovertebral bone. The latter connects the superior border of the scapula to the spinous processes or laminae of the lower cervical vertebrae, thus severely restricting scapular movement. A short humerus or femur, longitudinal deficiency of the radius or tibia, and cardiac and kidney anomalies have also been reported.

Klippel–Feil syndrome (KFS) is a congenital bone disorder characterized by abnormal fusion of two or more cervical vertebrae. It is characterized by a short, webbed neck, decreased range of movement in the cervical spine, and a low hairline. KFS and Sprengel's shoulder are closely associated (Figures 12.10 and 12.11).

Cavendish has classified the deformity into four grades, as shown in Table 12.2.

Treatment

The primary goals of treatment are to improve function and cosmesis. Disability is proportionate to the severity of the deformity. The outcome of surgery is better in early childhood, as the scapula is mobile.

Several surgical procedures have been described:

- The Woodward procedure (or its modifications) involves release of the trapezius and rhomboid muscles through a midline incision, excision of the omovertebral bone when present, and repositioning of the scapula (Figure 12.12).
- The modified Green scapuloplasty procedure involves two-staged operations; with the patient supine, a clavicle osteotomy is performed to protect the brachial plexus. Then the patient is positioned prone. The muscles are detached from their scapular insertion subperiosteally and the omovertebral bone, when present, is excised. The supraspinous fossa of the scapula is resected. The scapula is then displaced distally down to the level of the normal side, and the muscles are reattached in a certain order.
- Konig described an osteotomy within the scapula with the lateral portion pulled down to restore the shoulder joint to its appropriate position (Figure 12.13).
- Mears partial scapular resection (Figure 12.14) involves excision of the suprascapular fossa, a diagonal osteotomy from the superior border to the lateral border of the scapula. The shoulder is passively abducted fully, and the overlapped part excised from the body of the scapula. The two parts can then be sutured together and the layers are closed on top.

Scapular Winging

Scapula protruding from the chest wall, 'winging of the scapula', is a relatively uncommon condition, but a source of parental anxiety. Unilateral winging is common, and bilateral cases are often due to serious muscular dystrophies such as facioscapulohumeral dystrophy [4]. A useful clinical test is to ask the child to push hard against a wall, with the elbows locked in extension.

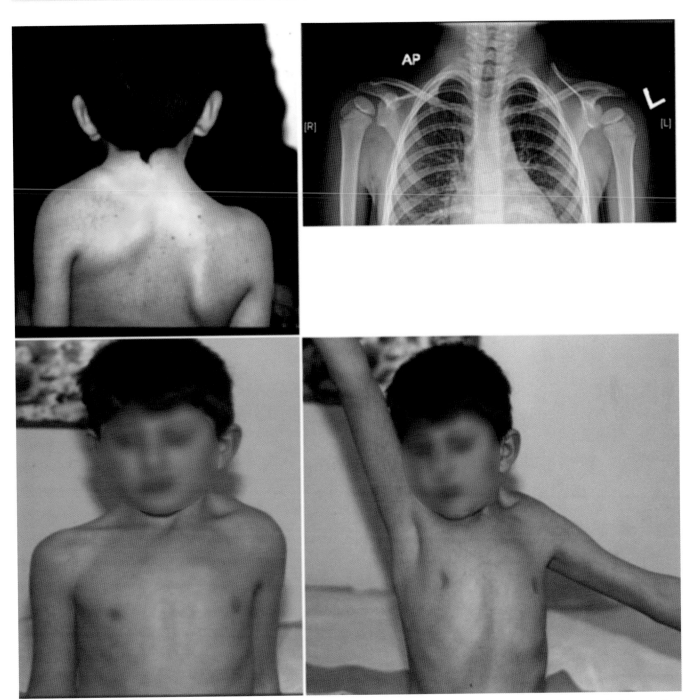

Figure 12.10 Sprengel's shoulder. Notice the high-riding scapula, webbing of the neck, and low hairline. There is limited shoulder abduction, which is caused by scapular–thoracic movement restriction. The glenohumeral joint is often normal.

A normal scapula abuts against the chest wall, but in winging, it stands out. Occasionally, convexity of the rib cage from scoliosis can be mistaken for a winging scapula and the above test helps to differentiate. The incidence of true scapular winging is low, and the importance lies in differentiating it from secondary winging due to neurological, muscular, and other causes. Differential diagnosis includes sequelae of brachial plexus palsy, long thoracic nerve palsy (serratus anterior paralysis) from trauma, and other causes such as scapular dyskinesia and osteochondroma (Figure 12.15).

Table 12.2 Cavendish grading of Sprengel's shoulder

Grade I	The deformity and functional deficits are very minor and no treatment is required
Grade II	The affected scapula is 1–2 cm higher than the normal side, and the superior border of the scapula is prominent. Extra-periosteal excision of the prominent superior border of the scapula is recommended
Grade III	The scapula is 2–5 cm higher, and lowering the scapula improves cosmesis dramatically, whilst function also improves
Grade IV	The scapula is high in the neck very near the occiput, and shoulder function is severely restricted. Surgical release and repositioning of the scapula improve the appearance, but there is often very little improvement in function in this group

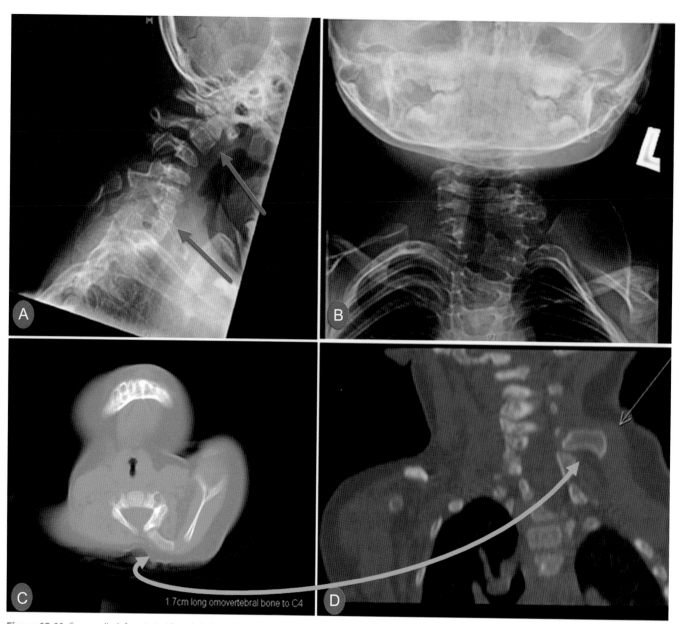

Figure 12.11 Sprengel's deformity in Klippel -Feil syndrome. Notice the cervical spine vertebrae fusion (A, red arrows) and the omovertebral bone (C and D, long and curved green arrow).(B) is AP view of the cervical spine,(C) shows the CT cross-sectional view and (D) the coronal section.

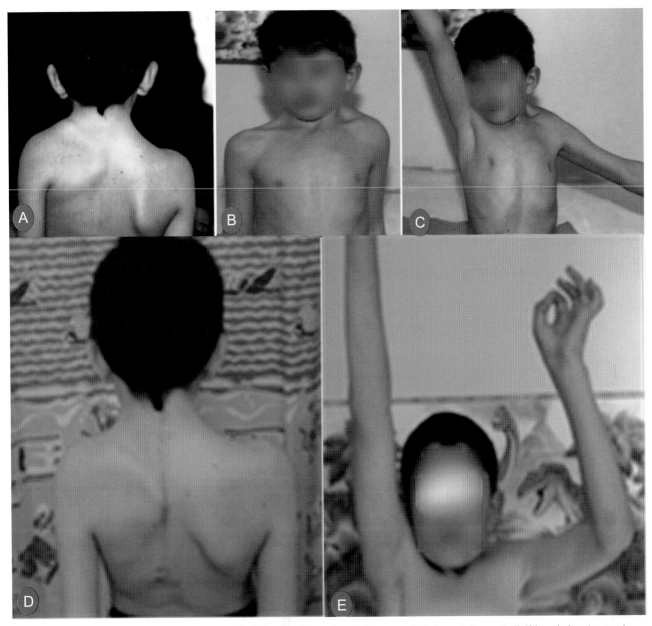

Figure 12.12 Sprengel's shoulder pre- and post-modified Woodward procedure (A-C) (same patient shown in Figure 12.10). Although there is a good cosmetic and functional improvements, they are never perfect (D,E).

Figure 12.13 Konig osteotomy for Sprengel's deformity.

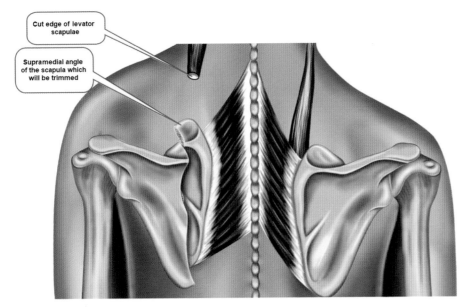

Cut edge of levator scapulae

Supramedial angle of the scapula which will be trimmed

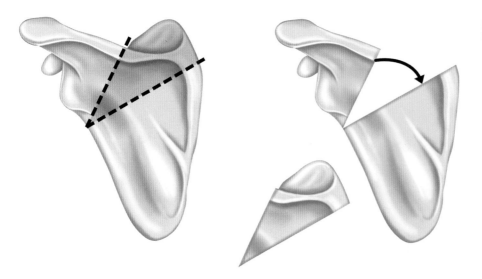

Figure 12.14 Mears partial scapular resection for Sprengel's deformity.

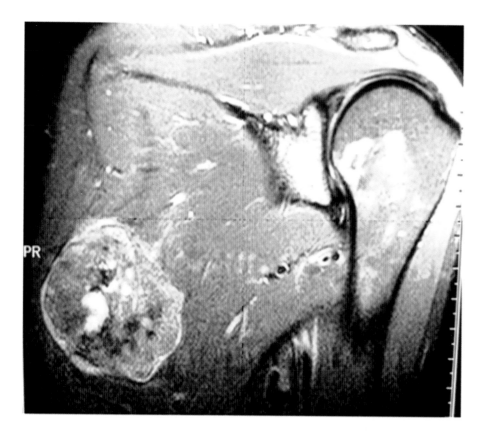

Figure 12.15 Osteochondroma of the ventral surface of the body of the scapula in a child with 'winging of the scapula'.

A good history and a thorough clinical examination are essential to differentiate between primary and secondary causes. Electromyography and MRI are helpful adjuncts. Treatment depends on the cause of winging.

Clavicle Pseudarthrosis

Congenital pseudarthrosis of the clavicle is a rare condition and is invariably seen on the right side, with left clavicle pseudarthrosis only associated with dextrocardia (Figure 12.16). Bilateral cases are very rare. The clavicle develops from fusion of two cartilaginous masses during the seventh week of life. Congenital pseudarthrosis develops due to failure of fusion of these two cartilage masses. With the heart on the left side, the subclavian artery is high on the right side and it is postulated that pulsations of the high subclavian artery hinder fusion of the two cartilage anlages, resulting in pseudarthrosis. The situation reverses in dextrocardia. Surgery is indicated for pain and shoulder deformity interfering with function. Reduction and internal fixation, with or without bone graft, are usually successful in achieving union (in contrast to pseudarthrosis associated with neurofibromatosis).

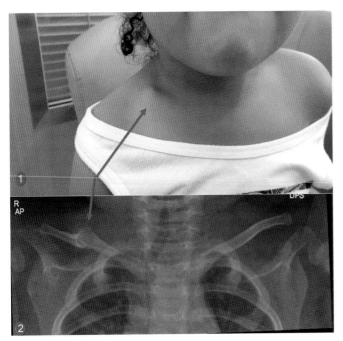

Figure 12.16 Clinical photograph (1) and plain radiograph (2) of a girl with clavicle pseudarthrosis. The X-ray of the right clavicle shows pseudarthrosis in the middle third of the clavicle and the adjoining ends of the clavicle which are rounded off.

Facioscapulohumeral Dystrophy

This is an autosomal dominant muscular dystrophy. It selectively affects the muscles of the face and shoulder girdle. Clinically, this manifests as a Bell's palsy-type droop to the face, with the classical sign of being unable to whistle.

In the shoulder, the scapula cannot be stabilized during abduction, preventing arm elevation despite good deltoid function. Marked winging is usually obvious, and treatment is scapulothoracic fusion using a plate and circlage wiring technique.

The differential for winging in children also includes localized nerve palsies (long thoracic nerve and spinal accessory nerve), Stanmore type 3 shoulder instability (scapula dyskinesia), and scoliosis.

Adolescent Shoulder Instability

The incidence of shoulder instability is poorly described in the paediatric population, although traumatic shoulder dislocation has been described in infants as young as 2 years old, and with increased participation in contact sports, the incidence is rising. It is widely acknowledged that younger patients have a higher risk of recurrence if treated non-operatively (up to 100% in some studies), with rates highest in boys and usually occurring within 2 years of the initial dislocation.

The high risk of further dislocations is caused by disruption of the surrounding structures during the initial event, such as tears to the joint capsule or the glenoid labrum, or damage to the glenoid or humeral head. Adolescents are at higher risk, owing to both their enthusiasm for reparticipating in high-risk activities (such as contact sports) and adolescent hyperlaxity. Recurrent shoulder dislocation in adolescence can go on to cause particular problems, such as glenohumeral joint degeneration, later in life.

Results for arthroscopic reattachment of the damaged labrum to reconstitute the inferior glenohumeral ligament are reasonable in adults. Adolescents have higher early redislocation rates following arthroscopic stabilization (up to a third), although this is lower than when managed non-operatively, and their satisfaction and return to sports are good. Such patients may be more suitable to have a primary coracoid transfer procedure if they wish to return to contact sports.

Non-operative management remains suitable for younger patients with low-level demands who have suffered one single episode of dislocation.

Atraumatic instability may result from congenital causes such as connective tissue disorders (e.g. Ehlers–Danlos syndrome) or glenoid dysplasia. It is often bilateral and referred to as 'born loose'. Its incidence and prevalence are difficult to establish but are generally much lower than for traumatic causes. However, overhead athletes, such as swimmers and gymnasts, have been found to have a higher incidence of multidirectional instability. The vast majority are treated successfully with a physical rehabilitation programme for strengthening and scapular stabilization. Surgery is often avoided though, and recent evidence from the literature suggests good results with an evolved arthroscopic technique in capsular shift for patients who fail conservative management.

Management of anterior dislocation in adolescent age groups, after initial closed reduction and immobilization, is controversial. Because of high recurrence rates, early surgical intervention may be warranted in athletic/active patients ≥14 years of age, with evidence of Bankart lesion on MRI. Management of younger children is controversial and literature supports non-operative treatment.

References

1. Annika J, Paul U, Anna-Lena L. Obstetric brachial plexus palsy – a prospective, population-based study of incidence, recovery and long-term residual impairment at 10 to 12 years of age. *Eur J Paediatr Neurol.* 2019;23(1): 87–93.

2. Olofsson PN, Chu A, McGrath AM. The pathogenesis of glenohumeral deformity and contracture formation in obstetric brachial plexus palsy: a review. *J Brachial Plex Peripher Nerve Inj.* 2019;14(1):e24–34.

3. Gilbert A, Tassin JL. [Surgical repair of the brachial plexus in obstetric paralysis]. *Chirurgie.* 1984;110(1): 70–5.

4. Klyce W, *et al.* Scapular winging in the pediatric patient. *JBJS Rev.* 2018;6(6):e8.

Introduction

Paediatric shoulder injuries are common and frequently associated with organized sports. Boys are more commonly affected, and injuries tend to occur as a consequence of contact with a surface, in sports such as rugby or wrestling, or in the overhead throwing athlete [1].

Accurate interpretation of injury and evaluation of plain radiographs require an understanding of the developing anatomy and sequential ossification of the immature shoulder. Growth plates and ossification centres can often be mistakenly interpreted as sites of injury if the treating physician is unaware.

Anatomy

At birth, the humeral diaphysis, mid shaft of the clavicle, and body of the scapula are ossified, whereas the remaining bones of the shoulder girdle are composed of non-ossified cartilage.

The clavicle is the first bone to begin ossifying in utero at 5 weeks' gestation, with the shaft ossification centre present at birth. The medial sternal physis is the last to close between 18 and 25 years of age, with the majority of clavicular longitudinal growth (80%) occurring through the medial physis. The lateral epiphysis fuses by the age of 18 years. Due to the persistence of physes into adulthood, true dislocations at the medial and lateral ends are rare and are usually physeal injuries which heal and remodel [2].

The majority of the scapula undergoes membranous ossification, and there are seven ossification centres that undergo endochondral ossification.

The proximal humerus begins to ossify at 3–6 months and is composed of three separate secondary ossification centres. The greater and lesser tuberosities appear at 1–2 years of age and fuse between 3 and 5 years. This gives the characteristic tent shape of the proximal humeral physis (Figure 13.1).

Eighty per cent of the longitudinal growth of the humerus occurs at the proximal humeral physis, and 20% at the distal humeral physis. This translates into significant remodelling potential in proximal humeral fractures (Figure 13.2) [3]. The proximal humeral physis fuses between the ages of 15 and 17 years in females and 18 years in males. The periosteum is usually much thinner anteriorly, then posteriorly, and this can lead to hinging of fragments posteriorly and possible entrapment of the periosteum anteriorly or even the long head of the biceps, which can impede fracture reduction.

Injuries to the Clavicle

Childhood clavicle fractures are the commonest fracture around the shoulder girdle, usually associated with competitive sports or a fall from standing height [4]. As with adults, the majority of injuries are midshaft (80%), with lateral (15%) and medial (5%) injuries being less frequent.

Midshaft Clavicle Fractures

In younger children, midshaft clavicle fractures are often incomplete (greenstick). In older active children, they can be completely displaced. The child frequently is seen supporting the elbow with the other hand, with the shoulder drooping, and usually lower, as compared with the normal side. Due to

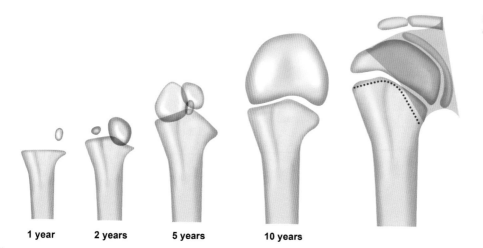

Figure 13.1 Appearance and fusion of the three ossification centres in the proximal humerus.

1 year   2 years   5 years   10 years

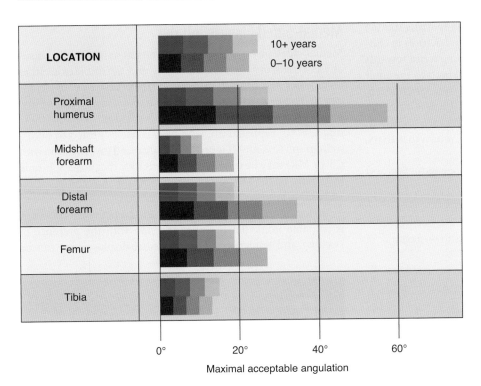

LOCATION	10+ years 0–10 years			
Proximal humerus				
Midshaft forearm				
Distal forearm				
Femur				
Tibia				
	0°	20°	40°	60°

Maximal acceptable angulation

Figure 13.2 Potential for remodelling among various long bones.

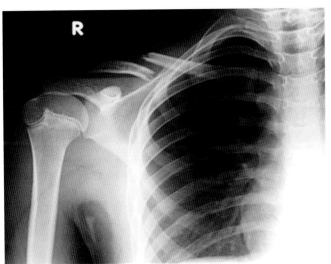

Figure 13.3 Standard anteroposterior radiograph including the full length of the right clavicle, demonstrating a displaced midshaft fracture.

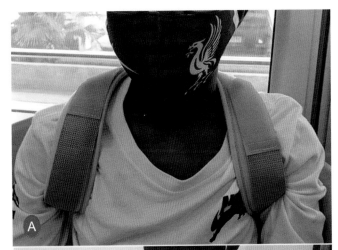

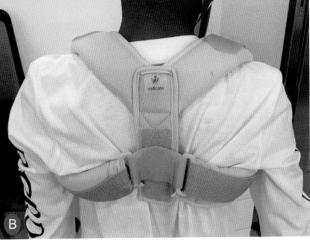

Figure 13.4 A figure-of-eight clavicle strap gives children the ability to use both hands(A,B). It is popular in Europe; the literature, however, shows no real difference in outcomes between patients treated with a figure-of-eight clavicle strap versus those treated with a sling.

tension in the sternocleidomastoid, the head is tilted towards the affected side, with the chin on the opposite side.

Midshaft clavicle fractures are easily identified on anteroposterior (AP) radiographs (Figure 13.3). Further dedicated clavicle views to assess for fracture displacement include a 10–45° cephalad angulation [5]. CT is the imaging modality of choice for identifying occult injuries and injuries involving the sternoclavicular joint.

Midshaft fractures heal well without complications and do not routinely require surgical intervention. Symptomatic treatment in the form of a sling or figure-of-eight clavicle strap helps take tension off the clavicle and provides comfort (Figure 13.4). Non-union of clavicle shaft fractures in children are infrequent (only 21 cases reported in 13 articles in the literature) [6]. Malunions of midshaft clavicle function well, with very little restriction of activities, including contact sports.

As a consequence, there is little evidence supporting routine surgical fixation of displaced midshaft clavicle fractures in children [7]. However, there has been an increasing trend towards surgical fixation, which has largely been influenced by the adult literature [4, 8]. There is evidence that even in older children, the initial fracture position may remodel [8]. There is currently no evidence that operative management of displaced midshaft clavicle fractures improves the time to union, return to activity, or overall complication rate [9].

Currently the only strong indication for open reduction and fixation in childhood are [5]:

- Neurovascular injury
- Open fracture
- Impingement of underlying structures due to posterior displacement
- Fracture fragment causing impending skin penetration.

Plates and screws are the traditional fixation of choice, although flexible nailing has become popular (Figure 13.5). Complications of surgery include anterior chest wall numbness, hardware irritation/prominence (59% of cases), and scar/wound issues.

Medial-Sided Clavicle Injuries

Medial-sided physeal separation are an uncommon injury, usually as a result of a high-impact injury, and can displace in either an anterior or a posterior direction. They can be difficult injuries to diagnose, so clinical evaluation and a high index of suspicion are key. Rockwood described a serendipity view for these injuries (40° cephalad tilt, with both clavicles projected onto a radiograph cassette) (Figure 13.6). Advanced investigation with CT or MRI may be required for a definitive diagnosis. Chronic instability of the sternoclavicular joint is a rare complication and may evade diagnosis.

In an anteriorly displaced injury, the metaphyseal fragment is palpable immediately under the skin with the presence of swelling and tenderness. Posteromedial displacement can be

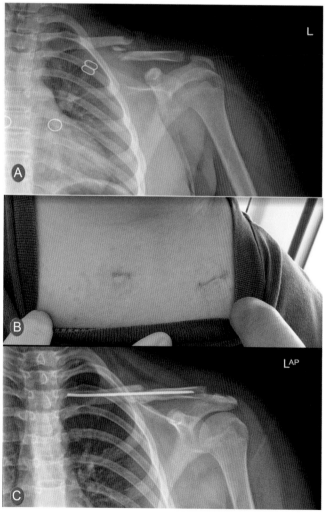

Figure 13.5 Midshaft clavicle fracture with impending skin puncture. AP shoulder radiograph demonstrating fracture(A) This was treated with open reduction and flexible nailing(B). Post op radiograph demonstrating flexible nailing(C). Postoperatively patient is encouraged to move the arm as much as tolerated. Immobilisation is not required. Extreme overhead activities usually limited for 3-6 weeks. Nail can be removed at 3 months.

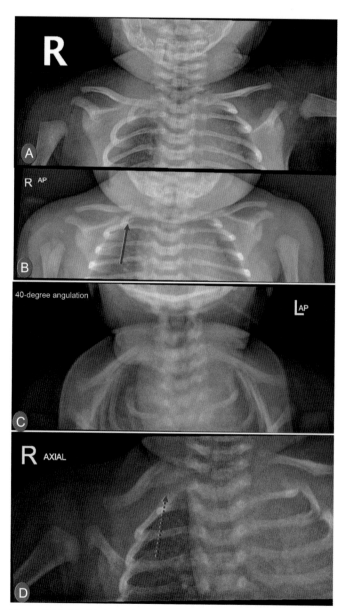

Figure 13.6 Medial clavicle fractures in children can be difficult to spot(A). This is due to the medial clavicle physis(B, solid red arrow). A serendipity view (C) (ultrasound and CT are good alternatives) can be very useful. (D) shows a large callus formation (dashed red arrow) due to macromotion at the fracture site.

life-threatening or can cause more serious injury due to compression of, or damage to, the underlying structures: trachea (dyspnoea and voice hoarseness), lung (pneumothorax), subclavian artery (vascular insufficiency), and brachial plexus (paraesthesia, numbness, or weakness).

In cases of both anteriorly and posteriorly displaced uncomplicated fracture patterns, immobilization with support of a sling usually results in a good long-term functional outcome. The presence of a robust periosteal sleeve usually results in effective remodelling at these sites. Unusual complications, such as thoracic outlet syndrome due to exuberant callus formation, have been reported but are extremely rare.

Where there is compromise of the overlying skin with an anterior dislocation, attempts at closed reduction are usually unsuccessful, with residual instability [10] (Figure 13.7). An anterior approach centred on the sternoclavicular joint allows for direct reduction, with options for subsequent stabilization. Various suture techniques are described, which adequately hold the reduced fragment [10, 11], avoiding the need for metalwork in this area in children.

In cases of posterior dislocation with associated neurovascular compromise, it is essential that a vascular or cardiothoracic surgeon is alerted prior to attempting reduction. Placing the child on a sandbag between the scapulae aids to elevate the medial end of the clavicle. Again, an anterior approach to the sternoclavicular joint is required, ensuring that this can be extended if vascular control is needed. Direct reduction of the posteriorly displaced fragment using a blunt clamp can subsequently be held and stabilized with suture techniques.

Lateral-Sided Clavicle Injuries

Lateral-sided injuries are sustained due to a direct blow to the shoulder. Symptoms depend on the type of injury and can mimic an acromioclavicular (AC) joint dislocation; the child complains of pain at the distal clavicle, with an inability to lift the arm. True AC joint dislocations are rare in the paediatric

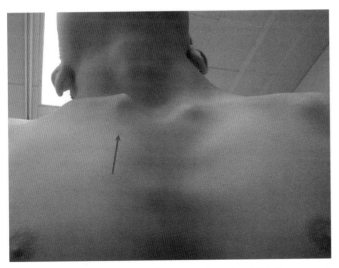

Figure 13.7 Anterior dislocation of the sternoclavicular joint that was caused by a fall from a horse. Although closed reduction was successful, the patient was left with anterior instability.

population, as the coracoacromial and AC ligaments usually stay attached to the inferior periosteal sleeve.

A number of subtypes of childhood injury have been described by Nenopoulos et al. (similar to modified Rockwood's classification) (Figure 13.8) [12], where fractures are classified from group I to V.

Once again, the adult literature has influenced the surgical management of these injuries, despite there being evidence to suggest that the majority of children do well without surgery [12] (Figure 13.9). Nenopoulos et al. suggested an algorithm for treatment, with all their children reported to have a good functional outcome, irrespective of treatment (Figure 13.10).

The Scapula

Fractures of the scapula are extremely uncommon injuries in both adults and children. As with adults, they are associated with high-energy injuries usually seen in addition to injuries to the chest, upper limb, and spine [21].

Diagnosis can often be difficult on standard AP and scapular Y plain radiographic views. CT with three-dimensional reconstructions may be helpful, and MRI can aid in the diagnosis of physeal fractures and avulsions.

The coracoid and AC joints are the most commonly injured areas of the scapula. Treatment is largely supportive, with analgesia and a supportive broad arm sling; functional outcomes are generally good. Surgery is usually described as part of individual case reports when associated with a significant mechanism of injury and surrounding structure compromise.

Injuries to the Humerus

The proximal humeral physis typically closes between 14 and 17 years in girls and between 16 and 18 years in boys. This physis contributes about 80% of the overall humeral length; therefore, injuries to this area at a young age may have long-term consequences. The biological activity of this physis, in conjunction with the mobility of the glenohumeral joint, allows for extensive remodelling of fractures.

Proximal Humeral Fractures

Proximal humeral fractures account for 3% of all physeal injuries. Although seen in children of all ages, they are common among adolescents. Most of them are Salter–Harris type I–II injuries. These fractures are sustained either by direct force on the shoulder or indirectly through the humeral shaft when the child falls onto an outstretched hand. In the newborn, physeal injuries can occur during birth. Fractures occurring under the age of 3 years need to be assessed for non-accidental injury.

Classification of these fractures is based on the type of physeal injury or displacement of the fracture, or both. Younger children usually have Salter–Harris type I physeal injuries. Older children can have Salter–Harris type II–IV physeal injuries. Fracture dislocations are rare.

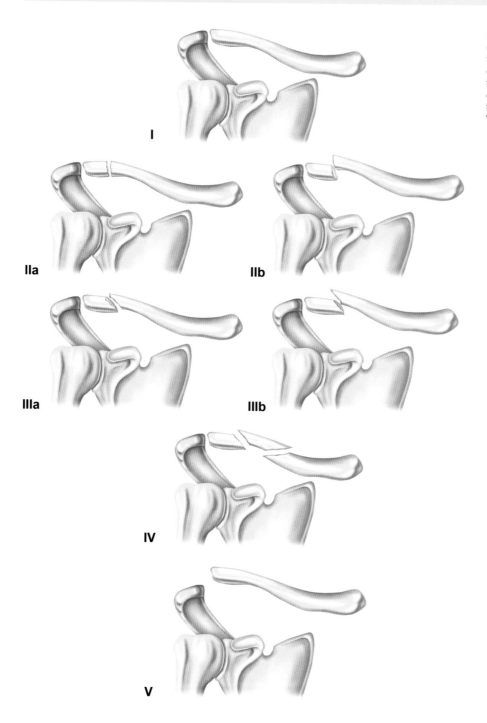

Figure 13.8 Nenopoulos *et al.*'s classification of lateral clavicle injury. Group I: greenstick fractures; group IIa: transverse fractures without displacement; group IIb: displaced transverse fractures; group IIIa: oblique fractures without displacement; group IIIb: displaced oblique fractures; group IV: comminuted fractures; group V: acromioclavicular dislocation.

Neer and Horwitz graded these fractures according to the amount of displacement (Table 13.1) [13].

Some amount of angulation is always associated with grade 3 and 4 injuries.

AP radiographs centred on the shoulder can identify the physeal fracture easily. The scapular Y view helps to assess the direction of displacement. Axillary views, although difficult to obtain in an acute injury, can be obtained with as little as 40° of abduction and can aid to judge the degree of displacement. CT scans can provide additional detail in cases of intra-articular injuries.

Most of these fractures heal extremely well with non-operative management.

Grade 1 and 2 injuries can be treated with a collar and cuff or a sling. Pendulum exercises can be started at 2–3 weeks as pain allows. Most of the children can start doing overhead activities at 6–8 weeks after injury.

Grade 3 and 4 injuries can be treated non-operatively in younger children. As the child's age increases, some surgeons are keen on managing them by operative methods. Many studies have shown no difference in functional outcomes in patients with grade 3/4 injuries who are treated non-operatively [14], whilst

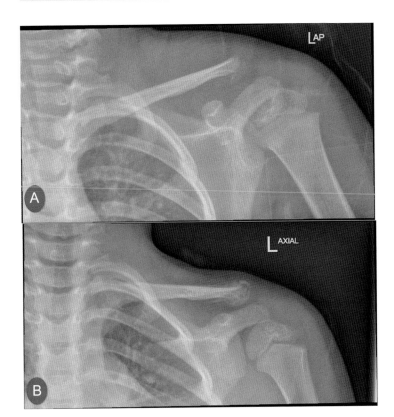

Figure 13.9 Type IIb with displacement of less than two cortices, treated with a sling(A,B).

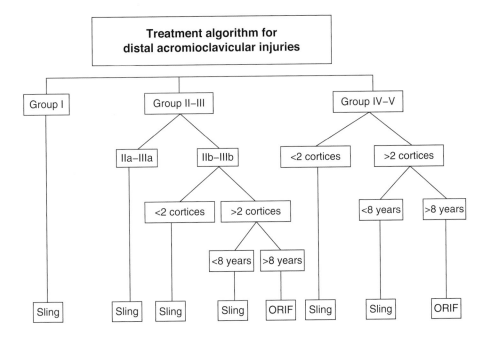

Treatment algorithm for distal acromioclavicular injuries

Figure 13.10 Treatment algorithm for lateral clavicle injuries, according to Nenopoulos *et al.* Open reduction and internal fixation (ORIF) is recommended when there is a displacement of more than two cortices in children above 8 years old (otherwise, non-operative treatment).

Table 13.1 Neer and Horwitz grading of proximal humeral fractures

Grade 1	<5 mm displacement
Grade 2	Displacement between 5 mm and one-third of the diameter of the humeral shaft
Grade 3	Displacement between one-third and two-thirds of the diameter of the humeral shaft
Grade 4	Displacement greater than two-thirds of the diameter of the humeral shaft

there have been reports of complications in patients treated surgically, including impingement of hardware requiring removal, osteomyelitis, and fractures through percutaneous pin sites.

Due to the tremendous potential of healing and great range of mobility of the glenohumeral joint, there is a tendency to accept deformity after union and reassure the parents that the bone will remodel with almost full functional range [15, 16].

Indications for surgery include:

- Intra-articular fractures (deltopectoral approach and anterior arthrotomy)
- Open fractures
- Neurovascular injury
- Neer–Horowitz grade 4 injury in patients nearing skeletal maturity
- Polytrauma patients to help in nursing (Figure 13.11).

Almost all fractures heal completely, giving a good functional range. Grade 4 injuries may damage the physis and hence cause stoppage of growth, resulting in a short arm. This does not affect the function though. Varus malunion is also reported; however, function of the glenohumeral joint is hardly affected. Osteonecrosis is reported in a few cases but is a rare complication.

Shaft of the Humerus

Humeral shaft fractures are the second commonest birth fractures. In children, they are not as common as they occur in adults. However, these humeral shaft fractures are often associated with radial nerve injuries, as they are in adults.

These humeral shaft fractures are straightforward injuries as a result of high-energy direct force on the arm. They can also occur due to indirect force, as transmitted after a fall on an outstretched arm, leading to spiral or oblique fracture patterns of the shaft. When fracture of the shaft of the humerus occurs after trivial or low-energy trauma, it should raise suspicion of a pathological fracture, as a unicameral bone cyst is quite common in this region, along with other benign bone conditions. In the setting of high-energy trauma, shaft fractures are part of multiple injuries and the fracture pattern often involves transverse, comminuted, or open injuries.

Clinically, these fractures are associated with pain, swelling, and crepitus, with deformity of the arm. The close relationship of the radial nerve to the shaft of the humerus makes it prone to injury. Careful examination is crucial in looking for sensation on the dorsum of the first web space of the hand and movements of the wrist, finger, and thumb extensors, as well as supination of the forearm. Ulnar and median nerve injuries are uncommon, and vascular injuries are very rare.

Plain AP and lateral radiographs help to assess the fracture pattern and alignment. CT is helpful in assessing fractures extending into the elbow or shoulder joint.

In older children, humeral shaft fractures are managed in a collar and cuff or a humeral brace to maintain the alignment for 4–6 weeks (Figure 13.12). Pendulum and circumduction exercises are begun once pain allows. Contrary to lower limb fractures, shortening and deformities are better tolerated.

Indications for open reduction and internal fixation are limited to open fractures/neurovascular injury or as part of treatment of multiple/polytrauma to help facilitate nursing of the patient. Methods of internal fixation include use of flexible intramedullary nails, locking/non-locking plates, and screws (Figure 13.13).

Humeral shaft fractures heal well with non-operative modalities. Complications associated with radial nerve injuries are often treated conservatively with serial casting and immobilization, as reports of complete severance of the radial nerve are rare [17]. The wrist and hand are maintained in functional position throughout the course of treatment. At 3 months, if recovery of radial nerve symptoms is poor, electromagnetic and nerve conduction studies may be warranted.

Non-unions of humeral shaft fractures are rare in children (none reported in the literature), and these are treated with open reduction and internal fixation using plates, along with bone grafting.

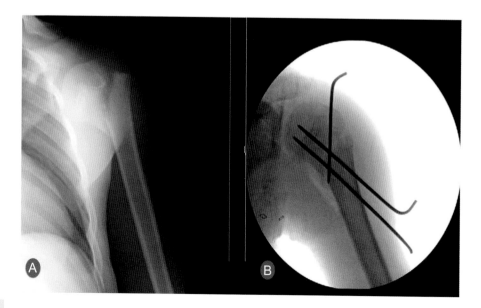

Figure 13.11 (A, B) Proximal humerus fracture that was treated with K-wires.

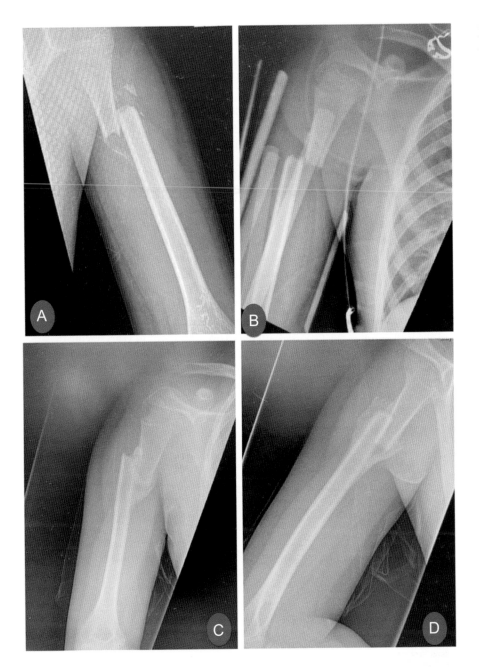

Figure 13.12 (A) Displaced humeral shaft fracture with good alignment. (B) Non-operative treatment using a humeral brace. (C, D) Bridging callus at 4 weeks.

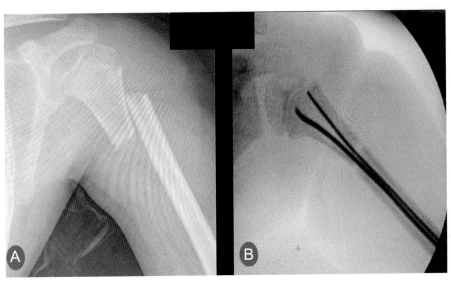

Figure 13.13 Proximal humeral shaft fracture(A) managed with flexible nailing (B).

Birth-Related Fractures of the Newborn

Rates of obstetric fractures are approximately 0.1% of all live births, with the clavicle and humeral shaft most commonly injured (Figure 13.14). These fractures are associated with high-birthweight babies and often occur during birth due to compression of the shoulder in the birth canal. Most of these are asymptomatic and many may have a delayed presentation with pseudoparalysis of the arm. An associated nerve injury can be present in up to 7.5%, and a comprehensive brachial plexus assessment must be carried out.

For neonatal clavicle injuries, plain radiographs may show an abundant periosteal reaction, which can discriminate this from the congenital condition, pseudarthrosis of the clavicle. Advice for the symptomatic newborn includes gentle handling of the baby. The limb can be supported by a tubular bandage or tucked inside the baby's vest to help reduce discomfort. Pain almost always subsides in 10–14 days, with return of normal shoulder range of motion.

Obstetric and infantile humeral shaft fractures are managed in swathe bandage, with the arm strapped across the thorax for 1–3 weeks. Parents are advised about skincare and cautioned about callus formation, which appears as a bump in the arm after about 6–8 weeks and which would eventually settle due to high remodelling potential. Follow-up is usually to detect any injury to the brachial plexus.

Paediatric Shoulder Instability

The glenohumeral joint has great mobility at the cost of its stability. The muscles of the rotator cuff supraspinatus, infraspinatus, teres minor, and subscapularis provide dynamic stability to the shoulder joint. The capsule and ligaments, along with bone components, provide static stability. The surface area of the capsule is almost twice that of the size of the humeral head. Anterior glenohumeral ligaments are condensations of the inner aspect of the capsule. Among these, the anterior glenohumeral ligament is the most important and most frequent area of pathology in anterior shoulder dislocation.

Glenohumeral dislocations have been reported in as young as a 2-year-old child. Dislocations associated with general hyperlaxity in childhood follow a more chronic course and will not be discussed further. Acute traumatic dislocations are more common among adolescents who are actively involved in contact sports, with males over the age of 14 years having the greatest incidence of recurrent problems [18].

The direction of the dislocation depends on the position of the arm at the time of the injury. An indirect force with the

Figure 13.14 Humeral fracture following difficult dystocia labour.(A) The fracture healed with abundant callus (B)

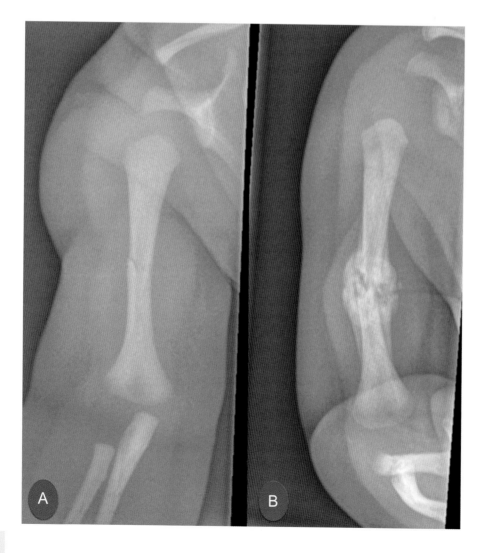

arm in a position of abduction, extension, and external rotation results in an anterior dislocation (90% of all dislocations of the shoulder joint). The child presents with severe pain and anterior shoulder swelling. The arm is held in slight abduction and external rotation, whilst supporting the affected elbow with the opposite hand. Clinically, the humeral head can be palpated anteriorly. Neurological examination to test the radial, ulnar, median, and axillary nerves is essential. The axillary nerve is the most commonly affected nerve in shoulder dislocations. Testing for shoulder abduction (deltoid) and sensation over the regimental badge area is key to ruling out axillary nerve injury.

For a posterior dislocation, the force required is usually larger, with a posteriorly directed force to the anterior aspect of the shoulder or arm in flexion, adduction, and internal rotation. Posterior dislocation also occurs after contraction of large muscles, which occurs during seizures or electrocution. In posterior shoulder dislocations, the child will hold the arm in a fixed, internally rotated position.

Cases of inferior glenohumeral dislocations (luxatio erecta) in children have been reported and account for <1% of all reported shoulder dislocations. The injury results from force acting on the shoulder during hyperabduction. The clinical picture of severe shoulder pain, elevated fixed abduction of the arm, and flexion of the elbow is classical. Nerve injury has been reported in up to 50% of these cases [19].

Standard plain radiographs – AP, scapular Y, and axillary views – can aid in the diagnosis of the direction of dislocation and more usefully exclude associated bony injury. The position of the humeral head in the subcoracoid position confirms an anterior dislocation. Posterior dislocations are often missed on radiographs, as the internal rotation, or 'light bulb sign', may be subtle on AP views. The inferior position of the humeral head, with the diaphysis directed superiorly and parallel to the scapular spine, confirms luxatio erecta.

A reduction should be attempted immediately after diagnosis. The commonest methods are a traction–countertraction technique in line with the humeral shaft, with a folded sheet across the torso of the patient helping in countertraction. The arm is then placed in a sling and immobilized for 2–3 weeks, and gentle pendulum exercises are started thereafter to prevent stiffness. A post-reduction neurovascular examination is mandatory to clear any iatrogenic injury. Post-reduction plain radiographs are essential to ensure a concentric reduction, with no evidence of any fractures.

CT with three-dimensional reconstructions is helpful for assessing bony lesions – bony Bankart, Hill–Sachs lesions, and glenoid bone loss in cases of recurrent dislocations. Magnetic resonance arthrography (MRA) can identify the spectrum of intra-articular pathologies that have been described in children: labral tears, anterior labral periosteum sleeve avulsions (ALPSAs), glenolabral articular disruptions (GLADs), rotator cuff tendon injuries (partial articular supraspinatus tendon avulsions, or PASTAs), and humeral avulsions of the glenohumeral ligament (HAGLs) [20].

There is a high risk of recurrence of instability in children due to inherent capsular laxity and disruption of surrounding capsuloligamentous structures. Younger patients may not be compliant with rehabilitation and have higher enthusiasm for reparticipation in contact sports or high-risk activities. Redislocation rates can be as high as 50–70% of children under 18 years of age and may require surgical stabilization in up to 20% of cases [21, 22].

The outcomes for surgery in children after a shoulder dislocation are variable, and surgical options are usually offered when non-operative treatment fails. However, there is some evidence that there is a high chance of recurrence, even after a first-time dislocation, and some authors advocate surgical stabilization at this stage [23].

A systematic review of surgical stabilization in anterior shoulder instability demonstrated that either an arthroscopic or an open Bankart repair is the most commonly performed procedure [24]. It is notable that there is double the risk of recurrent dislocations/subluxations in adolescents, compared to adults, after surgical stabilization. The presence of glenoid bone loss can lead to failure of surgical stabilization and may be underappreciated. Recurrent dislocations with associated glenoid bone loss of >20–25% may benefit from a primary bone block procedure such as coracoid transfer [25].

Given the high rates of failure associated with surgery, a more non-surgical approach in children with regard to intense physiotherapy and activity modification is usually followed. There is a high-level return to activities and sports, usually between 12 and 28 weeks, irrespective of treatment.

References

1. Kirkwood G, Hughes TC, Pollock AM. Results on sports-related injuries in children from NHS emergency care dataset Oxfordshire pilot: an ecological study. *J R Soc Med*. 2019;112(3):109–18.

2. Hughes JL, *et al*. The clavicle continues to grow during adolescence and early adulthood. *HSS J*. 2020;16(Suppl 2):372–7.

3. Staheli L. *Fundamentals of Pediatric Orthopaedics*, 4th ed. Philadelphia, PA: Lippincott Williams & Wilkins; 2008.

4. Ellis HB, *et al*. Descriptive epidemiology of adolescent clavicle fractures: results from the FACTS (Function after Adolescent Clavicle Trauma and Surgery) prospective, multicenter cohort study. *Orthop J Sports Med*. 2020;8(5):2325967120921344.

5. Herring JA. *Tachdjians' Pediatric Orthopaedics*, 5th ed. Philadelphia, PA: Saunders Elsevier; 2014.

6. Hughes K, *et al*. Clavicle fracture nonunion in the paediatric population: a systematic review of the literature. *J Child Orthop*. 2018;12(1):2–8.

7. Ahearn BM, *et al*. Factors influencing time to return to sport following clavicular fractures in adolescent athletes. *J Shoulder Elbow Surg*. 2021;30(7):S140–4.

8. Pennock AT, *et al*. Changes in superior displacement, angulation, and shortening in the early phase of healing for completely displaced midshaft clavicle fractures in adolescents: results from a prospective, multicenter study. *J Shoulder Elbow Surg*. 2021;30(12):2729–37.

9. Nawar K, *et al*. Operative versus non-operative management of

mid-diaphyseal clavicle fractures in the skeletally immature population: a systematic review and meta-analysis. *Curr Rev Musculoskelet Med*. 2020;13(1):38–49.

10. Swarup I, *et al*. Open reduction and suture fixation of acute sternoclavicular fracture-dislocations in children. *JBJS Essent Surg Tech*. 2020;10(3):e19.00074.

11. Siebenmann C, *et al*. Epiphysiolysis type Salter I of the medial clavicle with posterior displacement: a case series and review of the literature. *Case Rep Orthop*. 2018;2018:4986061.

12. Nenopoulos SP, *et al*. Outcome of distal clavicular fracture separations and dislocations in immature skeleton. *Injury*. 2011;42(4):376–80.

13. Neer CS, Horwitz BS. Fractures of the proximal humeral epiphysial plate. *Clin Orthop Relat Res*. 1965;41(1):24–31.

14. Chaus GW, *et al*. Operative versus nonoperative treatment of displaced proximal humeral physeal fractures. *J Pediatr Orthop*. 2015;35(3):234–9.

15. [No authors]. Towards evidence-based emergency medicine: best BETs from the Manchester Royal Infirmary. BET 2: Is ultrasound or plain film radiography a more sensitive diagnostic modality for diagnosing slipped capital femoral epiphysis? *Emerg Med J*. 2014;31(1):78.

16. King ECB, Ihnow SB. Which proximal humerus fractures should be pinned? Treatment in skeletally immature patients. *J Pediatr Orthop*. 2016;36(Suppl 1):S44–8.

17. O'Shaughnessy MA, *et al*. Management of paediatric humeral shaft fractures and associated nerve palsy. *J Child Orthop*. 2019;13(5):508–15.

18. Olds M, *et al*. In children 18 years and under, what promotes recurrent shoulder instability after traumatic anterior shoulder dislocation? A systematic review and meta-analysis of risk factors. *Br J Sports Med*. 2015;50(18):1135–41.

19. Stensby JD, Fox MG. MR arthrogram findings of luxatio erecta in a pediatric patient—arthroscopic confirmation and review of the literature. *Skeletal Radiol*. 2014;43(8):1191–4.

20. Edmonds EW, Roocroft JH, Parikh SN. Spectrum of operative childhood intra-articular shoulder pathology. *J Child Orthop*. 2014;8(4):337–40.

21. Yapp LZ, *et al*. Traumatic glenohumeral dislocation in pediatric patients is associated with a high risk of recurrent instability. *J Pediatr Orthop*. 2021. doi: 10.1097/BPO.0000000000001863.

22. Longo UG, *et al*. Epidemiology of paediatric shoulder dislocation: a nationwide study in Italy from 2001 to 2014. *Int J Environ Res Public Health*. 2020;17(8):2834.

23. Bonazza NA, Riboh JC. Management of recurrent anterior shoulder instability after surgical stabilization in children and adolescents. *Curr Rev Musculoskelet Med*. 2020;13(2):164–72.

24. Shanmugaraj A, *et al*. Surgical stabilization of pediatric anterior shoulder instability yields high recurrence rates: a systematic review. *Knee Surg Sports Traumatol Arthrosc*. 2020;29(1): 192–201.

25. Sofu H, *et al*. Recurrent anterior shoulder instability: review of the literature and current concepts. *World J Clin Cases*. 2014;2(11):676–82.

14

Orthopaedic Elbow Disorders

Om Lahoti and Matt Nixon

Radioulnar Synostosis

Radioulnar synostosis refers to the bony bridge between the radius and the ulna. This can be either congenital or post-traumatic. The precise cause of congenial synostosis is unknown. Embryologically, the elbow forms from the three cartilaginous parts representing the humerus, radius, and ulna. A programmed cavitation process leads to formation of the elbow joint; if this process fails, endochondral ossification results in a bony synostosis. Because the forearm bones differentiate at a time when the fetal forearm is in pronation, almost all forearm synostoses are fixed in this position.

Moreover, this process occurs at a time when all organ systems are forming; therefore, synostoses are seen in conjunction with, for example, Apert syndrome (acrocephalosyndactyly), Carpenter syndrome (acropolysyndactyly), arthrogryposis, and Klinefelter syndrome.

Congenital radioulnar synostosis is bilateral in 60% of cases. Like tarsal coalition, although it is a prenatal condition and present at birth, it is often undetected until early childhood, when lack of forearm rotation (i.e. pronation or supination) interferes with day-to-day activities. Children with congenital radioulnar synostosis may have difficulty in using a spoon and pencil, fastening buttons, and grasping small objects.

In severe cases, there is hyperpronation with a 'back-handed grasp'. In these situations, early realignment is indicated to allow proper hand development. In cases with minor restriction of forearm rotation, minor trauma is often blamed for such restriction, but the X-ray findings are often typical (Figure 14.1). Occasionally, synostosis may be post-traumatic, secondary to abnormal healing of combined radius and ulna fractures.

Treatment

Treatment depends on the degree of pronation fixation and functional difficulties. Painful snapping of the elbow has been reported but is extremely rare.

Generally, no treatment is required if the forearm is held in a neutral position. Similarly, unilateral cases are usually not disabling and often do not need treatment.

Fixed pronation of 45° or more is disabling, particularly in bilateral cases, and surgery is an option to improve function. There is broad agreement that only one side should be corrected, but in certain cultures, bilateral correction is desirable. In western cultures, the dominant hand is left in a pronated position and the non-dominant hand is corrected into various degrees of supination. Rotational osteotomy is the preferred surgery, and

excision of synostosis and fat interposition graft are reserved for post-traumatic synostosis only.

Site of osteotomy, single- or both-bone osteotomies, extent and mode of correction, and fixation methods remain controversial. Neurovascular compromise and compartment syndrome are important complications of acute rotational correction. Gradual correction in a circular frame is an option to minimize acute neurovascular compromise. Similarly, single-bone (radius diaphysis) osteotomy is also a safer alternative. Both-bone osteotomy is preferred for >45° rotational correction. The optimal position after osteotomy is also controversial, but 30–45° supination appears to be in the satisfactory range.

The reverse Sauve–Kapandji procedure has been promoted recently, with some promising results (Figure 14.2) [1].

Congenital Radial Head Dislocation

Congenital radial head dislocation is a rare condition, with an estimated incidence of 0.06–0.16%, but it generates considerable interest in paediatric orthopaedic clinics because it can be confused with traumatic dislocation of the radial head – particularly when the child presents after a minor incident. Distinguishing between the two clinical entities is important to avoid unnecessary anxiety and surgery. Good clinical history and clinical examination, and careful assessment of radiographs often help to differentiate. Posterior dislocation of the radial head is commoner in congenital dislocation than in traumatic dislocation. Although children with congenital radial head dislocation usually have reasonable elbow function and satisfactory pain-free supination and pronation, some of them become symptomatic during adolescence. An audible click and a radial head prominence are other presenting symptoms (Figure 14.3).

Congenital radial head dislocation is often associated with radioulnar synostosis and syndromes such as Larsen syndrome and nail–patella syndrome, so careful assessment is essential.

Radiology

Radiographs of the elbow are often characteristic, with posterior dislocation and loss of concavity of the radial head and convex shape of the capitellum and ulna. In some cases, it may be necessary to take comparison X-rays of the other elbow.

Treatment

Most congenital cases are asymptomatic or minimally symptomatic, and a simple explanation and reassurance are all that is necessary. In some cases, the clicks can be painful and the

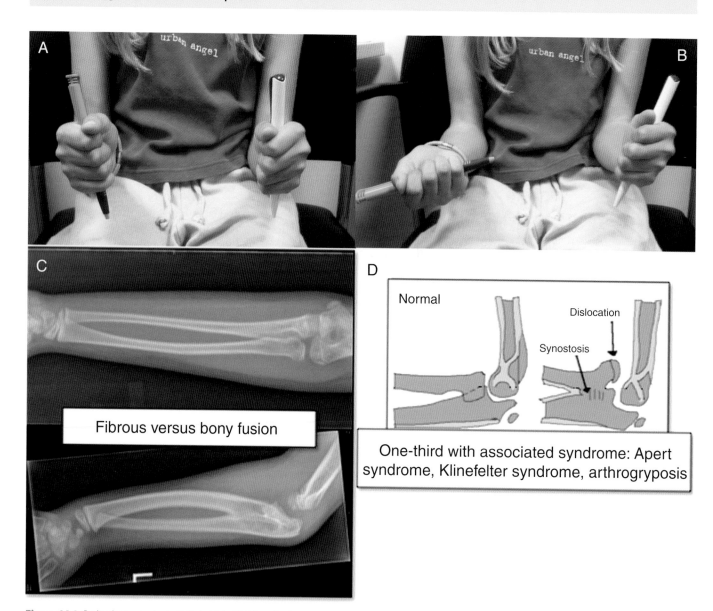

Normal

Dislocation

Synostosis

Fibrous versus bony fusion

One-third with associated syndrome: Apert syndrome, Klinefelter syndrome, arthrogryposis

Figure 14.1 Radioulnar synostosis. (A, B) A child with left radioulnar synostosis; there a restriction of supination. (C) Fibrous synostosis (top) and bony synostosis (bottom). (D) Diagrammatic features of synostosis with and without radial head dislocation.

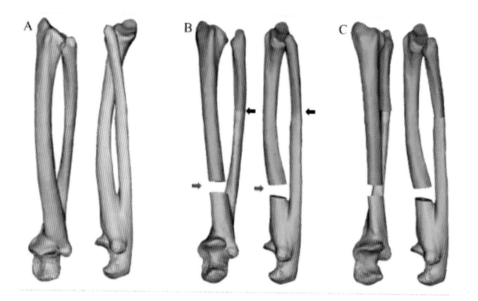

Figure 14.2 Reverse Sauvé–Kapandji procedure for congenital radioulnar synostosis.

A B

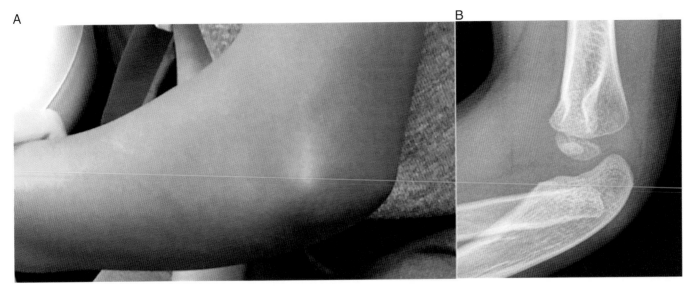

Figure 14.3 Congenital radial head dislocation. (A) Radiograph of the left elbow showing a typical posterior dislocation of the radial head. (B) Clinical picture of a prominent radial head.

prominent dislocated radial head needs intervention. Radial head relocation and reconstruction of the annular ligament are generally not advised in cases of congenital radial head dislocation because of a high rate of failure.

Radial head excision has been shown to improve rotational movement and elbow pain. Proximal migration of the radius and secondary effects on the wrist remain a concern in the long term, although satisfactory results have been reported in the medium term. Parents should be alerted to the possibility of some degree of residual stiffness, cubitus valgus, and wrist pain after radial head excision.

Madelung Deformity

Madelung deformity (MD) (Figure 14.4) is a rare deformity that results from asymmetric growth arrest of the volar and ulnar aspects of the distal radial physis. Although it is often described as congenital, this has never been proven at birth or even in early childhood.

The cause(s) is still unknown. Most patients with MD have an abnormal band of ligament between the radius and the lunate, called the Vickers ligament. It is 5–7 mm thick and histologically consists of fibrous tissue, fibrocartilage, and some areas of hyaline cartilage. It is found under the pronator quadratus and extends from the physis on the ulnar side of the anterior corner of the radius to the lunate. This ligament has been connected with the aetiology of idiopathic MD [2]. Ligament tethering results in increased volar and ulnar tilt. The ulna grows normally, thus becoming longer than the radius. This causes the ulnar head to be prominent and the carpus migrates proximally into the gap between the radius and the ulna. In addition, the forearm is shorter than normal.

Although it is frequently associated with Leri–Weill dyschondrosteosis and Turner's syndrome, it also presents as an isolated condition. It is common in females, with a 4:1 ratio, and is often bilateral, but not always symmetrical. Subtle deformity may be noticeable in childhood, but it becomes more noticeable

during growth. Many patients with MD have good wrist function and very little pain, and the main concern is cosmetic. However, the wrist can become painful after skeletal maturity.

There are several conditions that mimic MD. Multiple epiphyseal dysplasia, Ollier disease, and multiple hereditary or solitary exostoses (Figure 14.5) cause pseudo-Madelung or Madelung-type deformity. Post-traumatic or infective partial growth of the distal radius can also mimic it. In this regard, distal radial physeal trauma from repetitive loading of the wrist in female gymnasts is particularly interesting. Although radiological changes mimic MD, they are completely different entities with different aetiology.

Radiology

Radiographs confirm the diagnosis but also help determine the degree of deformity and assess the remaining growth potential. Radiographic features that characterize true MD are ulnar tilt of the distal radial articular surface, lunate subsidence causing 'pyramidalization' of the carpus on the posteroanterior view, and palmar displacement of the carpus on the lateral view. MRI is gaining importance in early management of this condition because of the importance of Vickers ligament (thickened radiolunate ligament) in causing the deformity and early encouraging results after its release.

Treatment

Treatment depends on age (growth remaining in the distal radius), degree of deformity, and symptoms such as pain and distal radioulnar joint (DRUJ) instability. Patients with minimal symptoms and acceptable deformity can be managed nonoperatively but should be carefully followed up until skeletal maturity. If deformity starts to increase, and if there is sufficient growth remaining in the distal radial physis, then release of Vickers ligament and physiolysis of the distal radius can be considered (Figure 14.6). This approach does not correct the pre-existing deformity, and either a guided growth procedure (on

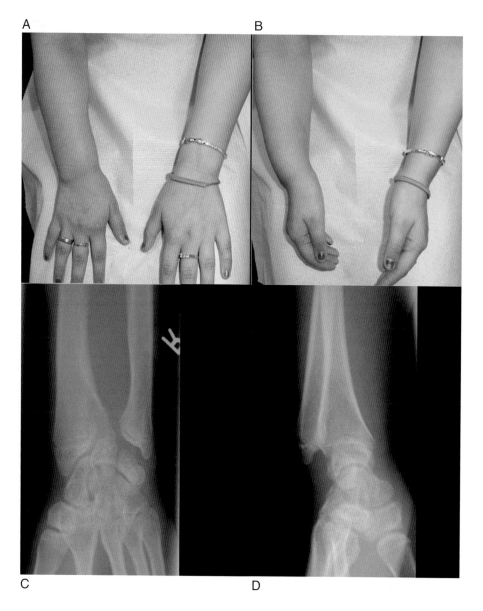

A   B

C   D

Figure 14.4 Madelung deformity.

the radial side) or acute correction of deformity through a dome osteotomy of the distal radius can be considered.

In the skeletally mature patient, the radial deformity can be acutely corrected with a radial osteotomy, and the length discrepancy treated with ulnar shortening. Alternatively, the ulna can be neglected, and the radius lengthened and realigned with Ilizarov distraction osteogenesis (Figure 14.6). Both these strategies aim to restore normal anatomy at the DRUJ. Salvage procedures, including excision of the distal end of the ulna (Darrach procedure), fusion of the distal ulna to the radius, and excision of a segment proximal to the fusion (Sauve–Kapandji procedure), are appropriate. These, however, address the wrong bone (i.e. the ulna, which is non-pathological).

Osteochondritis Dissecans

The elbow is the second commonest location for osteochondritis dissecans (OCD), following the knee, with the capitellum of the dominant arm as the commonest site. It occurs in adolescents and is commoner in boys. Repetitive overhead and upper extremity weight-bearing activities, gymnastics, and throwing are known risk factors. The aetiology is similar to that in the knee joint. Repetitive microtrauma to the immature capitellum and/or vascular insufficiency have been implicated as causes.

Diagnosis can be made with plane radiographs, but MRI studies can be helpful to evaluate the size of the lesion and the extent of bony oedema. Based on radiographic and arthroscopic findings, three grades are recognized:

- Grade I: intact covering cartilage. Bony stability may or may not be present
- Grade II: cartilage fracture with bony collapse or displacement
- Grade III: loose bodies present in the joint (Figure 14.7).

Treatment

It depends on the symptoms, size of the lesion, stability of the lesion, and presence of loose bodies (see Chapter 6, Figure 6.30).

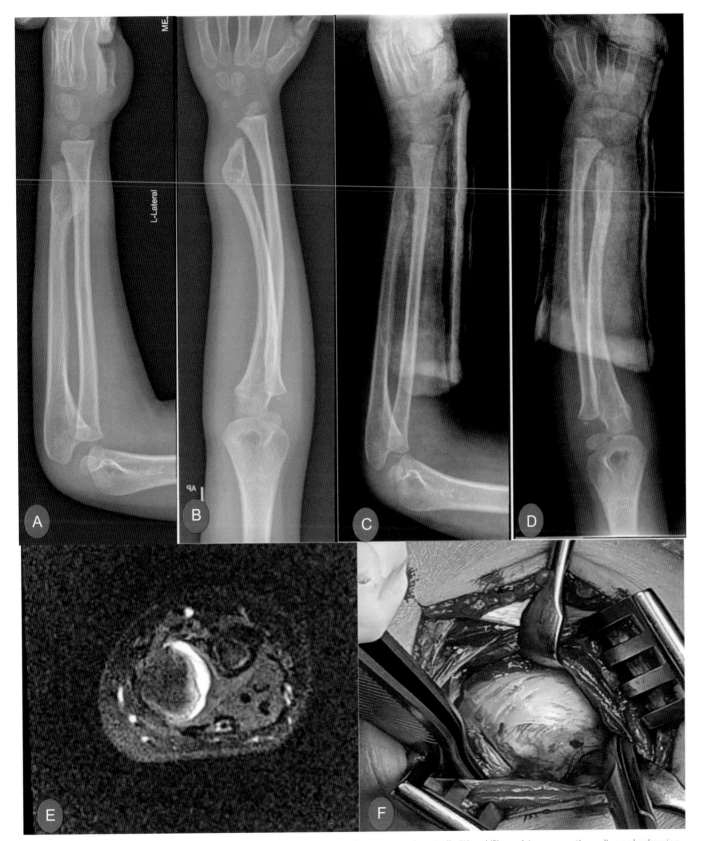

Figure 14.5 Pseudo-Madelung deformity caused by solitary osteochondroma that is removed surgically. (A) and (B) are plain preoperative radiographs showing the deformity that was caused by the osteochondroma. (E) shows an MRI scan confirming the diagnosis of osteochondroma. (F) is an intraoperative image of the osteochondroma.

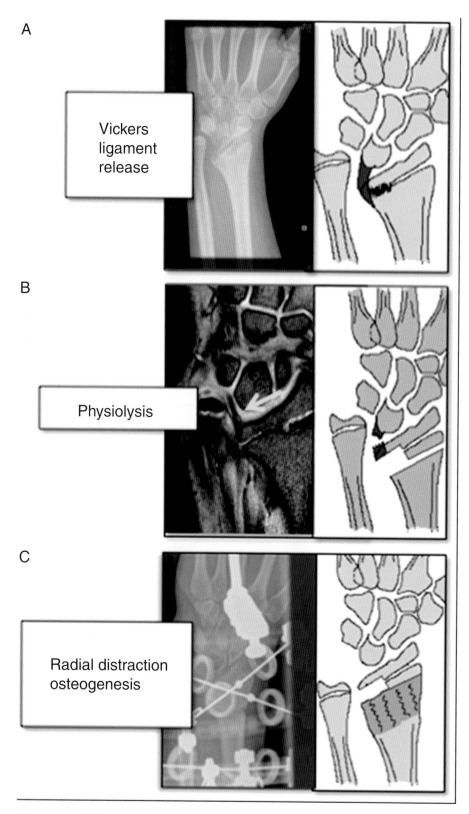

A

Vickers
ligament
release

B

Physiolysis

C

Radial distraction
osteogenesis

Figure 14.6 Madelung's deformity: treatment options.

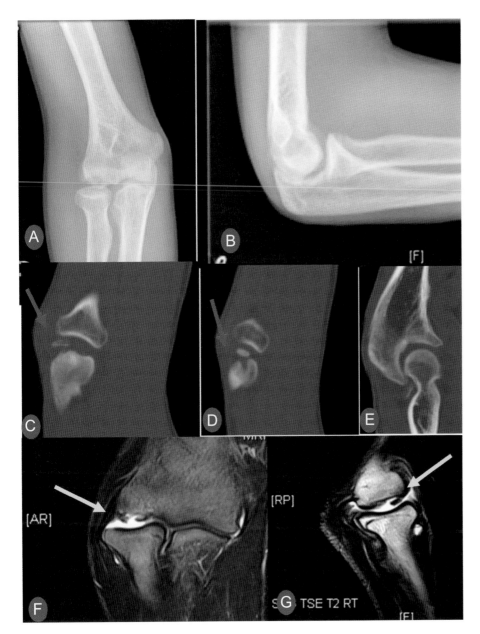

Figure 14.7 Grade III osteochonditis dissecans (OCD) of the elbow. It is difficult to visualize on plain radiographs (A, B) and high level of suspicion is required. Notice the flouting piece of bone (red arrow) on CT scans shown in (C) and (D). (F) and (G) are magnetic resonance scans showing the broken articular cartilage (yellow arrow).

Grade I

Non-operative treatment involves cessation of activity ± immobilization for 6 weeks, then gradual return to activities over the next 6–12 weeks. If no improvements, retroarticular drilling is performed.

Grade II

Arthroscopic microfracture or retroarticular drilling of the capitellum is performed. Large lesions that are incompletely displaced can be stabilized arthroscopically.

Grade III (and Unstable Grade II)

Treatment involves arthroscopic debridement and loose body excision. Osteochondral autograft or allograft is reserved for large grade II and III OCD.

Complications include elbow stiffness, persistent pain, inability to return to sports, and premature arthritis.

Panner's Disease

Panner's disease refers to osteochondrosis of the capitellum that occurs shortly after the appearance of the ossific nucleus before the age of 11 years, when the cells are considered vulnerable for ischaemia (Figure 14.8). It was first described by the Danish orthopaedic surgeon Dr Dane Panner in 1927 as an irregularity of the humeral capitellum on plain radiographs, which he attributed to osteochondrosis (i.e. similar to Legg–Calvé–Perthes disease) that was described 17 years earlier [3]. Panner's disease is a self-limiting disease and the majority of patients heal without clinical impairment. Surgery may be harmful for patients with Panner's disease. It should not be confused with elbow OCD, as they have significantly different aetiologies, treatments, and outcomes.

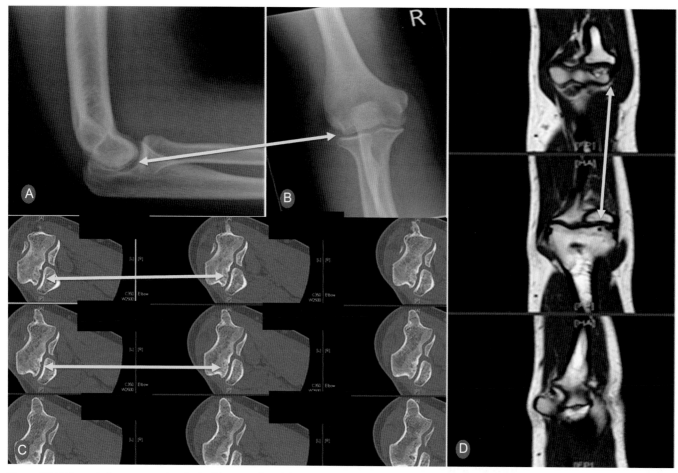

Figure 14.8 Panner's disease: osteochondrosis of the capitellum. (A) and (B) are plain radiographs of the elbow showing flattening of the capitellum. (C) shows CT sections depicting irregularity of the texture of the humeral capitellum. (D) shows MRI sections depicting abnormal signals.

References

1. Jiménez I, Delgado PJ. The reverse Sauvé–Kapandji procedure for the treatment of (posttraumatic) proximal radioulnar synostosis. *Eur J Orthop Surg Traumatol*. 2018;28(6):1225–9.

2. Herring JA. *Tachdjians' Pediatric Orthopaedics*, 5th ed, Vol. 1. Philadelphia, PA: Saunders Elsevier; 2014.

3. Claessen FM, *et al*. Panner's disease: literature review and treatment recommendations. *J Child Orthop*. 2015;9(1):9–17.

Traumatic Elbow Disorders

Thomas Dehler and John Davies

Introduction

Anatomy

The elbow is a combination hinge and pivot trocho-ginglymoid joint, formed by the ulno-humeral, radio-humeral, and proximal radioulnar articulations. The joint capsule is thickened medially and laterally to form the collateral ligaments, which are the major stabilizers of the elbow joint. Details of these ligaments are shown and described in Figure 15.1.

The medial (ulnar) collateral ligament complex has three bundles. The anterior bundle extends from the medial epicondyle to the coronoid process and serves as the main restraint to valgus overload. The posterior bundle arises from the posteroinferior medial epicondyle and inserts distally into the posteromedial margin of the trochlear notch, forming the floor of the cubital tunnel. The posterior bundle provides valgus stability in flexion of the elbow of >60°. The thin transverse ligament extends between the attachments of the anterior and posterior bundles, providing additional stability.

A posterior fat pad is present behind the upper part of the joint capsule and within the depths of the olecranon fossa, and an anterior pad overlies the coronoid fossa. Radiologically, the anterior fat pad is visible as a lucent crescent area just anterior to the coronoid fossa. The posterior fat pad is **not** normally visible on plain radiographs. Joint effusion distends the capsule and lifts these fat pads away from the bone, so that they become easily seen on X-ray (Figure 15.2). In the context of trauma, fat pad signs (a posterior fat pad sign or a ballooned anterior fat pad sign) suggest an occult non-displaced fracture – either a supracondylar humerus fracture (SCH) in children or a radial head fracture in adults [1].

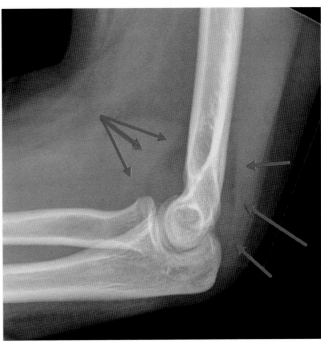

Figure 15.2 Fat pad signs (red arrows).

Lateral collateral ligament complex

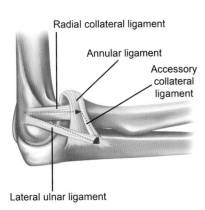

Radial collateral ligament

Annular ligament

Accessory collateral ligament

Lateral ulnar ligament

Medial collateral ligament complex

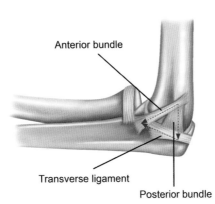

Anterior bundle

Transverse ligament

Posterior bundle

Figure 15.1 Collateral ligaments of the elbow. There are four elements of the lateral collateral ligament complex. The annular ligament encircles the radial head and provides primary stability to the proximal radioulnar joint in supination and pronation. The radial collateral ligament originates from the isometric point on the lateral epicondyle and blends anteriorly with the annular ligament. The important lateral ulnar (collateral) ligament is the primary restraint to varus and external rotation stress. It runs posterior to the radial head and inserts into the crista supinatoris of the proximal ulna. The accessory collateral ligament originates from the annular ligament and inserts into the supinator crest, providing additional stability to the annular ligament from varus stress.

The distal humeral epiphysis is entirely cartilaginous at birth, and in young children, this presents a challenge in precisely defining the exact anatomy of a fracture. Fundamental to this is the timing of the progressive appearance of the secondary ossification centres. The capitellum is the first to ossify in girls at around 12 months, and in boys at the age of 2 years. According to the mnemonic CRITOL, the ossification centres appear chronologically every 2 years in the sequence, as shown in Table 15.1.

In girls, the centres appear generally 6–12 months earlier than boys. As skeletal maturity approaches, the capitellum, trochlear, and lateral epicondyle coalesce into a single distal ossification centre, later fusing with the humeral metaphysis by the age of 14–16 years. The radial head, trochlea, and olecranon may also appear as more than one centre or have a fragmented appearance, which occasionally can be mistaken for an injury (Figure 15.3).

In terms of blood supply, the distal humerus is supplied by a collateral circulation, with the trochlea and capitellum supplied from non-anastomotic nutrient vessels entering posteriorly. Hence both are susceptible to avascular necrosis as a result of significant injury or excessive surgical dissection around the posterior aspect of the distal humerus. This is especially relevant in situations of non-union of a lateral condyle fracture, where extensive dissection of callus and fibrous tissue is often needed for adequate reduction of the fragment, with a high incidence of osteonecrosis.

Table 15.1 Timing of the appearance of secondary ossification centres (CRITOL)

Capitellum	2 years
Radial head	4 years
Internal (medial) epicondyle	6 years
Trochlea	8 years
Olecranon	10 years
Lateral epicondyle	12 years

Radiographic Anatomy

Radiographic examination should include an anteroposterior (AP) view, ideally with the elbow in extension, and a lateral view in 90° of flexion. As children are often reluctant to extend an injured elbow, the Jones view taken in maximal flexion is an alternative. However, due to superimposition of the proximal forearm onto the distal humerus, subtle fracture lines can be difficult to detect. Several useful radiological measurements have been proposed to assess abnormalities around the elbow, including:

1. Baumann's angle (Figure 15.4)
2. The radio-capitellar line (Figure 15.5)
3. Teardrop or hourglass (Figure 15.4)
4. The anterior and posterior humeral lines (Figure 15.4)
5. The shaft–condylar angle (Figure 15.4).

Supracondylar Fractures

Supracondylar fractures account for 50–70% of all elbow fractures in children, and are most commonly seen between the ages of 3 and 7. The articulating surfaces of the distal humerus are connected to the shaft by the medial and lateral columns, with a thin area of connecting bone between the coronoid and olecranon fossa (for an illustration of the teardrop, see Figure 15.4). When a force is applied, with the olecranon acting as a fulcrum, this leads to a fracture in this weak anatomical area. Hence, supracondylar injuries are caused by a fall onto the outstretched hand, with the elbow hyperextended in 95% of cases. Rarely, in flexion-type injuries, a posteriorly applied (anteriorly directed) force causes a fracture through this same area, with the distal fragment displacing anteriorly (Figure 15.6).

Assessment

Evidence-based guidelines from the American Academy of Orthopaedic Surgeons (AAOS) specify an accurate assessment of the child's neurovascular status on admission and

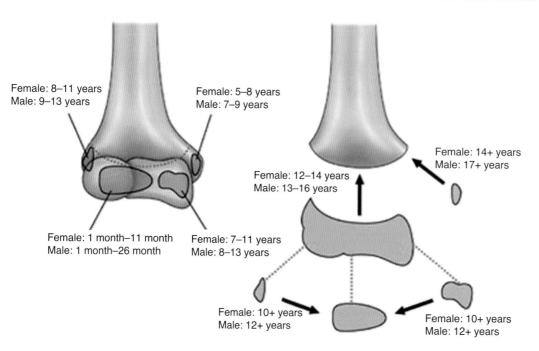

Figure 15.3 Timing of appearance and fusion of ossification centres around the elbow. ♀, girls; ♂, boys.

Female: 8–11 years
Male: 9–13 years

Female: 5–8 years
Male: 7–9 years

Female: 14+ years
Male: 17+ years

Female: 12–14 years
Male: 13–16 years

Female: 1 month–11 month
Male: 1 month–26 month

Female: 7–11 years
Male: 8–13 years

Female: 10+ years
Male: 12+ years

Female: 10+ years
Male: 12+ years

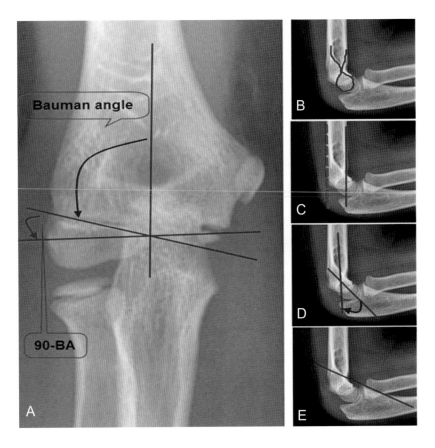

Figure 15.4 Radiographic anatomy of the elbow. (A) Baumann's angle (BA) formed by the capitello-physeal line and the long axis of the humerus (normally 75–80°); Baumann believed the reciprocal angle (90°-BA) equalled the carrying angle. (B) Teardrop or hourglass; the narrowest part represents the coronoid fossa. The inferior portion of the teardrop is the ossification centre of the capitellum. On a true lateral projection, this teardrop should be well defined (a useful sign of true lateral projection). (C) The anterior humeral line (solid red line) drawn along the anterior border of the distal humeral shaft; this should pass through the middle third of the ossification centre of the capitellum. The dashed blue line is the posterior humeral line. (D) The shaft–condylar angle is the angle between the long axis of the humerus and the long axis of the capitellum (normally 40°). (E) The coronoid line, which is directed proximally along the anterior border of the coronoid process, should barely touch the anterior portion of the lateral condyle.

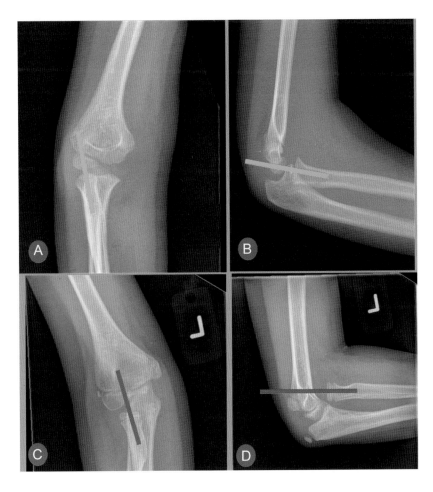

Figure 15.5 The radio-capitellar line. A line along the neck of the radius (not the shaft of the radius) should intersect the capitellum on the AP and lateral views, as shown in (A) and (B). (C) and (D) demonstrate an anterior dislocation of the radio-capitellar joint.

post-operatively [2]. The presence or absence of a radial pulse and capillary refill time, as well as function of all three peripheral nerves plus that of the anterior interosseous branch of the median nerve, should be documented:

- Anterior interosseous nerve, most commonly injured: check contraction of the flexor pollicis longus and the flexor digitorum profundus to the index and middle fingers. If the child cannot make the ring sign, it indicates anterior interosseous nerve palsy (and median nerve injury)

- Median: motor deficit in the thenar muscles and sensory loss on the palmar surface of the index finger
- Radial: check for wrist drop or lack of thumb interphalangeal joint extension and sensory loss in the first dorsal web space. The child cannot make a thumbs-up 'OK sign'
- Ulnar: check finger abduction and adduction for motor deficit in the interossei and for sensory loss on the palmar surface of the little finger. The child cannot cross the fingers 'for luck'.

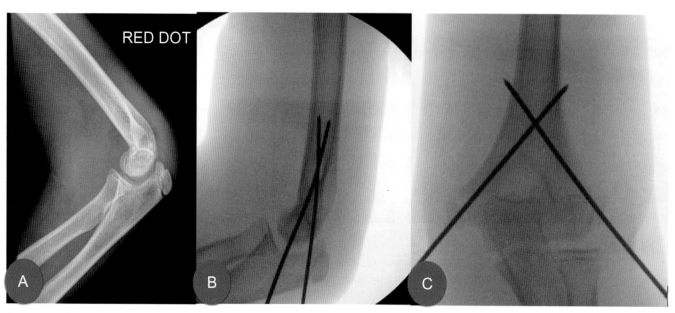

Figure 15.6 Flexion-type supracondylar fracture.

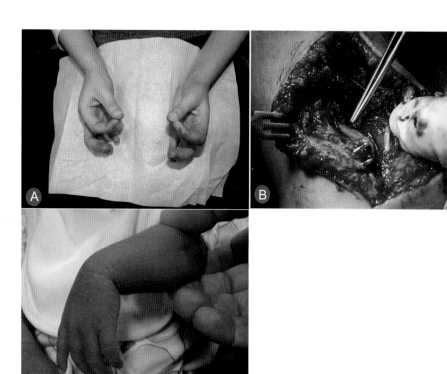

Figure 15.7 Neurological complications after supracondylar fractures. (A) A child who had an anterior interosseous nerve injury and was not able to make a ring sign. He made a full recovery and the image shows he is able to make a nice ring by flexing the index distal interphalangeal joint. (B) A child who was found to have an ulnar nerve palsy after stabilization. Unfortunately, the nerve status was not documented appropriately. Exploration showed two wires piercing the ulnar nerve. (C) shows a child with a wrist drop following a supracondylar fracture.

Gartland Classification

The Gartland classification (Figure 15.8) is probably the most commonly used classification in clinical practice to describe the severity of displacement for extension-type supracondylar fractures [3]:

- Type I: non-displaced; this is further subdivided into type 1A (no angulation in any plane) and type 1B (where there is medial column comminution, which can subsequently collapse into cubitus varus)
- Type II: angulated distal fragment with an intact posterior periosteal hinge; further subdivided into type 2A (no rotational abnormality) and type 2B (if there is a rotational abnormality)
- Type III: completely displaced; further subdivided according to coronal plane displacement of the distal fragment – whereby type IIIA is posteromedially, and type IIIB posterolaterally, displaced.

Treatment

Stable type IA and IIA injuries are suitable for conservative treatment with an above-elbow cast for 4 weeks. The other remaining unstable variants are treated by closed reduction and percutaneous pinning. The distal humerus has limited remodelling potential, as it only contributes to 20% of overall total growth of the bone. By 8–10 years of age, only 10% of longitudinal growth remains for remodelling of a supracondylar fracture to occur; hence it is difficult to expect reliable remodelling after significant deformity. The aim of treatment is to achieve adequate fracture reduction for healing without deformity, whilst avoiding morbidity from surgery and associated neurovascular injury. In general, sagittal plane deformity has a greater potential for remodelling with continued growth, as it is in the plane of motion of the elbow, whilst cubitus varus deformity in the coronal plane persists.

Controversies for Discussion

There are a number of controversies in displaced supracondylar management, with considerable interest around timing of surgery, associated vascular injury, and pin configuration for stable fixation.

Timing to Surgery

The timing of theatre for type III off-ended fractures is controversial. This is because of logistical problems of the time of day when children present, which often causes an inadequate fasting state, in combination with access to theatre and available skills of the out-of-hours team. Historically, surgery has been on the day

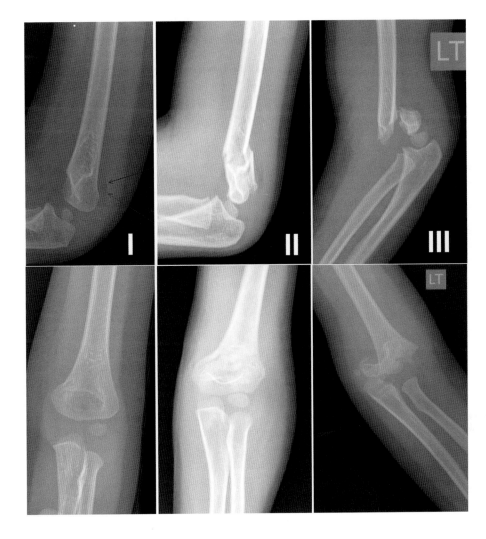

Figure 15.8 Gartland classification.

of admission. However, a delay (>12 hours) for uncomplicated displaced fractures has not been shown to cause adverse outcomes or to require open, rather than closed, reduction, whilst avoiding errors occurring with out-of-hours operating [4, 5]. In direct contradiction to this, good evidence also exists that a delay of over 8 hours increases the need for open reduction from 11.2% to 33.3% [6]. In situations where it is possible to get to theatre before midnight, this would seem a logical approach for proceeding with surgery out of hours and thereafter the child can be monitored closely overnight and undergo surgery first on the trauma list in the morning. Absolute indications for urgent intervention at any time during the night include associated neurovascular deficit, severe elbow swelling, anterior ecchymoses, and anterior skin compromise, which have been associated with evolution of compartment syndrome in the presence of excessive delay [7].

Vascular Compromise

Alteration of vascular status occurs in 10–20% of displaced fractures. It is important, when there is an absent radial pulse, to differentiate between a cold, poorly perfused hand and a warm, pink, well-perfused hand. A pink, well-perfused hand can be safely managed by accurate closed reduction, pinning, and subsequent careful observation for compartment syndrome, without formal exploration of the brachial artery (Figure 15.9). An absent pulse on discharge from hospital with a well-perfused

hand has not been shown to have any adverse effect on long-term functional outcome. However, if there is a neurological deficit with a pink, pulseless hand on admission, or if there is any evidence of ongoing ischaemia post-operatively, such as the presence of persistent and increasing pain, this mandates exploration [8, 9].

The cold, white, poorly perfused hand is a vascular emergency and requires immediate input from the vascular or plastics team. An expeditious closed reduction will restore circulation in cases where arterial inflow has been restricted due to direct compression from the fracture. However, if the fracture spike penetrates through the brachialis muscle causing a significant arterial injury such as transection, intimal tear or a thrombosed segment of vessel; microvascular anastomosis is required for restoration of arterial blood flow. After fracture stabilization, this is often by an interposition vein graft through an anterior approach. If there is significant ischaemic time or any concern for raised compartment pressures in the forearm, fasciotomies are required.

Nerve Injury

Peripheral nerve injury occurs in 10–15% of displaced supracondylar fractures, and most commonly the anterior interosseous nerve is injured. The anterior interosseous nerve is a pure motor nerve innervating the flexor pollicis longus and the deep flexors to the index and middle fingers. A clinical deficit can

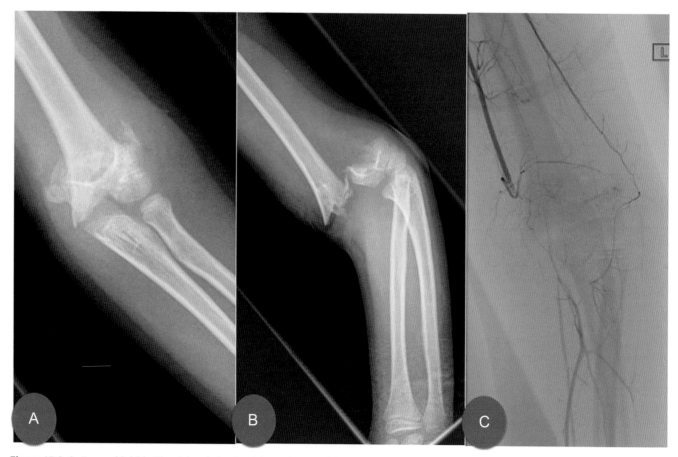

Figure 15.9 An 8-year-old child with a pink, pulseless hand. On application of traction, the hand became white. The vascular surgeon performed angiography, demonstrating a thrombosed segment, and immediate exploration of the brachial artery was done through an anterior approach and revascularization by a reverse saphenous vein graft.

be difficult to diagnose in an acutely distressed, uncooperative child. With type IIIA posteromedially displaced fractures, the radial nerve is most often injured. In type IIIB posterolaterally displaced fractures, median nerve injury occurs by stretching as the proximal fragment spike displaces anteriorly, whilst the median nerve is tethered distally at the pronator teres. The majority of traumatic nerve injuries involve neurapraxia, which can be expectantly observed. However, if function does not return within 6 weeks, a plastic surgery opinion should be sought and nerve conduction studies performed. Nerve transection from the initial injury, or iatrogenic injury as a result of entrapment during an imperfect fracture reduction or pin penetration, should be suspected (Figure 15.7).

Pin Configuration

Several biomechanical studies have shown crossed pins have the most stable configuration, although these are associated with an increased risk of iatrogenic ulnar nerve injury. However, whilst the crossed pin technique might be the most stable biomechanically, no significant difference clinically has been shown when comparing torsional stiffness of crossed versus three laterally placed wires [10]. The incidence of ulnar nerve injury can be reduced by selective use of a medial wire, reserved for fractures that remain unstable after provisional fixation with laterally based pins. This allows the medial wire to be placed with the arm in a safer extended position, and reduces the incidence of ulnar nerve injury from 15% to 2% [11]. In approximately 50% of children, when the elbow is flexed beyond 120°, anterior subluxation of the ulnar nerve occurs over the medial epicondyle. By initially fixing unstable fractures with either parallel or divergent lateral wires (Figure 15.10) before placement of a medial wire, this avoids medial pin placement with the elbow in flexion.

The goals of fixation are to achieve maximum spread of the pins at the fracture site and to engage both the medial and lateral columns, as well as to engage adequately the proximal and distal fragments. Sankar *et al.* published a paper in 2007 about pinning errors [12], recognizing three main types of technical error:

1. Type A errors occurring with failure to engage both fragments by two pins

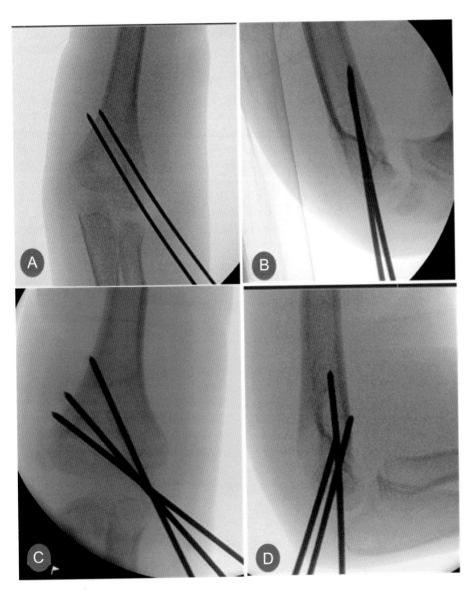

Figure 15.10 Parallel and divergent lateral entry wires.

2. Type B errors which occur with failure to achieve bicortical fixation with two pins or more

3. Type C errors which occur with inadequate pin spread-controlling rotation.

The presence of medial comminution in type IB fractures places them at risk of subsequent collapse into cubitus varus in the coronal plane and a resulting gunstock deformity. Whilst remodelling occurs in the plane of motion and some sagittal plane remodelling of flexion–extension deformities can be expected, angular malunion causing varus–valgus deformities typically remains constant until skeletal maturity. This highlights the importance of adequate fixation preventing subsequent collapse and shortening of the medial column.

Reduction and Fixation

Set-up and proper positioning are important to achieve an accurate closed reduction. Before starting, it is worthwhile asking the anaesthetist to give a muscle relaxant during general anaesthesia (GA), as well as to use a head ring. The child is positioned with the shoulder at the edge of the table, and the arm on the radiolucent arm table attachment. A high tourniquet is applied in case open reduction is needed. The first critical step is to ensure the image intensifier C-arm can access the elbow, with the screens positioned in clear view.

Closed reduction is by application of traction, with the elbow slightly flexed at 15–20°, reducing the distal fragment in line with the proximal fragment, which is controlled by the assistant holding the upper arm. In most cases, gentle sustained traction will disengage and align the fragments. Fluoroscopic screening with the image intensifier confirms the fracture is out to length. Medial and lateral translations and varus/valgus displacements are corrected by adjusting the direction of pull, with medial or laterally directed counterpressure. Posterior displacement is corrected by flexing the elbow, whilst firm pressure is applied on the humeral condyles and olecranon. To obtain a lateral image, the humerus, elbow, and forearm are moved as one, internally or externally rotating the entire arm at the shoulder. Often rotation in one direction yields a better reduction by correcting rotational alignment at the fracture site. For fixation, a minimum of two 2.0-mm wires are inserted from the radial side first, with the trajectory marked by placing a wire against the skin and drawing with a sterile marker pen. If a medial wire is required, the elbow is extended to bring the ulnar nerve away from the medial epicondyle, and a mini-open incision used to confirm safe entry of the wire into the bone. The wires are left proud of the skin, with dressings applied and an above-elbow backslab, with the elbow flexed at 90° in full supination. The cast is later completed at 1 week in clinic, with a check X-ray, and thereafter the wires can be removed at 4 weeks in clinic. (See Video 15.1.)

 Video 15.1 Supracondylar fracture reduction and stabilisation.

Corrective Osteotomy for Malunion

Several types of deformities have been described following SCH fractures (Figure 15.11). Cubitus varus is the commonest deformity after supracondylar fracture, arising from incomplete reduction or loss of fixation. The distal fragment is typically rotated internally, which allows it to heal with a varus tilt and typically in slight hyperextension. The varus tilt reverses the normal carrying angle of the elbow and is associated with prominence of the lateral condyle. Although there is no functional disability associated with cubitus varus, it causes most parents to opt for surgery to correct the appearance.

The simplest method to correct a cubitus varus 'gunstock' deformity is a laterally based closing wedge supracondylar osteotomy, with medial translation of the distal fragment to reduce the lateral prominence. Although it is possible to address the hyperextension and rotational components of the malunion, this increases the complexity of the osteotomy, and has minimal resulting effect on the carrying angle, which is the principal problem. A lateral incision to access the epicondylar ridge is used, avoiding the radial nerve, and K-wires are used as a guide for the oscillating saw when making the osteotomy (Figures 15.12 and 15.13). Fixation is with 2.0-mm K-wires in younger children, and with a 2.7-mm plate and screws in older children.

Lateral Condyle Fractures

Lateral condyle or lateral mass fractures are the second commonest elbow injury in children. They are often problematic because of involvement of the unossified physis and distal humeral articular surface. They arise either as a result of a traction 'pull-off', or a compression 'push-off', mechanism, which causes an oblique fracture through the cartilaginous hinge of the distal humerus. Classification and treatment depend upon the path of the fracture line, which begins at the posterolateral humeral metaphysis. Whilst the Milch classification system is more established, it has been deemed unreliable by some authors and of limited help in terms of management.

A Milch type I fracture is lateral to the ulno-humeral articulation, extending from the metaphysis into the capitellar physis, and anatomically does not cross the lateral ridge of the trochlea (equivalent to a Salter–Harris type IV injury). A Milch type II fracture extends into the trochlear sulcus (crossing the lateral trochlear ridge), which is considered a physis – hence it is equivalent to a Salter–Harris type II injury, so that the ulno-humeral articulation is unstable posterolaterally [13] (Figure 15.14).

The more useful Jakob system, later expanded by Weiss, is based upon the presence of an intact cartilaginous hinge and the amount of displacement [14]:

- Type I: fracture displaced <2 mm, does not fully disrupt the cartilaginous epiphysis; the cartilaginous hinge is intact

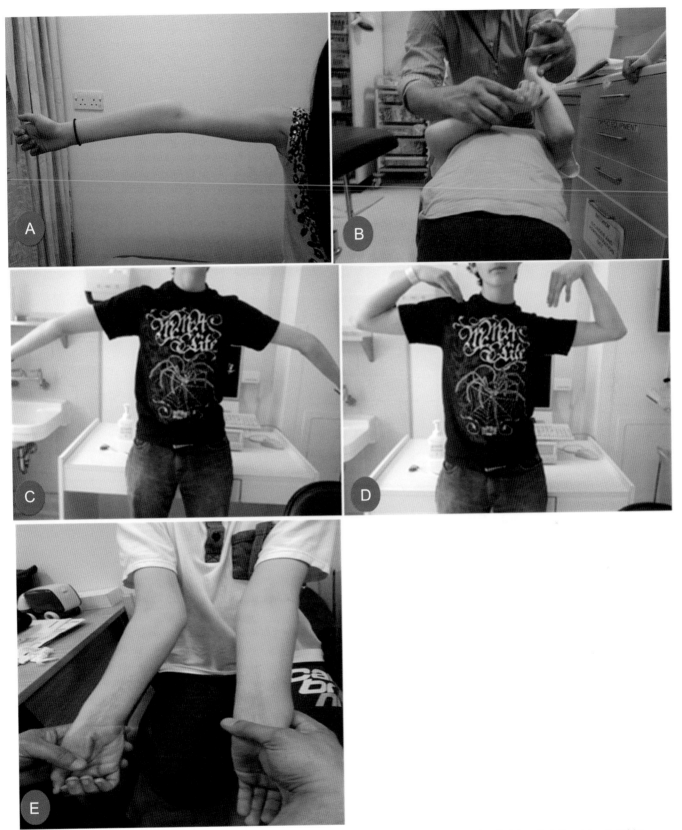

Figure 15.11 Fracture deformities following supracondylar humeral fractures. (A) Gunstock deformity. (B) Assessing the internal rotation deformity of the humerus (the Yamamoto test). (C, D) Extension deformity of the elbow. (E) Valgus deformity of the elbow.

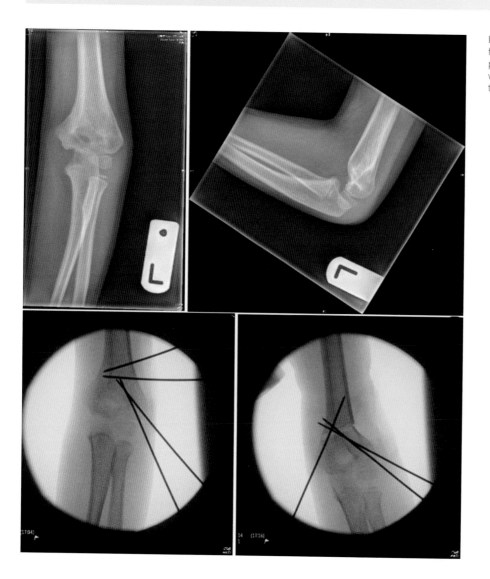

Figure 15.12 Lateral closing wedge osteotomy for correction of cubitus varus. Initially K-wires are placed as a guide before osteotomy, and a lateral wire is used to hold the fragments as the definitive treatment.

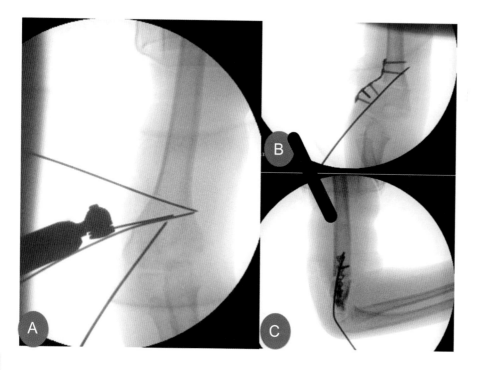

Figure 15.13 Lateral closing wedge osteotomy, stabilized using a contoured plate if K-wires alone are not sufficient(A-C). Note the initially increased Baumann's angle, reduced to the same value as the contralateral elbow from preoperative templating. A prominent lateral ridge persists, as the distal fragment is not medially translated.

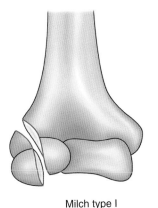
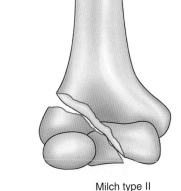

Milch type I   Milch type II

Figure 15.14 Milch classification.

- Type II: fracture displaced 2–4 mm, disrupting the epiphysis and cartilaginous hinge with a capitellum that may be displaced, but not rotated out of joint
- Type III: fracture displaced >4 mm and rotated out of joint, with an incongruous radio-capitellar joint.

Treatment

Jakob type I fractures are usually stable and can be treated non-operatively with a well-fitted above-elbow cast and X-ray monitoring. However, type II fractures are not stable and may displace. It is not possible to differentiate between type I and type II fractures clinically or on plain radiographs. Undisplaced type II fractures can be treated in a well-fitted above-elbow cast, with X-ray monitoring at 1, 2, and 3 weeks in clinic. However, in up to 30% of type II fractures that are initially considered to be stable, further displacement was found on X-ray by 15 days and subsequent fixation was needed. Often an extended period of 6 weeks of immobilization in cast is required for healing (Figure 15.16).

Several methods have been proposed to differentiate between type I and type II fractures, but none have been found clinically effective. Ultrasound is useful and does not require GA, but it is operator-dependent and requires a cooperative child who is not in pain. MRI in this age group often requires GA to keep the child still for the time needed to obtain a diagnostic scan. Intra-articular arthrography requires GA, and there is a valid argument that it is quicker and more efficient to stabilize an undisplaced type II fracture, rather than performing arthrography under GA to confirm whether it will displace or not.

Displaced fractures are inherently unstable, particularly when the fracture line is medial to the lateral ridge, or crista, of the trochlea. Lateral translation of the olecranon at the ulno-humeral joint is often seen, and in type III fractures, the fragment is rotated laterally, as well as being proximally displaced. In displaced Jakob type II and any type III fractures, open reduction via a lateral approach and divergent pins crossing laterally to the fracture site are used for fixation. Typically, one pin is directed medially towards the epicondyle, and the other more proximally above the coronoid fossa (Figure 15.17). If there is insufficient fixation in the metaphysis from pinning alone, a cannulated screw can be used to achieve interfragmentary compression and rigid fixation (Figure 15.18). As these are intra-articular fractures, it is important to ensure a perfect reduction of the joint surface, and this can be confirmed visually (accurate) or by using an arthrogram (less accurate), or both.

The main complications from lateral condyle fractures are delayed union or non-union and problems with growth arrest. Non-union arises because the fracture is intra-articular in an area of thin, less active periosteum, with possible interference from the synovial fluid in bone healing. This can lead to progressive cubitus valgus and potentially tardy ulnar nerve palsy. Growth disturbance or growth arrest can occur due to malalignment of the lateral condylar and medial trochlear ossification centres in the distal cartilaginous hinge. This causes formation of a bony physeal bar either centrally (with a resulting fishtail deformity) or laterally (causing cubitus valgus). Osteonecrosis

Figure 15.15 Jakob's classification.

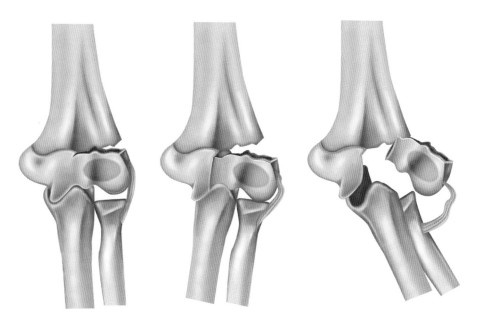

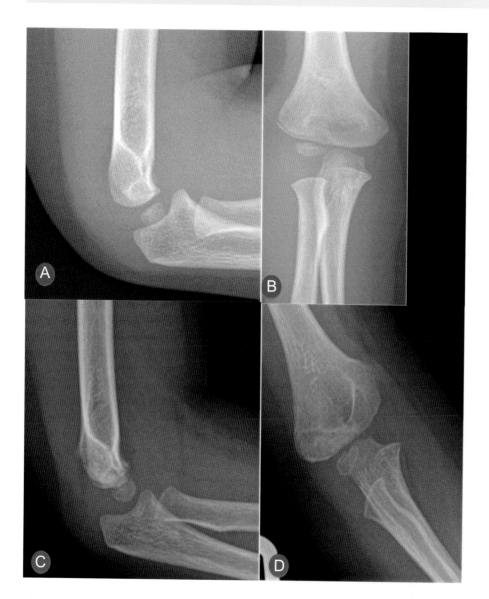

Figure 15.16 A minimally displaced lateral condyle fracture in a 3-year-old child treated with a cast for 6 weeks and X-ray monitoring in clinic(A,B). The final X-rays showed the fracture was healed (C, D).

occurs typically from iatrogenic extensive dissection needed in the setting of a late reduction or non-union, or from loss of blood supply at the time of initial injury.

Medial Epicondyle Fractures

The medial epicondyle is a traction apophysis and the origin of the flexor pronator muscle mass, as well as the ulnar collateral ligament and part of the elbow capsule. Injuries usually arise as a result of an avulsion, with a peak incidence at 9–12 years. Approximately 50% are associated with an elbow dislocation, and in some cases, the dislocation spontaneously reduces and the medial fragment remains entrapped in the joint (Figure 15.19). There is considerable debate about the best management of displaced fractures, with the results of conservative versus operative treatment being the subject of an ongoing study (SCIENCE: Surgery or Casts for Injuries of the EpicoNdyle in Children's Elbows: A Randomised Controlled Trial).

An absolute indication for surgical treatment is an entrapped fragment in the joint, when closed manipulation has failed to extract it and an open procedure is needed to retrieve it. If there is ulnar nerve dysfunction, this also mandates exploration and fixation of the fragment under direct vision. Relative indications for fixation include displaced fractures in children participating in high-demand athletic activities to prevent later symptomatic valgus instability (Figure 15.20).

These have a peak incidence in the 7- to 12-year age groups and occur from a fall onto a hyperextended elbow, with resulting valgus stress and axial compression. Mild radial neck angulation may be expected to remodel in younger children and heals with little functional deficit. However, 50% of all children who sustain a displaced radial neck fracture have evidence of permanent limitation of forearm rotation on follow-up. O'Brien classified radial fractures into three types, depending on the degree of angulation [15]:

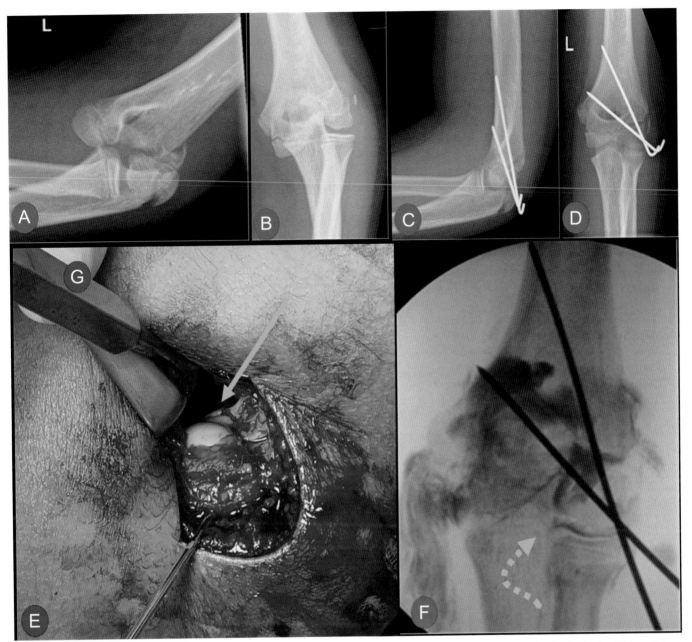

Figure 15.17 (A) and (B) show a displaced lateral condyle fracture and ulno-humeral instability. (C,D) shows displaced fracture fixed with 2 k-wires.(E) shows intra-operative anatomical reduction of the broken fragments (solid green arrow), and (F) shows confirmation of restoration of the joint surface (curved, dashed green arrow). In a few exceptional cases, displaced fractures undergo closed reduction and are pinned percutaneously when arthrography confirms a congruent restoration of the joint surface; however, this is the exception to the rule and type III injuries almost always mandate open reduction.

- Type I: angulation <30°
- Type II: angulation 30–60°
- Type III: angulation >60°.

Factors associated with a poor prognosis include age >10 years and angulation >30°. These two factors are often reasonably seen as threshold criteria for intervention. Closed reduction yields a better outcome than open reduction, which generally has a worse prognosis due to the associated incidence of stiffness, avascular necrosis, and non-union.

During closed reduction of an angulated radial neck fracture, it is important to determine the plane of maximum angulation by fluoroscopic screening (the forearm is rotated until maximum angulation is visible). This is important as the amount of actual displacement of the radial head is difficult to be determined accurately on standard AP and lateral views. The overall aim of intervention is to restore the arc of forearm pronation and supination to near normal.

Multiple techniques are described, with the Patterson and Israeli techniques being the two most commonly favoured. The Patterson technique involves traction with the elbow extended and varus force applied. Whilst the forearm is fully supinated, digital pressure is applied to the radial head to push it back medially, typically with the thumb. If the reduction is successful, the arm is rotated through a range of motion, with

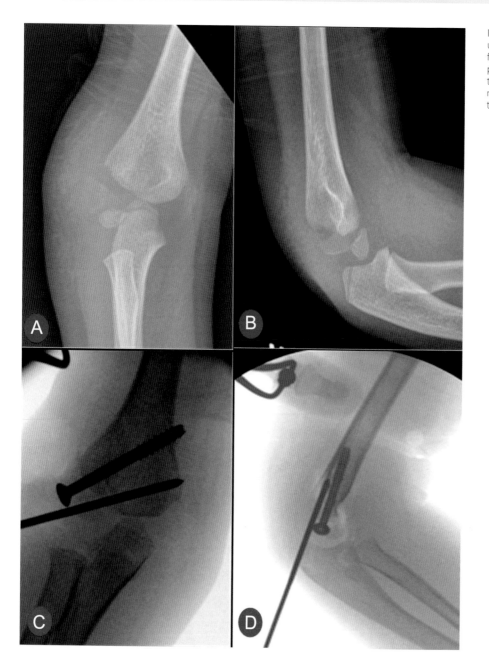

Figure 15.18 A 3-year-old child with an unstable and displaced type III lateral condyle fracture and a subtle undisplaced fracture of the proximal ulna. This was treated by open reduction and a 3.5-mm cannulated screw into the metaphyseal component, with K-wire fixation of the distal articular portion.

screening to check for stability. In the Israeli technique, the arm is initially supinated and the elbow flexed, with pressure over the head, before then pronating the forearm to bring the radial shaft up into alignment with the radial neck. Failure to achieve an angulation of <30° or >45° arc of pronation and supination (90° combined) is an indication for progressing to percutaneous reduction.

The main structure at risk during percutaneous reduction is the posterior interosseous nerve, which enters the arcade of Frohse at the level of the radial neck below the annular ligament. A small stab incision is made posteriorly at the fracture site, as close to the olecranon as possible, and by pronating the forearm, the nerve is brought anteriorly away from the incision. A stout K-wire is carefully directed as a joystick under screening, to relocate the radial head back onto the shaft. Usually the head

is stable on screening after reduction, but if additional internal fixation is required, either K-wire transfixation (Figure 15.21) or an intramedullary Metaizeau titanium elastic nail (TEN) can be used (Figure 15.22). This is introduced retrograde from the bare area of the radius or from the distal radial metaphysis, and advanced up to the fracture site, before engaging the head and neck fragment with the tip of the nail. The nail can also be used as a reduction device, by rotating the tip to reduce the head back onto the radius.

Monteggia Fracture Dislocations

Described by Giovanni Monteggia in 1814, this is a fracture of the ulna in association with a radial head dislocation, with a peak incidence between the age of 4 and 10 years. The majority

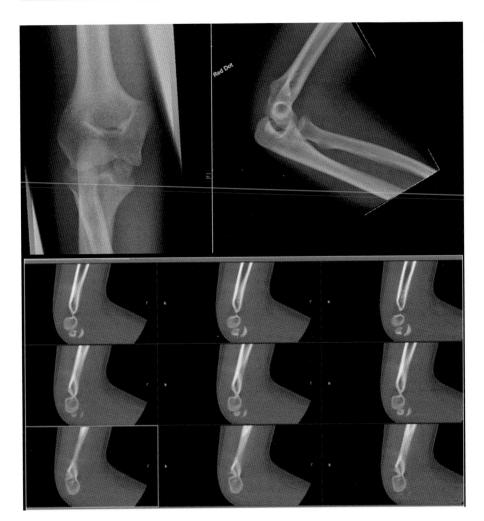

Figure 15.19 Medial epicondyle fracture with an entrapped fragment in the joint.

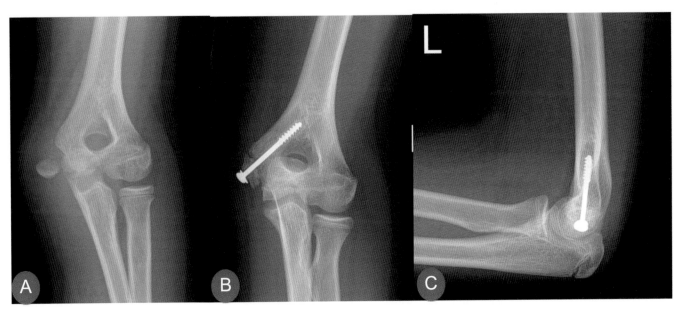

Figure 15.20 Fixation of a displaced medial epicondyle fracture in an 11-year-old gymnast with a slight valgus deformity. A single partially threaded cannulated screw with a washer was used. This was subsequently removed because of irritation. Lysis is visible at the tip of the screw, with evidence that the fracture was incompletely healed. After removal of the screw, the symptoms fully settled and the patient returned to her pre-injury level of activities.

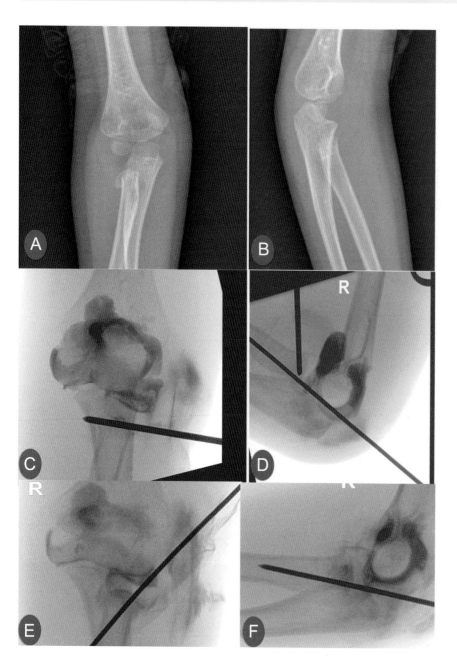

Figure 15.21 (A) and (B) show a displaced radial head fracture. As the child was 3 years old, the radial head had not ossified yet and was barely visible. Arthrograms outlined the radial head very well (C–F). A stout K-wire (size 2 mm) was used to reduce the fracture, and the radial head was transfixed with a smaller K-wire.

of problems are encountered in dealing with cases of late presentations, arising because of failure to diagnose them initially. They can be easily missed on X-ray if the fracture of the ulna is minimally angulated or there is subtle plastic deformation of the ulna.

The Bado classification system classifies these into four original types (Figure 15.23):

- Type I: anterior dislocation of the radial head, with an apex anterior fracture of the ulnar diaphysis, the commonest type in children
- Type II: posterior dislocation of the radial head, with an apex posterior fracture of the ulnar diaphysis or metaphysis, commoner in adults and rarely seen in children

- Type III: lateral or anterolateral dislocation of the radial head, with an associated fracture, typically greenstick, of the ulnar metaphysis, resulting in a varus deformity. This is the second commonest type (23%) in children
- Type IV: anterior dislocation with combined fractures of both the radius and the ulna at the same level, or the radial fracture distal to the ulnar fracture. This is the least common of all types.

There are other equivalent types to the four original, based on radiographic appearances and the mechanism of injury. This includes the subtle type I equivalent, whereby plastic deformation of the ulna accompanies an anteriorly dislocated radial head. When the posterior border of the ulna deviates from a straight line on a lateral forearm radiograph, the

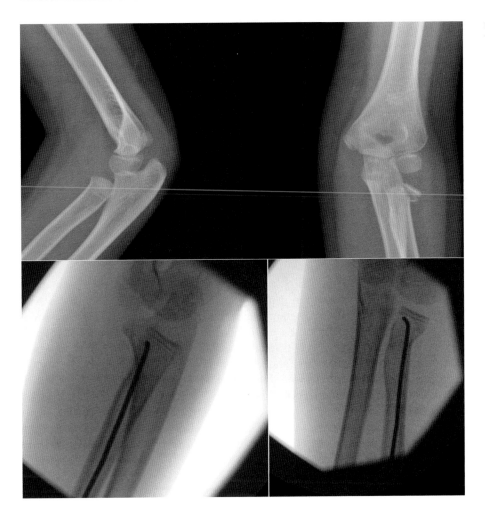

Figure 15.22 An intramedullary Metaizeau titanium elastic nail (TEN) used to stabilize a radial neck fracture.

Figure 15.23 Bado classification of Monteggia fractures.

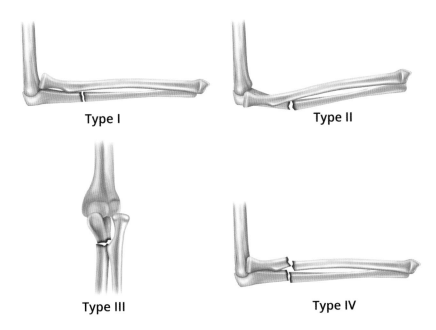

Type I

Type II

Type III

Type IV

'Mubarak ulnar bow line', a radial head dislocation should be suspected. Dedicated elbow views should always be requested when assessing any forearm injury, and on a true lateral elbow X-ray, the radio-capitellar line should be examined (Figure 15.5).

In general, treatment of these injuries depends on whether the ulnar length and alignment can be corrected by closed means and the accompanying reduction of the radial head is concentric and stable under fluoroscopic screening. Typically, this is the case in young children who undergo closed manipulation under anaesthesia of an acute Bado type I or III injury. It is important in these cases to fully correct any plastic deformation in the ulna that could result in late subluxation. Weekly follow-up X-rays, with the patient in an above-elbow moulded cast, are performed until 4–6 weeks when the fracture has united, and thereafter mobilization can safely commence.

Operative stabilization of the ulna is more likely to be required if there is a long oblique fracture or delayed presentation. This can be done by intramedullary pinning with a single ulnar TEN or by plating of the ulna if the fracture is inherently longitudinally unstable or the nail does not adequately control angular deformity. If ulnar length and alignment are restored, and the radio-capitellar joint does not concentrically reduce, open reduction of the radial head is required as the radial head may be dislocated out of the intact annular ligament, which, in turn, blocks reduction. This can be done either through the Kocher approach or the more extensile, posterolateral Boyd approach, with protection of the posterior interosseous nerve. Following this, the annular ligament can be reconstructed using a lateral strip from the triceps tendon or other tissue such as a palmaris longus tendon graft. If the ulnar plastic deformation is not correctable by closed means, an acute ulnar extension

osteotomy is needed to obtain a concentric radial head reduction (Figure 15.24).

Management of late-presenting injuries is challenging. However, children presenting within 3 weeks of injury with a persistent radial head dislocation can still be taken to theatre with an attempt at successful closed reduction. Beyond this time, open reduction is typically needed. It can be difficult to differentiate a late-presenting neglected injury from a congenital radial head dislocation incidentally found on X-ray following an innocuous elbow injury. The radiographic signs of a congenital radial head dislocation include a hypoplastic capitellum and a dysplastic radial head with a convex articular surface, and almost always these are posterior as well as bilateral.

In chronic, neglected dislocations presenting within 3 years after injury in children <12 years of age, good long-term outcomes are still seen after open reduction combined with ulnar osteotomy. Due to proximal migration of the radius, however, there is a much higher chance of posterior interosseous nerve palsy, and a more judicious approach for late reconstructive surgery is gradual reduction of the radial head, using an external fixator and lengthening of the ulna (Figure 15.25). In children in whom the radial head remains persistently dislocated, long-term problems include development of radial head hypertrophic changes, elbow pain and stiffness, and excessive valgus deformity, as well as radio-capitellar osteoarthritis. Salvage in this situation is by radial head excision at maturity (Figure 15.26).

Olecranon Fractures

This is an uncommon paediatric elbow injury, comprising only 5% of all fractures that occur around the elbow. Anatomically, fusion of the apophysis to the metaphysis of the olecranon

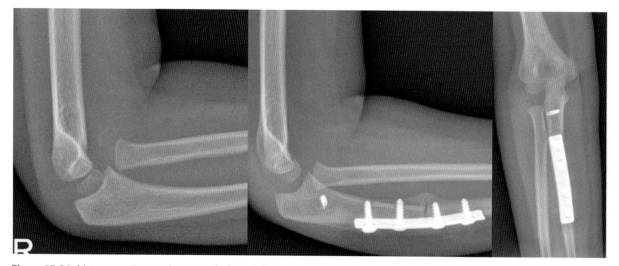

Figure 15.24 A late-presenting type I variant with plastic deformation of the ulna and an anteriorly dislocated radial head. Note the appearance of faint anterior calcification around the annular ligament at 4 weeks. An open reduction via the Boyd approach was performed, with reconstruction of the interposed annular ligament, after it was cut to allow the radial head to be reduced. To reduce the radial head, an opening wedge ulnar osteotomy (apex posterior) slightly overcorrecting the deformity was done.

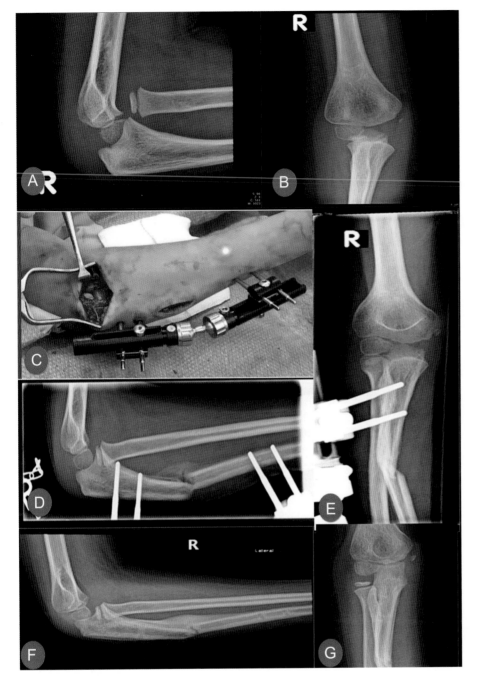

Figure 15.25 Use of an external fixator in fine-tuning an ulnar deformity to optimize radial head stability. (A) and (B) show preoperative X-rays of a child with Monteggia fracture dislocation. (C) is an intraoperative image showing open reduction of a radial head dislocation, a mini-incision ulnar osteotomy, and an external fixator in situ. (D) and (E) are immediate post-operative images. (F) and (G) are images taken 6 weeks post-operatively. *Source:* Images are courtesy of Marc Sinclair, Mediclinic City Hospital, Dubai.

occurs from anterior to posterior, with an average age of closure between 15 and 17 years. A partial closure of the ossification centre can sometimes be mistaken for an acute fracture on X-ray. Olecranon fractures can be associated with certain pathological conditions, such as osteogenesis imperfecta, where a sleeve-type fracture occurs.

The mechanism of injury is typically due to a fall on an outstretched hand, with an extension-type injury sometimes leaving the posterior periosteum intact (Figure 15.27), and a flexion-type injury causing disruption of the periosteum and avulsion of the proximal fragment (Figure 15.28).

The management algorithm is as follows.

1. Minimally displaced fractures can be treated with a long arm splint or casting, provided the integrity of the posterior olecranon periosteum is maintained. Typically, a period of 3–4 weeks of immobilization is needed, with repeat imaging at 7–10 days to ensure no significant displacement.

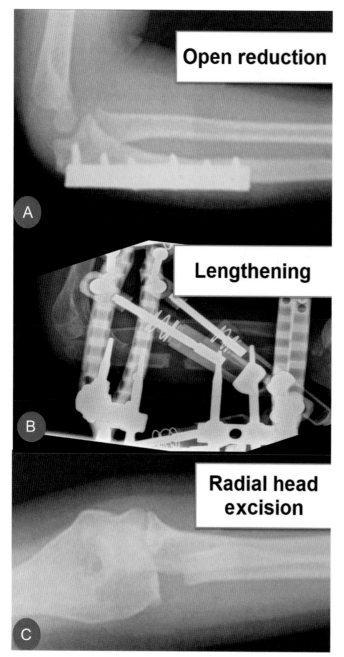

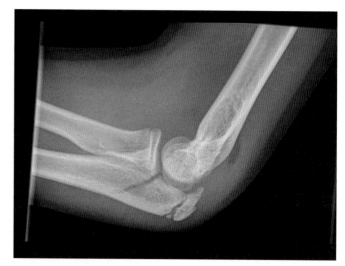

Figure 15.27 Extension-type olecranon fracture.

Figure 15.26 Three options for neglected Monteggia fracture.

2. Open reduction and internal fixation are indicated in displaced fractures. A tension band suture using a heavy suture, or conventional tension band wiring, is used with avulsion fractures (where the proximal fragment is at, or above, the level of the radio-capitellar joint); plate fixation is needed for comminuted fractures.

Elbow Dislocations

These are the second commonest traumatic major joint dislocations, after shoulder dislocations, occurring in children (Figure 15.28). They account for approximately 10–25% of all elbow injuries, predominantly in 10- to 20-year olds or in the second decade of life. Elbow dislocations are classified according to the position of the proximal radioulnar joint in relation to the distal humerus. Posterior or posterolateral dislocations are commonest (80%), followed by medial, lateral, and anterior dislocations, which occur rarely.

Typically, the elbow is held in flexion due to pain; the forearm appears short, and the distal humerus can be palpable in the antecubital fossa. It is essential to perform a neurovascular examination.

Initial radiographs include AP and lateral views of the affected elbow. As ossification centres may be difficult to interpret, X-rays of the contralateral elbow should be considered. Often there is an associated fracture of the medial epicondyle, coronoid, or proximal radius. In very young children under 3 years age, a high index of suspicion should exist for a transphyseal fracture or distal humeral epiphyseal separation, which occurs more frequently in this age group.

Closed manipulation and reduction are successful in the majority of cases, and subsequent cast immobilization should be minimized to 1–2 weeks to reduce the risk of post-operative stiffness. Post-reduction, it is important when children return to clinic for cast removal to obtain further good-quality X-rays to demonstrate the ossification centres of the elbow are correctly located and to exclude entrapped intra-articular fragments. Open reduction is indicated in cases of incarcerated fragments (typically of the medial epicondyle or coronoid process) in a joint that does not reduce. Failure to obtain or maintain adequate closed reduction, together with significant joint instability, is another indication, as well as late-presenting elbow dislocations, which often require open reduction.

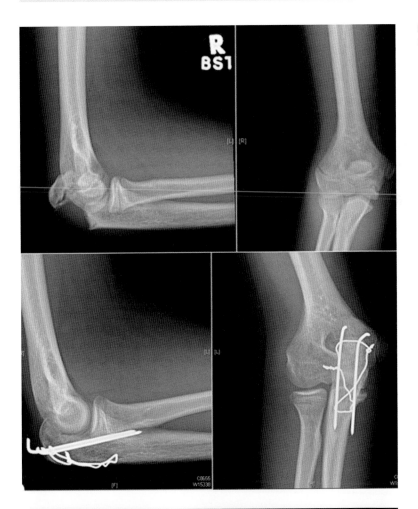

Figure 15.28 Displaced avulsion-type olecranon fracture stabilized using tension band wires.

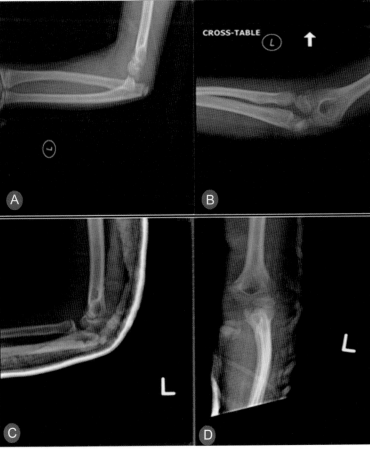

Figure 15.29 Left elbow dislocation in a child (A,B) treated by closed reduction(C,D).

References

1. Goswami GK. The fat pad sign. *Radiology*. 2002;222(2):419–20.

2. Howard A, Mulpuri K, Abel MF, *et al.* The Treatment of pediatric supracondylar humerus fractures. *J Am Acad Orthop Surg*. 2012;20(5):320–7.

3. Gartland JJ. Management of supracondylar fractures of the humerus in children. *Surg Gynecol Obstet*. 1959;109(2):145–54.

4. Leet AI, Frisancho J, Ebramzadeh E. Delayed treatment of type 3 supracondylar humerus fractures in children. *J Pediatr Orthop*. 2002;22(2):203–7.

5. Sibinski M. Early versus delayed treatment of extension type-3 supracondylar fractures of the humerus in children. *J Bone Joint Surg Br*. 2006;88-B(3):380–1.

6. Walmsley P, Kelly M, Robb J, *et al.* Delay increases the need for open reduction of type-III supracondylar fractures of the humerus. *J Bone Joint Surg Br*. 2006;88(4):528–30.

7. Ramachandran M, Skaggs DL, Crawford HA, *et al.* Delaying treatment of supracondylar fractures in children. *J Bone Joint Surg Br*. 2008;90-B(9):1228–33.

8. Blakey CM, Biant LC, Birch R. Ischaemia and the pink, pulseless hand complicating supracondylar fractures of the humerus in childhood. *J Bone Joint Surg Br*. 2009;91-B(11):1487–92.

9. Mounsey EJ, Howard A. Evidence-based treatments of paediatric elbow fractures. In: Alshryda S, Huntley JS, Banaszkiewicz P, eds. *Paediatric Orthopaedics: An Evidence-Based Approach to Clinical Questions*. Cham: Springer; 2016. pp. 305–15.

10. Kocher MS. Lateral entry compared with medial and lateral entry pin fixation for completely displaced supracondylar humeral fractures in children. A randomized clinical trial. *J Bone Joint Surg Am*. 2007;89(4):706.

11. Skaggs DL, Hale JM, Bassett J, Kaminsky C, Kay RM, Tolo VT. Operative treatment of supracondylar fractures of the humerus in children. *J Bone Joint Surg Am*. 2001;83(5):735–40.

12. Sankar WN, Hebela NM, Skaggs DL, Flynn JM. Loss of pin fixation in displaced supracondylar humeral fractures in children. *J Bone Joint Surg Am*. 2007;89(4):713–17.

13. Milch H. Fractures and fracture dislocations of the humeral condyles. *J Trauma*. 1964;4(5):592–607.

14. Jakob R, Fowles JV, Rang M, Kassab MT. Observations concerning fractures of the lateral humeral condyle in children. *J Bone Joint Surg Br*. 1975;57(4):430–6.

15. O'Brien PI. Injuries involving the proximal radial epiphysis. *Clin Orthop Relat Res*. 1965;41:51–8.

Chapter 16

Orthopaedic Hand and Wrist Disorders

Sara Dorman and Dean E. Boyce

Congenital Hand Differences

Introduction

The development of the upper limb begins during the fourth week of in utero life, when a limb bud consisting of undifferentiated mesenchymal cells encased in ectoderm develops. By 9 weeks, the bud has developed into an arm and hand with identifiable digits, and by 12 weeks, the digits have differentiated. Growth and differentiation are under the control of signal regions at the tip of the developing limb, with complicated interactions and feedback systems (Figure 16.1). Induction of mesenchymal cells in the 'progress zone' at the tip of the developing limb occurs under the influence of specific zones. The apical ectodermal ridge (AER) is the director of growth in the proximo-distal axis (excision of the AER results in a limb stump only, and transplantation may result in a duplicate limb). Differentiation in the radioulnar axis is under the control of the zone of polarizing activity (ZPA) (transplantation of the ZPA can give rise to a 'mirror hand'). Digits become 'ulnarised' the futher they are away from the ZPA. Differentiation in the volar–dorsal axis is under the control of the dorsal ectoderm (excision and rotation of this zone cause the dorsal muscles to form ventrally). Thus, there is a complicated interaction between the genes and the proteins they encode, which induces cells of the AER, ZPA, and dorsal ectoderm, driving limb development and patterning. Anomalies in these processes result in anomalies in limb development and can be the result of genetic mutation, interruption of a pathway at the molecular level, or gross insult. The aetiology of such insults can be environmental such as radiation, infection, and chemicals (including drugs), or be hereditary as part of a syndrome.

Congenital hand deformities have traditionally been classified using the 'Swanson classification' [1]:

1. Failure of formation (e.g. phocomelia, radial longitudinal deficiency)
2. Failure of differentiation (e.g. syndactyly)
3. Duplication (e.g. radial and ulnar polydactyly)
4. Overgrowth (e.g. macrodactyly)
5. Undergrowth (e.g. thumb hypoplasia)
6. Constriction ring syndrome
7. Generalized skeletal abnormalities

This classification is by no means perfect. For example, is central polysyndactyly (Figure 16.2) failure of differentiation or duplication? Some conditions such as polydactyly are relatively common, whereas a cleft hand is rarely encountered. The Oberg–Manske–Tonkin (OMT) classification allows upper-extremity anomalies to be specifically placed as malformations, deformities and dysplasias. Malformations are subclassified according to the axis of formation and differentiation affected and whether it involves the entire limb or just the hand plate [2]. The commonest and most important congenital conditions are described below.

Figure 16.1 Important zones in the developing limb bud.

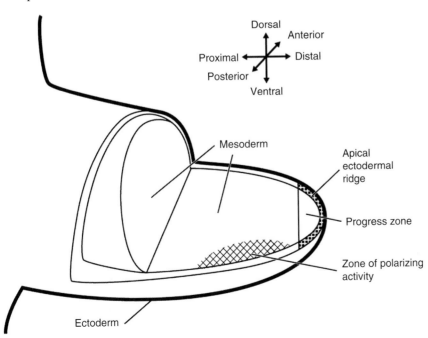

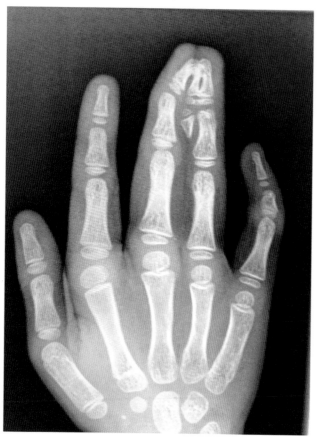
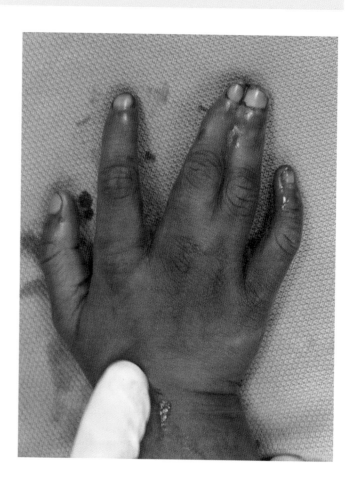

Figure 16.2 Central polysyndactyly.

Polydactyly

Polydactyly translates literally as 'many fingers' and is one of the commonest congenital hand deformities. It presents as a wide spectrum of disorders but is best thought of as digital 'duplication', with both components often being of abnormal morphology and hypoplastic [3].

The pattern of transmission is autosomal dominant, with variable penetrance and reported racial incidence for all types of polydactyly. Post-axial polydactyly is commoner in Africans, whereas pre-axial polydactyly is commoner in Caucasians.

Polydactyly is broadly categorized, in order of frequency, as **post-axial** (ulnar), pre-axial (radial), or central (Figure 16.3).

Post-axial Polydactyly

Post-axial duplication is duplication of the little finger. It is eight times commoner than any other polydactyly, often **bilateral**, and is commoner in Africans (1:150) than in Caucasians (1:300) where it is more commonly syndromic.

Post-axial polydactyly is classified as follows (Stelling classification), with type 1 the commonest, followed by types 2 and 3 in decreasing order of frequency:

- Type 1: soft tissue mass, no skeletal structure
- Type 2: duplicate digit/part digit articulating with normal/ bifid metacarpal/phalanx
- Type 3: duplicate digit, including duplicate metacarpal.

Diagnosis and Examination

Careful examination should include the range of movement (ROM) of bilateral hands and feet. Radiographs are not mandatory for simple type 1 duplications but may be warranted for types 2 and 3 to examine for shared epiphysis and the morphology of 'a normal digit', and to exclude symphalangism (fused phalanges), complex polysyndactyly, or deformity with angulation.

Management

Type 1 duplications can be managed simply with deletion/excision. This can be performed easily under local anaesthesia when <3 months of age, and timed after a feed when the child is most docile. Suture ligation is falling out of favour, as it leaves an ugly stump and sometimes can bleed or get infected.

Types 2 and 3 require excision and reconstruction of functional components, including the ulnar collateral ligament (UCL) (aided by a retained periosteal strip from the deleted digit) and reinsertion of the abductor digiti minimi.

Central Polydactyly

Central polydactyly refers to a duplication of the index, long, or ring finger. This is the least common polydactyly. It is commonly associated with syndactyly, only becoming apparent on preoperative radiographs and representing a 'hidden' central polydactyly between the syndactylized digits (Figure 16.2). Central

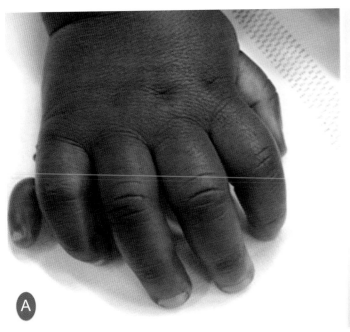

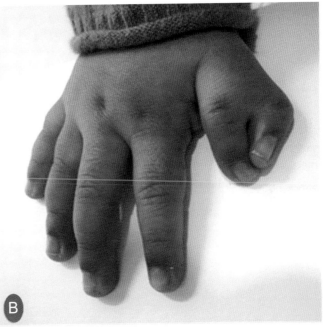

Figure 16.3 Polydactyly is broadly categorized as post-axial (A), pre-axial (B), or central (Figure 16.2).

polydactyly is frequently bilateral, with ring finger duplications the commonest, followed by the middle and index fingers.

They are classified using the *Stelling* classification, with type 2 duplications the commonest, followed by types 1 and 3 in decreasing order of frequency.

Diagnosis and Examination

Diagnosis is clinical and radiographic. Clinical assessment should include ROM, posture, and function. Classify the type and presence and degree of syndactyly. Indications and cautions with radiographs are the same as for post-axial polydactyly.

Management

An individualized approach is adopted, depending on the patient, state and extent of the duplicate digit, and presence of syndactyly.

In general, early surgical treatment, with excision of duplicate digit and complex bone and soft tissue reconstruction, is indicated. Exact procedures are case-specific and may vary from simple ray resection with intermetacarpal ligament reconstruction to complex redistribution of tendinous, ligamentous, and skeletal elements.

Pre-axial Polydactyly

Pre-axial polydactyly is duplication of the thumb. It has an incidence of 0.8 per 1000 live births and may have a dominant inheritance pattern. There is a female-to-male ratio of 2.5:1 and it is commoner in Caucasians.

Although a triphalangeal thumb is historically linked to maternal thalidomide ingestion, pre-axial polydactyly has numerous syndromic associations, including Holt–Oram, Fanconi pancytopenia, thrombocytopenia absent radii (TAR),

and Carpenter and Bloom syndrome. Abnormalities in the sonic hedgehog protein, which is expressed as part of radial–ulnar limb development, and abnormal expression of other morphogens, such as *Hox* genes, bone morphogenetic protein, and Gli-3, have been implicated in the development of thumb duplications.

Diagnosis and Examination

Syndromic causes involving every organ system necessitate careful examination and thorough workup. This should include multidisciplinary team involvement, including paediatricians, and management-specific focus on cardiac and haematological investigations before undertaking surgical correction.

Clinical examination to assess for ROM at all joints of both duplicate, as well as overall, upper limb function. Specific care should focus on the presence of thumb functional tendon units and the presence of angulation. Radiographs are mandatory.

Classification of pre-axial polydactyly is, in fact, radiographic and based on the presence of complete/incomplete duplication of each phalanx (**Wassel classification**) (Figure 16.4):

- **Type I**: bifid distal phalanx
- **Type II**: duplicate distal phalanx
- **Type III**: bifid proximal phalanx
- **Type IV**: duplicate proximal phalanx – commonest
- **Type V**: bifid metacarpal
- **Type VI**: duplicate metacarpal
- **Type VII**: triphalangism.

Type IV is the commonest (>40%) (Figure 16.4), and type I the least common. Type VII is the most complex and many consider it a separate entity.

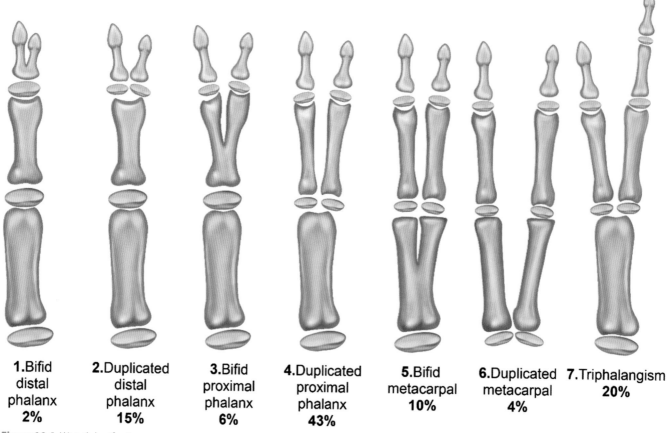

1. Bifid distal phalanx 2% **2.** Duplicated distal phalanx 15% **3.** Bifid proximal phalanx 6% **4.** Duplicated proximal phalanx 43% **5.** Bifid metacarpal 10% **6.** Duplicated metacarpal 4% **7.** Triphalangism 20%

Figure 16.4 Wassel classification.

Management

Surgical management is usually delayed until after 12 months, as this reduces the overall anaesthetic risk, allows for a full and thorough preoperative assessment, and eases surgery, thanks to a larger hand size. Only the unclassified '*pouce flottant*' (floating thumb) on a narrow skin-only stalk is managed earlier with simple excision or ligation (as for post-axial type 1 duplications).

The surgical principles are to produce a well-aligned, normally sized, and stable thumb before the age of 2, whilst preserving the epiphyseal plates where feasible. Despite this, the reconstructed thumb is nearly always smaller than the normal contralateral thumb.

Overall, nail appearance and joint motion are less important to a successful outcome, with stiffness at one thumb joint being functionally well tolerated.

Surgical treatment depends largely on classification but ranges from total ablation of one thumb to reconstruction using half components from each duplicate. In general, the ulnar-sided digit is preserved in favour of the radial duplicate, in order to save the ulnar collateral and provide metacarpophalangeal joint stability.

Types I and II: Symmetrical Duplication

Consider excision of the central composite tissue segment from both thumbs and approximation of the outer halves – **the Bilhaut–Cloquet procedure** (Figure 16.5).

Significant limitations include joint stiffness, wide distal phalanx, angular deformities, nail ridging, and poor cosmesis.

The modified Bilhaut–Cloquet procedure alleviates some of the limitations with the nail bed by using the nail bed of only one thumb.

Types III–VI: Asymmetrical Duplication

Consider deletion/excision of smaller duplicate. A deleted thumb is usually (and preferably) the radial digit due to preservation of the more functionally important UCL.

Deletion of radial duplicate usually involves (Figure 16.6):

- Racquet-shaped incision ± proximal and distal Z-plasty extensions
- Preservation of the abductor pollicis insertion
- Preservation of the radial collateral ligaments from the deleted thumb for later radial collateral ligament reconstruction
- Assessment and centralization of extrinsic tendons
- Reduction of the radial condyle, with preservation of the UCL
- Preservation of the growth plate
- Excision/fillet of the duplicate ulnar digit ± wedge osteotomy of the retained digit if angulation is present
- Looking for pollex abductus (an abnormal connection between extensor and flexor structures)

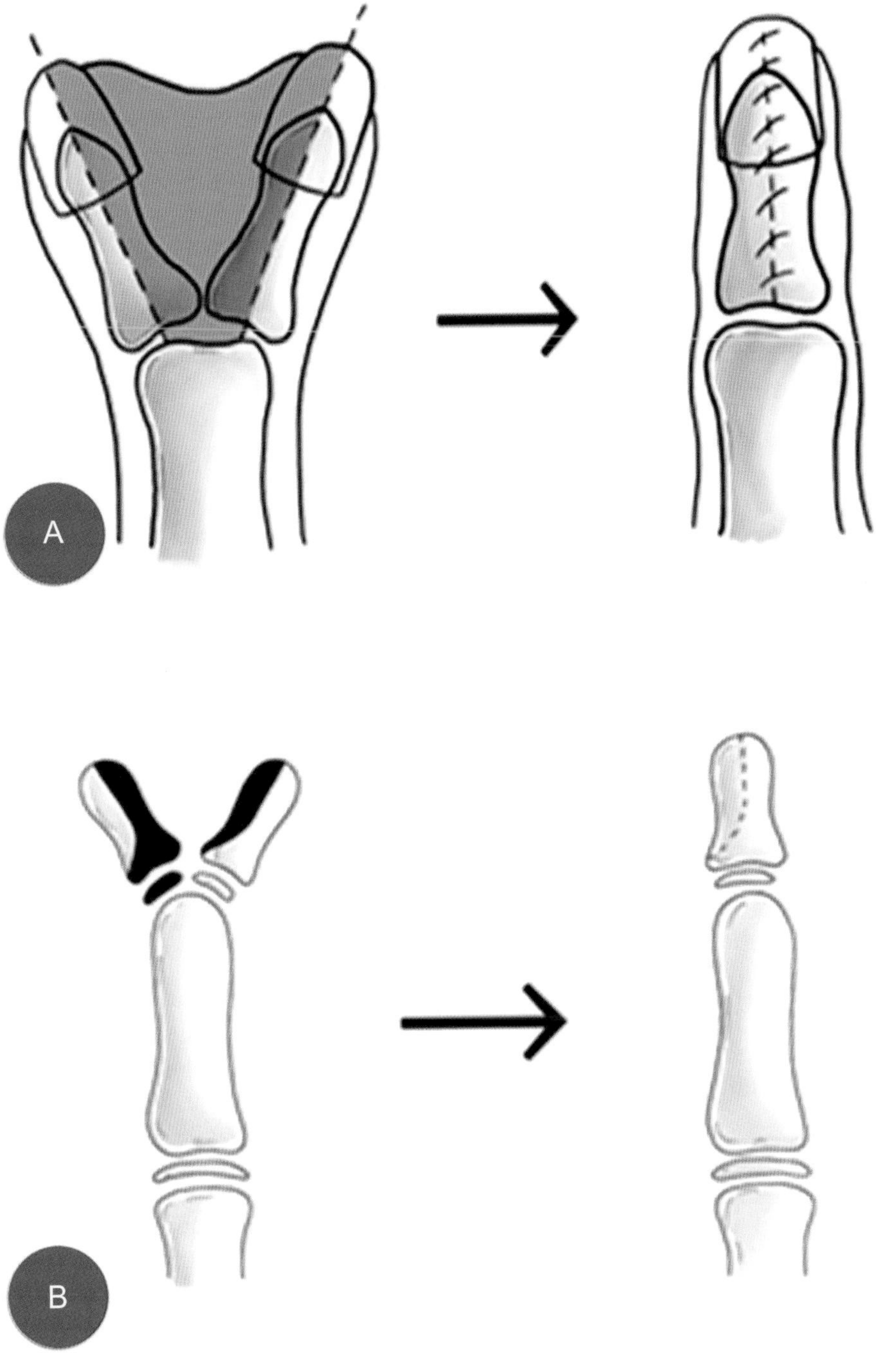

Figure 16.5 (A) Bilhaut–Cloquet procedure. (B) Modified Bilhaut–Cloquet procedure.

• Deleted digit soft tissue components can be further used to augment extrinsic tendons and soft tissue as required.

Combination Procedure

Very rarely, in complex cases, a combination procedure may be required. This may occur when asymmetry exists within each of the duplicated digits. Surgery is tailored to the individual, using the least hypoplastic components from each duplicated digit.

An example is when one digit has a better developed proximal component, and the other digit has a better developed distal fragment. In these cases, an 'on-the-top plasty' can be performed where the developed distal segment is dissected as a neurovascular island flap and fixed with a reciprocal osteotomy.

Syndactyly

Syndactyly, literally translated as *together* 'Syn', *finger* 'dactyl', is one of the commonest congenital hand deformities, with 1 per 2000 live births [4]. It carries an autosomal dominant pattern, with variable penetrance, although up to 40% have a positive family history. The pathological process is not precisely understood. Syndactyly is thought to arise from failure of apoptosis (programmed cell death) in interdigital tissue.

267

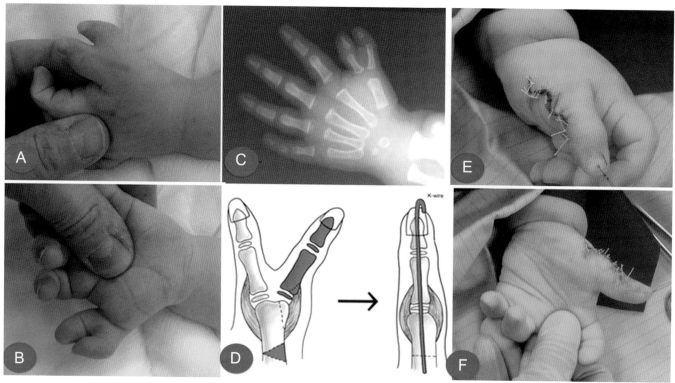

Figure 16.6 Wassel type IV thumb polydactyly (A,B). AP radiograph of thumb polydactyly(C). Ligamentoperiosteal flap raised to reconstruct radial collateral ligament MP joint. Metacarpal head was excised partially to fit base of dominant proximal phalanx. Corrective osteotomy was added to make a straight thumb (D) Deletion of radial duplicate (E,F).

It is bilateral in 50% of cases. Caucasians have the highest racial predilection and there is a male-to-female ratio of 2:1. Although often non-syndromic, associated syndromes include:

- Poland syndrome: unilateral chest and upper limb hypoplasia with symbrachydactyly typically affecting central digits, with relative sparing of the thumb and little finger (Figure 16.7)
- Trisomy 21
- Craniosynostosis syndromes such as Carpenter, Pfeiffer, and Apert – although the Apert hand is more properly termed acrosyndactyly and is sometimes referred to as a 'rosebud'. It is associated with symphalangism, radioulnar synostosis, craniosynostosis, and hypertelorism (Figure 16.8)
- Holt–Oram syndrome: also known as atrio-digital syndrome due to presence of cardiac and limb defects.

The commonest web involved is the third web (50%), with the first, second, and fourth webs accounting for 5%, 15%, and 30%, respectively. The second web is the most commonly involved in the foot, but this may represent referral bias.

Syndactyly is classified, based on completeness of web involvement, as either **complete**, with fusion at least up to the distal interphalangeal joint (DIPJ), or **incomplete**. It is further classified as skin-only syndactyly, termed **simple**, or as **complex**, involving both bony fusion and skin. A final category of '**complicated**' is reserved for cases where both syndactyly and polydactyly are present (Figure 16.9).

In summary, the commonest presentation is a Caucasian male with bilateral simple incomplete syndactyly of the middle/ring finger web.

Diagnosis and Investigations

Clinical examination should assess the number of rays involved and completeness of syndactyly, as well as identify syndromic features, and include a basic assessment of upper limb function. Examination should include passive ROM to assess associated symphalangism (stiff digits) and compare the digit lengths with the contralateral hand for brachysyndactyly. The pectoralis major should be examined: this will be hypoplastic in brachysyndactyly associated with Poland syndrome (Figure 16.9).

Syndactyly may also affect the toes. Most surgeons would not advocate surgical release due to the risk of painful hypertrophic scars. An exception, however, is the first web (Figure 16.10).

An X-ray is mandatory to evaluate for bony involvement and assess for the presence of transverse bars or more complicated hidden duplications. Both false positives and false negatives may result due to incomplete ossification. Arteriography is rarely indicated.

Management

Most hand function is learnt between 6 and 24 months. Consequently, syndactyly release is usually performed between 12 and 24 months. Exceptions to this are syndactyly involving the border digits (i.e. first and fourth webs) and in the complex Apert hand. The rationale for early surgical release (at <1 year of age) is where digital length discrepancy or complex bony involvement would, with continued growth, be expected

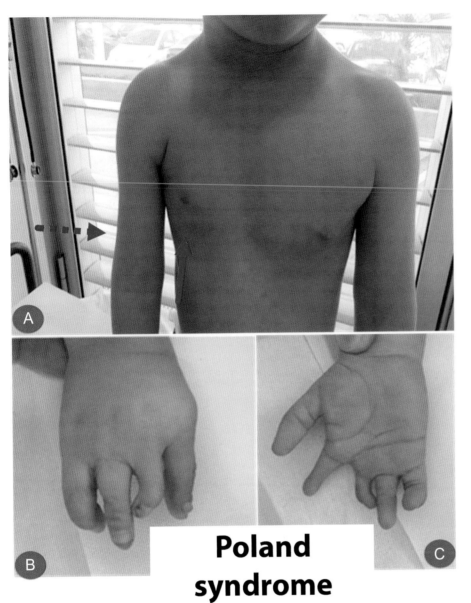

Figure 16.7 Brachysyndactyly, pectoralis major hypoplasia (solid red arrow), and upper limb hypoplasia (dashed red arrow) associated with Poland syndrome(A).Undeveloped hand and fingers (B,C)

Poland syndrome

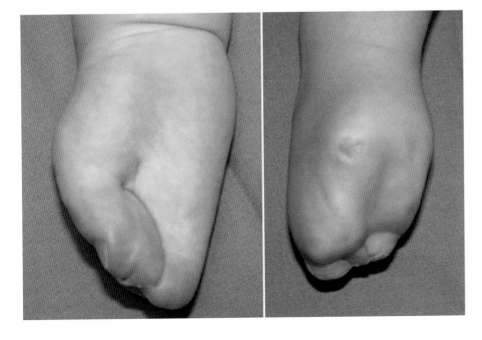

Figure 16.8 The rosebud hand. This is the most severe acrosyndactyly associated with Apert syndrome.

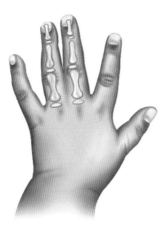

Single incomplete

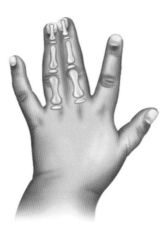

Simple incomplete

Figure 16.9 Classification of syndactyly.

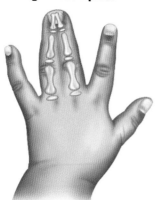

Complex

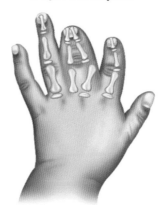

Complicated

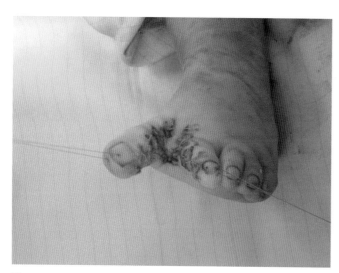

Figure 16.10 Release of the first and second toes using full-thickness skin grafts.

to cause tethering, impede development, or adversely affect future digital growth.

Relative contraindications include:

1. A minor degree of webbing (which is not cosmetically or functionally significant)

2. Hypoplastic digits (where one digit functions better than two would)

3. Feet (little functional benefit is offered, but painful hypertrophic scarring may result).

Surgical release at 12–18 months involves the following principles:

- Release only one side of the digit at a time to prevent vascular compromise.
- Avoid straight line scars or scars/incisions in the web.
- Use a dorsal skin flap for web space reconstruction.
- Use large, simple ulnar and radially based interdigitating flaps.
- Many cases can be completed without using grafts if properly planned, but always reserve the option of full-thickness grafts with preservation of the paratenon (Figure 16.11).
- Identify the neurovascular bundle proximally and volar, dissecting from the level of bifurcation.
- Address bony elements with excision, preserving joints and tendon slips, and covering exposed bone and joint with flap, as opposed to graft.
- Plan tip and lateral nail fold reconstruction with pulp plasty and Buck–Gramcko flaps (Figure 16.12).

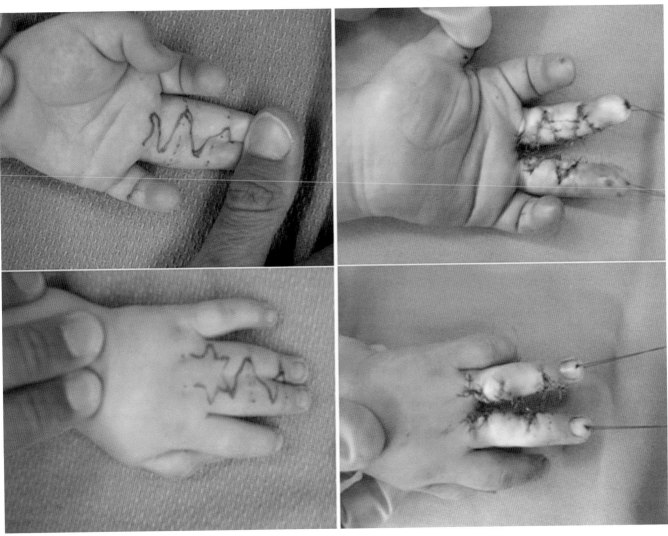

Figure 16.11 Release of the ring and little fingers without using skin grafts.

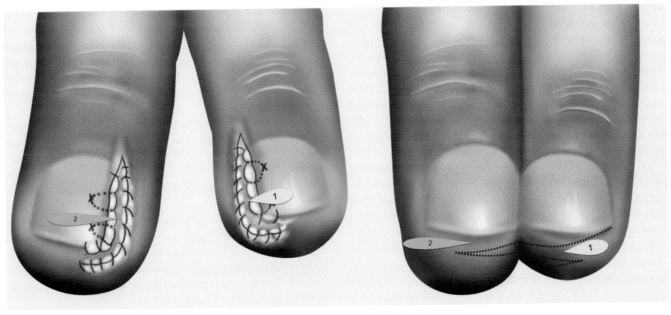

Figure 16.12 Buck–Gramcko pulp flaps. Flap arrangement for best coverage.

Camptodactyly

Camptodactyly is a congenital flexion deformity of the digit involving the proximal interphalangeal joint (PIPJ) and can be found in approximately 1% of the population. The incidence is likely an underestimate due to underreporting, and some literature quotes up to 20% among adolescent females. The term is derived from the Greek '*kamtos*' (arched) and '*dactyl*' (finger).

Camptodactyly has an autosomal dominant inheritance pattern, with variable penetrance, and tends to have a bimodal distribution. It is commonly bilateral and is classically defined as involving the little finger (although all digits may be involved, with an order of frequency of the little finger > ring finger > middle finger > index).

It is classified by its distribution into:

1. Infantile (at or soon after birth)
2. Preadolescent (can be more severe and progressive)
3. Syndromic (often severe and multiple digits involved).

In infancy, the male-to-female ratio is 1:1, whereas the adolescent variant has a female predominance. This has led some to believe they represent separate entities.

The aetiology remains poorly understood, with almost all structures crossing the volar aspect of the PIPJ being implicated. Abnormalities found on exploration include abnormal lumbrical insertion, short or tethered superficialis tendon, anomalous fibrous tissue, and abnormalities in the retinacular or extensor system. The DIPJ is not pathological but may develop late compensatory changes.

Diagnosis and Examination

Presentation of an abnormal posture involving the PIPJ requires careful history taking to help rule out non-congenital or traumatic aetiologies. Details on duration and progression of deformity allow for classification of camptodactyly if appropriate.

Clinical assessment is focused on the digits affected and assessment with measurement of both passive and active ROM, classifying the **PIPJ as either reducible or irreducible**.

To aid in localizing the abnormality, examination should include assessment for intrinsic tightness, which may indicate lumbrical pathology. Furthermore, if there is increased extension on the metacarpophalangeal joint (MCPJ) flexion, this may indicate deforming or tight volar structures. Careful examination must also look at overall finger morphology and the presence of flexion creases, as associated brachydactyly with very stiff PIPJ and absent creases may represent a diagnosis of symphalangism.

When the PIPJ flexion deformity is irreducible, the suggestion is of significant joint pathology and is not likely to be correctable by surgery. DIPJ involvement is not diagnostic of camptodactyly and may represent other aetiologies, including trauma.

Radiographic examination is mandatory, as pathological changes involving the PIPJ are a poor prognostic sign, that is, flattening out of the base of the middle phalanx and hypoplasia of the proximal phalangeal head, with volar notching of the neck

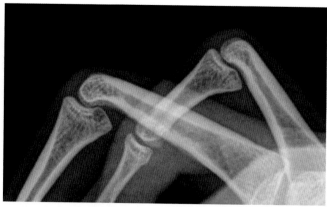

Figure 16.13 Camptodactyly. Bony changes associated with camptodactyly: flattening of the base of the middle phalanx, hypoplasia of the head, and notching of the neck of the proximal phalanx.

and loss of joint space (Figure 16.13). Lateral radiographs will further rule out congenital synostosis.

Management

Camptodactyly rarely affects function and most can be managed conservatively, particularly when contracture is <40°. Serial splintage and physiotherapy are the mainstays of treatment. If early correction is achieved, further splinting may be necessary in adolescence due to recurrent deformity during growth spurts [5].

In general, surgery should be avoided if the deformity is mild and not progressive. Therefore, relative indications for surgery are functional problems (with PIPJ flexion deformity ≥40°) and progressive disease when conservative therapies have failed. However surgical correction is never complete, particularly when radiographic evidence of PIPJ pathology is present.

The principles of surgery if no skeletal abnormalities are present include exploration of all volar structures around the PIPJ and release of abnormal/anomalous tissue. This should include examination of the flexor digitorum superficialis (FDS) and intrinsics through a Brunner-type incision or a midline incision with secondary Z-plasty.

After identification and release of the causative structure, capsular contracture release, with stepwise release of the flexor sheath, accessory collateral, 'check-rein' release, and volar capsulotomy may be performed until satisfactory correction is achieved.

Numerous procedures have also been described to rebalance the volar deforming forces across the PIPJ, including tendon transfer (FDS/lumbrical) to the lateral band/central slip. If passive MCPJ stability during examination allows active extension at the PIPJ, a 'lasso' procedure using a superficialis slip may be indicated.

The principles of surgery if skeletal abnormalities are present include the above exploration, as well as opening/closing wedge osteotomies, but will sacrifice functional flexion for extension without increasing the arc of motion, and are thus rarely performed. Arthrodesis is reserved for only the most severe cases when no useful function at the PIPJ can be attained.

Clinodactyly

Clinodactyly is characterized by radioulnar curvature of the digit distal to the MCPJ and has a reported incidence of between 1% and 19% of live births. It is derived from 'clino' (sloped) and 'dactyl' (finger). It can follow an autosomal dominant pattern, with variable penetrance, although it may be syndromic with associated syndromes, including Poland syndrome, Treacher Collins syndrome, Klinefelter syndrome, and trisomy 21 (with up to 80% of trisomy 21 patients having clinodactyly). It is often bilateral and most commonly affects the little finger (Figure 16.14) and involves the middle phalanx.

The aetiology of clinodactyly is unclear. However, clinical deformity results from abnormalities in growth plate morphology. Abnormalities include a C-shaped physeal plate, previously termed a bracketed epiphysis, but more correctly termed a longitudinal epiphyseal or diaphyseal bracket. Growth in the longitudinal portion of the epiphysis leads to asymmetrical growth and progressive abnormal phalangeal morphology. A delta phalanx is the name of the triangular-shaped bone that results from this abnormal growth pattern.

History and Examination

Assessment of a clinodactyly patient should start with a general review and identification of syndromic features. The involved digit should be assessed for the degree of deformity, based on the degree of angulation and the presence of shortening. Limited ROM is common with a bracketed epiphysis. Clinodactyly is generally painless, with painful deformity suggesting trauma.

Radiographic assessment in at least two views is mandatory to assess skeletal maturity and the degree of bony involvement, the presence of abnormal epiphysis, and the morphology of the phalanges.

Classification is based on the degree of angulation and physeal and phalangeal morphology:

I: minor angulation, normal length (very common)

II: minor angulation, short phalanx, associated with Down syndrome

III: marked deformity, associated with delta phalanx (wedge-shaped) with C-shaped physis.

Management

As the majority of clinodactyly patients have no functional deficit, reassurance is all that is required and surgery should be avoided for cosmesis only.

The indication for surgery is severe angulation with shortening or thumb involvement.

Treatment options depend on skeletal maturity, with the immature skeleton (<6 years of age) allowing for bracket resection and prevention of future angulation and shortening.

In the skeletally immature with mild shortening and minimal angulation, resection of abnormal bracket epiphysis and interposition fat grafting (Vicker's procedure) allow for longitudinal growth catch-up over a 2-year period (Figure 16.15).

In the skeletally mature, corrective osteotomies remain the mainstay, with both opening wedge and reverse wedge available. These are preferred over closing wedge osteotomy, which will further sacrifice phalangeal length. Any skin deficiencies after correction may require Z-plasty, and K-wires are used to hold corrections in place.

Trigger Thumb

Trigger thumb is described as a congenital deformity, but often there is no evidence that it is present at birth and may be best termed 'paediatric trigger thumb'. Twenty-five per cent of trigger thumbs are bilateral, and the estimated incidence is 3 in 1000, although this is likely underestimated.

Diagnosis and Examination

The typical presentation is with the thumb fixed and flexed at the interphalangeal joint (IPJ), although some cases are intermittent. There is usually a palpable nodule (Notta's node) at the level

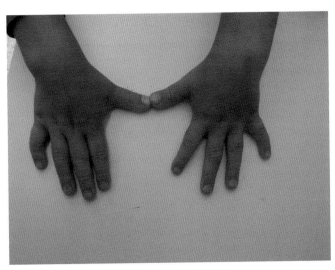

Figure 16.14 Clinodactyly of the little fingers. Parents sought orthopaedic opinion, admitting that there are no functional or aesthetic issues with them.

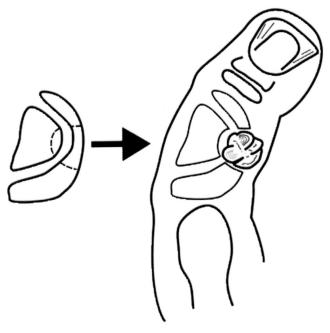

Figure 16.15 Vicker's procedure for delta phalanx causing clinodactyly.

of the MCPJ. Clinical catching or triggering is more difficult to elicit than adult triggering.

Management

Depending on the age of presentation, initial management is usually conservative, with 30% resolving before the age of 1. Flexion contractures do occur but correct spontaneously if trigger resolves or if surgical release is performed during childhood. Steroid injection is of no benefit.

Surgery is indicated if there is no resolution at 2–3 years of age (Figure 16.16). Surgical release involves release of the A1 pulley through a volar approach via a small transverse incision between MCPJ flexion creases. Release is generally performed on the radial side to avoid injury to the oblique pulley. Release of the pulley should be performed only enough to allow full extension at the IPJ.

Trigger Finger

Paediatric trigger finger is a completely separate entity to paediatric trigger thumb and adult trigger finger. It is uncommon and, when seen, should prompt further examination to rule out features of mucopolysaccharidosis (MPS) or other causes. MPS is a metabolic disorder causing accumulation of glycosaminoglycans and has a recognized association with paediatric trigger finger and paediatric carpal tunnel syndrome. Other reported causes include abnormal association between FDS and flexor digitorum profundus (FDP) tendons, anomalous FDS, tendinous nodules, calcific tendonitis, and constriction of the A2 and A3 pulleys.

Watchful waiting and splinting may be successful in many cases. If surgery is required, release of the A1 pulley alone is unlikely to resolve paediatric trigger finger, as typically the problem lies distal to the A1 pulley. After A1 pulley release, intraoperative assessment is undertaken, with a stepwise approach, until there is no longer any evidence of triggering. This may include division of the A3 pulley and partial division of the A2 pulley, widening of FDS chiasm, resection of one or both slips of the FDS, and tenodesis to the remaining FDP tendon.

Congenital Clasped Thumb

Clasped thumb is a deformity associated with a heterogenous group of congenital anomalies and is characterized by a persistent flexed and adducted thumb. It is due to weakness or deficiency of the extensor pollicis brevis or longus, or both, and is usually accompanied by a degree of first web space contracture.

There is a high incidence of clasped thumb patients with associated anomalies, including generalized musculoskeletal malformations, arthrogryposis, digito-talar dysmorphism, and Freeman–Sheldon syndrome.

The male-to-female ratio is quoted to be between 1 and 2.5:1. Although a third of cases are sporadic, with differing modes of inheritance from associated syndromes, a genetic defect is the likely causative factor, and inheritance follows an autosomal dominant pattern with variable penetrance.

History and Examination

Diagnosis of clasped thumb is often delayed, with infants frequently holding the thumb in the palm for the first 3–4 months of life. However, assessment of the clasped thumb patient should start with a general review of limb posture and function, with identification of syndromic features. Clinical examination should focus on assessment of thumb posture, passive ROM, and the first web space. The clasped thumb is usually rested in the palm, with an extension lag (most commonly at the MCPJ, which is suggestive of extensor pollicis brevis (EPB) deficiencies). Simultaneous lag at the IPJ indicates deficiency of the extensor pollicis longus (EPL), with adduction of the metacarpal implying abductor insufficiency. An important differential diagnosis is with the trigger thumb where the abnormality is localized at the IPJ and associated with Notta's node.

Radiographic assessment is not mandatory but is commonly undertaken to assess joint morphology.

Tsuyuguchi classified clasped thumb into:

- Type I: supple clasped thumb – the thumb can be passively abducted and extended against the resistance of thumb flexors ± other digital anomalies (Figure 16.17)

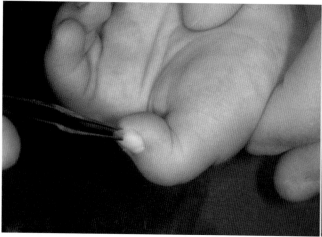
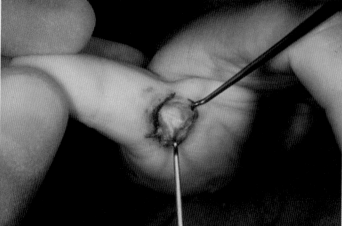

Figure 16.16 Trigger thumb release.

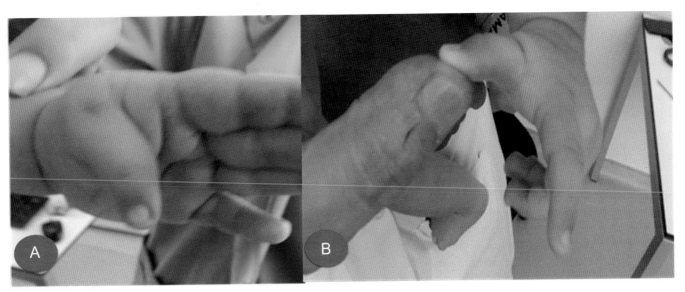

Figure 16.17 Type I supple clasped thumb. (A,B)

- Type II: clasped thumb with hand contractures – the thumb cannot be passively extended and abducted ± other digital anomalies
- Type III: clasped thumb associated with arthrogryposis.

Management

If the extensor tendons are present and the joint supple (type I), non-operative treatment is the mainstay and consists of thumb splinting (in extension) for at least 6 months, followed by night splinting for a further 6 months once active extension of the thumb is achieved. Surgery is indicated if conservative treatment fails or there is functional impairment.

If there is significant adduction contracture or more severe deformity (types II and III), operative treatment is indicated. Surgery should be individualized according to the degree of narrowing of the first web, stability of the MCPJ, and muscle deficiency.

The main aims of surgery are improvement in thumb span with release of the first web and tendon transfers to overcome the tendon deficiencies.

Soft tissue augmentation is achieved with simple Z-plasty, four-flap plasty, or rotation or transposition flaps, depending on the degree of deficit. If full passive extension and abduction cannot be achieved after adequate skin release, stepwise exploration and release may include release of the adductor pollicis insertion, the first dorsal interosseous muscle, and the carpometacarpal joint (CMCJ) capsule, plus K-wire stabilization and MCPJ chondrodesis for MCPJ instability.

Tendon transfers may be performed to restore active extension of the stable or stabilized MCPJ, with the extensor indicis (EI) as the preferred tendon for transfer. If absent, one slip of the FDS muscle can transfer to the vestigial remnant of the deficient thumb extensors.

Joint fusion remains an option in severe cases with fixed deformities.

Thumb Hypoplasia

Thumb hypoplasia represents a spectrum of deformity – from mild deficiency to complete thumb adactyly. It is best considered as part of radial deficiencies in terms of both its genetic cause and associated syndromes [6].

The overall incidence is approximately 1 per 100 000 live births, with an equal male-to-female distribution, and it is bilateral in 60% of patients. Associated syndromes include:

- Holt–Oram syndrome
- TAR
- VACTERL (vertebral defects, anal atresia, cardiac defects, tracheo-oesophageal fistula, renal anomalies, and limb abnormalities)
- Fanconi's anaemia.

Inheritance varies with associated syndromes – it is dominant with Holt–Oram syndrome, but recessive with TAR and Fanconi's anaemia.

History and Examination

Although more severe adactylies or 'floating thumbs' are diagnosed early, mild thumb hypoplasia may go unnoticed by medical teams and parents until fine motor skills begin and the thumb is noted to be ignored or smaller than the contralateral side. All thumb hypoplasia patients should be managed by a multidisciplinary team, including paediatricians, due to associations with blood dyscrasias and cardiac abnormalities.

Bilateral inspection and palpation are the mainstays of examination, comparing thumb size, consistency, thenar muscle bulk, and first web space. General assessment should include ipsilateral elbow, wrist, and index finger for associated radial longitudinal deficiencies and to assess the index finger in case of future pollicization. Good function in an index finger makes for good function after pollicization.

Gentle lateral stress is applied for assessment of MCPJ and CMCJ stability, which is vital in determining the surgical options for thumb reconstruction versus ablation and pollicization.

Pollex abductus, an abnormal insertion or communication between the FPL and the extensor mechanism, should be actively assessed and is suggested when there is abduction on thumb flexion.

Radiography is mandatory and should include bilateral hands, wrists, and forearms.

Classification (Blauth) is based on the degree of thumb hypoplasia, intrinsic and extrinsic hypoplasia, skeletal hypoplasia, and joint stability:

- Type 1: minor generalized hypoplasia
- Type 2: absence or hypoplasia of intrinsic muscles, first web contracture, and MCPJ instability
- Type 3: type 2 plus hypoplastic extrinsic muscles/tendons and greater skeletal deficiency; subdivided into:
  - 3a: stable CMCJ
  - 3b: unstable CMCJ
- Type 4 – '*pouce flottant*' or floating thumb: rudimentary appendage with small skin bridge
- Type 5: thumb adactyly.

Management

A normal-sized thumb with normal ROM should not be expected or promised, and treatments are aimed at function, not cosmesis. Surgical treatment is largely governed by Blauth classification, with type 1 hypoplasia usually having good function and requiring no treatment.

If the CMCJ is present and stable (types 2 and 3a), reconstruction of the thumb is advocated. Reconstructive options include MCPJ stabilization with UCL reconstruction, exploration and release of pollex abductus abnormalities (if present), deepening of the web space (usually with four-flap plasty), and augmentation of the intrinsic musculature with opponensplasty – most commonly ring finger FDS or abductor digiti minimi (ADM) (Huber) transfer. In type 3a thumbs, extrinsic extensor hypoplasia can be augmented with EI transfer.

If the CMCJ is absent or unstable (type 3b) and in type 4 and 5 thumbs, pollicization is preferred to reconstruction. This may be a difficult decision to explain to parents, as often the surgeon will need to discard a very reasonable-looking thumb (Figure 16.18).

Pollicization techniques have been refined over the last century but remain a complicated procedure requiring attention to detail. Although a detailed description is beyond the scope of this text, the basic principles are as follows.

- Dorsal skin flap from the radial side of the index finger, with transposition to create the first web
- Intrafascicular dissection of the index finger common digital nerves to the second web level, with preservation of accompanying digital vessels
- Excision of the index finger metacarpal, with resection of the metacarpal epiphysis (preserving the metacarpal head to act as a neo-trapezium)
- Extension of the index MCPJ (as can hyperextend), then rotation of the metacarpal head in 120° pronation, and securing in 45° palmar abduction

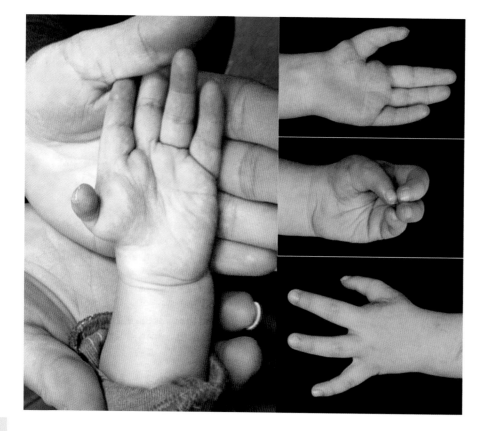

Figure 16.18 Pollicization of the index finger – clinical pictures.

- Shortening of the extensor and repositioning of:
    - EI → EPL
    - Extensor digitorum communis index → abductor pollicis longus
    - First palmar interosseous → adductor pollicis
    - First dorsal interosseous → abductor pollicis brevis (Figure 16.19).

Pollicization often provides improved cosmesis, as well as an opposable digit.

Macrodactyly

The term macrodactyly is derived from 'macros' meaning large and 'dactyl' meaning finger. It is characterized by enlargement of both soft tissue and osseous elements, and is a group of heterogenous disorders grouped as class IV overgrowth (Figure 16.20). Macrodactyly is of unknown aetiology, with the commonest theories relating to a nerve-stimulated overgrowth mediated by abnormal neural control or a localized form of neurofibromatosis. This observation has led to popularization of the term 'nerve territory-orientated macrodactyly'.

Macrodactyly is rare, with no clear inheritance pattern (Figure 16.17). There is a male predilection, and it most commonly involves the index finger; it can also involve the upper and lower limbs, with multi-digit involvement present in about half of cases.

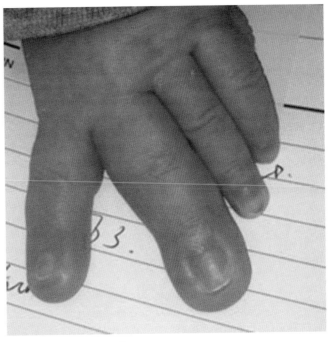

Figure 16.20 Macrodactyly.

Figure 16.19 Pollicization of the index finger – surgical technique.

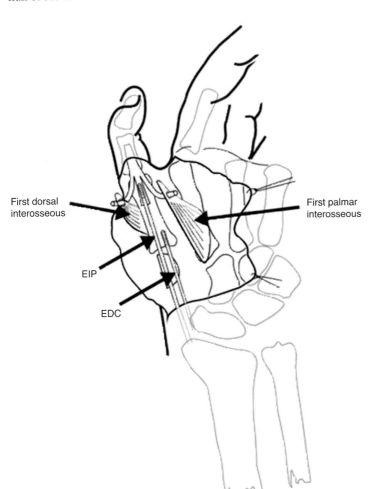

First dorsal interosseous

First palmar interosseous

EIP

EDC

History and Examination

Not all overgrowths are macrodactyly, and the condition should be distinguished from other conditions such as haemangiomas, vascular malformations, and Ollier disease. History is therefore based on the chronology of the overgrowth (static versus progressive), localization of the abnormality to the anatomical area and nerve territory, presence of features suggesting vascular abnormality (compressibility, warmth, thrill), degree of osseous involvement or overgrowth, and systemic features including those of neurofibromatosis.

Comparison radiographs are mandatory to document growth and assess for osseous involvement. Magnetic resonance or arteriography may be required to rule out vascular abnormality.

Macrodactyly can be classified simply by its evolution into either *static* or *progressive* type, with Upton further classifying into:

- **Type 1**: macrodactyly with lipofibromatosis
  - Static subtype: born with large digit, enlarges proportionally with age
  - Progressive subtype: near normal at birth, progressive growth until epiphyseal closure
- **Type 2**: macrodactyly with neurofibromatosis
- **Type 3**: macrodactyly with hyperostosis
- **Type 4**: macrodactyly with hemihypertrophy.

Management

Surgery for macrodactyly is often complex and unsatisfactory; yet psychological consequences can be severe. Social counselling and family involvement are imperative. The goals of surgery are control or reduction in deformity, with maintenance of sensibility and function [7].

Surgical option depends on aetiology, anatomical location, severity, and subtype, but include soft tissue reduction, epiphysiodesis, neurolysis, nerve excision and grafting, corrective osteotomies, arthrodesis, and, in severe cases, amputation. In general, it is best to perform a few definitive procedures, rather than multiple ones. Epiphysiodesis should be performed when the digit approaches adult size.

Arthrogryposis

The term arthrogryphosis is derived from 'Arthos' meaning joint and 'Gryposis' meaning curved or hooked.

Arthrogryposis is a congenital disorder affecting the muscles and is thought to be secondary to abnormality in the motor nerves. It is properly termed 'arthrogryposis multiplex congenita', literally meaning a congenital anomaly in the newborn involving multiple curved joints.

The overall incidence is approximately 1 per 10 000 live births.

It is important to note that arthrogryposis is essentially a descriptive term, and not an exact diagnosis. It has numerous underlying pathologies, which broadly fall into three groups:

- **Type 1**: classical arthrogryposis multiplex congenita, primarily involving the limbs with deficient or absent muscles

- **Type 2**: arthrogryposis associated with major neurogenic or myopathic dysfunction
- **Type 3**: arthrogryposis associated with other major anomalies and syndromes.

Pathologically, there is always a defect in the motor unit as a whole or at some point between the anterior horn cells and the muscle itself. Therefore, it can also be classified as neurogenic or myogenic. The aetiology is unclear, with theories postulating inflammatory or infective causes or maldevelopment secondary to increased immobility in utero. Some of these include structural abnormality of the uterus, oligohydramnios, increased intrauterine pressure or mechanical compression of the fetus, and breech presentation or prematurity.

Examination

Clinical examination remains the best modality for establishing the diagnosis, with classical presentation involving all four limbs, with multiple rigid joint deformities and defective/fibrosed or absent muscle groups, but normal sensation. Muscle and joint contractures result in cylindrical-appearing limbs lacking skin creases. Adducted and internally rotated shoulders, extended knees or elbows, and club-like hand and wrists are typical, although isolated distal variants may occur (Figure 16.21). Clasped thumb and thin, waxy skin are often present.

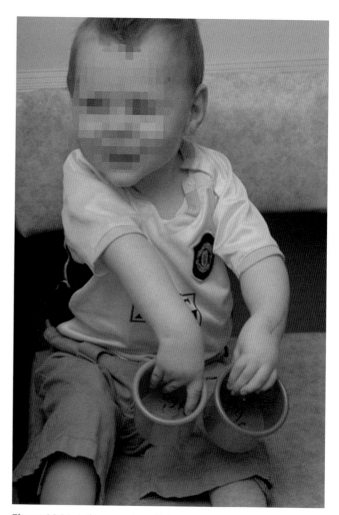

Figure 16.21 Arthrogryposis multiplex congenita.

In arthrogryposis, unlike paralytic disorders, joint deformities are stiff or rigid from birth and there is a tendency for symmetrical involvement, with increasingly severe contractures as one moves more distally on the affected limb.

Radiographs of the limbs are mandatory and may demonstrate osseous abnormality, with loss of subcutaneous fat and muscle. CT/magnetic resonance and muscle biopsy are rarely indicated, unless central nervous system involvement or a myopathic disorder is suspected.

Management

Arthrogryposis children should be managed in a multidisciplinary team involving surgeons, therapists, paediatricians, and geneticists. Early use of splints and serial casting is the mainstay of treatment to encourage elbow flexion and wrist extension, with prevention of contracture being preferred to surgery.

Surgery may be reserved for cases of failed splintage or late presentation, and aims to address posture and limb function, achieving improved position of the shoulder, elbow, wrist, and hand posture. Historically, one limb was aimed at perineal toilet, and the other for 'hand to mouth' use. However, this destroys the very useful bimanual function, as demonstrated in Figure 16.21. In principle, whatever is done to one upper limb should also be done to the other. Hand to mouth function and bimanual hand use are the key goals.

Surgery, when indicated, can be staged, with initial correction of deformity and contractures and later muscle transfers to achieve elbow flexion. The aim of wrist surgery is to put the wrists in a good position for keyboard use and it is usually achieved by carpal wedge osteotomy and tendon transfer (Figure 16.22). Recurrence is common, and ongoing splintage is required to maintain the correction until skeletal maturity.

Transverse Arrest

Transverse arrest is characterized by either complete absence of the upper limb distal to some point, producing an amputation stump (complete type), or absence of one portion of the limb (intercalated type).

Complete arrests (also known as congenital amputation, failure of development, terminal absence, and transverse amelia) can occur at any level but are commonest in the forearm at the junction of the proximal third and the middle third. The incidence is unknown and appears to not be inherited.

Intercalated variants (most commonly related to maternal thalidomide ingestion → phocomelia) can present as 'complete' with the hand attached directly to the torso, 'proximal' with a normal hand and forearm attached to the torso, or 'distal' with the hand attached to a normal upper arm at the elbow. The prevalence of intercalated variants is 0.6 per 100 000 births, with the majority of cases being isolated, although syndromic associations include musculoskeletal, cardiac, and intestinal abnormalities (Figure 16.23).

Complete and intercalated arrests are therefore postulated to be separate entities with differing aetiologies, despite being grouped together as 'transverse failure of formations'.

History and Examination

Maternal drug history taking and clinical examination for classification are the main aims, despite classification having no practical role in management thereafter.

In complete transverse arrest, examination should entail palpation of the distal portions, assessing for any ROM of the distal portion which may represent buried vestigial metacarpals or digits with the potential for independent function.

Management

Prosthetics is the mainstay of treatment, with limited possibilities for surgical intervention.

In complete transverse arrest, surgery is indicated in only exceptional cases where some functional distal remnant exists and could be expected to allow pincer function after release or improve prosthetic fitting or function. In these rare cases, distraction manoplasty or free phalangeal transfers may be occasionally indicated.

In intercalated variants, prosthetic fitting is required for most phocomelic patients who may activate the device using digits. Surgery is only indicated to achieve prosthetic fitting or improve function of the terminal digits. Many patients choose to do without prosthetics.

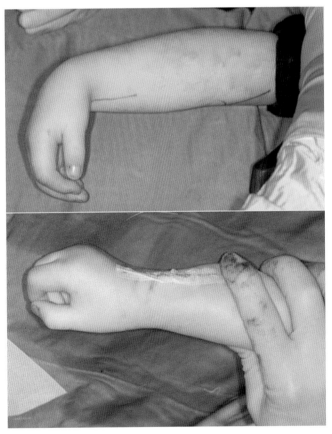

Figure 16.22 Position of the wrist before and after dorsal wedge osteotomy of the carpus and flexor carpi ulnaris/flexor carpi radialis transfer.

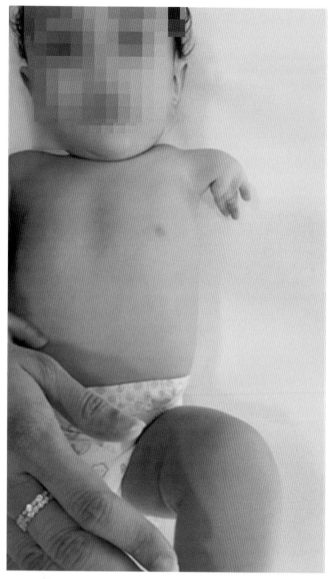

Figure 16.23 Phocomelia.

Brachydactyly

Brachydactyly is a general term ('*brachy*' meaning short, and '*dactyl*' meaning finger) that refers to disproportionately short fingers or toes and can occur either as an isolated malformation or as part of a complex malformation syndrome. In the majority of cases of isolated brachydactyly (and some syndromic forms), genetic abnormalities have been isolated. In isolated brachydactyly, inheritance is mostly autosomal dominant with variable penetrance.

Brachydactyly is therefore a general term and encompasses a number of pathological entities, including:

1. A distal form of *true transverse arrest*, with the more proximal part being *relatively* well developed (note: fingernails are absent)

2. Amputations as part of constriction ring syndrome, with proximal structures being *entirely* normal (note: fingernails are absent)

3. *Symbrachydactyly*, with significant reduction in bone and soft tissue elements and severely hypoplastic digits or nubbin-like remnants. There is hypoplasia of the more proximal hand, wrist, and forearm (note: fingernails/remnants are present on hypoplastic digits, or nubbins).

Symbrachydactyly

Symbrachydactyly is an important clinical entity, which Blauth has further subdivided into four descriptive types (Figure 16.24):

- **Peromelic type**: absence of all digits and metacarpals
- **Short finger type**
- **Cleft hand type**: absence of one or more central digits
- **Monodactylous type**: absence of all digits other than the thumb.

History and Examination

The severity of digital shortening is variable, with mild shortening only apparent due to loss of normal cascade. Careful examination, including the length and function of brachydactylous digits and the presence of remnant nail plates, is mandatory for diagnosis.

Examination of the shoulder, chest wall, and contralateral limb is required, as chest wall abnormalities are likely part of Poland syndrome. Associated abnormalities may include syndactyly, clinodactyly, and symphalangism.

Management

The functional and aesthetic aspects of symbrachydactyly can range from mild to severe, depending on the degree of shortening, status of the digital remnant and number of digits involved. Hence surgical intervention varies likewise.

When in an isolated form, the indication for surgery is function. Lengthening of the brachydactylous digit, either as a single stage, with step-cut osteotomy, or as a multistaged procedure and distraction osteogenesis, can be fraught with problems (particularly in the digit, as opposed to the metacarpal). Soft tissue release, lengthening, or ligamentous reconstruction may be required and result in an aesthetically unpleasing, stiff, and contracted digit with reduced function.

In general, with regard to lengthening of the brachydactylous digit, the preferred treatment for short phalanges is to avoid surgery, whereas for short metacarpals, lengthening, particularly with distraction osteogenesis, responds more favourably. Free phalangeal transfer (taking a non-vascularized toe middle phalanx and transferring to the digit) yields disappointing long-term results, and often a significant deformity in the donor toe.

Functional improvements are more predictable with soft tissue procedures, including widening of web space, Z-plasty lengthening of constriction bands, and ablation of short, useless

Figure 16.24 Symbrachydactyly classification.

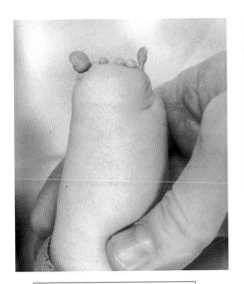

Peromelic type

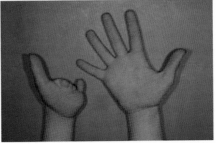

Short Finger type

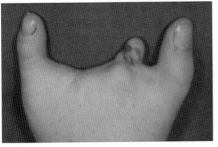

Atypical cleft type

Monodactylous type

nubbins, especially from the first web. Segments of one digit may be used to augment another. Often microvascular toe transfer will be the best option to restore a degree of pinch in a digitless or monodactylous hand.

Radial Longitudinal Deficiencies

Radial deficiencies consist of a spectrum of abnormalities that are classified as longitudinal deficiencies, as part of *type 1 'failure of formation'*. Although skeletal hypoplasia can occur in the whole arm, including humeral and ulnar elements, there is characteristic radial deviation of the wrist secondary to reduced radial support for the carpus (Figure 16.25).

The prevalence is approximately 1 in 30 000 live births, with radial deficiencies frequently bilateral and asymmetrical. Both environmental causes (including maternal use of thalidomide) and syndromic associations are well documented. Associated syndromes include VACTERL, Holt–Oram syndrome, TAR, Fanconi's anaemia, and trisomies 13 and 18. Inheritance patterns follow their syndromic causes when present, being recessive in Fanconi's anaemia and TAR, dominant in Holt–Oram syndrome, and sporadic in VACTERL and trisomies 13 and 18.

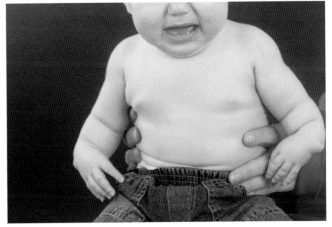

Figure 16.25 Radial longitudinal deficiency.

History and Examination

Due to associated syndromes, children with radial longitudinal deficiencies should be managed as part of a multidisciplinary team involving paediatricians and therapists. Haematological testing, cardiography, renal ultrasound, and genetic screening are also mandatory.

Complete physical examination is undertaken to assess for syndromic associations, and examination used to assess shoulder, elbow, and hand function. Serial examination of both upper limbs is undertaken, with mild forms of radial deficiencies being subtle.

Careful examination should be made to the elbow, with severe forms of radial deficiencies being associated with poor elbow function. In theory, hand to mouth function may be worsened by correcting the radial deviation in a child with a stiff elbow.

Stiffness or flexion contractures are common, especially of the index and middle fingers, along with thumb hypoplasia or aplasia, in up to 60% of patients with total radial absence. Careful examination of movement and function of the index finger in those with thumb aplasia is required, as a stiff and ignored index finger will not make a good pollicized thumb.

Radiography is mandatory and should be bilateral, including the digits, hand, wrist, and forearm (including the elbow):

Classification is based on radiographic severity, as outlined by Bayne:

- **Type 1**: short distal radius (>2 mm shorter than the ulna, with a normal proximal radius)
- **Type 2**: hypoplastic distal and proximal radius
- **Type 3**: partial absence of the radius
- **Type 4**: complete absence of the radius.

A fibrocartilaginous radial remnant, or *anlage*, may be identified at surgery.

Management

Treatment is broadly based on the severity of deformity, although functional impairment, secondary to forearm length, wrist instability, and thumb hypoplasia, is the main indication for treatment. Physiotherapy is required in all but the most minor of cases and helps to prevent progression of stiffness.

In **types 1 and 2**, management is primarily with stretching and splintage. Severe type 2 deficiencies occasionally require soft tissue release or tendon transfers. Centralization of the carpus on the ulna is rarely warranted.

In **types 3 and 4**, wrist instability with more severe radial deviation necessitates preoperative stretching followed by surgical realignment of the carpus on the ulna. Contraindications include major organ defects, making anaesthetic risk unacceptable, inadequate elbow flexion (as discussed above), or firmly established functional patterns in adults.

Preoperative stretching through use of serial casting has now been largely superseded by *external distraction*. Distraction offers both osseous realignment, making wrist stabilization easier, and soft tissue lengthening, reducing the requirement for local skin flaps to cover radial shortages and reducing the need for tendon lengthening procedures. Tendon transfer and rebalancing are still required to help maintain the carpus in its new position.

Once adequately distracted, the realignment procedure can either be '*centralization*', with the carpus repositioned over the ulna (usually by making a notch in the carpus) and stabilized

with pin fixation through the third metacarpal, or '*radialization*' with the scaphoid placed over the ulnar head and secured through the second metacarpal. The decision is usually based on expected outcomes and the presence of adequate radial carpus stock for a carpal slot to fit the scaphoid. Radialization is preferred, if possible, as there is less injury to growth plates, thus maximizing potential longitudinal growth.

Surgery is often followed by pollicization to reconstruct an absent or hypoplastic thumb (Figure 16.25).

Ulnar Longitudinal Deficiencies

Ulnar deficiencies are far less common than their radial counterparts and occur in approximately 1 in 100 000 live births. Occurrence is sporadic, more commonly unilateral, and is associated with systemic conditions.

History and Examination

Ulnar deficiencies differ from radial-sided deficiencies with marked elbow pathology, but a stable wrist. Despite this, the hand and carpus are always abnormal, with most associated with adactyly, a third with syndactyly, and over two-thirds with thumb hypoplasia. Examination is therefore based on assessing bilateral upper limbs, with focus on elbow and wrist function and identification of associated abnormalities. Bilateral radiography is mandatory for comparison and diagnosis.

Classification is into four types depending on the degree of ulna hypoplasia:

- **Type 1**: hypoplastic ulna
- **Type 2**: partial absence of the ulna
- **Type 3**: partial absence of the ulna, with a normal radio-humeral joint
- **Type 4**: total absence of the ulna, with synostosis of the radio-humeral joint.

Management

The commoner unilateral ulnar deficiency patients usually function well, preferring the normal limb for one-handed tasks and adapting well for bimanual function.

Surgical treatment depends on severity, with better outcomes in types 1 and 2. In such cases, surgery for associated thumb hypoplasia or syndactyly is all that is usually required.

Indications for surgery in progressive or unstable type 2 and 3 deficiencies remain controversial. Excision of the ulna *anlage* (fibrocartilaginous remnant) has been advocated by some for progressive deformity. Realignment and formation of a one-bone forearm have been described but risk sacrificing forearm rotation for forearm stability.

Type 4 deficiencies result in marked internal rotation of the limb, which severely limits limb function. If functional compensation is not achieved through conservative measures, osteotomy with corrective external rotation is occasionally indicated.

Central Longitudinal Deficiency

Central ray deficiencies typically involve aplasia of the central digits, forming what is also known as split hand/foot malformation (Figure 16.26). It is characterized by partial or complete

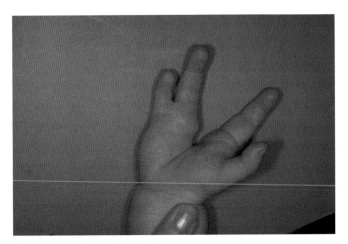

Figure 16.26 A 'typical' cleft hand.

Table 16.1 Differentiation between the typical and the atypical cleft hand

Typical	Atypical
Autosomal dominant	Sporadic
Bilateral	Unilateral
V-shaped	U-shaped
Feet involved	Nubbins/nails present
No finger 'nubbins'	Thumb present if monodactylous
Little finger present if monodactylous	

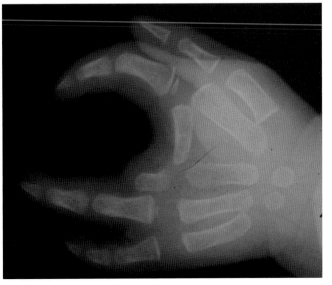

Figure 16.27 Transverse bar in a cleft hand.

absence of a central ray, forming a deep v-shaped cleft. It is often bilateral and may involve both hands and feet, and a family history is common. Incidence is estimated at 1 in 10 000 live births. Bones are either absent or malpositioned, but never hypoplastic.

Central ray deficiencies can present as part of a syndrome or as an isolated abnormality. It is thought to result from abnormalities of the AER in utero, with multiple genetic loci identified for non-syndromic variants. Associated conditions include ectrodactyly–ectodermal dysplasia–clefting syndrome, acrorenal syndrome, Cornelia de Lange syndrome, and ectrodactyly and craniofacial syndromes.

History and Examination

The characteristic appearance is a deep v-shaped cleft associated with absence or deficiency of a central ray. Associated first web syndactyly should be addressed.

There are a number of significant characteristics which differentiate *true* from *atypical* cleft hands (Table 16.1).

Radiographs are mandatory and may demonstrate transverse bony elements within the cleft, which will require excision (Figure 16.27).

Management

In the absence of first web space contractures, hand function is often remarkably good. This has led it to be labelled as a '*functional triumph but a social disaster*' [8].

Indications for early surgical intervention include border syndactyly and the presence of transverse bones within the cleft. Marked length discrepancies between the syndactylized digits can severely affect growth potential, and transverse bone growth within the cleft results in progressive cleft widening.

Closure of the cleft is the mainstay of surgical management and may involve transfer of the second metacarpal to the third metacarpal base and reconstruction of the transverse metacarpal ligament, with skin adjustment to provide a good first web.

Congenital Constriction Band Syndrome

The precise aetiology of congenital constriction band syndrome (CCBS) remains a matter of debate, with theories including intrinsic defects in the germ cell layer or vascular disruption.

Physical disruption in utero by constriction from amniotic tissue, however, remains the commonest theory and one borne out by clinical findings (Figure 16.28). The principal defect in CCBS is distal ischaemia caused by the ring; thus, proximal bone and soft tissue structures are normal.

Clinical features are varied. These may include partial or complete circumferential constrictions, mimicking the appearance of skin creases and sometimes extending down to the bone; acrosyndactyly with distal digital fusion (Figure 16.29); or the more severe vascularly compromised or amputated limb or digits.

CCBS is rare, with an incidence of 1 in 15 000 live births, presents sporadically, and may be unilateral or bilateral, but rarely symmetrical. Associations include talipes equinovarus, cleft lip and palate, haemangioma, meningocele, and cranial or cardiac defects in 20–50% of cases. Imaging using modern ultrasound may permit prenatal diagnosis.

Classification of CCBS by Patterson is into four groups and descriptive in nature:

- **Group 1**: simple constriction
- **Group 2**: constriction and lymphoedema
- **Group 3**: constriction and acrosyndactyly
- **Group 4**: intrauterine amputation.

History and Management

All patients with CCBS should be managed within a wider multidisciplinary team. Given the prevalence of associated disorders,

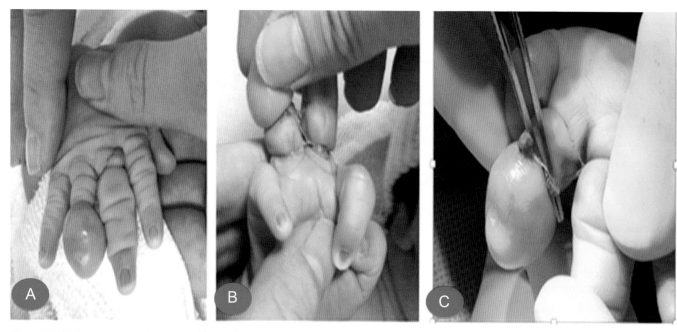

Figure 16.28 Constriction band syndrome affecting the digits, causing extreme lymphoedema of the ring finger(A). Amniotic strands are evident(B). These were removed and the constrictions excised as an emergency procedure the day after birth(C).

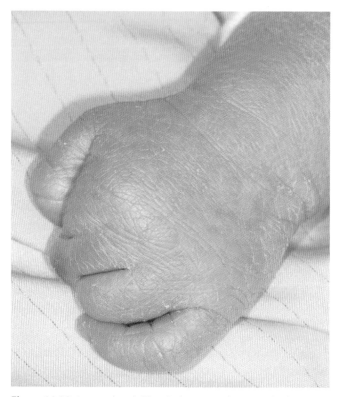

Figure 16.29 Acrosyndactyly. There is always a gap between the digits proximal to the syndactyly.

management should include careful preoperative assessment by paediatric and anaesthetic teams.

The first priority in CCBS assessment is to determine the need for emergent surgical release of a compromised limb or digit, as indicated by severe distal lymphoedema. A rare progressive presentation can occur with recurrent episodes of maceration or infection, leading to fibrosis without the pronounced distal lymphoedema. This too may require emergent release. Where emergent treatment is indicated, assessment should focus on observing for spontaneous movements and, where available, on sensation testing using a tactile adherence test. Severe constriction of nerves may be evidenced by severe pain and crying on motion or manipulation, in addition to evident nerve palsy (Figure 16.30).

Where a complete amputation is present, assessment should determine the level, assess passive and active motion in the proximal joints, and include appropriate radiographs. Nerve palsies have been associated with CCBS and should be observed for. Arteriography may also be indicated.

The most urgent of the congenital hand conditions is probably a severe constriction ring causing distal lymphoedema and circulatory compromise. Surgical release is indicated as an emergent procedure and involves exploration and excision of the ring, including involved subcutaneous tissue. Z-plasty release is not universally undertaken in the emergent setting. Nerve palsies associated with CCBS require exploration and excision of the constricting tissue to decompress. Surgical findings may include variable loss in nerve continuity and although full recovery has been reported, it is not universal.

In the non-compromised digit or limb, surgery should be undertaken at 6 months to 1 year of age. Traditional teaching has been to avoid circumferential release. However, this can be undertaken safely. An exception involves two rings that are closely adherent, in which case release should be staged. The skin may be closed by direct suture, but if elongation and reorientation are undertaken, Z- or W-plasty techniques may be used. Management of secondary soft tissue contour defects can be managed separately with a fat transfer procedure, but this is rarely necessary.

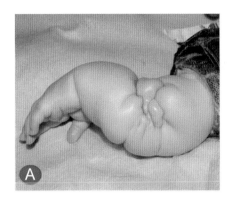
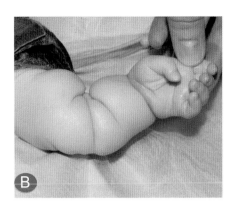

Figure 16.30 Complex constrictions affecting the forearm, with extreme pain on manipulation and an absent radial artery. The constriction extended down to the bone and compressed the median and radial nerves(A). Release of constriction and neurolysis completely resolved the pain.(B)

Acrosyndactyly associated with CCBS is managed using a similar principle to syndactyly, although early release of tethering constriction bands is indicated where digits are of unequal length and may compromise normal growth. Amputations associated with CCBS are managed similarly to transverse arrest. Furthermore, a normal proximal anatomy facilitates free toe transfer when appropriate.

References

1. Swanson AB. A classification for congenital limb malformation. *J Hand Surg*. 1983;8:693–702.

2. Goldfarb CA, Ezaki M, Wall LB, *et al.* The Oberg-Manske-Tonkin (OMT) Classification of Congenital Upper Extremities: update for 2020. *J Hand Surg Am*. 2020 Jun;45(6):542–7.

3. Marks TW, Bayne LG. Polydactyly of the thumb: abnormal anatomy and treatment. *J Hand Surg*. 1978;3:107–16.

4. Eaton CJ, Lister GD. Syndactyly. *Hand Clin*. 1990;6:555–75.

5. Siegert JJ, Cooney WP, Dobyns JH. Management of simple camptodactyly. *J Hand Surg (Br)*. 1990;15:181–9.

6. Blauth W. The hypoplastic thumb. *Arch Orthop Unfallchir*. 1967;62:225–46.

7. Tsuge K. Treatment of macrodactyly. *J Hand Surg (Am)*. 1985;10:968–9.

8. Flatt AE. Cleft hand and central defects. In: Flatt A, ed. *The Care of Congenital Hand Anomalies*. St Louis: Mosby; 1977. pp. 265–85.

Traumatic Hand and Wrist Disorders

Ehab Aldlyami and Khalid Alawadi

Wrist Fractures

Wrist fractures are the commonest paediatric fracture, comprising 20% of all fractures in children. The majority are simple torus fractures caused by compression forces acting along the main axis of the bone, with buckling of the cortices, often more pronounced on the concave side (Figure 17.1). Greenstick fractures occur from a bending force with a unicortical break of the convex side. These fractures are inherently stable and can be treated with a short period of immobilization (typically 3 weeks) in a cast or splint, with good outcome (Figure 17.2).

Bicortical metaphyseal fractures often are displaced and treated with closed reduction and cast immobilization (Figure 17.3). In children who are younger than 10 years, 20° of angulation and 40% of displacement can be accepted and do not require reduction (see Chapter 13, Figure 13.2) [1]. In general, remodelling potential is high, particularly closer to the physis, in the plane of motion, and with more remaining years of growth. Some displacement can be treated with plaster wedging (Figure 17.4).

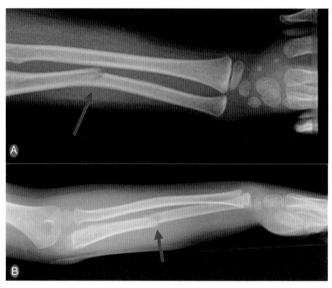

Figure 17.2 Plastic deformation of the ulna and greenstick fracture where one cortex remains intact. A true lateral view of the elbow joint is mandatory in these fractures.

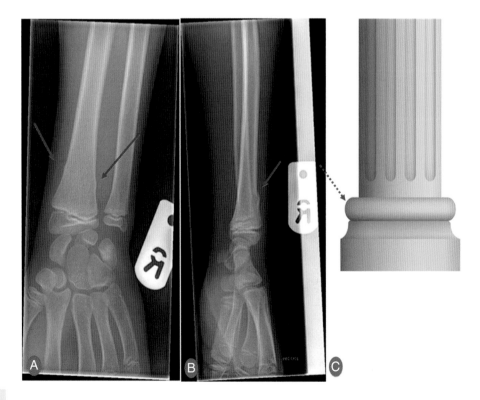

Figure 17.1 Torus fractures are caused by compression forces, with buckling of the bone cortices (solid red arrows) (A,B). The name was derived from the resemblance to a Roman column torus (dashed red arrow)(C).

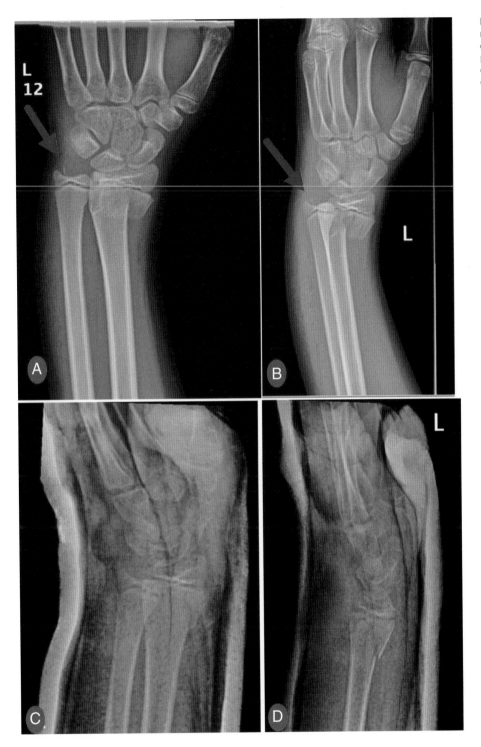

Figure 17.3 Displaced distal radius fracture managed with closed reduction and application of a well-moulded cast. Notice a small ulnar process avulsion fracture (A and B, red arrows); this could indicate avulsed triangular fibrocartilage complex.

Unstable or redisplaced fractures are indications for reduction and stabilization, often using K-wires. Complete displacement of both (radius and ulna) or a displaced radius fracture with an intact ulna has the reputation for displacement after closed reduction, and therefore, stabilization is recommended (Figure 17.5).

A bayonet fracture refers to a fracture in which the two bone fragments are aligned side by side, rather than in end-to-end contact (Figure 17.6). These have been traditionally reduced and stabilized. Reduction is not always easy and often requires open reduction (as high as 30%). However, there has been increasing evidence that these heal with a good clinical outcome, provided shortening is <1 cm and there is minimal angulation [2].

The distal radius physis grows by around 6 mm a year (75% of the radius growth and 40% of the whole upper limb growth). Physeal fractures of the radius are classified according to the Salter–Harris classification. Most are Salter–Harris type I or II fractures, and 20° angulation is acceptable for children who are under 10 years of age. A repeat X-ray within a week is required to ensure no further displacement has occurred. Remanipulation after a week is not recommended as it damages the growth plate.

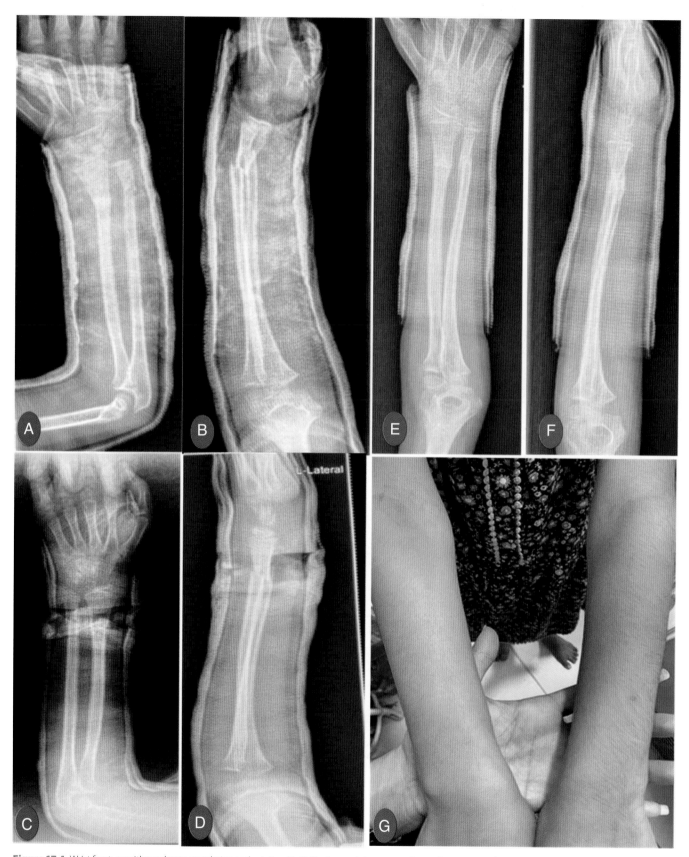

Figure 17.4 Wrist fracture with moderate angulation and rotation (A, B). Plaster wedging was performed to improve alignment (C, D), with good radiological and clinical outcome (E–G). Notice excessive hair growth on the left forearm, a frequent phenomenon following cast application.

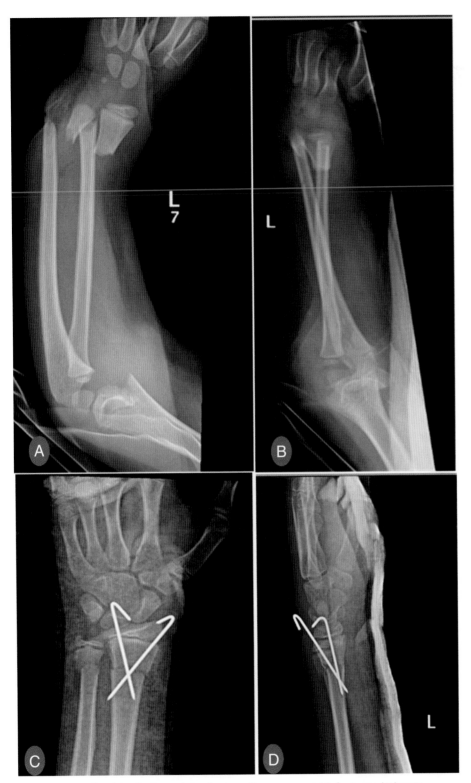

Figure 17.5 Displaced distal radius and ulnar fractures. These were unstable fractures which were reduced, closed, and stabilized with two K-wires. The surgeon avoided the growth plates, as there was enough metaphyseal fragment for wire purchase; this is not always possible. Crossing the physis is permissible in these fractures, but accuracy, minimal passes, cooling the wires, and burst drilling are essential to reduce damage to the growth plate. Have you noticed the concomitant supracondylar fracture?

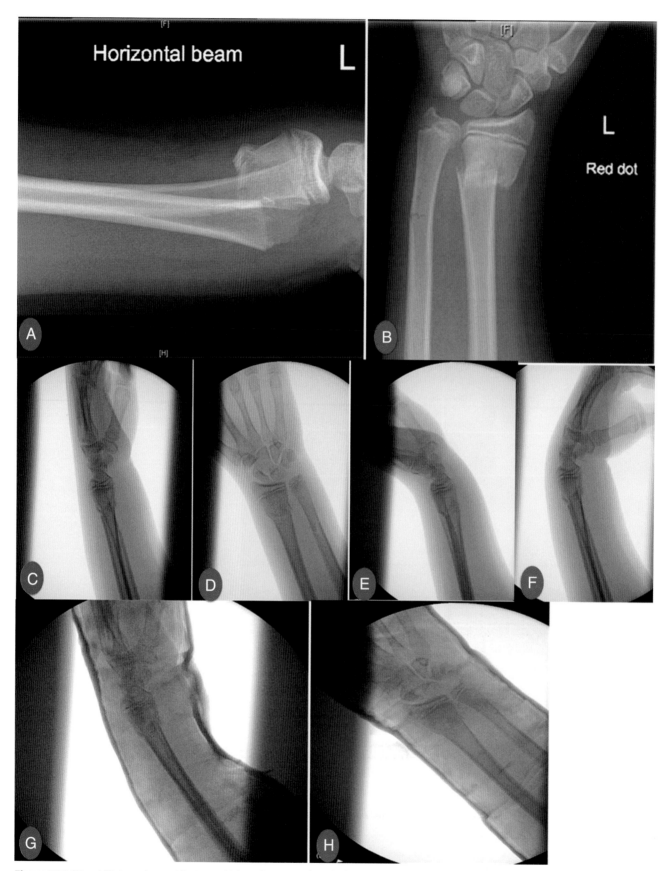

Figure 17.6 (A) and (B) show a bayonet fracture, with bony fragments aligned side by side, rather than in end-to-end contact. This was managed with closed reduction (C, D). Stability was tested by forced dorsiflexion and volar flexion (E, F), and was found to be stable. A well-moulded cast was then applied (G, H). The fracture healed well; however, the argument (which is supported by a growing body of evidence) is that this fracture could have healed with the same outcome even without reduction!

Type III and IV fractures are rare and often require open reduction and anatomical fixation to reduce the joint surface and decrease the risk of growth arrest. Type V fractures are often missed and diagnosed retrospectively when growth arrest has occurred. The overall risk of physeal arrest has been reported to be 4%.

Carpal Bone Fractures

Paediatric carpal fractures are uncommon and can be challenging to diagnose, partly because of their size and incomplete ossification of the carpal bones. As in adults, scaphoid fractures are the commonest fracture, followed by capitate fractures.

When suspected, immobilization is recommended, even when radiographs are normal. Children with persistent symptoms after 10 days following an injury merit a repeat X-ray and if this normal, MRI should be considered.

Scaphoid Fractures

Scaphoid fractures account for 0.45% of upper limb fractures, and 2.9% of all hand and wrist fractures in children, making them the commonest carpal fracture in children.

Historically, paediatric scaphoid fractures tend to occur at the distal pole and heal well with immobilization. However, with the rise in childhood obesity and involvement in more aggressive sports, adult-pattern scaphoid fractures are now seen in children.

Scaphoid fractures generally heal very well with cast immobilization – distal pole fractures for 4–8 weeks, and waist fractures for 5–12 weeks. Non-union is seldom seen in scaphoid fractures in children due to good blood supply of the bone and excellent healing potential (Figure 17.7). Even with a missed scaphoid fracture at first presentation with non-union and cystic changes, immobilization in a cast for 6–12 weeks may unite the fracture.

Persistent non-united fractures need CT confirmation, and open reduction and stabilization using a headless compression screw.

Metacarpal Fractures

Metacarpal fractures are common in children, particularly when close to skeletal maturity. Eighty per cent involve the little finger's metacarpal neck. Management of these fractures is similar to that for the adult population. The single most important indication for operative management is malrotation and scissoring. Angulation is better tolerated, particularly in the little finger and in younger patients. As a rough guide, a fracture angulation of 10°, 20°, 30°, and 40° of the index, middle, ring, and little metacarpal, respectively, is acceptable.

Phalangeal Fractures

Phalanges often fracture either at the base (as in physeal injuries) or at the neck (condylar fractures). Phalangeal shaft fractures are less common. Minimally or non-displaced fractures are treated with immobilization, with expected good outcomes. Displaced injuries, however, can compromise hand function and correction is indicated (Figures 17.8 and 17.9). Closed reduction and neighbour strap or cast often suffice; however, failing this, open reduction and fixation with K-wire or screws are required.

Neck fractures of the phalanges are common in toddlers; they happen when children violently withdraw their fingers that are trapped in a closing door. The serious nature of these fractures may be missed unless a true lateral radiograph is obtained (Figure 17.10). With no tendon attachment, sometimes, the

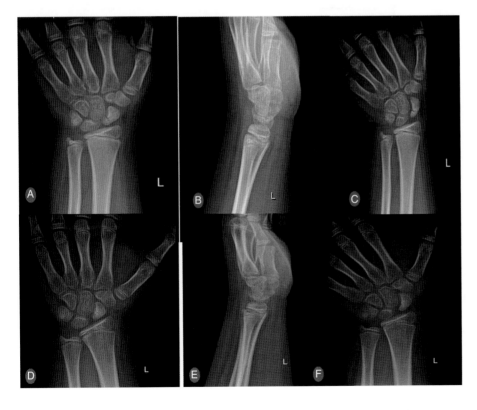

Figure 17.7 A child who presented a few weeks after an injury that caused a scaphoid fracture (A–C). Despite the fracture not uniting with the fracture sclerotic edges, the fracture healed after 8 weeks of immobilization.

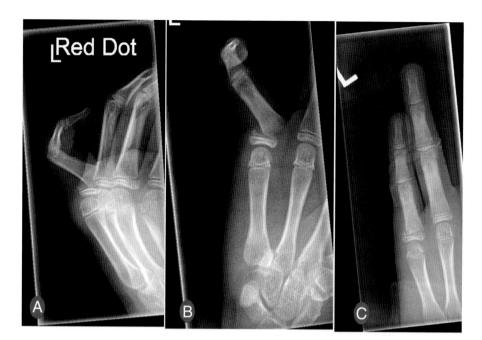

Figure 17.8 Salter–Harris type II fracture of the phalangeal base of the little finger, which was managed with a closed reduction and stabilized with a neighbour strap.

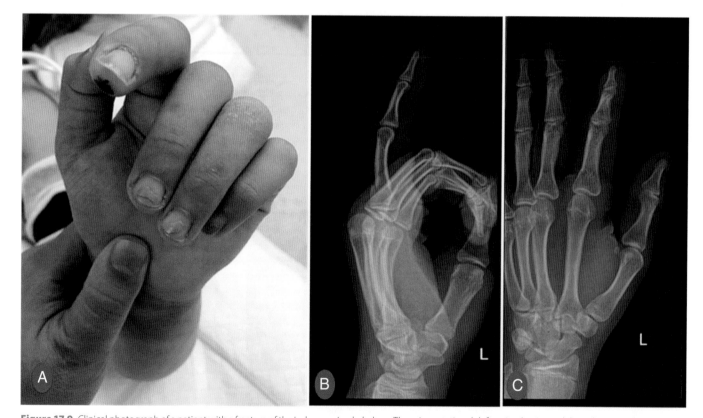

Figure 17.9 Clinical photograph of a patient with a fracture of the index proximal phalanx. There is a rotational deformity that is much less obvious radiologically. When the patient is asked to make a fist, loss of normal finger cascade would uncover rotational deformity. Care should be taken not to confuse finger abduction that is caused by the fracture swelling and true rotational deformity (look for the actual rotation, and not just the gap!)

head fragment displaces dorsally and rotates 90°. These fractures may also go into non-union (Figure 17.11).

They are inherently unstable, with poor remodelling potential due to its distance from the physis. The Al Qattan classification is the most commonly used [3]:

- Type I: displaced (non-operative treatment)
- Type II: displaced, with some bone-to-bone contact (operative treatment)
- Type III: displaced, with no bone-to-bone contact (operative).

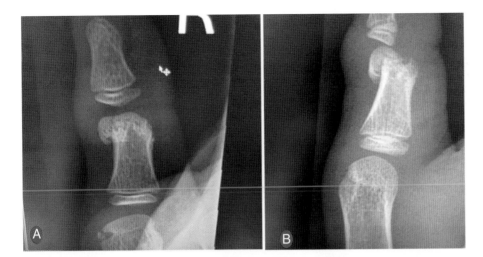

Figure 17.10 Condylar fracture of the phalanx. The amount of displacement is better appreciated on the lateral view (B).

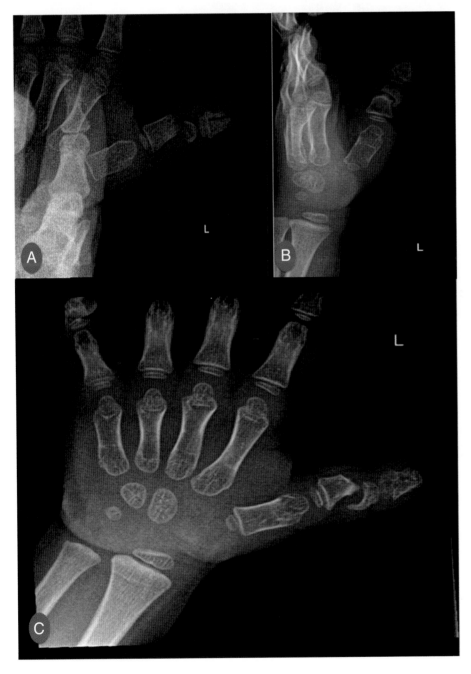

Figure 17.11 Radiographs of a 14-month-old child who presented with a crush injury to the thumb. The fracture went into non-union because of inability to immobilize the fracture properly.

Condylar Fractures

The condyles are a pair of tuberosities that form the distal articular surfaces of the proximal and middle phalanges. Condylar fractures are intra-articular in nature and often unstable. These fractures require meticulous reduction to ensure proper joint congruity.

Fractures involving the distal third of the proximal phalanx are approached by elevating the lateral bands through a curved dorsal skin incision, or by elevating a V-shaped slip of the extensor tendon, based on the central slip, which allows excellent visualization of the proximal interphalangeal joint. Fractures through the condyles are held by cross-pinning. Unicondylar or avulsion fractures are held by wires or screws inserted parallel to the joint (Figures 17.12 and 17.13).

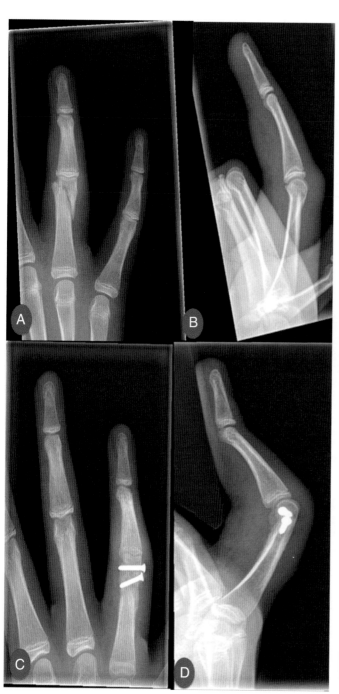

Figure 17.12 Condylar fracture of a displaced ring finger middle phalanx, which was treated with open reduction and stabilization using microscrews.

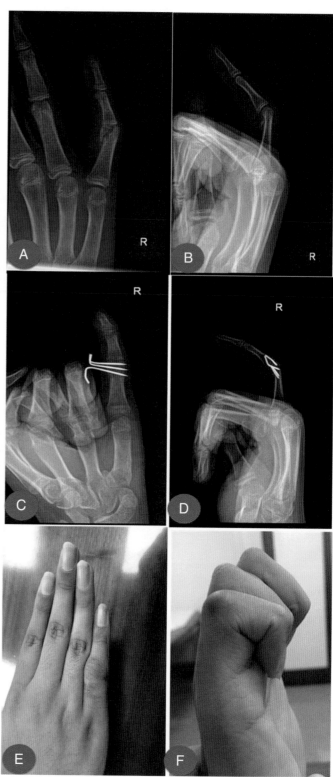

Figure 17.13 A 15-week-old condylar fracture that was treated with interfragment osteotomy and stabilization using three small wires. (E) and (F) show good clinical outcome.

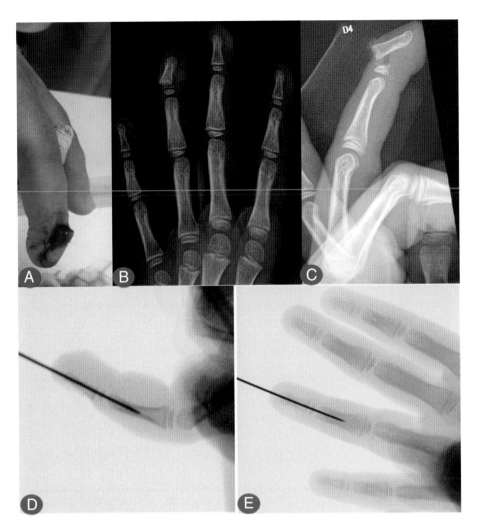

Figure 17.14 Seymour fracture. (A) Clinical photograph showing nail avulsion. (B) and (C) are preoperative radiographs. (D) and (E) are post-operative radiographs showing fixation using K-wire.

Seymour Fractures

In Salter–Harris type II epiphysial fractures of the distal phalanx, the injury may manifest as an open mallet and be mistaken for a distal interphalangeal joint dislocation, which is usually an apex dorsal angulation at the fracture site. There is almost always a transverse laceration of the nail matrix and an avulsed nail plate. Unless the nail plate is replaced in its correct position, the fracture cannot be reduced (Figure 17.14).

Ideal treatment consists of irrigation, debridement, fracture reduction, repair of the nail matrix, replacement of the nail plate beneath the proximal fold, and if the fracture is felt to be unstable, K-wire fixation.

Failure to recognize the injury or inadequate primary management may result in acute osteomyelitis or septic arthritis.

Salter–Harris type III and IV epiphyseal injuries can be reduced by extending the distal phalanx and gently massaging the displaced fragment back into position. The joint is immobilized in slight extension, with a volar, not dorsal, splint because of the risk of skin necrosis. Sometimes a large fragment of the epiphysis may be irreducible, so open reduction and K-wire fixation may be indicated.

Nail Bed Injuries and Tuft Fractures

A radiograph should be requested in all cases of nail bed injury to exclude a fracture. The nail bed is repaired by using 6/0 or 7/0 absorbable sutures. If the nail plate is undamaged, it should be cleaned, debrided, and sutured back into the nail fold to act as a splint. If damaged, then the foil from a suture is used back to keep the nail fold open.

Tuft fractures usually result from a crush injury, mostly from a door. These injuries often are associated with nail bed and pulp lacerations. If the nail is intact and adherent, then the fracture is managed non-operatively. However, if there is disruption of the nail plate, then nail plate removal, debridement and washout, and nail bed repair are indicated.

References

1. Shah AS, Caird MS. Upper extremity fractures. In: Weinstein SL, Flynn JM, eds. *Lovell and Winter's Pediatric Orthopaedics*, 8th ed, Vol. 2. Philadelphia, PA: Lippincott Williams & Wilkins; 2021. p. 5574.

2. Laaksonen T, *et al*. Cast immobilization in bayonet position versus reduction and pin fixation of overriding distal metaphyseal radius fractures in children under ten years of age: a case control study. *J Child Orthop*. 2021;15(1):63–9.

3. Al-Qattan MM. Phalangeal neck fractures in children: classification and outcome in 66 cases. *J Hand Surg Br*. 2001;26(2):112–21.

Neuromuscular Conditions/Lower Limbs

18a

Simon L. Barker and Sattar Alshryda

Introduction

Neuromuscular disorders (NMDs) constitute a major part of paediatric orthopaedic work. As most conditions are chronic and their management requires high-ordered thinking, they are generally considered good exam cases. The spectrum of such diseases is really wide and includes:

1. Brain disorders such as cerebral palsy (CP) and hereditary paraparesis
2. Spinal cord conditions such as spina bifida and syringomyelia
3. Peripheral nerve conditions such as hereditary sensory motor neuropathy (HSMN)"? (HMN)
4. Muscular conditions such as Duchenne muscular dystrophy (DMD).

This chapter covers the principles of managing NMD in children. These children should be managed by multidisciplinary teams involving:

1. Neurologists
2. Neurorehabilitation physiotherapists (hospital- and community-based)
3. Orthotists
4. Occupational therapists and speech therapists
5. Clinical psychologists
6. Play therapists
7. Orthopaedic surgeons
8. Neurosurgeons
9. Social workers and family support groups.

It is essential to recognize two distinctive groups of NMDs: progressive (or degenerative) and non-progressive (non-degenerative). In the former, the disease progresses relentlessly and often cause premature death, making decisions to operate on these children challenging. Non-progressive NMDs, such as CP, are more predictable and surgical interventions have become vital elements of improving the quality of life. Table 18a.1 summarizes common progressive and non-progressive NMDs that are encountered in orthopaedic practice. CP is by far the commonest NMD in paediatric orthopaedic practice (its incidence is 2 in 1000) and will be the focus of this chapter. Several aspects of managing children with CP have been utilized to treat other conditions (whether progressive or non-progressive), with variable success.

Key Points: Progressive and Non-progressive Disease Pitfalls

1. Progressive diseases are usually life limiting and the principles of orthopaedic treatments are to keep children comfortable. Surgical interventions are often avoided unless a condition causes signifcant symptoms. However, with a few exceptions, the average lifespan of children with these conditions vary considerably, rendering surgical decision even more difficult.
2. The rise of gene therapy has changed the outcome of some progressive NMDs, such as spinal muscular atrophy, which complicates decision-making even more.
3. Some conditions such as Rett syndrome do not fit well in either group.

Cerebral Palsy

Definition and Aetiology

CP is a disorder of movement and posture that results from permanent and non-progressive damage to the developing brain. Although brain damage is not progressive, the clinical findings and impact on function change with growth. CP is common, with an incidence of 2 per 1000 live births. The incidence has been increasing because more premature and unwell children survive with advancing healthcare worldwide. Table 18a.2 summarizes the known causes of CP.

Classification

Several classification systems exist, each describing a different aspect of the condition.

Anatomical

This refers to the number of limbs that are involved and includes (Figure 18a.1):

Table 18a.1 Common types of progressive and non-progressive brain disorders

Non-progressive brain disorders	Progressive brain disorders
1. Cerebral palsy	1. Leigh syndrome
2. Stroke	2. Canavan disease
3. Trauma	3. Lipofuscinosis
4. Some benign brain tumours	4. Some malignant tumours

Table 18a.2 Aetiology of cerebral palsy

Prenatal	Perinatal	Postnatal
1. Placental insufficiency	1. Prematurity (commonest)	1. Infection (meningitis, cytomegalovirus, rubella)
2. Toxaemia	2. Anoxia	2. Head trauma, including non-accidental injury
3. Smoking	3. Infection	3. Near drowning
4. Alcohol	4. Erythroblastosis fetalis and kernicterus	
5. Drugs	5. Birth trauma	
6. Infection such as toxoplasmosis, rubella, cytomegalovirus, herpes simplex type II, and syphilis (ToRCHeS)	6. Placental abruption	
7. Epilepsy		

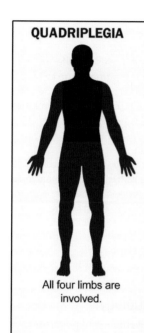

QUADRIPLEGIA

All four limbs are involved.

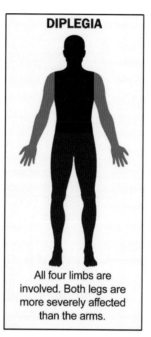

DIPLEGIA

All four limbs are involved. Both legs are more severely affected than the arms.

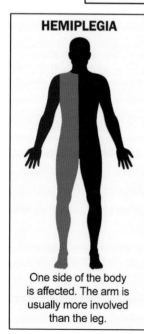

HEMIPLEGIA

One side of the body is affected. The arm is usually more involved than the leg.

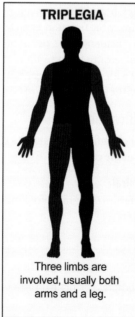

TRIPLEGIA

Three limbs are involved, usually both arms and a leg.

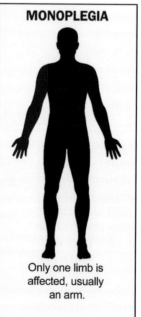

MONOPLEGIA

Only one limb is affected, usually an arm.

Figure 18a.1 Anatomical classification of cerebral palsy.

1. Monoplegia: a single limb
2. Hemiplegia: one side of the body – the upper limb is usually more involved than the lower limb
3. Diplegia (all four limbs are involved, but upper limb involvement is usually mild in comparison to lower limb involvement)
4. Triplegia – three limbs are involved
5. Quadriplegia or 'total body involvement'.

A fifth type (bilateral hemiplegic) has been described when all limbs are involved, but the upper limbs are worse than the lower limbs (i.e. the inverse of the diplegic type). However, this is rare and has not been widely adopted.

Physiological

This classification is based on the impact of brain injury on muscle and consequent abnormal movements:

1. Spastic type: this is the commonest type. Spasticity is defined as speed-dependent hypertonia. In this type, the muscle tone increases by increasing the speed of limb movement. Typically, limping becomes worse when the child is asked to run. This type is caused by damage to the motor cortex and pyramidal tracts in the brain
2. Dyskinetic type: this is characterized by abnormal movements caused by damage to the extrapyramidal system and basal ganglia. A few types have been described:
   a. Athetoid: slow, writhing movements of the fingers and hands, and the rest of the upper limbs. The mouth and lower limbs may also be involved
   b. Ballismus and hemiballismus: infrequent jerky, purposeless movements involving a single limb
   c. Chorea: random movements of the limbs that increase during rest and may improve with movement
   d. Dystonia: involuntary, sustained muscle contractions that result in an abnormal posture. The muscle tone fluctuates and often increases with effort and emotion (not the speed of movement)
3. Ataxic type: problems with balance and coordination caused by damage to the cerebellum
4. Mixed type.

Functional (GMFCS Levels)

The Gross Motor Function Classification System (GMFCS) is probably the most useful classification of CP. It consists of five levels, based on assessment of self-initiated movement, with emphasis on function with regard to walking (Figure 18a.2) [1–3]. These are:

- Level I: walks without limitations
- Level II: walks with limitations
- Level III: walks with a handheld mobility device (e.g. crutch)
- Level IV: self-mobility limited, may use powered mobility
- Level V: transported in a manual wheelchair.

The GMFCS classification should not be confused with the Gross Motor Function Measure (GMFM). The latter is an outcome measure designed to measure changes in gross motor function over time or after an intervention in children with CP. It covers five dimensions:

- A: lying and rolling
- B: sitting
- C: crawling and kneeling
- D: standing
- E: walking, running, and jumping

There are two versions of the GMFM, based on items that are covered in the above five domains: GMFM-88 and GMFM-66. The minimum possible GMFM score is zero, and the maximum score is 100. GMFCS, in comparison, is a classification system based on the ability to ambulate.

Naturally, children acquire new motor skills (whether they are normal or have CP) from birth until the age of 4–6 years. Therefore, the GMFCS is usually utilized after the age of 4–6 years. Figure 18a.3 illustrates the relationship between GMFCS levels, GMFM-66 scores, and age.

Pathology

CP is caused by damage to the developing brain. There is no consensus on when the human brain completes development, but most agree development finishes in around the second year of life. Brain damage leads to primary, secondary, and tertiary pathological changes.

Primary Pathological Changes

These changes are directly related to loss of function of the damaged part of the brain. These could be:

1. Intellectual impairment
2. Epilepsy
3. Visual problems
4. Hearing loss
5. Speech and communication problems
6. Swallowing difficulty
7. Feeding difficulty, failure to thrive
8. Respiratory problems
9. Incontinence
10. Musculoskeletal problems:
    a. Abnormal muscle tone
    b. Balance problems
    c. Loss of selective control
    d. Pathological reflexes or persistence of primitive infantile reflexes
    e. Loss of sensation.
11. Loss of sensation

GMFCS E & R between 6th and 12th birthday: Descriptors and illustrations

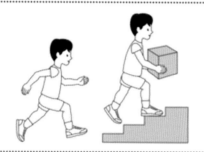

GMFCS Level I

Children walk at home, school, outdoors and in the community. They can climb stairs without the use of a railing. Children perform gross motor skills such as running and jumping, but speed, balance and coordination are limited.

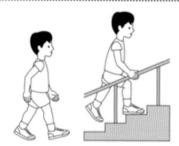

GMFCS Level II

Children walk in most settings and climb stairs holding onto a railing. They may experience difficulty walking long distances and balancing on uneven terrain, inclines, in crowded areas or confined spaces. Children may walk with physical assistance, a hand-held mobility device or used wheeled mobility over long distances. Children have only minimal ability to perform gross motor skills such as running and jumping.

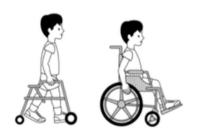

GMFCS Level III

Children walk using a hand-held mobility device in most indoor settings. They may climb stairs holding onto a railing with supervision or assistance. Children use wheeled mobility when traveling long distances and may self-propel for shorter distances.

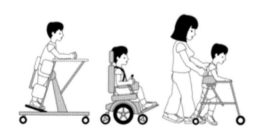

GMFCS Level IV

Children use methods of mobility that require physical assistance or powered mobility in most settings. They may walk for short distances at home with physical assistance or use powered mobility or a body support walker when positioned. At school, outdoors and in the community children are transported in a manual wheelchair or use powered mobility.

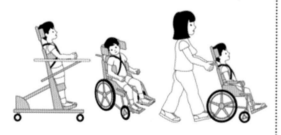

GMFCS Level V

Children are transported in a manual wheelchair in all settings. Children are limited in their ability to maintain antigravity head and trunk postures and control leg and arm movements.

GMFCS descriptors: Palisano et al. (1997) Dev Med Child Neurol 39:214-23
CanChild: www.canchild.ca

Illustrations Version 2 © Bill Reid, Kate Willoughby, Adrienne Harvey and Kerr Graham,
The Royal Children's Hospital Melbourne   ERC151050

Figure 18a.2 The Gross Motor Function Classification System for children with cerebral palsy. Source: Courtesy of Kerr Graham, The Royal Children's Hospital, Melbourne.

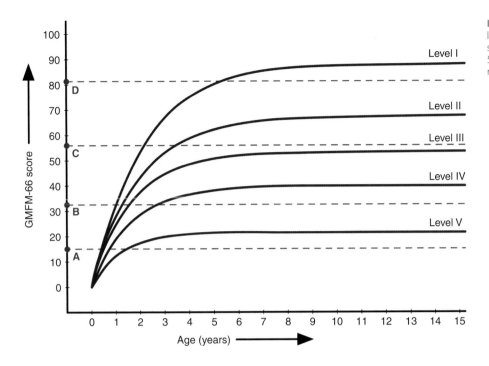

Figure 18a.3 The relationship between GMFCS levels, GMFM scores, and age. The average GMFM score for GMFCS level I is 87, level II 68, level III 54, level IV 40, and level V 20. These are usually reached between the ages of 4 and 6 years.

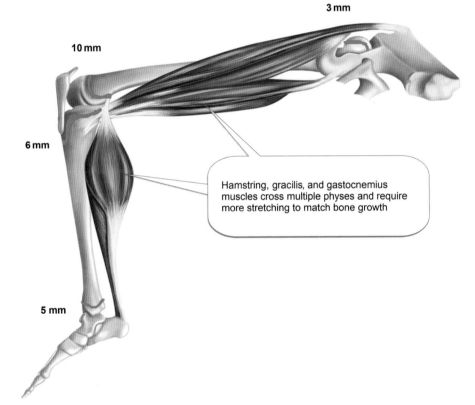

Figure 18a.4 Bone growth and muscle length underpin most of the secondary musculoskeletal changes in children with CP. Gastrocnemius muscles, for example, have to stretch 21 mm a year to match the growth of bones in front of them, whereas the soleus muscles needs to stretch 5 mm a year. That is why gastrocnemius tightness is commoner than soleus tightness.

Hamstring, gracilis, and gastocnemius muscles cross multiple physes and require more stretching to match bone growth

Secondary Pathological Changes

Most secondary pathological changes are related to length mismatch between growing bones and affected muscles. As bones actively grow through growth plates, muscles get stretched and elongated during children's walking, running, and playing. In children with CP, this process does not happen normally. The coordination of muscles is poor, the stretch may be less and resting tone greater. The more severe the CP, the more profound the length mismatch is. Muscles that cross multiple growth plates, such as the hamstrings, gracilis, and gastrocnemius are more affected than muscles that cross fewer growth plates such as the soleus and hip adductors (Figure 18a.4). This relative muscle shortening leads to joint contractures. In order for bones to continue growing against contracted muscles, they have to bend or dislocate from the joint above or below. Consequent clinical outcomes are joint contractures, bone deformity, joint dislocation, and scoliosis.

Hip dislocation is common in children with CP and the incidence is directly related to the severity (Figure 18a.5). Contracture of the hip adductors and flexors and the medial hamstrings causes abnormal hip positioning in adduction, flexion, and internal rotation. Hip adduction contracture of <30° is considered a risk factor for hip dislocation. As the femur gets longer, it exerts pressure on the acetabular rim, causing gradual damage and flattening of the rim posterosuperiorly [4]. Subluxation then develops gradually, with increasing lateralization and proximal migration of the femoral head.

The femoral head changes as well. Pressure effects from the capsule, rim of the acetabulum, hip abductors, and ligamentum teres cause the femoral head to lose its sphericity and become irregularly shaped, which further damages the articular cartilage (Figure 18a.6).

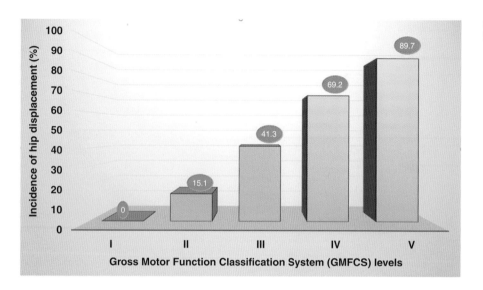

Figure 18a.5 The relationship between the incidence of hip displacement and GMFCS levels.

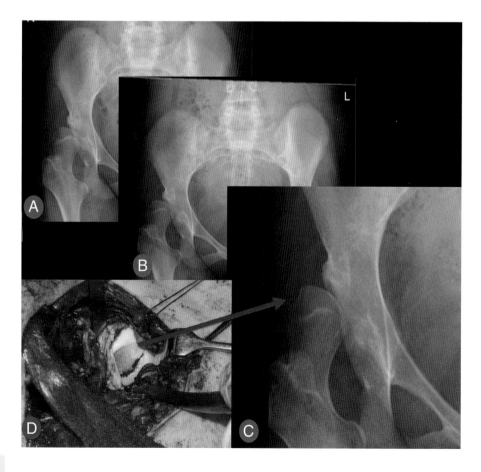

Figure 18a.6 Gradual damage to the femoral head.

The talonavicular joint and the metatarsophalangeal joint (MTPJ) of the big toe are other common examples of joint subluxation or dislocation in children with CP. Tightness in the gastrocnemius muscle causes them to walk on their toes, and with time, the weight of the child leads to planovalgus deformity with gradual subluxation of the talonavicular joint and the forefoot starts pointing outward and upward (Figure 18a.7). This, in turn, exerts an increasing force on the medial side of the forefoot and the big toe, pushing them laterally.

Lever Arm Syndrome

The concept of lever arm syndrome is very important to understand in ambulatory children (GMFCS levels I–III). Most joints function like levers. The centre of the joint is the axis (or

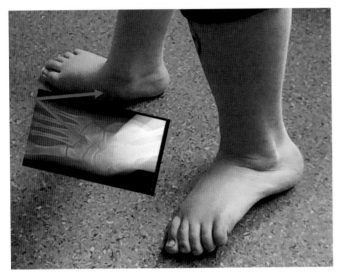

Figure 18a.7 A clinical photograph and plain foot X-ray (inset) showing talonavicular joint subluxation in a child with cerebral palsy.

fulcrum), whilst muscles crossing the joint produce the force and the weight of the limb or body is the resistance. Based on the position of the axis in relation to the force and weight, levers are classified into first class, second class, or third class. All three types are represented in the body (Figure 18a.8). These very well-optimised lever arm systems are affected in children with CP, undermining the functional capability of children with CP.

The hip abductors function well when their lever arm is longer. Coxa valga or a short femoral neck reduces this lever arm, weakening hip abduction. Correcting coxa valga or lengthening the femoral neck is possible surgically (Figure 18a.9).

Excessive femoral anteversion is very common in children with CP. The child has to turn their hip inward, so that the tip of the greater trochanter is lateralised. This increases the hip abductor lever arm to the maximum and eliminates the extensor component lever arm that could be caused by the tip of the greater trochanter staying behind the optimal coronal plane (Figure 18a.10). However, there is a limit to how much children can turn their hips inward, and in severe cases, in-toeing is not enough to optimize hip abductors. This can be corrected surgically by derotation femoral osteotomy which is often combined with varus osteotomy for aligned objectives.

In the knee, the body weight is balanced by the force that is generated by the quadriceps muscles. The knee centre of rotation is the axis. When the knee is fully extended, the body weight passes through, or just anterior to, the axis (the moment is almost zero). Therefore, the quadriceps muscles do not need to work to keep the body upright. However, when there is a knee flexion contracture, which is common in children with CP, the situation changes, as depicted in Figure 18a.11. Several surgical

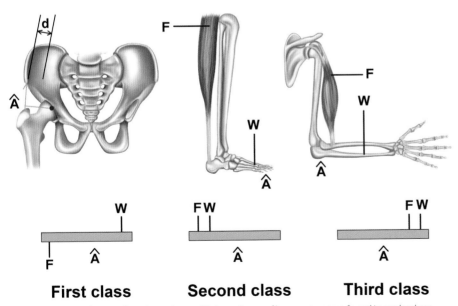

First class   Second class   Third class

Figure 18a.8 Body joints function as levers. All three classes of lever systems are found in our body, as shown in the three examples of lever systems.

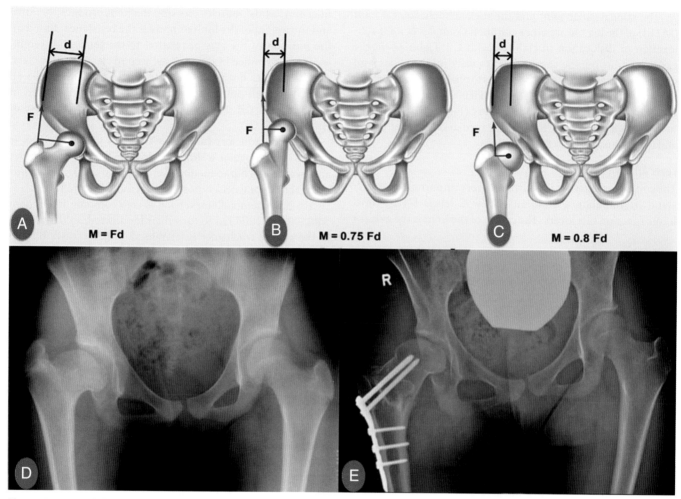

Figure 18a.9 Hip abductors' moment is directly related to its arm (d = distance between the centre of the femoral head and the insertion of hip abductors). The longer the arm, the greater the moment, and vice versa. True coxa valga or brevia reduces the effective arm (d) and causes a smaller moment, as shown in (B–D). Optimizing hip abductors functions by increasing the neck of the femur (E).

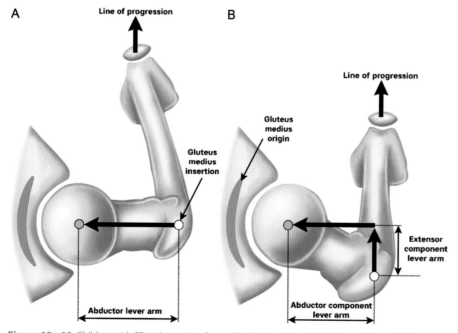

Figure 18a.10 Children with CP and excessive femoral torsion turn lower limbs inward (in-toeing) to increase the hip abductors' lever arms for better walking. If they do not, not only the hip abductors' moment will be less, but abductor muscles will extend the hip (extensor component lever arm) which reduces walking efficiency. However, excessive in-toeing can cause trips and falls. In the past, femoral de-rotation orthoses were used but clearly this was wrong as it interfere with their compensatory mechanism to improve hip abduction. Femoral de-rotation osteotomy is required to stop in-toeing and tripping and not interfering with the compensatory mechanism.

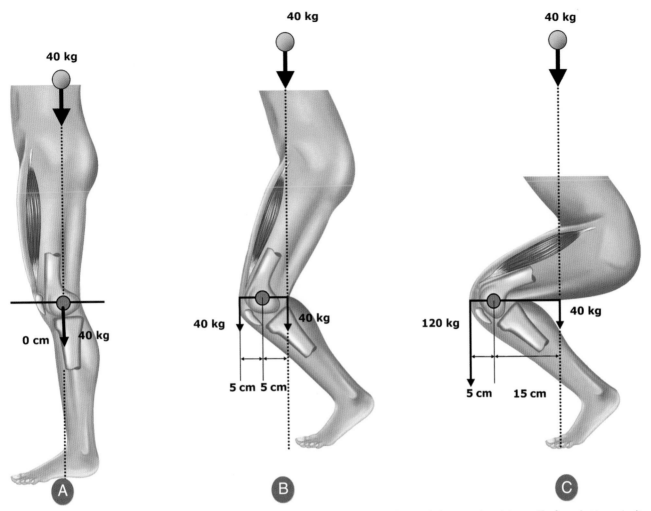

Figure 18a.11 The effect of knee flexion contracture on the required force to stand and walk. (A) The weight lever arm length is zero. The force that is required to keep the body upright will be zero. (B) and (C) show that in increasing the weight lever arm's length, proportionately increasing force is required to keep the body upright.

procedures have been advised to improve knee contractures, including (Figure 18a.12):

1. Hamstring lengthening (less popular because it worsens the anterior pelvis tilt)
2. Distal femur anterior hemi-epiphysiodesis (gradual and not immediate correction, so the benefit is not immediately visible. This cannot be used after growth has finished)
3. Distal femoral extension osteotomy
4. Patellar pull-down (shortening the patellar tendon in children with patella alta improves knee extension).

If the knee does not extend fully because of quadriceps weakness, rather than contracture, a ground reaction ankle foot orthosis (GRAFO) can be utilized to keep the knee straight (Figure 18a.13).

Talonavicular joint subluxation (and hallux valgus deformity) reduces the effective length of the foot as a lever arm, weakening the foot push-off strength (Figure 18a.14). This can be corrected using ankle foot orthosis (AFO) or surgically. Correcting foot deformity by reducing the talonavicular joint

and hallux valgus deformity improves the foot as a lever arm (Figure 18a.15).

Tertiary Pathological Changes

Tertiary changes arise from coping or compensatory mechanisms that help a child with CP to ambulate. One common example is that children with knee flexion contracture walk on their toes, even when they do not have any tendo Achilles contracture. This was commonly mistaken in the past for tendo Achilles contracture, and some children underwent unnecessary tendo Achilles lengthening, which led to the child being unable to walk. It is not always straightforward to differentiate between secondary and tertiary changes.

Multidisciplinary team

All children with NMD should be managed through multidisciplinary teams where various aspects of care are covered by the most expert in the team. Various centres have various settings on how the multidisciplinary team functions. The following is relevant to orthopaedic surgeons.

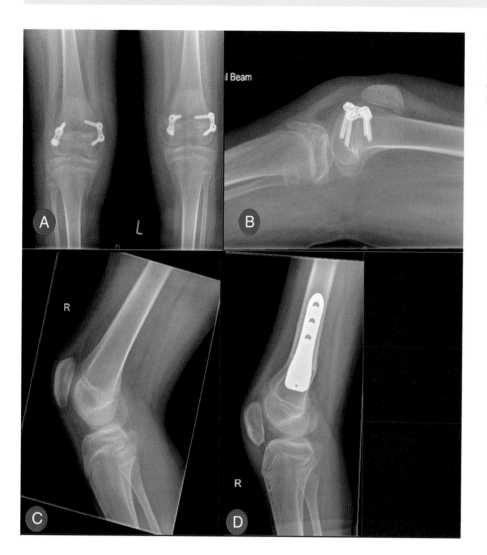

Figure 18a.12 Surgical intervention to straighten the knee in patients with knee fixed flexion contractures. (A) and (B) show distal femoral anterior hemi-epiphysiodesis. (C) and (D) show distal femoral extension osteotomy and patellar pull-down.

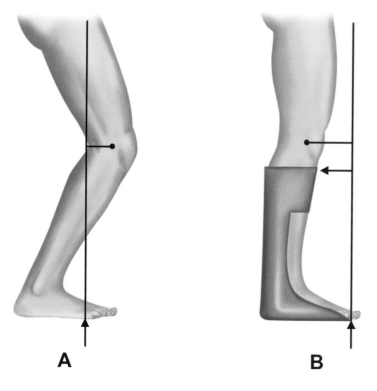

Figure 18a.13 Use of ground reaction ankle foot orthosis to straighten the knee. It converts an ankle dorsiflexion moment into a knee extending moment.

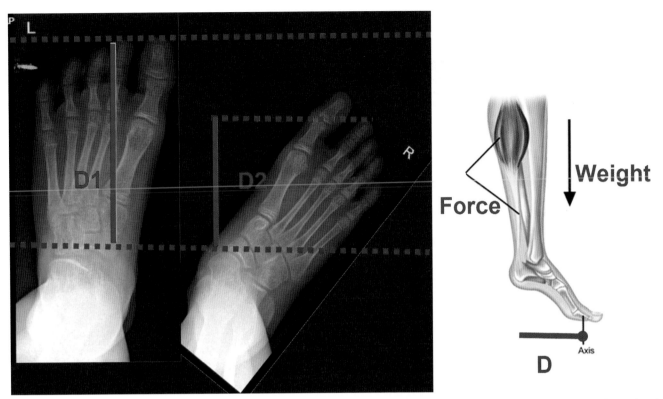

Figure 18a.14 Effect of talonavicular subluxation on the effective length of the foot as a lever (D). The right foot push-off lever arm (D2) is made shorter than the normal left side (D1) by talonavicular dislocation.

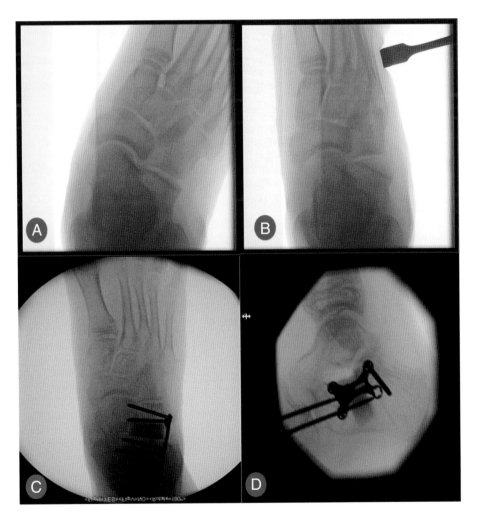

Figure 18a.15 Correcting talonavicular subluxation to improve foot length. (A) and (B) show the talonavicular joint can be reduced easily, but the calcaneocuboid joint opens up. By lengthening the calcaneum, this minimizes the risk of recurrence and supports the calcaneocuboid joint.

Comprehensive History

1. The current problem(s):
   a. What is it? And the impact on children and parents?
   b. What have been done to improve them? The outcome? (see management options below)
   c. What are the patient's and parent's expectations?
   d. What are the functional goals?
2. Current capabilities:
   a. Motor and social milestones
   b. GMFCS/Manual Ability Classification System (MACS) levels
   c. Use of medications, braces, sleeping system, seating systems, and standers
   d. Physiotherapy sessions (frequency, compliance, tolerance)
   e. Feeding (normal, modified, percutaneous endoscopic gastrostomy)
   f. Sleeping patterns
   g. Schools and education
3. Comorbidities and any previous surgery:
   a. See the above list of primary abnormalities.

Clinical Examination

Table 18a.3 summarizes a typical clinical assessment chart for a child with CP (and NMD). The tests are covered in Chapter 2 (the clinical examination) and Video 2.1. In the first instance, the chart may look very complicated, but with some practice, it is relatively simple and reproducible.

Investigations

Most investigations to confirm the diagnosis, such as MRI brain or ultrasound, and blood or genetic tests if required, are usually done by the neurologist. With respect to orthopaedic concerns, investigations are guided by examination and potential treatment. The following are typical:

1. Radiological tests:
   a. Pelvic X-rays to check for hip dysplasia (see details on the Cerebral Palsy Integrated Pathway (CPIP) in Surgical Treatment of Specific Pathologies below)
   b. Spine if scoliosis is suspected
   c. Feet if deformity is suspected
   d. CT if the pathoanatomy is not very clear (particularly in revision surgery)

Table 18a.3 Orthopaedic neuromuscular examination chart (sample)

Date	Joint	Sagittal		R (R1)	L (R1)	Coronal	R	L	Transverse	R	L
Range of motion	Ankle	Dorsiflexion (knee 0)		15	−10 (0)	Inversion	F	F	HBL	2IDS	2IDS
		Dorsiflexion (knee 90)		20	−5 (5)	Eversion	F	F	FTA	15E	15E
		Plantar flexion		F	F	Mid-foot break	No	Y	TMTA	NT	NT
		Plantaris		No	No	Hallux valgus	No	No			
	Knee	Extension		F	F						
		Flexion		F	F						
		Popliteal angle	1	60 (40)	60 (40)	Valgus					
			2			Varus					
			35°	<20	<20						
		Patella alta		No	No						
	Hip	Flexion		F	F	Abduction (knee 0)	45	45	Internal rotation	65	90
		FFD		No	No	Abduction (knee 90)	50	50	External rotation	30	0
		Extension		NT	NT	Adduction					
Strength	Ankle	Dorsiflexion		5	4	Inversion					
		Plantar flexion		5	5	Eversion	5	3			
	Knee	Flexion		5	5						
		Extension		5	5						
	Hip	Flexion		5	5	Abduction	5	5			
		Extension		5	5	Adduction	5	5			
Spasticity	Ankle	Dorsiflexion (knee 0)		1	2						
		Dorsiflexion (knee 90)		1	2						
	Knee	Hamstring		1	2						
	Hip	Rectus		0	0						

LLD = 0 (X-ray 4 mm). Galeazzi test: −ve. Spine: mild scoliosis. Confusion test: negative (good selective control)

Key   R = right; L = left; R = range of motion 2; R1 = range of motion 1; F = full; knee 0 = knee fully extended; knee 90 = knee flexed to 90; HBL = heel bisector line; FTA = foot–thigh angle; TMTA = transmalleolar–thigh angle; NT = not tested; LLD = leg length discrepancy. Red = worsened; uncoloured = unchanged; green = improved in comparison to last visit.

e. Dual-energy X-ray absorptiometry (DEXA) for multiple fragility fractures

2. Gait analysis:
   a. Indicated in ambulatory patients only
   b. Before surgery and 1 year after surgery
   c. Baseline gait analysis in children who are anticipated to need future surgery at around the age of 5 years (when GMFCS levels starting to plateau)

3. Blood tests:
   a. Pre- and post-operatively
   b. Vitamin D levels, particularly with fragility fracture.

Management of Cerebral Palsy

A multidisciplinary team approach for managing CP (and all NMDs) cannot be emphasized enough. Each team has a role to play. There are six treatment options that are often used in combination. These are:

1. Physiotherapy and occupational therapy
2. Orthoses
3. Equipment and assistive devices
4. Spasticity treatment
5. Serial castings
6. Surgery.

Key Points: Evidence for Treatment Modalities

Novak and colleagues conducted a systematic review of the treatment interventions and produced 'a state of evidence traffic lights' for treating children with cerebral palsy. It is worth reading to understand the strength of the evidence behind these interventions and to raise your marks to 8 in the exam [5].

Physiotherapy and Occupational Therapy

This is probably the most important line of treatment and it may be the only modality that is needed in a substantive proportion of patients. The key aims include posture management and maintaining active and passive ranges of movement. Strengthening, coordination, and functions are also important.

For best outcome, it is physiotherapist-led, but delivered by parents and patients. The physiotherapist team decide on the frequency at which they need to see the child, based on severity, growth, tolerance, and patients' and parents' compliance with physiotherapy exercises.

Due to the complex and varied presentations in CP, it is not possible to give a formula for management. There are, however, some interventions that are frequently employed. In each case, it is vital that physiotherapy is coordinated to make the most of any intervention. This list cannot be exhaustive and there is no substitute for attending several combined CP clinics to gain an appreciation of the decision-making process in the orthopaedic care of these children.

Orthoses

Orthoses are an essential part of CP treatment. They are used for various purposes, and these are covered in details in Chapter 18c.

Equipment and Assistive Devices

Devices to improve the quality of life in children with NMD have been advanced substantially to the extent that surgical approaches to these children are being re-evaluated.

The following are common variety of assistive devices that are used to improve and maintain the functional capabilities of children with CP (Figure 18a.16):

1. Canes and crutches (standard, forearm crutches, tripod and quad canes)
2. Walkers to help with balance – a rear walker is most often used, as it is easier to manoeuvre and promotes extension of the lower limbs and back. Some also has a folded chair in case the child gets tired
3. Hoists for easy transfer
4. Standers to maintain the child in an upright position, which facilitates social interaction and some mechanical loading
5. Wheelchair (manual or motorized)
6. Functional electrical stimulation (FES) uses low-energy electrical pulses to artificially generate muscle contraction and subsequent body movements. This is commonly used for the tibialis anterior muscle, instead of AFO, in children with foot drop
7. Robotic suit and powered exoskeleton – these devices overcome muscle weakness and balance problems that patients have and render a non-ambulatory patient to ambulatory (Figure 18a.17). However, they require functioning joints and reasonable learning ability.
8. Sleep systems – for posture

Treatment of Spasticity

Spasticity is the primary pathology that underlies most of the secondary pathological changes. Therefore, its treatment is important to minimize, slow down, or even prevent secondary musculoskeletal changes.

In addition to physiotherapy, several modes of treatments are available, including:

- Oral medications (baclofen, benzodiazepines, dantrolene, and tizanidine)
- Intramuscular (botulinum toxin A, phenol, and alcohol)
- Intrathecal baclofen
- Selective dorsal rhizotomy (SDR).

Baclofen

Baclofen acts by binding to gamma-aminobutyric acid (GABA) receptors. Side effects are common and include sedation, confusion, memory loss, dizziness, ataxia, and weakness, which are the causes of cessation. Oral baclofen is usually used in children who are too small or too young for a more effective treatment. Intrathecal baclofen has fewer systemic side effects (although there is significant local risk) and the therapeutic dose is only 1%

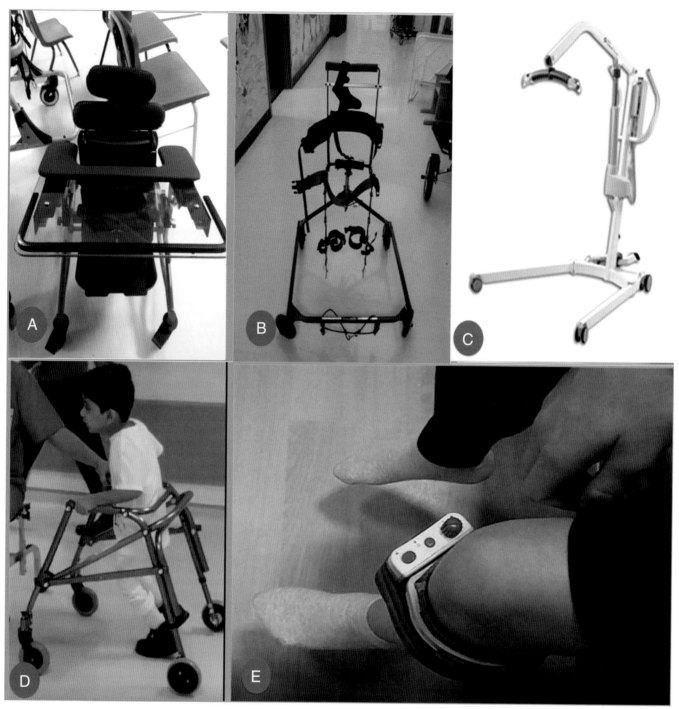

Figure 18a.16 Assistive devices for children with cerebral palsy. (A) and (B) show two types of standers. They are designed to help the child achieve various tasks whilst standing. (C) is a manual hoist for easy child transfer. (D) shows a child walking using a rear walker. (E) shows a functional electric stimulator for the tibialis anterior muscle in a child with foot drop.

of the oral dose. It is usually delivered through a programmable pump implanted under the skin. The dose is titrated based on clinical response. The pump must be refilled every 1–5 months. Children need to be a minimal size and weight to be suitable.

Botulinum Toxin A (BoNT, commonly known by its brand name Botox)

BoNT is a potent neurotoxin which presynaptically and irreversibly binds at the motor end plate, preventing acetylcholine release and thereby reducing muscle activity (both involuntary spasm and voluntary contraction). Muscle function (and spasticity) gradually recovers over a 3-month period, as new motor end plates replace those that have been irreversibly blocked. Medium- and long-acting Botox formulations are being developed. Ultrasound guidance and muscle stimulators are used to improve the accuracy of Botox injection.

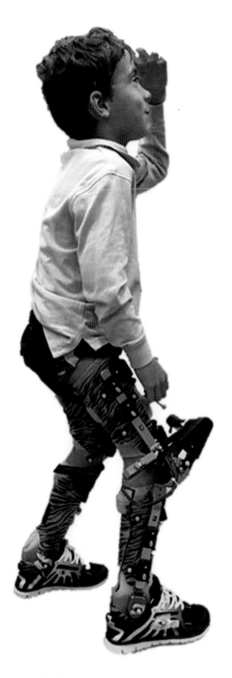

Figure 18a.17 A powered exoskeleton to overcome weakness. *Source:* Image is courtesy of Functional and Applied Biomechanics Section, Rehabilitation Medicine Department, National Institutes of Health Clinical Center.

Systemic side effects are rare in the CP setting. However, pain, generalized muscle weakness, blurred vision, ptosis, dysphagia, dysphonia, dysarthria, urinary incontinence, and breathing difficulties are described.

Indications and long-term benefits of BoNT have been debated [6]. BoNT is used in CP to reduce muscle spasm, typically in the hip adductors, hamstrings, and gastrocnemius. The controversy is whether spasm alone is the indication for using BoNT, or the presence of functional limitation that is caused by the spasm. Some authors give BoNT regularly every 6 months, and others only when there are functional needs.

BoNT is useful to predict the impact of a more permanent surgical tendon or muscle procedure such as tenotomy or tendon transfer.

Selective Dorsal Rhizotomy

SDR refers to selective division of sensory nerve roots from L1 to S1 or S2. Each rootlet is stimulated to identify the ones that contribute most to the spasticity, which are then divided. There are several variations in the technique, but the broad principle is the same in each case. There has been considerable debate about its value. The recent Commission through Evaluation (CtE) multicentre trial by NHS England led to the recommissioning of NHS-funded SDR on the basis of improvements demonstrated in children who met strict 'selection' criteria [7]. These included:

- Children with spastic diplegia
- MRI changes consistent with CP
- Dynamic spasticity interfering with function and mobility
- No dystonia
- Age 3–9 years
- GMFCS levels II–III with adequate anti-gravity muscle power.

Serial Casting

Serial casting is an effective way to stretch contracted muscles [8–10]. It involves stretching these muscles using casting on a weekly basis for an average of 3–4 weeks. The gastrocnemius, hamstrings, and hip adductors are the commonest muscles to benefit from serial casting (Figures 18a.18 and 18a.19). Although the principle and technique are simple, attention to details is required for best results.

Surgical Interventions

The principles of surgical treatments of children with CP (and indeed all NMD) are simple and not different from treatments used in other orthopaedic fields (Table 18a.4). However, they need careful consideration and thoughtful patient selection. The goals of surgical interventions are different between ambulatory and non-ambulatory children. In ambulatory children, the goals can be summarized as follows:

1. To optimize gait efficiency:
   a. To optimize energy conservation
   b. To preserve or improve physical function
   c. To preserve or increase activities and participation
2. Gait cosmesis: to improve the appearance of gait
3. Pain relief.

In non-ambulatory children, the goals are:

1. To prevent or relieve pain and discomfort
2. To facilitate caregiving
3. To preserve or improve quality of life.

Surgical Treatment of Specific Pathologies

The Hip

Hip adduction contracture of <30° heralds joint subluxation. This has become one of the criteria for hip screening in most national CPIPs. This is often supplemented with AP pelvic

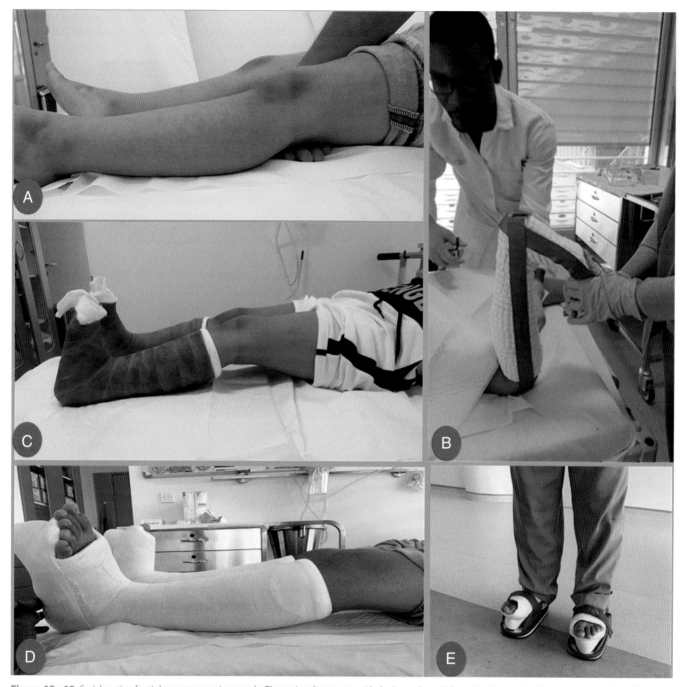

Figure 18a.18 Serial casting for tight gastrocnemius muscle. The patient lies prone, with the knees bent 90° to relax the muscle. Maximum stretch is applied, followed by casting (B). Effective stretching is manifested by flexed knees (A, C). The last set may require forefoot wedges to prevent crouching, which reduces the stretching efficiency (D, E).

radiographs to evaluate the hip using four radiographic parameters (Figure 18a.20):

1. Reimer's migration index (RMI)
2. Acetabular index (AI)
3. Femoral neck–shaft angle
4. Shenton's lines.

The RMI is the percentage of uncovered head (calculated as the width of the uncovered head divided by the width of the head, and multiplied by 100). A normal RMI is <30%. Recent evidence shows a migration percentage of >40 implies dislocation is inevitable without intervention.

Typical surgical treatments of neurological hip dysplasia could involve any of the following, depending on severity:

1. Adductor(s) release through a small medial incision. The adductor longus, gracilis, and adductor brevis can be released, whilst protecting the anterior division of the obturator nerve. In a non-ambulatory child, the psoas tendon can be released through the same approach to improve flexion contractures.

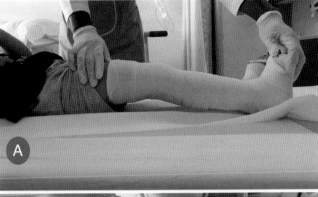

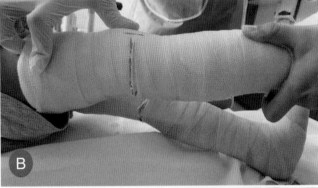

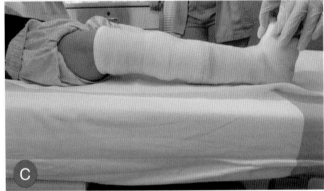

Figure 18a.19 Serial casting for hamstring tightness. Above-knee cast is applied in as full extension as possible, followed by open wedging behind the knee to increase the stretch.

2. Flexion contracture is improved by fractional lengthening (dividing the tendinous parts and leaving the muscle fibres intact) of the iliopsoas tendon over the pelvic brim through an anterior hip (Smith–Peterson) approach. This preserves muscle power and prevents excessive weakness associated with dividing the whole tendon (through a medial approach in a non-ambulatory child).

3. Femoral varus and derotation osteotomy (VDRO) through a lateral sub-vastus approach. This to improve the hip joint biomechanics (see Lever arm syndrome above) and minimize the risk of redislocation. Adding slight extension to the osteotomy has become a more popular technique to overcome mild to moderate hip flexion contracture, compared to psoas muscle release.

4. Pelvic osteotomy through an anterior hip approach. Dega pelvic osteotomy (or its modification such as San Diego) is the commonest type used in children with CP because

Table 18a.4 Surgical treatments of common pathologies in children with cerebral palsy

Pathology	Surgical treatment	Common pitfalls
Contractures	Releases/lengthening	Not a substitute for rehabilitation Interfering with compensatory changes
Bony deformity	Deformity corrections	Inappropriate selection Wrong timing
Joint dislocation and instability	Reduction/stabilization	Prevention is possible (Cerebral Palsy Integrated Pathway) Delaying treatment
Lever arm syndrome	All of the above	Birthday syndrome (correcting one problem every year)
Degenerative arthritis	Joint replacement (hips) Fusion (metatarsophalangeal joints) Excision (hips and proximal interphalangeal joint)	Avoidance of surgery

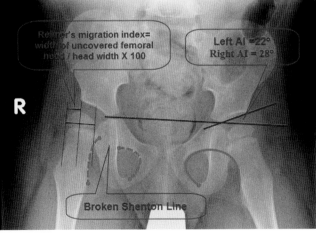

Figure 18a.20 Pelvis X-ray of a child with cerebral palsy. Right hip Reimer's migration index (RMI) is >45%; left hip RMI is <30%. Right acetabular dysplasia (acetabular index 28°), broken Shenton's line, and marked coxa valga. Some of the coxa valga may be apparent as there is usually significant femoral anteversion.

of the nature of the acetabular deficiency (posterolateral). A curved osteotomy is made 1 cm above, and parallel to, the acetabular margin, and is deepened medially and downwards towards the triradiate cartilage. It is important not to break through the medial wall or the triradiate cartilage. Then the acetabular rim is folded down to reduce the acetabular size and provide lateral and posterior wall cover (Figure 18a.21). The difference between the two osteotomies is minor, but important. The supra-acetabular bone is imagined as a box with long lateral and medial walls and narrow anterior and posterior walls. Dega osteotomy involves the lateral and anterior walls, whereas San Diego osteotomy involves the anterior, lateral, and posterior walls, allowing more coverage posteriorly and laterally. They differ from Pemberton osteotomy, in which the lateral, anterior, and medial walls are osteotomized (see Chapter 5) [11]. Other types of pelvic osteotomies, such as Ganz and triple osteotomies, have been used if the pathoanatomy is not typical. This is particularly frequent in hemiplegic CP (see Chapter 4, Figures 4c.24 and 4c.25).

5. Salvage procedures for non-reconstructable hip dislocation, particularly when the articular cartilage is badly damaged:

   a. Proximal femoral resection, with or without proximal valgus osteotomy, using a plate (Figure 18a.22). The risk of heterotopic ossification is significant.

   b. Prosthetic replacement in carefully selected patients (either total hip replacement or hemi-arthroplasty) in patients who can walk with good muscle strength and no pelvic obliquity

   c. Hip fusion (very unpopular and rarely used in CP).

The Knee

Two important deformities require orthopaedic surgical interventions: fixed flexion deformity and stiff knee in extension. The former was discussed earlier (see Lever arm syndrome).

In stiff knee gait, the tight rectus femoris interferes with knee flexion in the swing phase, which creates foot clearance problems. Sometimes, the muscle is not particularly tight, but it contracts at the wrong time (EMG studies during gait analysis can show this). The solution is either recession of the muscle or transferring it to the hamstring muscles. The alleged benefit of transferring the rectus is to increase knee flexion in the swing phase, aiding foot clearance. However, the evidence from gait analysis is still controversial.

The Foot and Ankle

Foot and ankle deformities associated with CP include equinus, equinovarus, equinovalgus, and hallux valgus.

Equinus

It is usually caused by gastrocnemius contracture with or without the soleus. The Silfverskiöld test is used to differentiate

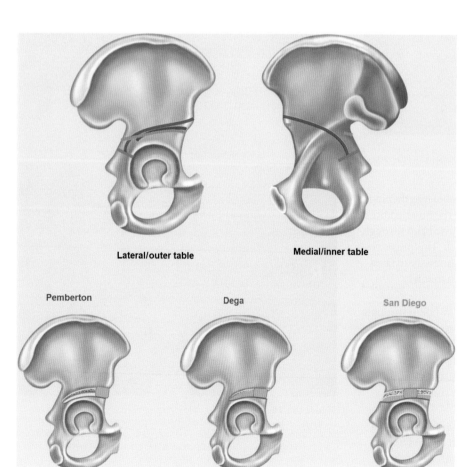

Figure 18a.21 Comparison of San Diego, Dega, and Pemberton pelvic osteotomies. In San Diego osteotomy, the lateral wall is cut fully and the cut extended to the inner wall at the front and back only (green cuts). In Dega osteotomy, the inner wall is untouched (purple cut). By contrast, in Pemberton osteotomy, both the inner and outer walls are cut, leaving only a small hinge near the triradiate cartilage (red cut). Pemberton (and Salter) osteotomies are not recommended for children with CP, as they increase the anterolateral coverage at the expense of the posterolateral coverage, which is already deficient in children with CP.

Lateral/outer table

Medial/inner table

Pemberton

Dega

San Diego

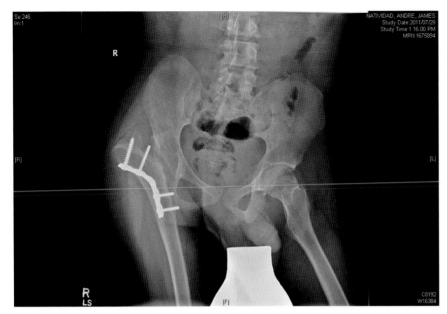

Figure 18a.22 Excisional arthroplasty with valgus osteotomy of the proximal femur.

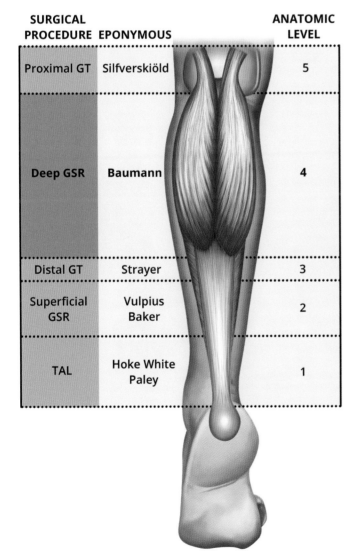

SURGICAL PROCEDURE	EPONYMOUS	ANATOMIC LEVEL
Proximal GT	Silfverskiöld	5
Deep GSR	Baumann	4
Distal GT	Strayer	3
Superficial GSR	Vulpius Baker	2
TAL	Hoke White Paley	1

Figure 18a.23 Surgical interventions for equinus deformity. GT, gastrocnemius tenotomy; GSR, gastroc–soleus recession; TAL, Tendo Achilles lengthening.

between the two. Lengthening the gastrocnemius alone preserves the power of push-off (by the soleus) and is less likely to result in overcorrection, which is more problematic. This may entail leaving some residual tightness from the soleus muscle. Several techniques have been described (Figure 18a.23):

1. The Silverskiöld procedure involves proximal gastrocnemius tenotomy.
2. Baumann described deep gastroc–soleus recession through the interval between the gastrocnemius and the soleus when approached medially.
3. Strayer lengthened the gastrocnemius selectively by dividing the tendon just proximal to where it blends with the soleus fascia. This is usually resutured at a higher level to the soleus fascia.
4. Superficial gastroc–soleus recession at the musculo-tendinous junction is described by Vulpius (Chevron-type cut) and Baker (tongue in groove-type cut).
5. Tendo Achilles lengthening by open Z-plasty or percutaneous techniques – White used two percutaneous cuts (anterior two-thirds divided at the distal incision. At the proximal exposure, the medial half to two-thirds of the tendon is divided (a useful mnemonic is DAMP: distal, anterior, medial, proximal). Hoke described a three-cut technique (proximal and distal medial and middle lateral). Video 18a.1 demonstrates how to perform Achillis tendon lengthening

Equinovarus

This is most often seen in hemiplegic CP. Treatment follows the same principle of correcting pes cavus deformity. If deformity is still flexible, soft tissue procedures are performed to balance the foot. This often involves:

 Video 18a.1 Achillis tendon lengthening.

1. Tendo Achilles and tibialis posterior lengthening
2. Split tendon transfer of either the tibialis posterior (to the peroneus brevis) or the tibialis anterior (to the lateral cuneiform) which may be required to balance the forces and prevent recurrence. The **confusion test** is proposed to help determine which muscle to transfer; with active hip flexion, if the forefoot is supinated, the tibialis anterior is likely involved, whereas pure dorsiflexion suggests involvement of the tibialis posterior. However, this has been contested based on EMG gait analysis studies, which are more valid [12]

If deformity is rigid, then bony surgery is required, which typically involves:

3. Lateral calcaneum slide osteotomy or lateral column shortening.

Equinovalgus

This is commoner in diplegics and quadriplegics and is usually caused by tight tendo Achilles, spastic peronei, and weak tibialis posterior, or in various combinations (Figure 18a.7).

The hindfoot valgus can occur at the subtalar and/or ankle joint. Radiographs are essential to establish the pathoanatomy. Surgical treatment involves lengthening the contracted muscles (tendo Achilles and peroneus brevis) and lateral column lengthening through the calcaneum. There are other alternatives, depending on severity of the deformity and the state of other joints.

Hallux Valgus

It is usually associated with an equinovalgus foot and external tibial torsion; hence it is important to evaluate and treat the entire limb. The most reliable procedure is arthrodesis of the MTPJ, as other procedures have a high recurrence rate (Figure 18a.24).

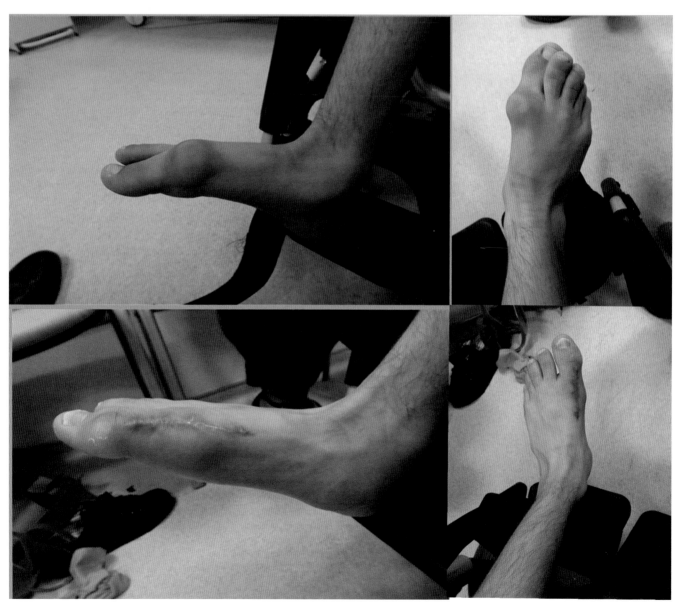

Figure 18a.24 Big toe metatarsophalangeal joint fusion in a child with cerebral palsy.

Spina Bifida

Neural tube defects comprise varying degrees of abnormalities, ranging from spina bifida occulta to the devastating rachischisis. The terminologies used by different authors for different categories of spina bifida are overlapping and can be confusing.

Spina bifida occulta is a developmental failure of the arch to close at one or more vertebral levels. It occurs in 10% of the asymptomatic population and is *not* a source of pathology.

Spina bifida cystica describes significant pathologies, with various subcategories:

1. **Meningocele** – the meninges protrude through a defect in the spine; the child is usually neurologically intact
2. **Myelomeningocele** – the meninges and cord protrude through a defect in the spine
3. **Rachischisis** – a fissure in the spine (Greek '*Rachis*' meaning spine; *schisis* meaning division). A severe form occurs when the neural elements are exposed (no coverings).

Lipomeningocele is a subcutaneous lipoma connected to an intraspinal lipoma through a fibro-fatty stalk; neurological deficits are common. Diastematomyelia is a split in the spinal cord with a bony or cartilaginous septum.

Embryology

The spinal cord develops in three phases:

1. Gastrulation (2–3 weeks in utero) involves the embryonic disc forming three distinct layers of ectoderm, mesoderm, and endoderm
2. Primary neurulation (3–4 weeks in utero) involves the notochord and overlying ectoderm forming the neural plate, which then folds along its long axis to form the neural tube, which closes proximally and distally
3. Secondary neurulation (5–6 weeks in utero) involves a secondary neural tube formed by the caudal cell mass. This cavitates eventually, forming the tip of the conus medullaris and the filum terminale by a process called retrogressive differentiation.

To explain the pathoaetiology of the spina bifida, two theories are proposed – von Recklinghausen proposed a primary failure of neural tube closure, whereas Morgagni proposed a rupture of the closed neural tube.

Aetiology

1. Failure of genes controlling neural tube closure – the risk of having a neural tube defect is 2–4% if one sibling is affected, and 10–25% if >1 are affected.
2. Environmental factors:
   a. Maternal insulin-dependent diabetes mellitus
   b. Maternal hyperthermia (e.g. saunas)
   c. Maternal valproate (antiepileptic medication)
   d. Maternal folate deficiency – grain product fortification with folic acid in the United States (begun in 1996) resulted in a 19–25% reduction in live births with spina bifida over 5 years.

Diagnosis

Maternal α-fetoprotein, antenatal ultrasound, and amniotic α-fetoprotein can diagnose this condition by 18 weeks of pregnancy.

Postnatal classification by neurosegmental level has prognostic implications; however, the level is seldom clear-cut and it may take to the age of 3 or 4 years to finally declare itself (Table 18a.5).

Annual assessment of muscle function should be undertaken, as deteriorating function may be caused by treatable conditions (tethered cord, syrinx, Arnold–Chiari malformation, malfunctioning shunt, or worsening hydrocephalus), and an MRI scan is indicated.

Management

Standard treatment of spina bifida is still urgent closure after birth. Surgery in utero has potential promise but carries a significant risk for child and mother.

Orthopaedic Issues

Spine

The incidence of scoliosis is related to the level of the lesion:

- <10% of sacral lesions
- 40% of low lumbar lesions
- >90% of high lesions.

Any developing curvature mandates an MRI scan in case of cord tethering or syringomyelia.

Bracing and/or surgical correction is considered when curves are progressing beyond a Cobb angle of 30°.

Kyphosis is common in higher lesions. There is no bracing solution; however, surgery is fraught with significant complications.

Hip

The hip may present with contractures, subluxation, or low tone dislocation. Contractures are generally addressed with surgical release of the offending muscle(s). Care must be taken not to weaken important muscles in barely walking children.

Dislocation is commoner with higher-level lesions (L2 and above). Although reduction is possible, redislocation is very common (where the underlying cause is not removed) and complications are common. Consideration is given to unilateral dislocation in lower-level lesions (i.e. in the ambulant); however, there is general agreement that bilateral dislocation is best left untreated.

Knee

Contractures are common; flexion contracture, extension contracture (recurvatum), and valgus deformities are the

Table 18a.5 Spina bifida classification by level

Anatomical level[a]	Functional level[a]	Ambulation	Notes on orthoses
High thoracic	No control of any muscles of ambulation	Non-walker	Cumbersome orthoses are available but require strong motivation and support THKAF and crutches or Swivel walker, which converts side-to-side motion of the thorax into forward motion, with a swivelling base
Low thoracic/high lumbar	Lack or weakness of hip muscles	Non-walker	Reciprocating gait orthoses (RGOs) abandoned by 99%; the rationale is when one hip flexes actively (L1), the other passively extends using a cord and pulleys HKAFO helps position the legs under the trunk, but most patients have flexion contracture, which renders it less functional
Low lumbar	Lack or weakness of quadriceps	Walker using (K)AFO and crutches	The quadriceps are important for ambulation, to extend the knee in the swing phase and keep it straight in the stance phase. Patients with weak quadriceps (L3–4) benefit from hinged KAFO with a drop lock to stabilize the knee. If the quadriceps are not significantly weak, but the tibialis anterior is weak, causing foot drop and impairing foot clearance in the swing phase, a rigid AFO alone suffices
High sacral	Lack or weakness of gastroc–soleus	Walker using AFO, no crutches 98% walkers, but gluteal lurch	Ground reaction AFO is open posteriorly and closed anteriorly over the tibia, with about 5° plantar flexion. During the stance phase, it produces a posteriorly directed force on the tibia, helping to compensate for weak gastroc–soleus There are other custom AFOs that are used to hold flexible deformity such as heel varus, valgus, supination, or pronation, and combined clinic with orthotics is the usual
Low sacral	Good gastroc–soleus function	Normal walkers	

[a] Anatomical and functional levels may not correlate and often there is a grey area. It is important to assess patient capabilities on an individual basis.THKAF, trunk–hip–knee–ankle–foot orthosis; RGO, reciprocating gait orthosis; HKAFO, hip–knee–ankle–foot orthosis; KAFO, knee–ankle–foot orthosis; AFO, ankle–foot orthosis.

commonest. The former two can be treated with serial casting and surgical releases of contracted muscles, depending on severity. Osteotomy is rarely necessary. Valgus deformity may accompany external tibial torsion. Knee–ankle–foot orthoses (KAFOs) are used to protect the knee from valgus stress in patients with a low lumbar level. Derotation osteotomy can be considered when torsion is significant (over 20°).

Night extension splints are also employed to reduce the development of contractures.

Foot and Ankle

More than three-quarters of children with myelomeningocele will develop a foot and ankle deformity. Several types of deformities have been associated with spina bifida (including club foot, calcaneus, calcaneovalgus, planovalgus, and cavus deformities; Figure 18a.25). A plantigrade braceable foot is the aim (Figure 18a.26). Casting is certainly a good starting point for most deformities; however, division of tendons (e.g. tendo Achilles) can be reasonably contemplated in the non-ambulant to address resistant deformity. A more aggressive approach in ambulant children may be warranted. Insensate skin is vulnerable and extra care is needed with splintage. Seating and wheelchairs need careful consideration to reduce pressure sores.

Intercurrent Issues

It is important to be mindful of the associated features of spina bifida:

- Hydrocephalus – 90% of children with myelomeningocele require shunting. Complications include infection and shunt blockage.
- Arnold–Chiari malformation – describes herniation of the hindbrain through the foramen magnum.
  - o Type I is limited to the cerebellar tonsils, and causes adolescent headaches, lower limb spasm, and upper limb pain.
  - o Type II (Figure 18a.27) presents in infancy and is commoner, with herniation of the brainstem, cranial nerve dysfunction (feeding problems), and hydrocephalus.
  - o Type III is an encephalocele.

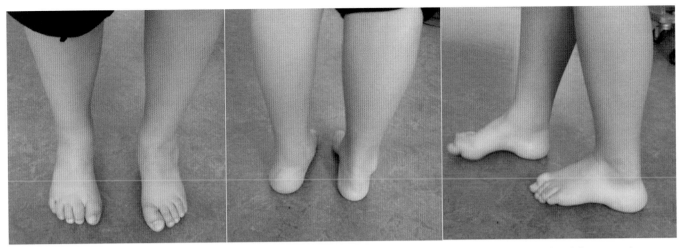

Figure 18a.25 Foot deformity in spina bifida. A child with lumbar spina bifida (namely lipomeningocele) developed asymmetrical foot deformities: right cavovarus foot and left calcaneovalgus deformity.

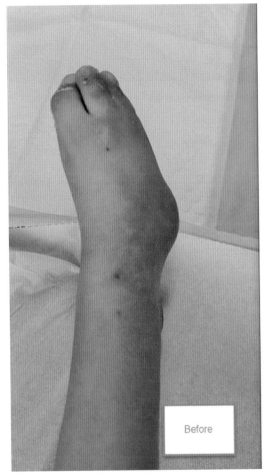
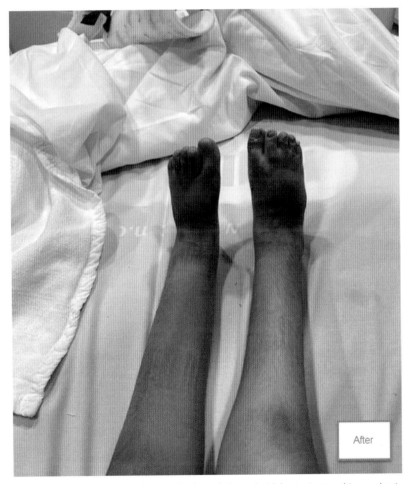

Before

After

Figure 18a.26 Cavovarus foot deformity in a child with spina bifida, which was treated with serial casting (eight sets), then cuboid shortening to achieve a plantigrade braceable foot.

- Tethered cord – this is a feature of myelomeningocele at birth, in which a fibrous band connects the conus medullaris to the bony sacrum, preventing normal cranial migration of the conus with growth. It frequently persists with scarring – demonstrable on MRI – but less than a third show clinically reduced motor function, spasticity, and/or scoliosis and bladder problems; hence neurosurgical release is only indicated when there is confirmed neurological deterioration.

- Syringomyelia – a fluid-filled cavity in the cord in up to half of patients. This may cause pressure problems with spasticity, weakness, and scoliosis.

A

B

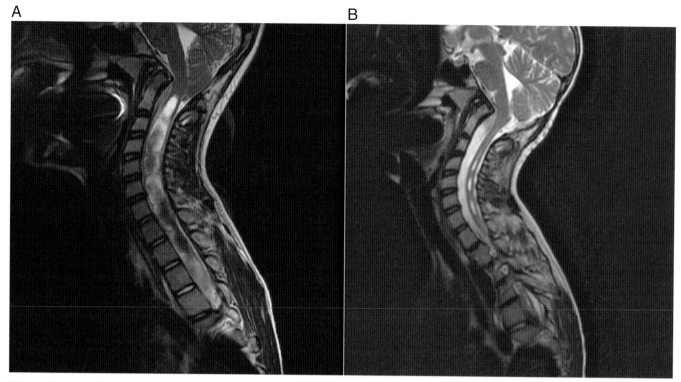

Figure 18a.27 Arnold–Chiari malformation and syrinx. Two MRI scans of the neck, with (A) showing the cerebellar tonsils projecting below the foramen magnum. There is expansile syringohydromyelia extending from the inferior aspect of C1, with multiple internal septations. (B) shows significant improvement after surgical decompression. Notice the position of the cerebellar tonsils, cerebrospinal fluid around the cord, and resolution of the syrinx.

- Urological problems – significant renal dysfunction (due to post-renal obstruction) has been significantly reduced in this patient group by close monitoring and early intervention (e.g. self-catheterization). Urinary tract infection should be considered, and antibiotic prophylaxis planned carefully when undertaking orthopaedic procedures.
- Latex – as many as 8 in 10 children with spina bifida have latex allergy, compared with 1% of the general population; this may be related to frequent catheterization or hospital contact.

Muscular Dystrophies

There are a series of conditions due to gene mutations on X chromosomes or autosomes involved in muscle protein production.

Duchenne Muscular Dystrophy

This is the commonest NMD (incidence 13–33 in 100 000). It is inherited in an X-linked recessive pattern, and hence males are affected and females are carriers. Muscle fibres are gradually replaced by fibro-fatty infiltrates. This causes significant muscle weakness despite an incongruous increase in muscle size (pseudohypertrophy). Steroid treatment has been shown to slow disease progression, including orthopaedic deformities.

The presenting history includes:

- 'Floppy infant'
- Delayed milestones
- Toe walking
- Clumsy, fatigable, waddling gait from 4 years of age.

Clinical features include:

- Pseudohypertrophy of the calf
- Scapular winging (facioscapulohumeral dystrophy – autosomal dominant inheritance)
- Scoliosis due to paraspinal muscle weakness
- Proximal weakness preceding distal weakness
- Gower's sign – climbing up the legs with the hands to rise from sitting (see Chapter 2, Figure 2.6)
- Cardiorespiratory failure in late teens.

Diagnosis involves the following:

- Clinical features
- Significantly raised creatine phosphokinase levels
- Genetic diagnostic testing
- EMG and muscle biopsy – diminished use since the advent of genetic testing when readily available.

Orthopaedic aspects of management include:

- Physiotherapy to maintain strength
- Orthotics to assist in maintaining ambulation and independence
- Contracture release for wheelchair seating (release in the ambulant child is controversial)
- Scoliosis – progressive in 90%; therefore, early consideration for surgery before respiratory compromise precludes it. Scoliosis is usually observed at around the age

of 2 years. Although scoliosis in the early stages gets worse slowly, it can deteriorate quite dramatically over a short period of time (30° per year; often referred to as spinal collapse). Indications for surgery are different from those for idiopathic scoliosis. Surgery should be performed once a curve reaches 30° and the patient is non-ambulatory. Preoperative planning must include cardiac evaluation and pulmonary function tests. There is some controversy on including the pelvis in scoliosis corrective surgery. There are pros and cons for either approach.

Becker Muscular Dystrophy

This is also inherited in an X-linked recessive pattern, but it is less severe and slower to progress, with longer survivorship into adulthood. Its onset occurs after 7 years of age. Its symptomatic management is as for DMD.

References

1. Rosenbaum PL, Palisano RJ, Bartlett DJ, Galuppi BE, Russell DJ. Development of the Gross Motor Function Classification System for cerebral palsy. *Dev Med Child Neurol.* 2008;50(4):249–53.

2. Rosenbaum PL, Walter SD, Hanna SE, *et al.* Prognosis for gross motor function in cerebral palsy: creation of motor development curves. *JAMA.* 2002;288(11):1357–63.

3. Wood E, Rosenbaum P. The Gross Motor Function Classification System for cerebral palsy: a study of reliability and stability over time. *Dev Med Child Neurol.* 2000;42(5):292–6.

4. Graham HK. Painful hip dislocation in cerebral palsy. *Lancet.* 2002;359(9310):907–8.

5. Novak I, Morgan C, Fahey M, *et al.* State of the Evidence Traffic Lights 2019: systematic review of interventions for preventing and treating children with cerebral palsy. *Curr Neurol Neurosci Rep.* 2020;20(2):3.

6. Carpenter C, Bass A. The value of gait analysis in decision making about surgical treatment of cerebral palsy. In: Alshryda S, Huntley JS, Banaszkiewicz P, eds. *Paediatric Orthopaedics: An Evidence-Based Approach to Clinical Questions.* Cham: Springer; 2016. pp. 361–7.

7. National Institute for Health and Care Excellence. Interventional procedure overview of selective dorsal rhizotomy for spasticity in cerebral palsy. 2006. Available from: https://www.nice.org.uk/guidance/ipg373/evidence/overview-pdf-316141021.

8. Adelaar RS, Williams RM, Gould JS. Congenital convex pes valgus: results of an early comprehensive release and a review of congenital vertical talus at Richmond Crippled Children's Hospital and the University of Alabama in Birmingham. *Foot Ankle.* 1980;1(2):62–73.

9. Booth MY, Yates CC, Edgar TS, Bandy WD. Serial casting vs combined intervention with botulinum toxin A and serial casting in the treatment of spastic equinus in children. *Pediatr Phys Ther.* 2003;15(4):216–20.

10. Churgay CA. Diagnosis and treatment of pediatric foot deformities. *Am Fam Physician.* 1993;47(4):883–9.

11. Caffrey JP, Jeffords ME, Farnsworth CL, Bomar JD, Upasani VV. Comparison of 3 pediatric pelvic osteotomies for acetabular dysplasia using patient-specific 3D-printed models. *J Pediatr Orthop.* 2019;39(3):e159–64.

12. Davids JR, Holland WC, Sutherland DH. Significance of the confusion test in cerebral palsy. *J Pediatr Orthop.* 1993;13(6):717–21.

Neuromuscular Conditions/Upper Limbs

Bavan Luckshman and Rachel Buckingham

Introduction

Upper limb involvement and impaired functional use of the hand is common in CP [1, 2]. It is typically evident by 1 year of age when infants fail to achieve certain motor milestones such as a refined pincer grasp. Neurological impairment can manifest with spasticity, weakness, or, in the case of dyskinetic CP, involuntary movement and fluctuations in tone [3]. Management of upper limb impairment in CP requires a comprehensive multidisciplinary team approach, with the goal of improving function, providing comfort, enabling good hygiene, or addressing cosmetic concerns.

Clinical Assessment

It is important to obtain a clear understanding of the patient's day-to-day functioning and create a comfortable environment for assessment. The examination must establish joint position, and active and passive range of motion. Sensation and power must also be carefully evaluated, and distinguishing voluntary from involuntary movement is essential [4, 5]. Spasticity is the main neuromotor impairment in the majority of patients with CP. It is necessary to differentiate spasticity from permanent muscle contracture, which, unlike spasticity, cannot be overcome. This is particularly relevant when considering treatment options, as contractures will persist following nerve blockade or botulinum toxin treatment. Validated objective tools can be used to quantify spasticity; these include the modified Ashworth Scale and the Tardieu Scale [6–9].

Patients can display varying patterns of spasticity, and presentation may not be symmetrical in individuals with bilateral involvement. The commonest upper extremity deformities observed are depicted in Figure 18b.1. Shoulder adduction and internal rotation occur secondary to spasticity of the pectoralis major, subscapularis, and latissimus dorsi. Flexion at the elbow is due to biceps and brachioradialis spasticity, and forearm pronation is often seen with pronator teres spasticity. Ulnar deviation at the wrist is most commonly due to flexor carpi ulnaris (FCU) involvement, although extensor carpi ulnaris (ECU) can be responsible if the wrist is in extension. A wrist flexion deformity can be the direct cause of weak grip strength due to loss of tension in the long flexors. Long flexor tendon tightness also contributes to wrist flexion, as well as to finger flexion, and can be assessed by measuring the Volkmann angle (Figure 18b.2). Passive extension of the proximal and distal interphalangeal

joints in isolation can differentiate flexor digitorum superficialis (FDS) from flexor digitorum profundus (FDP) involvement.

Release of tight digital flexors without an appreciation for intrinsic tightness can result in metacarpophalangeal (MCP) joint flexion and interphalangeal joint extension deformity. Intrinsic tightness can be evaluated by Bunnell's test (Figure 18b.3), and an ulnar nerve block can help differentiate spasticity from fixed contracture of the intrinsic muscles or proximal interphalangeal joints. Thumb involvement in CP is common, and typically the thumb will be flexed inside the palm, impairing grasp and use of the other digits. The underlying deformity is complex, and examination must evaluate potential spasticity

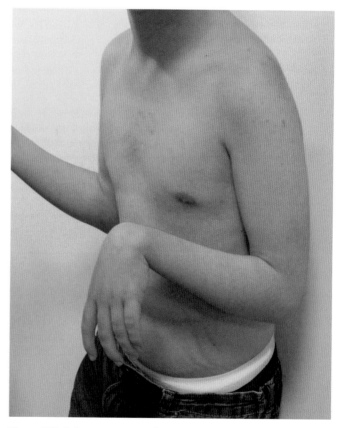

Figure 18b.1 Common pattern of upper limb deformity in cerebral palsy: shoulder adduction and internal rotation, elbow flexion, forearm pronation and wrist flexion, and ulnar deviation.

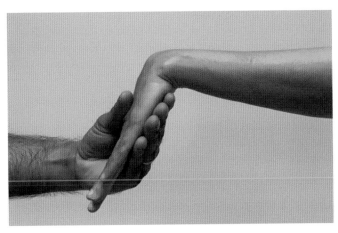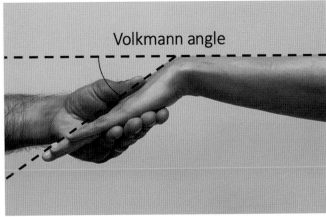

Figure 18b.2 Long flexor tendon tightness can be assessed by passively bringing the wrist from flexion to extension, with the digits held completely extended throughout. The wrist cannot be brought to neutral with digital flexor contracture.

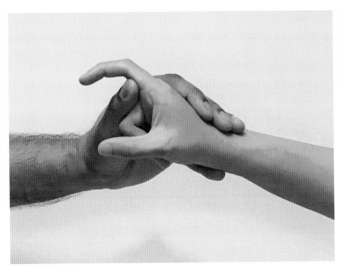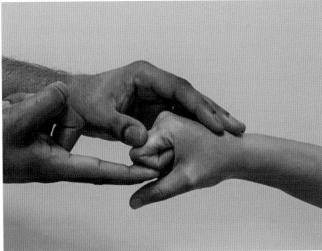

Figure 18b.3 The Bunnell's test involves assessing proximal interphalangeal joint range of movement, with the metacarpophalangeal joint in flexion and extension. A positive intrinsic tightness test demonstrates a relatively greater range in flexion.

of the adductor and flexor muscles (adductor pollicis, flexor pollicis brevis, first dorsal interossei, and flexor pollicis longus), weakness of the extensors and abductors, mobility of the MCP joint, and possible web space contracture [3].

Classifications and Grading of Function

A variety of systems allow us to classify upper limb function in patients with CP. The Manual Ability Classification System (MACS) is a widely used and validated tool [2, 10], aimed at classifying children between 4 and 18 years of age into five categories:

1. Handles objects easily and successfully
2. Handles most objects, but with somewhat reduced quality and/or speed of achievement
3. Handles objects with difficulty; needs help to prepare and/or modify activities
4. Handles a limited number of easily managed objects in adapted situations
5. Does not handle objects and has severely limited ability to perform even simple actions.

Other validated tools exist, which provide a more detailed assessment of upper limb function using structured assessments. These include the Assisting Hand Assessment (AHA), which measures use of the affected hand acting collaboratively with the unaffected hand during bimanual play [11]. Some tools can also help characterize the pathological mechanisms underlying functional deficiencies in a clinically useful way. The Shriners Hospital Upper Extremity Evaluation (SHUEE) objectively evaluates various domains of upper limb function, and is validated for use in assessment, treatment planning, and measurement of treatment outcomes [12]. It is a useful tool for the surgeon, as it assesses abnormal joint positioning during activity.

Non-operative Treatment

Range of motion and strengthening exercises can help maintain and improve function. Constraint-induced movement therapy and bimanual therapy are evidence-based strategies proven to improve dexterity, control, and coordination [13–15]. Serial casting and splinting can also help stretch out tight muscle groups. However, results tend to be short-lived and most splints are rarely suitable for everyday practical use [3].

Systemic anti-spasticity medications (e.g. baclofen, diazepam, tizanidine) can have a role in management of upper limb spasticity in CP. These medications can be helpful for more severely affected patients but can cause side effects such as weakness and hypotonia [16]. Targeted botulinum toxin injections can be a useful adjunct to physiotherapy, provide short-term improvements in spasticity, and help with predicting surgical outcomes [17].

Surgery

Assessment of suitability for surgery requires consideration of the patient's age, intelligence, motivation, and available support. There is no strict consensus on optimal timing of surgery, although it is largely accepted that the predominant patterns of arm use should be apparent, which is typically after 6 years of age. When possible, multilevel deformities should be addressed concurrently in a single stage to optimize functional outcomes and patient satisfaction [18]. SEMLS may not be suitable for all patients, and the practicalities of post-operative rehabilitation should be considered on an individual basis. It is generally recommended that features of dystonia and choreoathetosis are addressed prior to any operative intervention, and reports suggest that patients with dyskinetic forms of CP tend to have less predictable outcomes following surgery [19].

Muscle rebalancing procedures in the form of release, lengthening, and transfer can provide improvements in limb position and function for patients with spasticity, contracture, and weakness. Extensive release or lengthening can result in significant muscle weakening, and shortening osteotomies can be considered as an alternative. Tendon transfer procedures allow redirection of forces to improve joint position, and augment weaker agonists to improve dynamic hand function (Figure 18b.4). If joint contractures exist, capsular releases can be performed, and in some cases, corrective osteotomy, epiphysiodesis, and arthrodesis may be required. In cases where the hand has limited function, wrist fusion can be performed for pain relief, to improve hygiene, or to improve cosmesis. Careful examination of the hand with the wrist in neutral must be performed to determine if additional releases or transfers may be required [3, 16].

Whilst a detailed discussion on specific surgical options for treatment of upper limb spasticity is beyond the scope of this chapter, Table 18b.1 details established management options for common upper limb deformity and patterns of functional weakness seen in CP [3, 5, 16].

Table 18b.1 Summary of common surgical options for management of upper limb deformity or weakness in cerebral palsy

	Deformity	Surgical treatment options
Shoulder	Adduction and internal rotation	Subscapularis and pectoralis major lengthening or release
Elbow	Flexion	Biceps, brachialis, and brachioradialis lengthening or release
Forearm	Pronation	Pronator teres release or rerouting Flexor–pronator slide
Wrist	Flexion and ulnar deviation (extensor weakness)	Flexor carpi ulnaris to extensor carpi radialis brevis transfer Extensor carpi ulnaris to extensor carpi radialis brevis transfer Pronator teres to extensor carpi radialis brevis transfer Flexor carpi ulnaris/flexor carpi radialis lengthening or release Wrist arthrodesis
Hand	Digital flexion/clasp hand (extensor weakness)	Flexor digitorum superficialis lengthening Flexor digitorum superficialis to profundus transfer Flexor–pronator muscle slide Flexor carpi ulnaris to extensor digitorum communis transfer
	Swan neck	Intrinsic release Central slip release
	Thumb-in-palm	Web space contracture release Intrinsic release Flexor pollicis longus lengthening Extensor pollicis longus rerouting Brachioradialis to abductor pollicis longus transfer Metacarpophalangeal joint arthrodesis

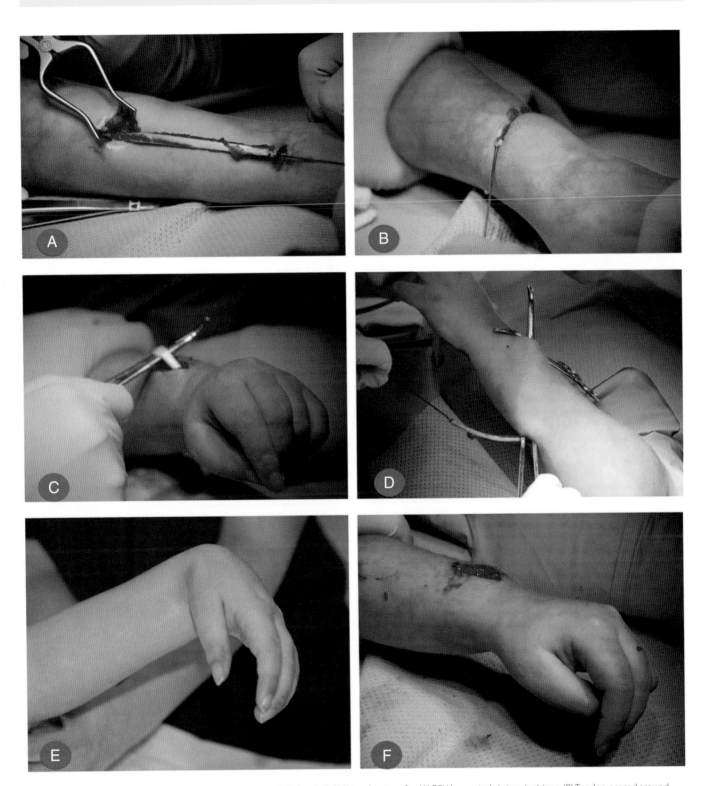

Figure 18b.4 Flexor carpi ulnaris (FCU) to extensor carpi radialis brevis (ECRB) tendon transfer. (A) FCU harvested via two incisions. (B) Tendon passed around to the dorsal aspect of the distal forearm to determine the site of attachment to the ECRB. (C) ECRB tendon identified. (D) FCU tendon tunnelled subcutaneously before attachment to the ECRB. Wrist position before (E) and after (F) tendon transfer.

References

1. Arner M, Eliasson AC, Nicklasson S, Sommerstein K, Hagglund G. Hand function in cerebral palsy. Report of 367 children in a population-based longitudinal health care program. *J Hand Surg Am*. 2008;33(8):1337–47.

2. McConnell K, Johnston L, Kerr C. Upper limb function and deformity in cerebral palsy: a review of classification systems. *Dev Med Child Neurol*. 2011;53(9):799–805.

3. Carlson MG, Athwal GS, Bueno RA. Treatment of the wrist and hand in cerebral palsy. *J Hand Surg Am*. 2006;31(3):483–90.

4. Rhee PC. Surgical management of upper extremity deformities in patients with upper motor neuron syndrome. *J Hand Surg Am*. 2019;44(3):223–35.

5. Tranchida GV, Van Heest A. Preferred options and evidence for upper limb surgery for spasticity in cerebral palsy, stroke, and brain injury. *J Hand Surg Eur*. 2020;45(1):34–42.

6. Bohannon RW, Smith MB. Interrater reliability of a modified Ashworth scale of muscle spasticity. *Phys Ther*. 1987;67(2):206–7.

7. Tardieu G, Shentoub S, Delarue R. [Research on a technic for measurement of spasticity]. *Rev Neurol (Paris)*. 1954;91(2):143–4.

8. Yam WK, Leung MS. Interrater reliability of Modified Ashworth Scale and Modified Tardieu Scale in children with spastic cerebral palsy. *J Child Neurol*. 2006;21(12): 1031–5.

9. Gracies JM, Burke K, Clegg NJ, *et al*. Reliability of the Tardieu Scale for assessing spasticity in children with cerebral palsy. *Arch Phys Med Rehabil*. 2010;91(3):421–8.

10. Eliasson AC, Krumlinde-Sundholm L, Rosblad B, *et al*. The Manual Ability Classification System (MACS) for children with cerebral palsy: scale development and evidence of validity and reliability. *Dev Med Child Neurol*. 2006;48(7):549–54.

11. Krumlinde-Sundholm L, Holmefur M, Kottorp A, Eliasson AC. The Assisting Hand Assessment: current evidence of validity, reliability, and responsiveness to change. *Dev Med Child Neurol*. 2007;49(4):259–64.

12. Davids JR, Peace LC, Wagner LV, Gidewall MA, Blackhurst DW, Roberson WM. Validation of the Shriners Hospital for Children Upper Extremity Evaluation (SHUEE) for children with hemiplegic cerebral palsy. *J Bone Joint Surg Am*. 2006;88(2):326–33.

13. Chen YP, Pope S, Tyler D, Warren GL. Effectiveness of constraint-induced movement therapy on upper-extremity function in children with cerebral palsy: a systematic review and meta-analysis of randomized controlled trials. *Clin Rehabil*. 2014;28(10):939–53.

14. Dong VA, Tung IH, Siu HW, Fong KN. Studies comparing the efficacy of constraint-induced movement therapy and bimanual training in children with unilateral cerebral palsy: a systematic review. *Dev Neurorehabil*. 2013;16(2):133–43.

15. Chiu HC, Ada L. Constraint-induced movement therapy improves upper limb activity and participation in hemiplegic cerebral palsy: a systematic review. *J Physiother*. 2016;62(3):130–7.

16. Koman LA, Smith BP. Surgical management of the wrist in children with cerebral palsy and traumatic brain injury. *Hand (N Y)*. 2014;9(4):471–7.

17. Farag SM, Mohammed MO, El-Sobky TA, ElKadery NA, ElZohiery AK. Botulinum toxin A injection in treatment of upper limb spasticity in children with cerebral palsy: a systematic review of randomized controlled trials. *JBJS Rev*. 2020;8(3):e0119.

18. Smitherman JA, Davids JR, Tanner S, *et al*. Functional outcomes following single-event multilevel surgery of the upper extremity for children with hemiplegic cerebral palsy. *J Bone Joint Surg Am*. 2011;93(7):655–61.

19. Monbaliu E, Himmelmann K, Lin JP, *et al*. Clinical presentation and management of dyskinetic cerebral palsy. *Lancet Neurol*. 2017;16(9): 741–9.

Gait Analysis and Orthoses

Jennifer Walsh, Syed Kazmi, and Tahani Al Ali

Gait Analysis

Gait analysis is an essential orthopaedic skill. It represents a *dynamic* complement to *static* clinical examination. It is important to remember that gait by observation requires no more equipment than stereoscopic vision. As with all other skills, it requires persistence, reflection, and experience to master.

There are several useful commonly used descriptors in any form of gait analysis. The five prerequisites of normal gait (Perry) are:

1. Stability in stance
2. Foot clearance in swing
3. Pre-positioning of the foot in swing
4. Adequate step length
5. Energy conservation.

Energy is conserved by:

1. Minimizing excursion of the centre of gravity
2. Control of momentum (eccentric contraction)
3. Transfer of energy between the limb and body segments.

The **gait cycle** describes distinct stages from the point when one foot strikes the floor to the point when that same foot next strikes the floor. It is usually described in ordinary walking but can be modified for running.

There are two phases:

- **Stance phase** – when the foot is in contact with the floor (60% of the cycle); starts with the initial contact
- **Swing phase** – when the foot is not in contact with the floor (40% of the cycle); starts from toe off and ends with the next initial contact.

Confusion often arises when considering the other foot – which is doing the same cycle of stance and swing, but offset so that the swing starts at 10% into the first leg's cycle and initial contact at 50%. Two periods of **double support** are described when both feet are in contact with the floor, each representing 10% of the cycle. Running is defined when double support gives way to **double float** when both feet are off the floor at the same time.

In the gait cycle, there are seven events which divide the gait cycle into seven periods, four of which occur in the stance phase and three in the swing phase (Table 18c.1; Figure 18c.1).

Gait analysis should be considered in the three-dimensional planes (sagittal, coronal, and transverse). Although the sagittal plane is probably the most important, where most of the movement takes place, some pathologies is evident in other planes such as the Trendelenburg gait in the coronal plane and in-toeing in the transverse plane (Figure 18c.2).

Gait by Observation

It is possible to assess gait by simple observation (Table 18c.2). It is good practice to assess posture (and balance) standing at rest and then the gait walking up and down a corridor (most clinic rooms are not large enough to establish a normal gait pattern). Assess gait both shod (with orthoses fitted where appropriate) and unshod.

The Three Rockers of the Foot

It is important to have a comprehensive understanding of the three rockers of the foot (a common exam question!). Be careful about casually commenting on them as a throw-away remark, especially if it is something you really know very little about.

During the stance phase, the foot progresses through three 'rocker' periods, beginning with the heel strike and ending with the toe-off (Figure 18c.3). In the first rocker, the heel touches the ground. Eccentric contraction of the ankle dorsiflexors allows the ankle to plantar flex in a controlled manner. In the second rocker, the tibia rolls forward over the talus to permit continued forward movement of the body. The foot remains planted throughout the second rocker. In the third rocker, the foot is planter flexed through the ankle and the MTPJs, culminating in the event of toe-off.

Table 18c.1 Gait cycle: seven events, seven periods, and two phases

Phases	Events	Periods
Stance phase	Initial contact	Loading response
	Opposite toes off	Mid stance
	Heel rise	Terminal stance
	Opposite initial contact	Pre-swing
Swing phase	Toe off	Initial swing
	Feet adjacent	Mid swing
	Tibia vertical	Terminal swing

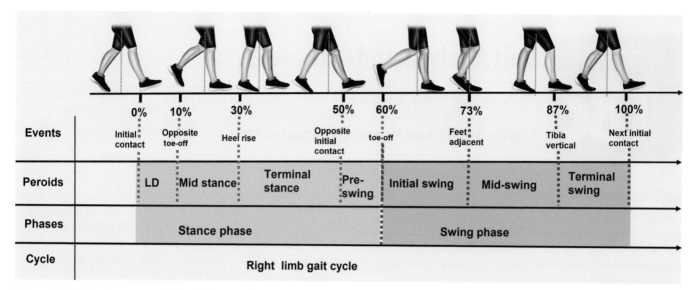

Figure 18c.1 Gait cycle events, periods, and phases. Initial contact: the first point of contact of a given foot with the floor, which denotes the start of the loading response period (LD), in which there is deceleration and energy absorption. This period represents the first double support (both feet on the ground) and ends when the opposite big toe leaves the ground. The mid-stance phase comprises the end of the first rocker and the whole second rocker, and ends with the heel rise. The terminal stance coincides with the third rocker of the foot and ends with the opposite initial contact. Pre-swing: this represents the second double support period and ends with the toe-off. Initial swing period: there is acceleration of the swinging leg (like a pendulum); it starts with the toe-off and finishes with the feet adjacent to each other. Mid swing: transition to the terminal swing – deceleration of the swinging leg, as it is pre-positioned for stance, and it finishes with the tibia vertical. The last period is the terminal swing which ends with the next initial contact.

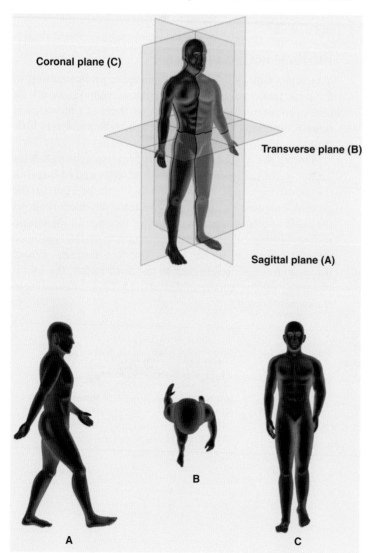

Figure 18c.2 Reprogramme your brain to think about gait analysis in the three dimensions: sagittal, coronal, and transverse. Start by learning the sagittal plane first!

Table 18c.2 A simple framework for observing gait

Parts	What to look for?		
	Sagittal	**Coronal**	**Transverse**
Foot and ankle	The three rockers of the foot		Foot progression angle
Knee	Does it bend as expected? Straight at initial contact and 60° Flexion at mid swing?	Is there lateral thrust?	Patellar progression angle
Hip	Does it bend as expected? Flexed to 40° at initial contact and extended at 20° at toe-off		
Pelvis		The swinging side should rise up?	
Body		No excessive lateral bend	
Arms	Swing straight, matching the opposite lower limb		

With a bit of practice, you can get all the above information within a minute of observing the gait.
The empty squares are not easy to analyse by observation; three-dimensional computerized gait analysis can help.
Does it fit the recognized pathological gait patterns? Then say it!
Always correlate between the gait observation and the subsequent clinical examination.

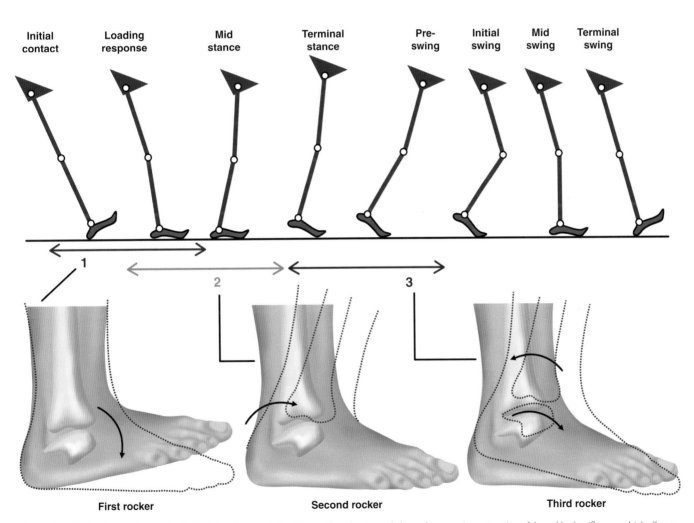

Figure 18c.3 The three rockers of the foot. First rocker (heel): the heel touches the ground, through eccentric contraction of the ankle dorsiflexors, which allows the ankle to plantar flex in a controlled manner. Second rocker (ankle): the tibia rolls forward over the talus to permit continued forward movement of the body. Third rocker (forefoot): the foot is plantar flexed through the ankle and the metatarsophalangeal joints, culminating in the event of toe-off.

The first (heel) rocker may be absent or shortened with a tight tendo Achilles (failure of heel strike) or weak tibialis anterior (poor control and a slapping foot, foot drop).

The second (ankle) rocker may be abnormal with ankle osteoarthritis, stiffness, or ankle fusion. It may be shortened in severe equinus. The third rocker may be abnormal if the gastro–soleus muscle is weak or there is forefoot pathology such as hallux rigidus.

Three-Dimensional Instrumented Gait Analysis

This involves the addition of technology to support gait by observation.

There are several proprietary systems. A compliant patient is essential – usually this means the child is at least 5 years old and 1 m tall (or taller).

Essentially the 'laboratory' is a predefined space through which the patient moves. Landmarks on the patient (such as the anterior superior iliac spine) are identified to the cameras around the room by means of markers attached to the skin. A computer program recreates an electronic three-dimensional image of the patient's movements, usually synchronously with orthogonal video image capture. Movement (kinematic) data are supplemented by data from force plates embedded in the floor of the laboratory to generate moments, powers, and ground reaction forces (kinetics). Kinetic data can only be reliably captured in those who are able to walk unaided. Once crutches or frames are used, the load distributed through the force plate becomes meaningless.

The technique can be further supplemented with EMGs to evaluate whether a given muscle is firing in a predicted fashion or not (e.g. the rectus femoris frequently exhibits inappropriate activity or 'cospasticity' in CP and is thought to be responsible for a 'stiff kneed gait' in such individuals).

Data generated from three-dimensional instrumented gait analysis are superficially bewildering but generally follow a conformed layout, often displayed in specially designed viewing software such as Polygon®. Data include:

1. Patient demographics
2. Temporal data:
   a. Velocity
   b. Step length (distance between the two feet)
   c. Stride length (distance between the two initial contacts of the same foot = sum of both step lengths)
3. Video footage – orthogonal video of walking – can be slowed and repeated as often as required; can be a very useful way to see more than the eye can comprehend at normal walking speeds
4. Kinematics – represent graphs of each limb motion captured in three planes (sagittal, coronal, and axial) (Figure 18c.4). The x-axis is time, and the y-axis is the magnitude and direction of the motion of a given segment when compared to the more proximal segment.

Traditionally, the pelvis, hip, knee, and foot and ankle are used. On each graph, there are two lines (one for each limb) and a normal range. Sometimes there are additional lines representing the use of orthoses or comparator data from previous gait laboratory sessions. Figure 18c.5 explains how to describe these kinematic charts in the exam, and Figure 18c.6 explains how abnormalities may look on these charts in a simplified way.

5. Kinetic graphs are usually displayed on a second screen (Figure 18c.7). The x-axis still represents time, but the y-axis demonstrates moments and power generated and absorbed. These charts help to examine the mechanisms that either control or produce the motion, developing a more comprehensive understanding of the motion. A detailed description is beyond the exam syllabus.

There remains significant scepticism in the orthopaedic community over the value of instrumented gait analysis. Much like an MRI scan, it is not self-interpretive and is dependent on observers for its analysis. Interpretation is hampered by:

- **Patient** variability of a given individual's gait pattern
- The **equipment** – reliability of marker placement (some output data are very vulnerable to magnified error due to misplaced markers; for example, when orthoses are worn, then landmarks are covered and marker placement error increases)
- The **interpreter** – there is an evolving understanding of 'what is normal?' and 'what does deviation from normal mean?'.

Nevertheless, it does represent an attempt to gather objective data where otherwise none exists. Attending a data gathering and analysis session is a useful introduction to the technique. Studying a set of normal walking data alongside the gait cycle will give a deeper appreciation of the data.

Orthoses
Terminology

Orthosis is derived from the Greek word 'Ortho' meaning straight, upright, or correct. Orthoses are externally applied devices used to modify the structural and functional characteristics of the neuromuscular and skeletal systems. Orthotics is the science and art involved in treating patients by use of an orthosis. An orthotist is a qualified professional having completed an approved course of education and training to clinically assess and prescribe the design, and measure and fit orthoses.

Orthoses are described by the joints they encompass. An orthosis that modifies the foot and ankle is called an ankle–foot orthosis (AFO). If the orthosis extends to the knee, it is called KAFO. HKAFO is the name of an orthosis that modifies the hip, knee, ankle, and foot. TLSO stands for thoracic, lumbar, and sacral orthosis, and so on.

KINEMATIC

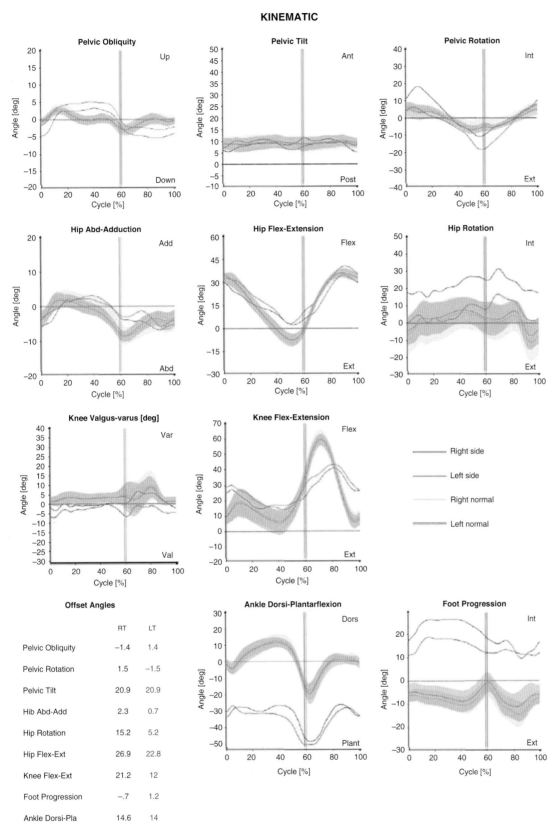

Figure 18c.4 Kinematic graphs for a child with cerebral palsy. In this example, the charts are displayed as coronal, sagittal, and transverse from left to right, respectively, and the pelvis, hip, knee, and ankle from top to bottom, respectively. Traditionally, the left limb is displayed as a red line, and the right limb as a blue line. The grey shaded area represents the normal range. The x-axis is the time in the gait cycle, with the 60% mark representing the start of the swing phase. The y-axis is the magnitude and direction of the motion of a given segment, with '0' denoting the neutral position of that particular segment. The charts show that this child walks on his toes with significant in-toeing, and he has a stiff knee gait and a Trendelenburg gait. Did you spot these?

A

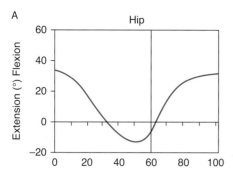

B

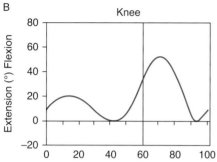

C

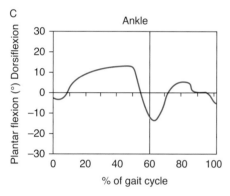

% of gait cycle

Figure 18c.5 Kinematic graphs of a hip, knee, and ankle in the sagittal plane. Each rectangle represents one gait cycle (100%), divided into the stance phase (60%) and the swing phase (40%). (A) represents the hip joint motion; the hip extends and flexes once in each gait cycle. At the initial contact (IC), the hip is flexed to 35° and starts extending to about −15° just before the swing phase starts, then flexes back to 35° as it approaches the next IC. (B) shows the knee motion, which involves two flexion and two extension peaks during each gait cycle. The knee is extended at the IC, flexes during the loading response (LR), reaching a peak of about 20° in the mid-stance phase, then extends fully again at the end of the mid stance, before starting to flex again, reaching a peak of about 60° during the initial swing phase. It extends again prior to the next IC. (C) represents the ankle joint movement, which is a bit more complex than that of the other two joints. It is neutral at the IC, followed by plantar flexion to bring the foot flat on the ground (first rocker). During the mid stance, the tibia moves forward over the foot and the ankle joint becomes dorsiflexed (second rocker). Towards the end of the stance phase, the ankle joint plantar flexes to propel the body forward, using the forefoot as a fulcrum (the third rocker). During the swing phase, the ankle dorsiflexes again to clear the ground, after which it plantar flexes to the neutral position, preparing the foot for the next IC.

Key Points: Old Terminology

- Braces – a device fitted to a weak or injured part of the body to give support (French 'bracier' meaning embrace)
- Corset – a tightly fitting laced or stiffened outer bodice (eighteenth-century diminutive of 'corps' or body, from the Latin word 'corpus')
- Splint – a strip of rigid material used for supporting and immobilizing a broken bone when it has been set (German 'splinte' meaning metal plate or pin)
- Calipers – a metal support for a person's leg (sixteenth century).

These devices are identified by names – or eponyms – derived from the place of origin, the developer, or others. A similar plethora of names are used for braces applied to other parts of the body.

These eponyms frequently do not give the site of application and often give no indication of the function provided. Two braces ordered by one eponym from two suppliers may result in two braces which are significantly different, not only from each other, but also from the description of the original developer. Because the terminology is illogical, use of these named braces can only be learnt by rote.

Indications

Orthoses are used to achieve several objectives:

1. To relieve pain
2. To compensate for abnormalities of the segment length or shape
3. To manage deformities (prevent, reduce, or stabilize a deformity)
4. To prevent an excessive range of joint motion
5. To increase the range of joint motion
6. To reduce or redistribute the load on tissues and promote healing
7. To compensate for weak muscle or control hyperactive muscle.

Duration of use depends on the indications to use them and tolerance to their use. Several problems can be caused by orthoses that may preclude their use. The following are examples:

1. Discomfort
2. Skin breakdown
3. Muscle atrophy with prolonged use

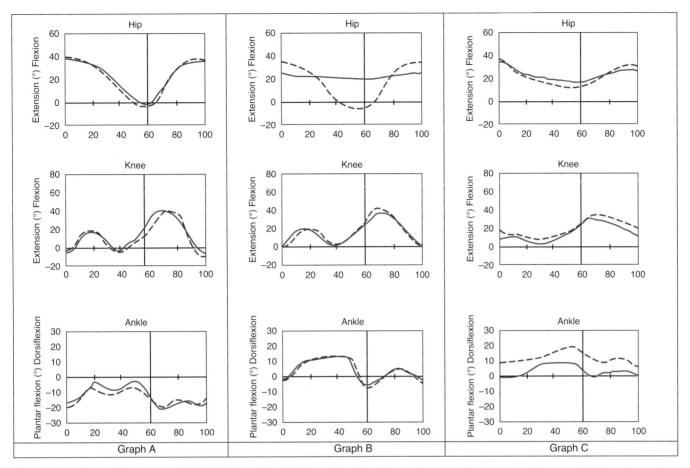

Figure 18c.6 Abnormal kinematic graphs. Graph A shows the ankle does not dorsiflex. Although the range of knee movement is reasonable, there is hyperextension of the knee at the IC and at the end of the mid stance. The hip movement is normal. These features are those of a toe walker. Graph B shows the left hip movement remains constant at around 25°, giving the impression that the hip is fused. Graph C shows all joints (hip, knee, and ankle) are flexed throughout the gait cycle and the range of movement is reduced – features of the crouch gait. These have to be correlated with the history, examination, video analysis, moment, and power graphs, as well as electromyography.

4. Local pain
5. Nerve compression
6. Possible increase in energy expenditure with ambulation
7. Difficulty with transfers
8. Difficulty with donning and doffing of orthosis
9. Psychological and physical dependency
10. Poor patient compliance.

Design Characteristics

The design of orthosis must be based on the concept of 'FUNCTION WITHOUT DYSFUNCTION'. It means there must be:

- Improved function
- Less energy expenditure
- Increased endurance.

The orthosis can be:

- Prefabricated – available off the shelf
- Customized – designed for a specific problem
- Static – without any option to change the angles
- Dynamic – offering joint movement control within ranges.

Several considerations are taken when choosing a specific design:

1. Cosmesis
2. Cost
3. Adjustability
4. Durability
5. Materials
6. Ability to fit various sizes of patients
7. Ease of putting on and taking off
8. Access to surgical sites for wound care
9. Aeration to avoid skin breakdown.

The following section covers the most commonly used orthoses in the neuromuscular orthopaedic clinic that may feature in the FRCS exam.

Ankle–Foot Orthosis

Four different types of AFOs are commonly used: solid AFO, hinged AFO, posterior leaf spring AFO, and GRAFO (Figure 18c.8).

The effect of solid AFOs on gait is summarized in Table 18c.3.

KINETICS

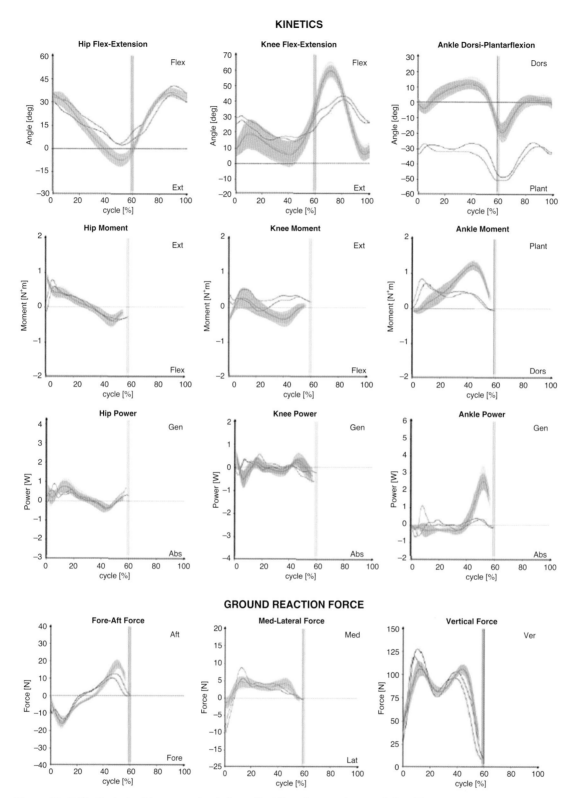

Figure 18c.7 Kinetic charts of the same patient in Figure 18c.4. These focus on the sagittal plane. The top row represents kinematic charts (see above); the middle row represents moments (N.m) and the power generated or absorbed. These are calculated through complex physical equations, utilizing the ground reaction forces measured by the force plate.

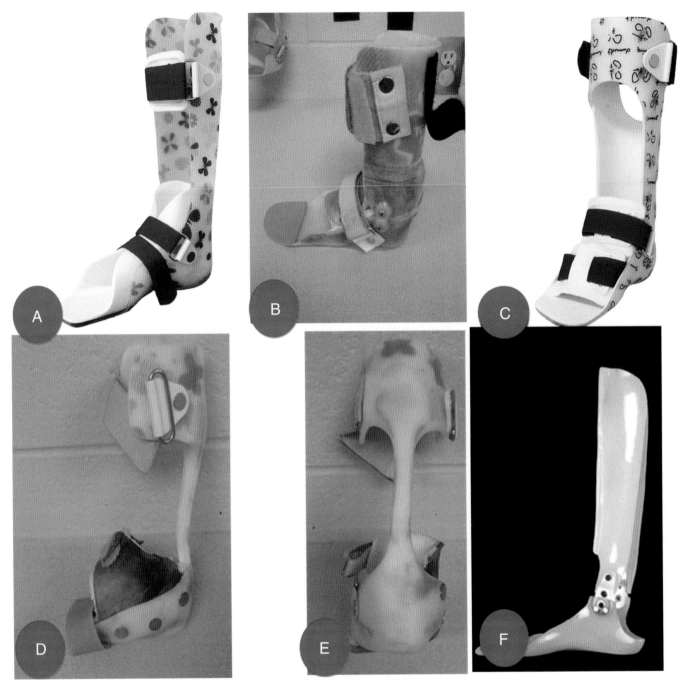

Figure 18c.8 Various types of ankle–foot orthoses (AFOs). (A) Solid AFO. (B) Hinged AFO. (C) GRAFO. (D, E) Posterior leaf spring AFO. (F) Hinged GRAFO. Notice that a hinged AFO allows ankle dorsiflexion, whereas a hinged GRAFO allows plantar flexion.

Table 18c.3 Effect of solid AFOs on gait

Ankle range of motion	Block dorsiflexion Block plantar flexion Block inversion and eversion	
Foot rockers	First rocker	Blocked
	Second rocker	Blocked
	Third rocker	Blocked
Effect on knee	Provide limited knee extension moment (useful in mild crouch gait)	

Table 18c.4 Effects of hinged AFOs on gait

Ankle range of motion	Allow dorsiflexion	
	Block plantar flexion	
	Resist inversion and eversion	
Foot rockers	First rocker	Blocked
	Second rocker	Allowed
	Third rocker	Blocked
	Swing phase	1. Maintain plantar grade
		2. Resist plantar flexion spasm
		3. Provide heel strike
Effect on knee	1. Resist hyperextension (prevent knee recurvatum deformity associated with equinus deformity or spasticity)	
	2. Reduce plantar flexion, knee extension couple (make crouch gait worse)	

Use of solid AFOs has many useful functions in children with CP. They cause passive stretching of the gastrocnemius muscle, protect against mid-foot deformity, and provide knee extension moment to improve crouch gait. In spina bifida, they support flail or calcaneus feet. Contraindications for solid AFOs include:

1. Severe crouch gait
2. Fixed varus
3. Fixed equinus.

Use of hinged AFOs is similar to solid AFOs, but they are preferable when the equinus is correctable or in swing only (better stretching for the gastrocnemius muscle than with solid AFOs). Hinged AFOs do not cause knee hyperextension deformity. They are contraindicated in crouch gait or fixed equinus (Table 18c.4). Posterior leaf spring AFOs are the first choice for pure foot drop secondary to tibialis anterior weakness with no deformity or spasticity, as they strike the right balance between size, weight, and the desired objective (Table 18c.5).

GRAFOs provide the same functions as solid AFOs in the frontal plane. However, in the sagittal plane, they provide significant knee extension moment during the weight-bearing/stance phase (Table 18c.6). These can be an excellent alterative to a KAFO design for patients with weak quadriceps, as they can achieve knee stability whilst maintaining efficiency by reducing weight and bulkiness. The main indication is crouch gait.

The hinged designs may help in allowing for a more normal gait by not unnecessarily blocking plantar flexion. The following are important considerations/contraindications for GRAFOs:

1. Recurvatum or unstable knee
2. Knee extension moment compromised with external foot rotation in excess of 25°
3. Presence of knee flexion contractures exceeding 15°
4. Must be able to get the ankle to a neutral or slight plantar flexion
5. Minimum of fair quadriceps strength needed if applied bilaterally (because the sound side allows the patient to know where they are placing the affected side)
6. Presence of some trunk balance needed or ability to use the walking side.

Supramalleolar Foot Orthosis

The supramalleolar foot orthosis (SMO) supports the foot just above the ankle bone (malleoli, hence the name) (Figure 18c.9). It is less bulky than the AFO and often preferred by parents and patients with mild CP. It is designed to maintain a vertical, or neutral, heel whilst protecting against mid-foot break.

Table 18c.5 Effects of posterior leaf spring AFOs on gait

Ankle range of motion	Allow dorsiflexion	
	Resist plantar flexion	
Foot rockers	First rocker	Resisted
	Second rocker	Allowed
	Third rocker	Partially blocked
	Swing phase	1. Control foot drop
		2. Provide toe clearance
Effect on knee	None	

Table 18c.6 Effects of posterior ground reaction AFOs on gait

Ankle range of motion	Block dorsiflexion	
	Block plantar flexion (unless hinged GRAFOs)	
	Resist inversion and eversion	
Foot rockers	First rocker	Blocked
	Second rocker	Blocked
	Third rocker	Blocked (unless hinged GRAFOs)
	Swing phase	1. Maintain plantar grade
		2. Resist PF spasm
		3. Provide heel strike
Effect on knee	Provide knee extension moment, increasing plantar flexion, knee extension couple	

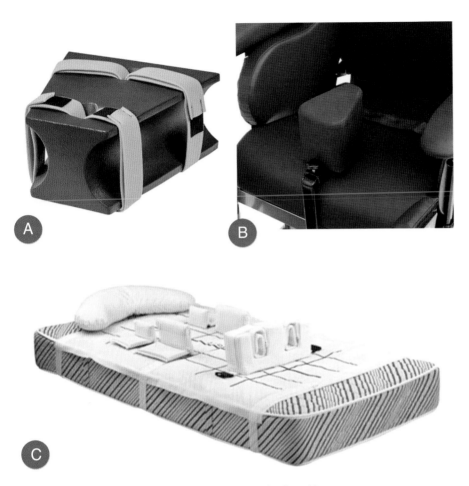

Figure 18c.9 Abduction wedges and sleeping systems to maintain position.

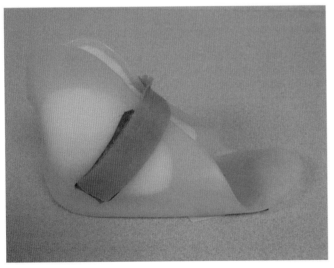

Figure 18c.10 Supramalleolar foot orthosis. This can be worn alone or inside an AFO.

Knee Braces (Hinged or Non-hinged)

These are often used after knee surgery on a temporary basis until healing is achieved or strength is regained.

Hip Abduction Wedges

These are designed to keep the hips in an abducted position to minimize hip dislocation (Figure 18c.10). They can be used during sleep, or built in the chair whilst sitting. Several commercially available sleeping systems that incorporate various orthoses to maintain different body part positions are now available. However, their use is hampered by the inconvenience and discomfort they cause to patients.

19

Musculoskeletal Infection

Mark Gaston, Richard Gardner, and Simon Kelley

Background

Bone and joint infections in children are often surgical emergencies. The following will be discussed in this chapter:

1. Septic arthritis and the differentiation from transient synovitis
2. Acute and chronic osteomyelitis.

Septic Arthritis

Septic arthritis is an intra-articular microbial infection of the joint. It typically affects large joints, such as the hip (35%), knee (35%), and ankle (10%), although other joints may be affected. Usually only one joint is affected, but multiple joint involvement has been reported.

It is commoner in the younger child (50% are <2 years), although children of all ages may get septic arthritis. Premature and immunocompromised children are at greater risk, as are children in the ICU who may have multiple lines and other sources of infection.

Aetiology

Septic arthritis may be the result of:

1. Haematogenous spread from an infective focus elsewhere in the body via the bloodstream (commonest mechanism)
2. Local spread from adjacent bone or soft tissue infection (i.e. osteomyelitis)
3. Direct seeding into a joint following surgery or penetrating trauma.

In early infancy, before the formation of the growth plate, the transphyseal blood vessels may act as a route for transfer of bacteria into the joint. In the hip, elbow, and shoulder joints, septic arthritis may develop after metaphyseal osteomyelitis, as the metaphysis of these joints is intra-articular. This is not the case for the knee.

The organisms that cause septic arthritis are depicted in Table 19.1 [1]. *Staphylococcus aureus* is the commonest (56%) and group A *Streptococcus* is usually observed after chickenpox [2].

Clinical Features

- Constitutional upset (fever, malaise, anorexia)
- Joint effusion, overlying erythema, restricted range of movement
- Loss of function: if a lower limb joint is involved, the child may limp or be unable to walk. In the infant, the only positive local sign may be 'pseudoparalysis'– a lack of active movement of the affected limb.

Investigations

Clinical suspicion should be combined with blood tests and imaging to confirm the diagnosis.

Blood Tests

Tests for full blood count with differential, erythrocyte sedimentation rate (ESR), and C-reactive protein (CRP) should be taken, and blood cultures obtained. The latter should be repeated during any temperature spikes. The white blood cell count may be raised in only 30–60% of cases. The level of CRP is elevated early

Table 19.1 Causative organisms in septic arthritis

Group	Causative organism[a]	
Neonates	Group B *Streptococcus*, *S. aureus*[b], *Escherichia coli*, *Haemophilus influenzae* (now rare due to immunization)	
Early childhood (up to 3 years)	*S. aureus*, *Kingella kingae*[c], *Streptococcus pneumoniae*, *Neisseria meningitides*	
Childhood (3–12 years)	*S. aureus*, group A β-haemolytic *Streptococcus*	
Adolescence (12–18 years)	*S. aureus*, group A β-haemolytic *Streptococcus*, *Neisseria gonorrhoeae*	
Other groups[d]	Sickle cell	*Salmonella* species
	Foot puncture	*Pseudomonas aeruginosa*
	Following varicella infection (chickenpox)	Group A *Streptococcus*

[a] There is an increasing incidence of methicillin-resistant *S. aureus* (MRSA) across all age groups.
[b] *S. aureus* is the commonest cause of musculoskeletal infections of all types in all age groups.
[c] *K. kingae* is a fastidious, aerobic, Gram-negative bacillus that is increasingly noted to be a major cause of osteomyelitis and septic arthritis in children under 4 years. It can be cultured in aerobic blood culture bottles and PCR techniques have been described to aid diagnosis [3].
[d] The mentioned organisms should be considered, although there is evidence that they may not be the commonest.

on in the disease process and normalizes within a week of effective treatment; hence, this marker is effective in monitoring response to treatment. In contrast, ESR may take 24–48 hours to elevate and 3 weeks to normalize.

Procalcitonin (PCT) is another infection marker that has become increasingly popular in musculoskeletal infection. PCT has greater specificity than CRP in identifying patients with bacterial infection. It is still expensive and not widely available [4, 5].

Ultrasonography

This is the first-line imaging modality for septic arthritis. It is useful in determining the presence of a joint effusion (Figure 19.1). Findings of intra-capsular debris and synovial and capsular thickening can help to differentiate septic arthritis from transient synovitis [6, 7], although this is not reliable enough to determine treatment [8].

X-rays

In septic arthritis, plain radiographs help to exclude other diagnoses but may also show indirect evidence of an effusion, for example, joint space widening of the hip or fat pad sign (Figure 19.2). Soft tissue swelling may be seen early on, but bone changes often take 2 weeks or longer to become evident (Figure 19.3).

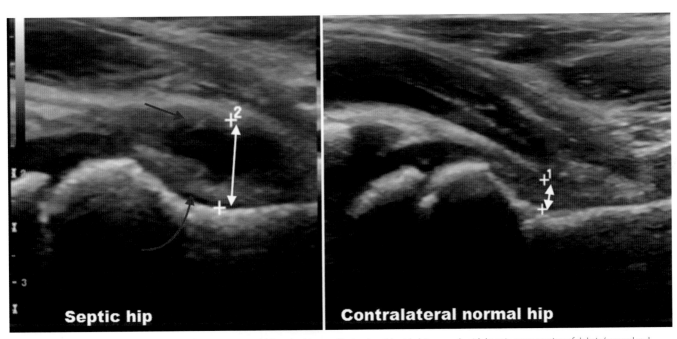

Figure 19.1 Ultrasound images of the right hip in a 3-year-old female. A large effusion is evident (white arrow), with layering suggestive of debris (curved red arrow). Capsular thickening (straight red arrow) is also evident.

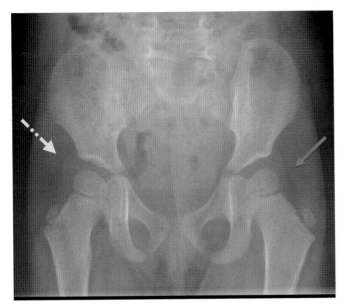

Figure 19.2 Plain X-ray of a limping child. She was not able to put weight on the right hip. The X-ray shows that the bones are normal-looking. There is ballooning of the hip fat pad on the right side (dashed yellow line) in comparison to the left (solid blue arrow).

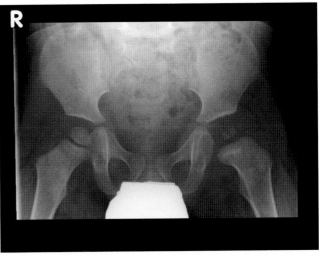

Figure 19.3 Septic arthritis of the left hip, with bony changes of the ossific nucleus. Subluxation or dislocation of the joints can also be seen when there is delayed treatment.

Magnetic Resonance Imaging

MRI should be considered if the clinical picture is not convincing or ultrasonography fails to reveal a joint effusion, as it may reveal features of osteomyelitis or other abnormalities such as a tumour.

Aspiration

Joint aspiration should be performed when joint sepsis is suspected, and ideally prior to administration of antibiotics (but it should not delay antibiotic administration if the child is very sick). Aspiration of the hip must be done with sterile precautions, ideally in the operating room, with use of ultrasonography or an image intensifier (Figure 19.4 and Video 19.1).

 Video 19.1 Joint aspiration.

Gram staining may confirm the presence of organisms. Cell counts of >50 000/ml, with >75% of white polymorphonuclear (PMN) cells in the aspirate are suggestive of sepsis. Positive Gram staining is noted in only 30% of cases of confirmed joint sepsis (Table 19.2).

 Video 19.2 The string test.

Differential Diagnosis

1. Transient synovitis
2. Osteomyelitis
3. Juvenile rheumatoid arthritis (JRA).

Transient synovitis (aseptic inflammation of the synovium) often has a similar presentation to that of septic arthritis in the early stages, but typically runs a benign course and does not require treatment. It is therefore essential to differentiate it from septic arthritis.

In a study of 282 patients, Kocher and colleagues identified four independent predictors to differentiate between transient synovitis and septic arthritis [9]. These are:

1. Fever (>38.5°C)
2. Inability to weight-bear
3. ESR >40 mm hr^{-1}
4. WBC >12 000/μl.

This was a retrospective study comparing patients with septic arthritis (defined as either a positive finding on culture of the joint fluid or a WBC in the joint fluid of at least 50 000 cells/mm³, with or without positive findings on blood culture) to those with transient synovitis (defined as a WBC in the joint fluid of <50 000 cells/mm³, with negative findings on culture and resolution of symptoms without antimicrobial therapy).

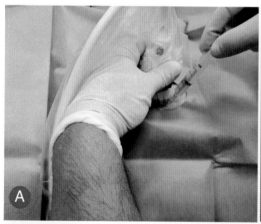
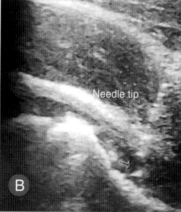
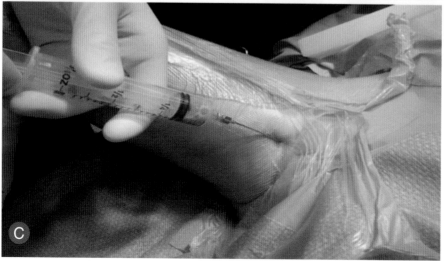

Figure 19.4 Hip aspiration under ultrasound guidance (A, B) and under fluoroscopy screening (C). The patients in (A) and (B) did not have septic arthritis, but the patient in (C), in whom a purulent fluid was obtained, had confirmed *S. aureus* septic arthritis.

Table 19.2 Characteristics of synovial fluids in different conditions

Characteristics	Normal	Non-inflammatory	Inflammatory	Septic[a]
Clarity[b]	Transparent	Transparent	Cloudy	Cloudy
Colour	Clear	Yellow	Yellow	Yellow
Viscosity[c]	Normal	Normal	Low	Low
WBC/ml	<200	200–2000	200–50 000	>50 000
PMN cells (%)	<25	<25	>50	>75
Cultures	Negative	Negative	Negative	Positive (in <50% of cases
Crystals	None	None	Multiple or none	None
Associated conditions		OA, trauma	Gout, pseudogout, JRA	Infection

[a] There is an overlap in composition between conditions. High lactic acid and low glucose levels (50 mg dl^{-1} less than blood levels) have been associated with septic arthritis.
[b] The fluid is considered turbid when the writing on the syringe or container cannot be seen through it (Figure 19.5).
[c] String test: synovial fluid dripping from a syringe in the form of a long string (10–15 cm) indicates normal viscosity, whereas fluid falling as free droplets indicates low viscosity (Figure 19.5 and Video 19.2).WBC, white blood cell count; PMN, polymorphonuclear; OA, osteoarthritis; JRA, juvenile rheumatoid arthritis.

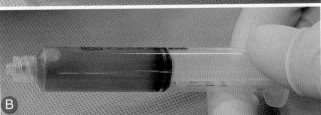

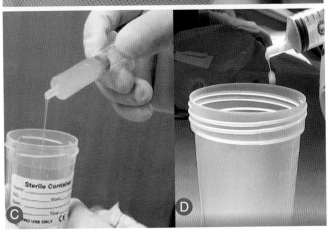

Figure 19.5 Synovial fluid characteristics. (A) and (B) show a turbid synovial fluid where the syringe writing cannot be seen through the fluid. (C) shows normal viscosity of the synovial fluid, whereas (D) shows infected synovial fluid that was aspirated from a child's elbow with septic arthritis (string test).

The predicted probability of septic arthritis with one predictor was 3%, two predictors 40%, three predictors 93%, and four predictors 99.6%. Kocher *et al.* validated their criteria prospectively in a later study and showed relatively similar findings [8, 10]. Caird *et al.* noted that the level of CRP (>20 mg l^{-1}) was another independent predictor for septic arthritis of the hip [11]. Table 19.3 summarizes the findings from these three studies. Other authors have used these criteria and found the predictive value to be less reliable [12].

A rare, but important, differential diagnosis is JRA, which is an autoimmune disease with an incidence of about 5 in 100 000. It is not unusual for patients to present initially with single joint involvement. The WBC and inflammatory markers are usually raised. The synovial fluid is usually turbid, but sterile. The WBC in the synovial fluid is usually high, but often <50 000, with high lymphocyte counts. Uveitis is a serious associated problem in JRA and may affect the child's vision; therefore, having a high degree of suspicion and making an early referral to a rheumatologist and an ophthalmologist are regarded as good practice.

Treatment

Management of septic arthritis is considered an orthopaedic emergency. Joint destruction is closely associated with time to treatment. Bacteria and leucocytes release proteolytic enzymes (matrix metalloproteinases), resulting in rapid cartilage breakdown, inflammatory effusion, and joint destruction.

Once the diagnosis is confirmed, prompt surgical drainage and administration of intravenous antibiotics are required to prevent permanent damage to the joint (Figure 19.6 and Video 19.3) A delay in acquiring an ultrasound scan should not delay surgical drainage. Open surgical lavage remains the gold standard; however, this may be done arthroscopically.

The initial antibiotic coverage should be broad-spectrum, in line with local microbiology guidelines. This is administered once joint fluid has been acquired for urgent Gram staining, unless the child is haemodynamically unstable, in which case the child should be resuscitated with fluids and antibiotics commenced immediately. Positive Gram staining is observed in about 30% of cases of septic arthritis.

 Video 19.3 Hip joint septic arthritis washout.

Table 19.3 Predictors for septic arthritis

Predictors	Number of predictors	Predicted probability of septic arthritis *(%)*		
		Kocher *et al.*, 1999 [9]	Kocher *et al.*, 2004 [10]	Caird *et al.*, 2005 [11]
Fever (>38.5°C)	0	0.2	2	16.9
Inability to weight-bear	1	3	9.5	36.7
ESR >40 mm hr⁻¹	2	40	35	62.4
WBC >12 000/µl	3	93.1	72.8	82.6
Fever (>38.5°C)	4	99.6	93	93.1
CRP (>20 mg l⁻¹)	5			97.5

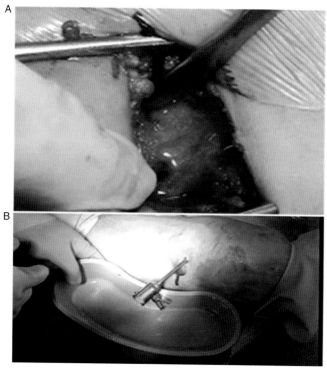

Figure 19.6 Joint washout. (A) shows open washout of the hip joint, and (B) shows arthroscopic washout of the knee joint.

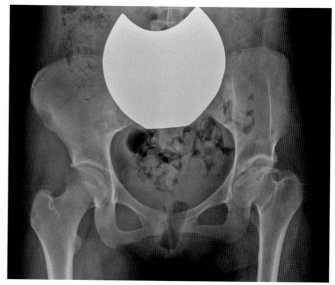

Figure 19.7 Long-term complication of septic arthritis with osteoarthritic changes, including an abnormally shaped head, narrowing of joint space, subchondral bone sclerosis, and bone cysts.

The initial antibiotic regimen is altered, based on culture sensitivities. Drains and immobilization of the joint are not advisable. Antibiotics are administered for a period of 3–6 weeks, depending on response to treatment and local antimicrobial policies.

If the response is not as good as expected or worsens after treatment, the following must be considered:

1. Associated osteomyelitis (get an MRI scan)
2. Resistant organism (chase culture, consult a microbiologist)
3. Ineffective washout and debridement
4. Immunocompromised child (consult an immunologist)
5. Coexistent or untreated deep tissue infection/pyomyositis (MRI scan needed)
6. Haemophagocytic lymphohistiocytosis (HLH) – rare, but can be fatal (consult a haematologist)

Sequelae of septic arthritis include:

1. Chondral damage

2. Avascular necrosis
3. Growth arrest, angular deformity, leg length discrepancy
4. Degenerative arthritis.

Key Points: Septic Arthritis

1. Early diagnosis is essential for a successful outcome.
2. Although Kocher's criteria and investigations are important, diagnosis is clinical as all investigations may be normal. If in doubt, wash out!

Osteomyelitis

Osteomyelitis usually occurs in the first decade of life and predominantly involves the lower extremities: 27% of cases occur in the femur, 26% in the tibia, 9% in the pelvis, and 8% in the humerus [13]. It may be acute, subacute (<3 weeks), or chronic (Figure 19.8).

Pathogenesis

Children have a predisposition to developing osteomyelitis. Reasons include:

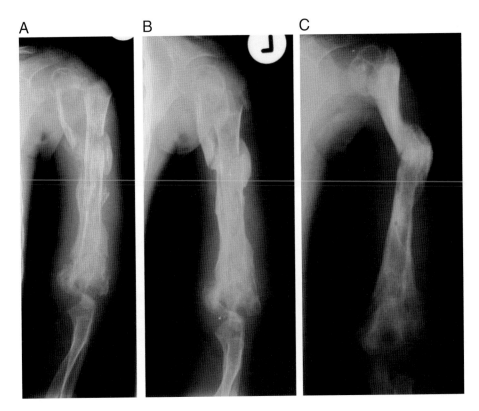

Figure 19.8 Chronic osteomyelitis of the humerus in a 4-year-old boy. The entire diaphysis was sequestrated. The involucrum can be seen to develop in (A) and (B). The sequestrum was removed when the involucrum was deemed to offer structural support.

1. Turbulent, sluggish blood flow due to vascular loops in the metaphysis
2. Relative paucity of reticulo-endothelial cells adjacent to the physis
3. Increased blood flow.

Acute haematogenous osteomyelitis has a predilection for the metaphysis of long bones where sluggish blood flow causes blood-borne organisms to be deposited. A collection may form in the metaphysis, resulting in thrombosis of the endosteal blood vessels. Localized bone is resorbed through a combination of osteoblast death and osteoclast activation. The release of prostaglandin E_2 stimulates further resorption [14].

The metaphyseal cortex is thin and pus may penetrate it, resulting in a subperiosteal abscess. This, in turn, deprives the cortex of periosteal blood supply. If effective management is not instituted, the segment of the cortex becomes necrotic and forms a sequestrum. The periosteum, however, retains osteogenic properties and new bone is laid down – the involucrum. The sequestrum and involucrum are the hallmarks of chronic osteomyelitis.

In the neonate, vascular channels from the metaphysis link into the epiphysis. Osteomyelitis in the metaphysis can result in thrombosis of these vessels, leading to severe osteonecrosis of the epiphysis. With development of the femoral ossific nucleus, both the epiphyseal and metaphyseal blood supply become independent, with the physis providing a barrier to spread [15, 16].

Clinical Features

These are similar to those of septic arthritis, with pain, limp, and difficulty with weight-bearing. The child, however, does appear toxic and osteomyelitis may be more difficult to differentiate from septic arthritis than from transient synovitis.

Investigations

Blood

These are as for septic arthritis. CRP is the most useful test and its level will be elevated in 98% of cases. It will decline rapidly with response to treatment, and failure to decline should initiate investigations for an alternate diagnosis. ESR will decline more slowly and can be more useful over the longer term or for chronic osteomyelitis. Blood cultures are less often positive, compared to septic arthritis [17].

X-rays

This is often the first imaging investigation done for osteomyelitis. However, bone changes often take 2 weeks or longer to become evident [13], so X-rays are often not helpful in the early stages They are useful for longer-term follow-up.

Ultrasonography

In osteomyelitis, ultrasonography can detect subperiosteal abscesses and help to determine whether surgical intervention is required.

Magnetic Resonance Imaging

This is the gold standard for osteomyelitis and is increasingly used in its detection and for determining treatment (Figure 19.9). It is very helpful when the diagnosis is not clear and importantly it can help to differentiate infection from tumours and other important diagnoses. Careful correlation with the clinical picture is needed, as fractures, bone bruising, and bone infarcts can have a similar appearance. Fat suppression sequences obtained

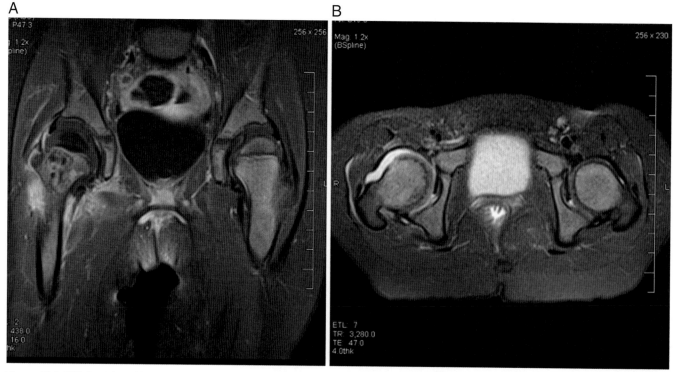

Figure 19.9 MRI of an infected hip. (A) Coronal image demonstrating osteomyelitis in the proximal femoral metaphysis. Reduced signal in the right epiphysis is suggestive of avascular necrosis. (B) Axial view demonstrating right hip effusion.

with gadolinium as a contrast agent highlight marrow changes, whereas abscesses demonstrate rim enhancement [16].

Bone Scan (Technetium-99m)

This is rarely done nowadays but is a good investigation for localizing osteomyelitis. It is especially useful in neonates and in children with multifocal osteomyelitis. Results may be negative in the first 24 hours [18].

Aspiration

Aspiration may be performed in suspected osteomyelitis. Fluid may be aspirated from a subperiosteal abscess, and a large-bore spinal needle can be used to perforate the thin metaphyseal cortex and aspirate a purulent intramedullary collection.

Differential Diagnosis of Osteomyelitis

Osteomyelitis may be mistaken for neoplasia. Leukaemia has similar radiological findings, as well as a frequent presentation of fever, raised ESR/CRP levels, and increased leucocyte counts. A blood film is essential if leukaemia is suspected. Eosinophilic granuloma, Langerhans cell histiocytosis or chronic recurrent and multifocal osteomyelitis (if multiple lesions), Ewing's sarcoma, and osteosarcoma should also be considered.

Treatment

Acute Haematogenous Osteomyelitis

In the absence of an identified collection, intravenous antibiotic therapy is the first-line treatment and, unlike septic arthritis,

this is started empirically. Most centres will have an agreed protocol, and liaison with paediatricians who have an interest in infectious diseases and microbiologists with bone and joint expertise is invaluable [19].

Antibiotic treatment is initially administered intravenously, followed by a period of oral antibiotic treatment. Evidence for the duration of antibiotic therapy is lacking. Traditionally, this is 6 weeks, but decisions on duration will depend on the bacteria identified, response of the patient, temperature, and CRP level [20]. Conversion to oral antibiotics similarly depends upon the resolution of clinical signs. Again, liaison with paediatricians and microbiology colleagues is very helpful [13, 21].

Failure to show signs of improvement with antibiotics suggests either inappropriate antibiotics or the presence of an abscess or a collection. MRI in this situation is very helpful. Attempts should initially be made to confirm that the microorganism is sensitive to the selected antibiotic, especially in this era of increasing methicillin-resistant *S. aureus* (MRSA) and virulent form of *Streptococcus*.

Bone aspiration may be considered to obtain a sample for culture if this is proving elusive. However, these samples will not always yield results, particularly if the patient has already been on broad-spectrum antibiotics.

Identification of a collection or an abscess is an indication for surgery (Figure 19.10). Deep pelvic abscesses (>2 cm) should also be considered for drainage, but assistance from paediatric abdominal surgeons may be needed for these [13, 22].

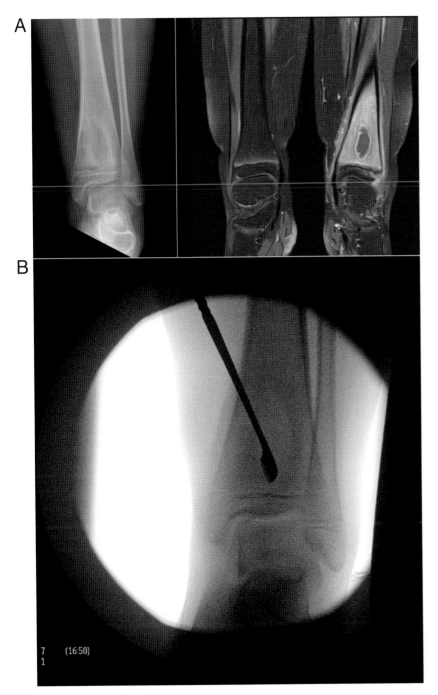

Figure 19.10 Bone abscess (often called Brodie's abscess). (A) shows bony changes in the distal tibia, with MRI revealing a rim-enhanced abscess. (B) shows incision and drainage with careful protection of the growth plate.

Chronic Osteomyelitis

As discussed, the hallmarks of chronic osteomyelitis are the presence of dead bone, the 'sequestrum' and new bone formation from the periosteum, the 'involucrum'. In the majority of cases, chronic osteomyelitis is a surgically managed condition requiring debridement and removal of the sequestrum. Prolonged administration of antibiotics alone will usually not resolve the infection. Careful timing of the sequestrectomy is needed, waiting for the involucrum to provide structural support to the diseased bone. The sequelae of segmental bone loss, limb shortening, physeal growth arrest and recurrent infection are a challenge and often needs reconstructive surgery.

Key Points: Chronic Osteomyelitis

The best treatment for chronic osteomyelitis is prevention by aggressively treating acute bone infection.

References

1. Herring JA. *Tachdjians' Pediatric Orthopaedics*, 5th ed, Vol. 1. Philadelphia, PA: Saunders Elsevier; 2014.

2. Russell CD, *et al.* Microbiological characteristics of acute osteoarticular infections in children. *J Med Microbiol.* 2015;64(Pt 4):446–53.

3. Ceroni D, *et al. Kingella kingae* osteoarticular infections in young children: clinical features and contribution of a new specific real-time PCR assay to the diagnosis. *J Pediatr Orthop.* 2010;30(3):301–4.

4. Maharajan K, *et al.* Serum Procalcitonin is a sensitive and specific marker in the diagnosis of septic arthritis and acute osteomyelitis. *J Orthop Surg Res.* 2013;8:19.

5. Zhao J, *et al.* Serum procalcitonin levels as a diagnostic marker for septic arthritis: a meta-analysis. *Am J Emerg Med.* 2017;35(8):1166–71.

6. Dorr U, Zieger M, Hauke H. [The painful hip – diagnostic possibilities of sonography]. *Rofo.* 1988;148(5):487–91.

7. Dorr U, Zieger M, Hauke H. Ultrasonography of the painful hip. Prospective studies in 204 patients. *Pediatr Radiol.* 1988;19(1):36–40.

8. Zamzam MM. The role of ultrasound in differentiating septic arthritis from transient synovitis of the hip in children. *J Pediatr Orthop B.* 2006;15(6):418–22.

9. Kocher MS, Zurakowski D, Kasser JR. Differentiating between septic arthritis and transient synovitis of the hip in children: an evidence-based clinical prediction algorithm. *J Bone Joint Surg Am.* 1999;81(12):1662–70.

10. Kocher MS, *et al.* Validation of a clinical prediction rule for the differentiation between septic arthritis and transient synovitis of the hip in children. *J Bone Joint Surg Am.* 2004. 86-A(8):1629–35.

11. Caird MS, *et al.* Factors distinguishing septic arthritis from transient synovitis of the hip in children. A prospective study. *J Bone Joint Surg Am.* 2006;88(6):1251–7.

12. Luhmann SJ, *et al.* Differentiation between septic arthritis and transient synovitis of the hip in children with clinical prediction algorithms. *J Bone Joint Surg Am.* 2004;86-A(5):956–62.

13. Dartnell J, Ramachandran M, Katchburian M. Haematogenous acute and subacute paediatric osteomyelitis: a systematic review of the literature. *J Bone Joint Surg Br.* 2012;94(5):584–95.

14. Speers DJ, Nade SM. Ultrastructural studies of adherence of *Staphylococcus aureus* in experimental acute hematogenous osteomyelitis. *Infect Immun.* 1985;49(2):443–6.

15. Trueta J. The normal vascular anatomy of the human femoral head during growth. *J Bone Joint Surg Br.* 1957;39-B(2):358–94.

16. Herring JA. Infection of the musculoskeletal system. In: Herring JA, ed. *Tachdjians' Pediatric Orthopaedics*, 4th ed, Vol. 3. Philadelphia, PA: Saunders Elsevier; 2008. pp. 2089–146.

17. Stans AA, Schoenecker JG. Musculoskeletal infection. In: Weinstein SL, Flynn JM, eds. *Lovell and Winter's Pediatric Orthopaedics*, 8th ed, Vol. 1. Philadelphia, PA: Lippincott Williams & Wilkins; 2021. p. 396.

18. Pennington WT, *et al.* Photopenic bone scan osteomyelitis: a clinical perspective. *J Pediatr Orthop.* 1999;19(6):695–8.

19. Megan Mignemi M, Lawson Copley M, Schoenecker JM. Evidence-based treatment for musculoskeletal infection In: Alshryda S, Huntley JS, Banaszkiewicz P, eds. *Paediatric Orthopaedics: An Evidence-Based Approach to Clinical Questions.* Cham: Springer; 2016. pp. 51–75.

20. Jagodzinski NA, *et al.* Prospective evaluation of a shortened regimen of treatment for acute osteomyelitis and septic arthritis in children. *J Pediatr Orthop.* 2009;29(5):518–25.

21. Peltola H, *et al.* Short- versus long-term antimicrobial treatment for acute hematogenous osteomyelitis of childhood: prospective, randomized trial on 131 culture-positive cases. *Pediatr Infect Dis J.* 2010;29(12):1123–8.

22. Connolly SA, *et al.* MRI for detection of abscess in acute osteomyelitis of the pelvis in children. *AJR Am J Roentgenol.* 2007;189(4):867–72.

Chapter 20

Musculoskeletal Tumours

Richard Gardner, Gino R. Somers, and Sevan Hopyan

Background

This chapter aims to cover the commonest benign and malignant bone tumours in paediatric orthopaedics practice (and exams). Table 20.1 summarizes bone tumours and their cells of origin, and Table 20.2 summarizes bone tumour-like conditions. The selected tumours in this chapter are those that are most frequently addressed in the FRCS exams. The current evidence is discussed, and the identifiable radiological and histological features are illustrated. To this aim, we have also included the soft tissue tumour rhabdomyosarcoma.

Benign Tumours

- Unicameral bone cyst (UBC)
- Aneurysmal bone cyst (ABC)
- Fibrous dysplasia (FD)
- Osteochondroma/multiple hereditary exostosis
- Osteoid osteoma
- Chondroblastoma.

Malignant Tumours

- Ewing's sarcoma
- Rhabdomyosarcoma
- Osteosarcoma.

Grading System

The Enneking classification (Table 20.3) is used to stage malignant tumours of bone and soft tissue. It is used to guide prognosis and evaluate the results of treatment. Tumours are categorized according to their grade, their containment within the compartment, and whether metastases are present.

A low-grade tumour (e.g. chondrosarcoma) is well differentiated, with minimal atypia and few mitotic figures. A high-grade tumour (e.g. osteosarcoma, Ewing's sarcoma) is poorly differentiated, with cellular atypia and mitotic figures, and have a higher rate of metastasis. Grading is described as G1 (low grade) and G2 (high grade). Low-grade bone tumours metastasize in 10% of cases, intermediate grade in 10–30%, and high grade in >50%.

Table 20.1 Bone tumours and their cells of origin

Cells	Benign	Malignant
Haematopoietic		1. Myeloma 2. Lymphoma
Chondrogenic	1. Osteochondroma 2. Chondroma 3. Chondroblastoma 4. Chondromyxoid fibroma	1. Primary chondrosarcoma (LG) 2. Secondary chondrosarcoma (LG) 3. Dedifferentiated chondrosarcoma (mixed) 4. Mesenchymal chondrosarcoma 5. Clear cell chondrosarcoma
Osteogenic	1. Osteoid osteoma 2. Osteoblastoma	1. Osteosarcoma (HG) 2. Parosteal osteosarcoma (LG) 3. Periosteal osteosarcoma (IG)
Unknown origin	1. Giant cell tumour (fibrous) 2. Histiocytoma	1. Ewing's tumour (HG) 2. Malignant giant cell tumour (HG) 3. Adamantinoma (LG)
Fibrogenic	1. Fibroma (metaphyseal fibrous defect, non-ossifying fibroma) 2. Desmoplastic fibroma (LG)	1. Fibrosarcoma (HG) 2. Malignant fibrous histiocytoma (HG)
Notochordal		Chordoma
Vascular	Haemangioma	1. Haemangioendothelioma (LG) 2. Haemangiopericytoma
Lipogenic	Lipoma	
Neurogenic	Neurilemmoma	

LG, low grade; mixed, mix of high and low grades; HG, high grade; IG, intermediate grade.

Table 20.2 Bone tumour-like conditions

Conditions	Description
1. Eosinophilic granuloma[a]	Highly destructive lesion with well-defined margins; cortex may be destroyed and there is soft tissue swelling Self-limiting, steroid, radiotherapy, C&B
2. Osteomyelitis	
3. Avulsion fracture	
4. Aneurysmal bone cyst	75% in <20 years, eccentric, lytic, expansile in the metaphysis Treated with C&B or radiotherapy
5. Fibrous dysplasia[b]	Highly lytic or like ground glass. There is sometimes a well-defined rim of sclerotic bone around the lesion; 'shepherd's crook' sign Observation, corrective osteotomy + ORIF, bisphosphonate
6. Osteofibrous dysplasia	<10 years, tibia, X-rays are needed to make the diagnosis and a biopsy may be needed where the diagnosis is in doubt; biopsy will show fibrous tissue stroma and a background of bone trabeculae with osteoblastic rimming
7. Heterotopic ossification	
8. Unicameral bone cyst	Central lytic and symmetrical; thinning of the cortex; active when touching the physis. Commonly affects the humerus Aspirate and methylprednisolone injection, C&B ± IF
9. Giant cell reparative granuloma	
10. Exuberant callus	

[a] Lichtenstein classified histiocytosis X (Langerhans cell histiocytosis) into three types: (1) eosinophilic granuloma (monostotic bone disease); (2) Hand–Schüller–Christian disease (multiple bone lesions and visceral disease); and (3) Letterer–Siwe disease (a fulminating condition in young children).

[b] Fibrous dysplasia is caused by a genetic mutation which causes activation of the G_s alpha surface protein, resulting in increased production of cyclic adenosine monophosphate (cAMP). This causes failure of production of normal lamellar bone. Clinically, there is a developmental abnormality of bone – either monostotic or polyostotic involvement. The name of McCune–Albright syndrome refers to the association of fibrous dysplasia and endocrine abnormalities.

C&B, curettage and bone grafting; IF, internal fixation.

Table 20.3 Enneking classification of malignant tumours of bone and soft tissue

Stage	Subgroup	GTM	Description
I	IA	G1T1M0	Low grade, intracompartmental, no metastases
	IB	G1T2M0	Low grade, extracompartmental, no metastases
II	IIA	G2T1M0	
	IIB	G2T2M0	High grade, extracompartmental, no metastases
III	IIIA	G1/2T1M1	Any grade, intracompartmental, with metastases
	IIIB	G1/2T2M1	Any grade, extracompartmental, with metastases

Table 20.4 Classification of benign tumours of bone

Stage	Group	Characteristics
1	Inactive (latent)	Refers to lesions which are not causing pain and show no evidence of active growth. Stage 1 lesions are generally treated with observation only
2	Active	Refers to lesions which are causing pain or some form of disability. If a lesion has weakened the structure of the bone such that a fracture may occur, the lesion would also be considered a stage 2 lesion
3	Aggressive	Refers to lesions which are large, have broken into soft tissues, or have caused a pathologic fracture. These lesions are usually prone to local recurrence and have the potential of causing a major problem for the patient

The site of the tumour is confirmed by further imaging, typically MRI. The lesion is considered intracompartmental (T1) if it is contained within the bone or if it is a soft tissue mass within the fascial compartment. If these boundaries are breached, the tumour is extracompartmental (T2). If metastases are present, the annotation M1 is used; when no metastases are present, M0 is recorded.

The system for benign lesions is divided into three groups: inactive (latent), active, and aggressive (Table 20.4).

Unicameral Bone Cyst

It is a common benign lesion of bone. The true incidence is unknown, as many are asymptomatic. It is described as a unicameral (single chamber) or simple bone cyst. There is a male:female preponderance of 3:1. Diagnosis is typically made in the first decade.

It is predominantly located centrally in the metaphysis of bones, most commonly in the proximal humerus and proximal femur (90%). The aetiology is unknown. A few theories have been postulated:

- The vascular theory – suggested a localized blockage to interstitial fluid drainage
- Entrapped synovial tissue or intraosseous synovial cysts – both synovial type A and B cells were found in the lining of the UBC
- Recently genetic abnormalities have been described in children with simple bone cysts [1, 2].

The cyst contains straw-coloured serous fluid. High levels of prostaglandin have been found [3]. The lesions are frequently an incidental finding on X-ray, or may present with dull ache (possibly secondary to a microfracture) or secondary to a pathological fracture.

Cysts can be considered to be in a latent or an active phase. The cyst is 'active' when immediately adjacent to the physis, often with a thin, partially expanded cortical shell. It is considered latent when it grows away from the physis. The cortex becomes more substantial; there are no signs of progression, and there is evidence of metaphyseal remodelling.

Imaging

A UBC appears as a central, well-defined, lucent metaphyseal lesion. Cortical thinning may be present, with ballooning/expansion of the metaphysis, but rarely exceed the width of the adjacent physis (unlike an ABC). No soft tissue swelling or periosteal reaction is evident in the absence of a pathological fracture. The 'fallen fragment sign' may be present (Figure 20.1). This represents a pathological fracture (a small flake of bone that settles in the base/dependent region of the lesion), indicating the cystic, rather than solid, nature of the lesion [4]. Use of MRI is not necessary when findings are typical. Features are characteristic and summarized in Figure 20.2.

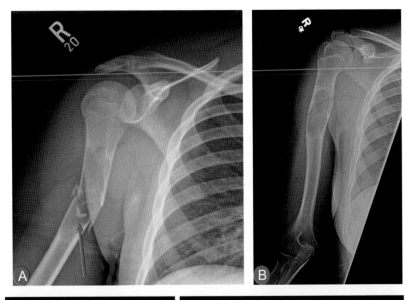

Figure 20.1 A pathological fracture through a unicameral bone cyst of the humerus. A fallen fragment, or the leaf sign, is evident (A, red arrow). (B) Two months later following fracture union, demonstrating persistence of the cyst.

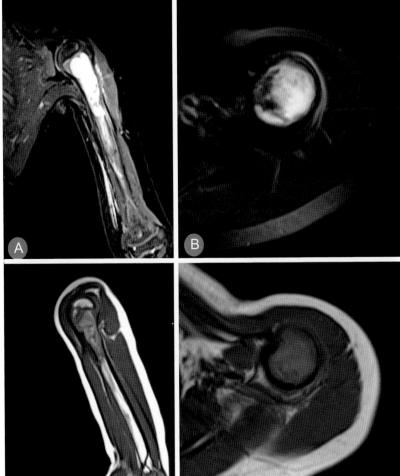

Figure 20.2 MRI scan of a unicameral bone cyst. On T2-weighted images (A, B), the cyst exhibits a high signal intensity because of its fluid content. There is no fluid level (unless there is a complicated fracture). On T1-weighted images (C, D), the cyst has a low to intermediate signal intensity, when compared to the adjacent skeletal muscles. There is usually no septations or loculations. There should be no extraosseous soft tissue mass, periosteal reaction, or callus, unless it is complicated by a fracture.

Natural History of Unicameral Bone Cysts

The natural history of UBCs is to heal in late adolescence, although the incidence is unclear. Moreover, children with a UBC could sustain up to five fractures before the cyst heals. This could have substantive social and physical impact on the children and their families [5].

Healing is not often well defined, even after intervention. Wright *et al.* [6] introduced a reasonable grading system of cyst healing:

1. Not healed:
    a. Grade 1: clearly visible cyst
    b. Grade 2: cyst that is visible, but multilocular and opaque

2. Healed:
    a. Grade 3: sclerosis around or within a partially visible cyst
    b. Grade 4: obliteration of the cyst (complete healing).

Contrary to common advice, UBCs do not routinely heal after a fracture. Whilst abundant callus may initially form, it tends to resorb after 6 months and there is a low likelihood of the cyst healing post-fracture. The true incidence is unknown, but likely to be 5–15% (Figure 20.3) [7].

Management

A pragmatic approach to treat UBCs is advisable. The following factors are to be considered [8]:

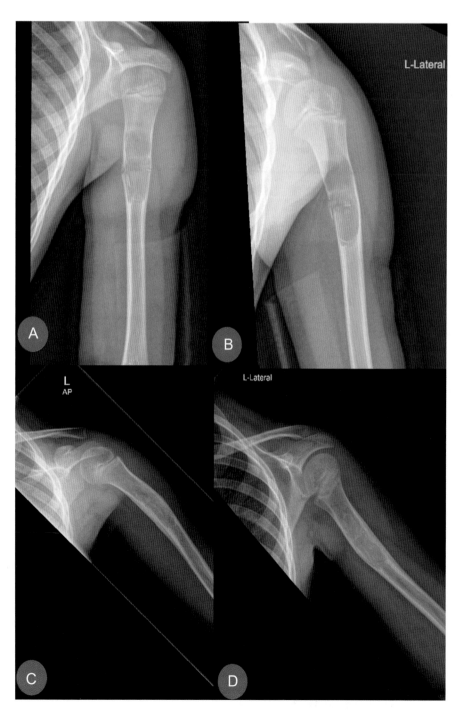

Figure 20.3 Although not common, unicameral bone cysts can heal after a fracture.

1. Site of the cyst: upper versus lower limbs. Pathological fractures in the lower limbs can be more serious than those in the upper limbs
2. Age: younger children heal more quickly and are more amenable to lifestyle restrictions than older adolescents
3. General health of the child
4. Available expertise and equipment
5. The child's and family's preferences (risk of fractures versus risk of surgery).

A small, asymptomatic UBC in the humerus with good cortical thickness can be observed; however, a large UBC in the peri-trochanteric area in a very active adolescent is better treated surgically.

Several surgical interventions have been advocated, with variable success rates. Currently, the following are in practice (Figure 20.4):

1. Intralesional injection
2. Trepanation and decompression
3. Curettage with or without bone or artificial graft
4. Curettage with or without bone or artificial graft, with stabilization using metalwork.

Reported healing rates following intralesional steroid injection was 60% [9]. The rationale for steroid use is the high level of prostaglandin noted in the cyst fluid [3]. However, successful healing may require multiple injections of methylprednisolone. A higher healing rate of 76% was reported after aspiration and a single autologous bone marrow injection [10].

Curettage–mechanical disruption of the cyst has been shown to be an effective treatment. In a retrospective study of 46 patients with UBC treated with isolated curettage ($n = 10$), methylprednisolone injection ($n = 17$), or autologous bone marrow injection ($n = 19$), the healing rates were 70%, 41%, and 21%, respectively ($P = 0.08$) [11].

Other studies showed addition of drainage, whether through a cannulated screw or intramedullary flexible nailing, improved success rates. Intramedullary flexible nailing also provided extra strength to the bone, preventing or minimizing the risk of fractures [8, 12].

Aneurysmal Bone Cysts

These are benign, expansile vascular lesions that usually involve the metaphyses of long bones but have been identified throughout the skeleton. ABCs represent the commonest benign aggressive tumour in the paediatric population. They predominantly occur in the first two decades of life [13], most commonly in the humerus, femur, and tibia. The spine is involved in 20% of cases and can cause neurological compromise that may even be acute due to vertebral collapse [15]. Seventy per cent present as a primary tumour, whereas 30% are secondary [16], forming a cystic part of osteosarcoma, giant cell tumour, osteoblastoma, or chondroblastoma.

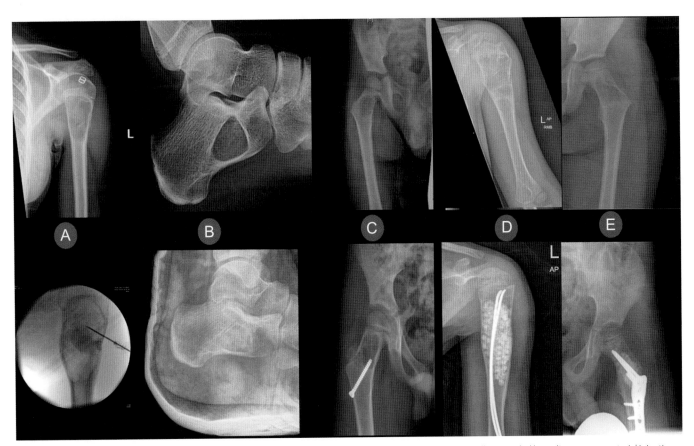

Figure 20.4 Various treatment methods for a simple bone cyst. (A) Steroid or bone marrow injection. This is usually preceded by radio-opaque material injection to ensure accuracy. (B) Curettage and bone grafting. (C) Decompression using a cannulated screw. (D) Artificial bone grafting and intramedullary stabilization. (E) Curettage, artificial bone grafting, use of cannulated screw as a drainage system, and extramedullary stabilization.

Aetiology

A chromosomal translocation t(16;17) is thought to be the cause of ABCs. This fuses the *CDH11* (osteoblast cadherin 11) gene to *USP6*, an oncogenic promoter [17]. High levels of insulin-like growth factor have been found in ABCs, suggesting a role in the pathogenesis [18]. Theories of historical interest include the presence of a localized vascular disturbance resulting in increased intraosseous pressure [16].

Clinical Presentation

Whilst the clinical course is heterogenous in children, ABCs usually present with swelling, discomfort, and occasionally a pathological fracture. They can grow rapidly, with extensive expansion and osteolysis of the host bone. When they are spinal in origin, neurological deficit may occur.

Imaging

Plain radiographs demonstrate an expansile, often eccentric metaphyseal lesion. Depending on the active nature of the cyst, the cortex is thinned or the cyst is lined by a thin shell of subperiosteal new bone formation (Figure 20.5). ABCs may be described as:

- Inactive (when the periosteal 'shell' is intact, with sclerotic margins)
- Active (incomplete periosteal shell, but with a defined border)
- Aggressive (no periosteal shell or evidence of bone formation) [18].

MRI demonstrates 'fluid–fluid' levels and contrast-enhancing walls of the cyst (Figure 20.5). The fluid–fluid level is not a pathognomonic feature, as it is also seen in telangiectatic osteosarcoma, giant cell tumour, and simple bone cysts following a fracture [13].

ABCs are difficult, if not impossible, to differentiate from telangiectatic osteosarcoma; therefore, bone biopsy is mandatory.

Histology

ABCs are cavitary lesions with fibrous septae, filled with haemorrhagic tissue (Figure 20.6). There may be evidence of osteoid formation [13]. The presence of malignant cells indicates that

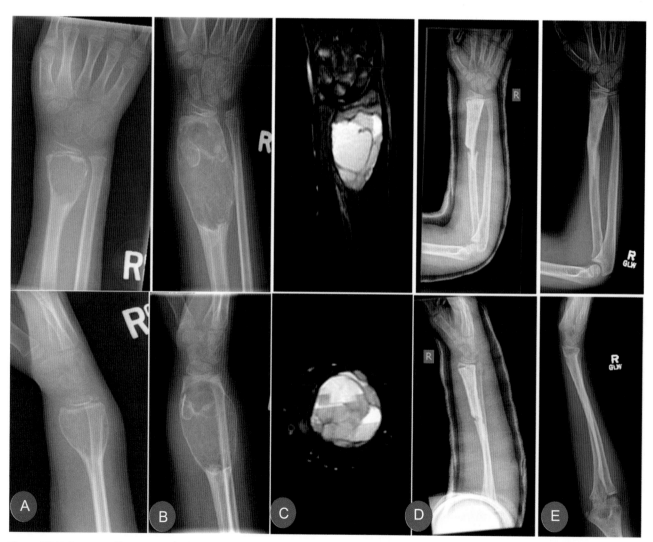

Figure 20.5 Aneurysmal bone cyst in the distal radius. (A) This 9-year-old boy presented with pain and swelling of the distal radius due to ABCs. (B) He underwent unsuccessful curettage, with subsequent expansion of the ABCs after 1 year. (C) MRI demonstrated a fluid–fluid level and no other pathologies. (D) The cyst was saucerized; the membrane was resected with a curette and high-speed burr, and a distal radius allograft was inserted. (E) Incorporation of an allograft 6 months post-operation.

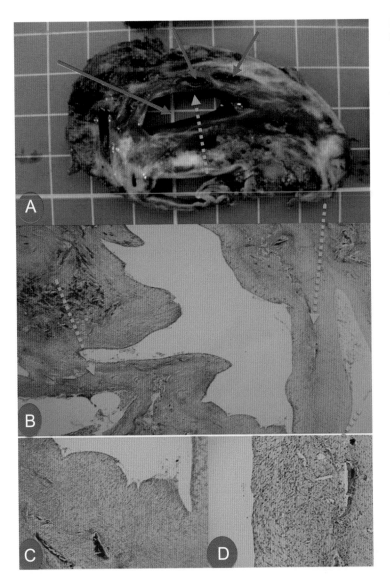

Figure 20.6 Aneurysmal bone cyst. (A) Macroscopic picture demonstrating blood-filled cavities of different sizes (red arrows), separated by fibrous septae (dashed green arrows). (B) Cystic spaces filled with blood and separated by fibrous septae (haematoxylin and eosin (H&E), ×25). (C) Fibrous septae containing giant cells, haemosiderin-laden macrophages, and osteoid (H&E, ×50). (D) Cysts and septae lined by fibroblasts, myofibroblasts, and histiocytes, but not endothelium (H&E, ×100). *Source:* Courtesy Edmund Cheesman, Royal Manchester University Hospital.

the ABC is secondary to another tumour rather than primary. Primary ABCs often have rearrangement of the *USP6* gene, detectable by a variety of molecular methods [14].

Treatment

Active treatment is recommended due to the risk of further bone destruction, fracture, and infrequent rates of spontaneous healing [15]. The options are (Figure 20.7):

1. Curettage and bone grafting. This is the traditional choice, but there is a high recurrence rate. Combining curettage with high-speed burring of the surrounding bone has been reported to result in healing rates of 90% [1]
2. Cryotherapy and sclerotherapy have been used successfully
3. Arterial embolization may be used as an adjunct to surgery, as well as in areas where surgical management is challenging (e.g. the pelvis and spine) [19, 20]

4. En bloc resection may be considered where the bone is expendable (e.g. the rib and fibula) [15].

Fibrous Dysplasia

FD is a benign condition that is characterized by expansile fibro-osseous tissue in one or more bones. The bone has a disordered woven appearance, as opposed to adult lamellar bone. It is not thought to be hereditary.

Classification

- Monostotic: only one bone involved.
- Polyostotic: several areas of the skeleton may be affected. Commonly, the metaphyseal and diaphyseal regions of the long bones, skull, and mandible are involved.
- McCune–Albright syndrome: polyostotic FD with endocrine abnormalities (e.g. precocious puberty).

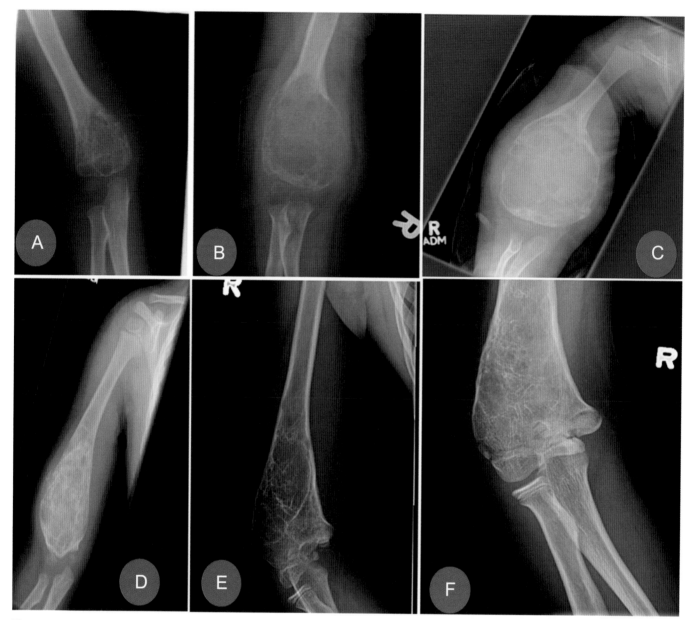

Figure 20.7 Aneurysmal bone cyst of the distal humerus. (A) Initial presentation with pain and restriction of movement at 2 years and 9 months of age. (B) Continued expansion with pathological fracture despite intralesional sclerotherapy at age 3 years. (C) Curettage attempted, but further expansion evident at age 3 years and 3 months. (D) Combination therapy with repeat curettage and embolization, demonstrating cortication of the ABC and early remodelling (age 3 years and 8 months). (E, F) Final remodelling and healing of the cyst with valgus deformity at age 9 and 11 years. Later corrective osteotomy restored the carrying angle.

Aetiology

The exact cause of FD is not known [19], although there is an association with a mutation in the α subunit of the Gsα binding protein. GTPase is inhibited, increasing cyclic adenosine monophosphate (cAMP) production. It is postulated that mutation early in embryogenesis results in the mosaicism that accounts for the variable skeletal and cutaneous manifestations. Increased production of cAMP has been shown to increase interleukin-6 (IL-6) production, which increases the number of osteoclasts and resultant bone resorption. There is thus failure of maturation of immature woven bone to lamellar bone [21]. The woven bone fails to adapt to mechanical stress (the trabeculae are inappropriately orientated and

encased in fibrous tissue) and does not mineralize appropriately [22].

Clinical Presentation

The incidental finding of an asymptomatic lesion is not unusual, but patients usually present with pain, deformity, or a pathological fracture. Bone pain is due to fatigue fractures in the involved bone. Deformity is particularly seen in the polyostotic form, commonly involving the proximal femur (the 'shepherd's crook' sign), tibia, and humerus. Deformity may progress following skeletal maturity with polyostotic FD, but not in the monostotic form [23]. Café-au-lait spots with a ragged border (Coast of Maine) pattern are observed, rather than

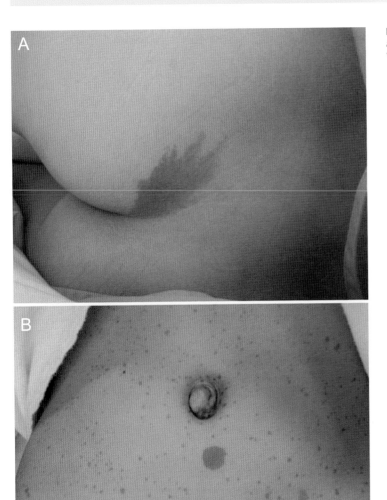

Figure 20.8 (A) Ragged border 'Coast of Maine' pattern café-au-lait spots in a patient with fibrous dysplasia. (B) Smooth border 'Coast of California' pattern seen in neurofibromatosis.

with the smooth border (Coast of California) seen in neurofibromatosis (Figure 20.8).

Imaging

The radiographic findings may demonstrate an expansile lesion with cortical thinning/endosteal scalloping with a 'spreading flame' appearance. The involved bone is described as having a 'ground-glass' quality due to the homogenous appearance and absence of trabeculae. The classic deformity in the proximal femur is termed a 'shepherd's crook' deformity when repeated areas of microfracture through pathological bone result in a progressive varus deformity.

Histology

FD has a very distinctive histological appearance. Under low magnification, it looks like low to moderately cellular fibrous stroma surrounding irregular, curvilinear trabeculae of woven bone, which is arranged in a pattern commonly referred to as 'resembling Chinese alphabet characters' (Figure 20.9). In challenging cases, demonstration of missense mutations in GNAS gene can help confirm the diagnosis of fibrous dysplasia [24].

Management

- **Observation**: non-operative treatment is the mainstay. Asymptomatic lesions may be monitored for progression. An endocrinology workup should be performed when polyostotic FD is diagnosed.
- **Bisphosphonates**: these have been used successfully to treat bone pain and have been reported to improve cortical thickness in pathological bone.
- **Operative management**: this is considered when progressive deformity (or fracture) occurs or is anticipated, typically with more severe polyostotic involvement.
- Curettage and grafting have a relatively high rate of failure due to recurrence. Autogenous cancellous grafts resorb quickly, in contrast to cortical strut grafts.
- If the deformity is diaphyseal, intramedullary stabilization should be used (e.g. Fassier–Duval growing rod insertion in the femur) (Figure 20.10). If the deformity is localized to the proximal femur, corrective osteotomies are required, with internal fixation.

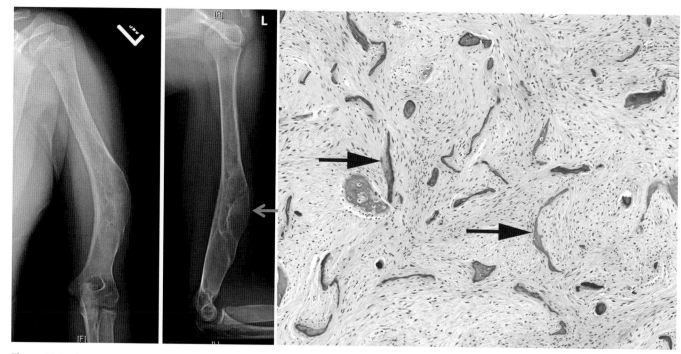

Figure 20.9 Fibrous dysplasia of the humerus. An 11-year-old female with polyostotic fibrous dysplasia. The deformity of the left humerus is evident, with localized cortical expansion and endosteal scalloping. It has a homogenous 'ground-glass' appearance. The 'spreading flame' is marked by the blue arrow. Histologically, fibrous dysplasia shows a variably cellular fibrous stroma, throughout which are scattered irregular trabeculae of unmineralized osteoid of variable shapes and sizes (black arrows). The appearance has been termed 'Chinese alphabet soup'. The trabeculae are not lined by osteoblasts and there is no significant atypia. Haematoxylin and eosin staining, original magnification ×100. The gross macroscopic appearance has a yellowish colour and a gritty texture.

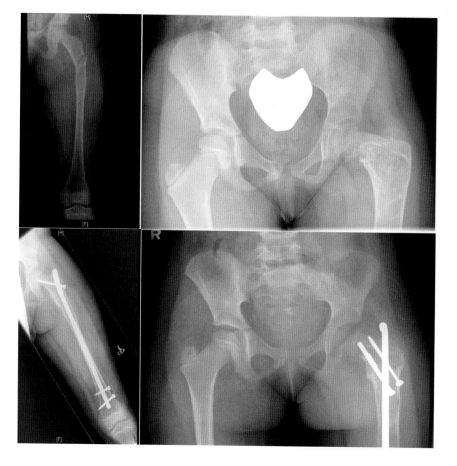

Figure 20.10 Fibrous dysplasia: surgical stabilization. Two different patients with fibrous dysplasia treated with intramedullary stabilization. The implant choice depends on bone size and age of the patient (remaining growth and weight).

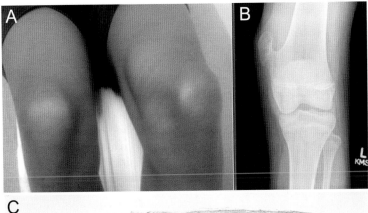

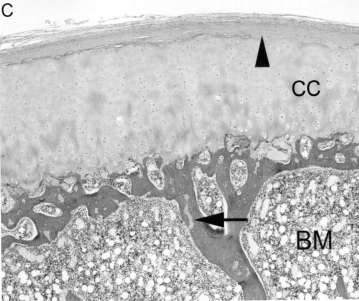

Figure 20.11 Osteochondroma. (A, B) Pedunculated distal femoral osteochondroma. Notice that the lesion is growing away from the physis and has cortical and medullary continuity with the femoral diaphysis. (C) Photomicrograph of osteochondroma, showing the cartilage cap (CC) with orderly chondrocyte growth, lined on its surface by pink periosteum (arrowhead). Also seen is evidence of endochondral ossification, with cartilage within the underlying bony trabeculae (arrow) and underlying bone marrow (BM). The cartilage cap is typically 1–3 mm thick (can be 10 mm thick in younger patients). Haematoxylin and eosin stain, original magnification ×40.

Osteochondroma/Exostosis

This is the commonest benign bone tumour. It is thought to be due to aberrant growth of the physis at the perichondral ring. The lesion grows by endochondral ossification of the cartilaginous cap, with the cortex and medulla continuous with the normal bone. It typically assumes a sessile or pedunculated appearance, with the latter directed away from the physis towards the diaphysis (Figure 20.11). Predominant locations are the metaphysis of the distal femur, proximal tibia, and proximal humerus.

Osteochondroma can be discovered incidentally and presents as swelling, pain, and pressure effect on an important structure or as a deformity. Sarcomatous change is rare (<1%), with conversion to well-differentiated chondrosarcoma. Signs include: irregularity of the margin, inhomogenous mineralization, increase in size after skeletal maturity, and soft tissue mass. A cartilage cap >20 mm in thickness is also suggestive. Following wide excision, disease-free survival can be achieved [25].

Treatment

Symptomatic osteochondromas can be excised. Delaying surgery, where possible, until late adolescence minimizes the risk of recurrence and physeal injury.

Multiple Hereditary Exostosis

Multiple hereditary exostosis is an autosomal dominant condition with high penetrance (approximately 96%). The exostosin (*EXT*) family of genes encode glycosyltransferases, which are responsible for heparan sulfate biosynthesis. Mutations in *EXT1*, *EXT2*, and *EXT3* (chromosomes 8, 11, and 19, respectively) are associated with multiple hereditary exostosis. Reduction or absence of heparan sulfate results in disturbed chondrocyte signalling and abnormal endochondral ossification. The majority of mutations involve *EXT1* and are associated with a greater burden of exostoses, deformity, and risk of malignant transformation to chondrosarcoma relative to those mutations in *EXT2* [26].

Prevalence is around 1:100 000, with 10% of individuals having no family history [27]. Most patients have evidence of multiple exostoses in the first decade of life.

Clinical Presentation

The most commonly involved sites are the metaphyses adjacent to the knee (>90%), proximal humerus, forearm, ribs, and scapula. Short stature is common, and 10% have a leg length discrepancy, with genu valgum being the commonest limb abnormality. Forearm asymmetry with increased radial inclination and negative ulnar variance is common (Madelung's appearance). Subluxation of the radial head occurs. The spinal canal may be involved, with occasional neurological symptoms. Pain due to mechanical symptoms from prominent exostosis is a common feature, with a significant impact on the quality of life (Figure 20.12).

Malignant Transformation

Variable rates are quoted in the literature (from 0.9% to 10%) but are likely to be approximately 1%. Features of concern are identical to those for an isolated osteochondroma.

Treatment

Regular assessment is required for leg length discrepancy or angular malalignment. At skeletal maturity, an X-ray of the pelvis is advised to identify any axial and non-palpable exostosis.

Options and indications for surgery are:

1. Excision of symptomatic lesions (overlying irritation, pressure on neurological structures)
2. Correction of angular limb deformity and leg length discrepancy may be required
3. Forearm involvement may be addressed by excision of the exostosis, combined with ulnar lengthening or radial shortening, although significant recurrence rates are reported [5].

Osteoid Osteoma

Osteoid osteoma is a common, benign osteoblastic lesion of uncertain aetiology. It has a 2:1 male predilection. It is characterized by several features, as detailed below.

Symptoms

There is a chronic, dull, aching pain, which is typically worse at night and responsive to non-steroidal anti-inflammatory drugs (NSAIDs). The pain has been attributed to the presence of high levels of prostaglandins within the nidus (hence the efficacy of NSAIDs), as well as to histological evidence of unmyelinated axons.

Location

Osteoid osteomas are typically present in the diaphyses and metaphyses of the long bones and are frequently, but not always, intracortical. They also occur in the posterior elements of the spine where they are associated with painful scoliosis (the lesion is often on the concave side, possibly secondary to local muscle spasm). Occasionally, they are found in an intra-articular (with less reactive bone) or subperiosteal location.

Imaging

Plain radiographs often demonstrate a radiolucent nidus, surrounded by dense sclerotic bone. The nidus is typically <1.5 cm and may have a central region of mineralization. These may

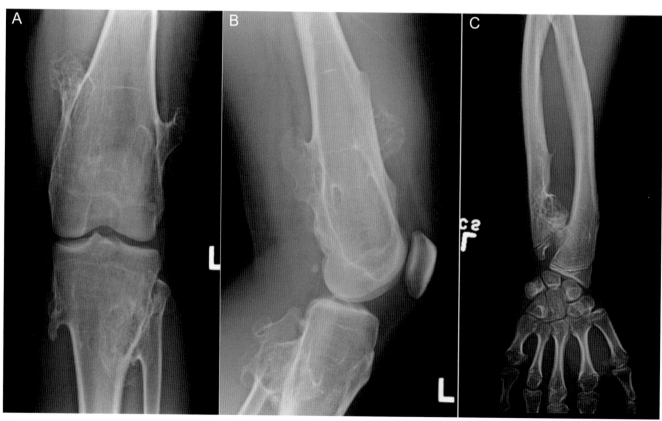

Figure 20.12 Multiple hereditary exostosis. A patient with multiple hereditary exostosis affecting the metaphyses adjacent to the knee and distal ulna. The large osteochondroma of the distal ulna has resulted in negative ulnar variance, incongruity of the distal radioulnar joint, and resultant restriction in forearm rotation.

only be seen on CT axial images (Figures 20.13 and 20.14). Bone scans are a reliable investigation to localize the tumour, as technetium-99m is preferentially taken up by the nidus. Differential diagnosis includes stress fracture, Brodie's abscess, and osteoblastoma.

Histologically, **osteoblastomas** are identical to osteoid osteomas, but they are usually much larger (2–10 cm). They usually occur in patients aged 10–25 years. Unlike osteoid osteomas, 30–40% of osteoblastomas are found in the spine where they most often affect the posterior elements, including the spinous processes, transverse processes, laminae, and pedicles. Treatment consists of curettage or local excision. The risk of recurrence after such treatment is approximately 10–20%.

Treatment

Osteoid osteoma is self-limiting, but spontaneous improvement may take several years. Options are:

- CT-guided radiofrequency ablation – the treatment of choice. Under CT guidance, a radiofrequency probe is inserted into the lesion and the nidus is heated to 80°C for 4 minutes, with the skin protected. This reliably induces a 1-cm zone of necrosis. Treatment is successful in 95% of cases, but no histological analysis is possible.

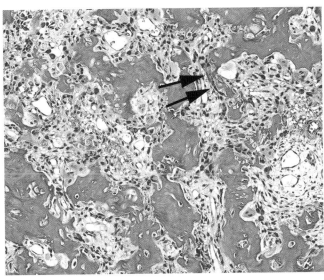

Figure 20.14 Osteoid osteoma histology. Photomicrograph showing a nidus of an osteoid osteoma. There are bland, pink bony trabeculae and osteoid matrix intermixed with cellular fibrovascular stroma. Osteoblasts line up along some of the osteoid (arrows). No atypia is seen. Haematoxylin and eosin, original magnification ×200.

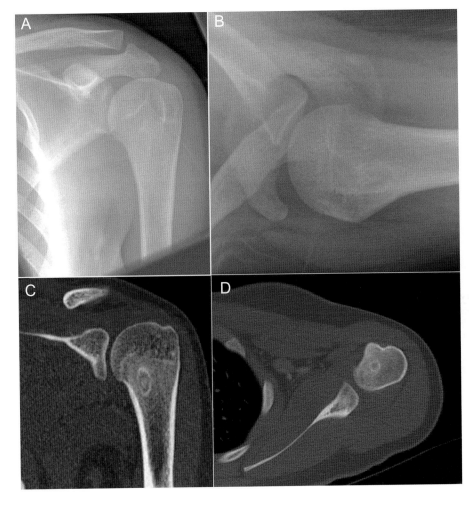

Figure 20.13 Osteoid osteoma of the proximal humerus. The lesion is subtle on the plain radiographs (A, B), but the sclerotic margin, nidus, and central mineralization are clearly evident on the CT scans (C, D).

- Open surgical resection – generally not recommended but may occasionally be preferred when adjacent neurovascular structures are at risk. It has the advantage of histological confirmation of the lesion. Disadvantages include resection of normal bone, potentially requiring grafting or stabilization, and the risk of fracture.

Chondroblastoma

This is an uncommon, benign cellular cartilage tumour that is most often located in the epiphyses of the long bones. The commonest locations are the proximal humerus, distal femur, and proximal tibia. The male:female ratio is 2:1. The majority of patients present before 30 years of age, and the aetiology is still debated [15].

Symptoms are usually mild and consist of pain and localized tenderness. Pain may be present for many years before a diagnosis is made. Because the lesion is epiphyseal, the adjacent joint may be swollen and have a limited range of motion.

Histologically, chondroblastoma is characterized by polygonal cells (chondroblasts), giant cells, islands of chondroid or hyaline cartilage, 'chicken-wire' calcification, and nodules of calcification in the stroma [4]. Chicken-wire calcification results when lace-like deposits of calcium are intermixed on the intercellular chondroid matrix (Figure 20.15).

Imaging

Radiological features are often diagnostic (Figure 20.16). The lesion is typically located in the epiphysis. It is usually eccentric, involving less than half of the entire epiphysis. The lesion is rimmed by a sclerotic margin, and small punctate calcifications are present. Commonly, the physis adjacent to the lesion is present at the time of diagnosis.

Differential diagnosis includes giant cell tumours (mature skeleton), clear cell chondrosarcoma, enchondromas, synovial

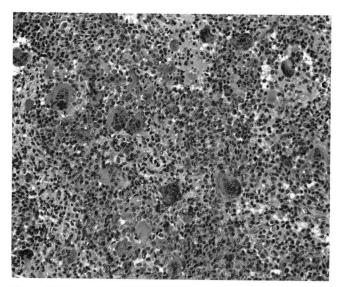

Figure 20.15 Chondroblastoma histopathology. Photomicrograph of a chondroblastoma showing a cellular tumour composed of sheets of polygonal cells with slightly irregular nuclei (coffee-bean like). Numerous osteoclast-like giant cells are present and a small amount of pale pink stroma is seen. This slide does not show chicken-wire calcification. Hematoxylin and eosin, original magnification ×200.

lesions (e.g. pigmented villonodular synovitis, rheumatoid arthritis), and atypically located eosinophilic granuloma. Fine-needle aspiration yields satisfactory material for interpretation and confirmation of the diagnosis. Demonstration of mutations in the H3-3B or H3-3A histone genes is helpful in confirming the diagnosis in challenging cases [28].

Complete curettage and excision of the lesion (using high-speed burring) are often successful, with 80% local control. Preservation of the joint surface and physes is important for functional outcome. The defect is filled with either autogenous or allograft bone. Two per cent of chondroblastomas may metastasize to the lung.

Osteosarcoma

This is the commonest malignant tumour of bone. The aetiology is unknown, but genetic predispositions have been established. Patients with Li–Fraumeni syndrome (*p53* tumour suppressor gene mutation) and hereditary retinoblastoma (mutation of the *RB* gene) have a high incidence of developing osteosarcomas.

There is a bimodal age distribution, with the majority of cases in the second decade and a second peak in the elderly, usually secondary to Paget's disease (Paget's sarcoma). The histological hallmark is the presence of malignant osteoblasts with osteoid production.

Subtypes

- **Intramedullary osteosarcoma.** The classical form. Typically, high grade and arising from the metaphysis. The remainder of this discussion will focus on the management.
- **Parosteal osteosarcoma.** Arises from the periosseous tissues, commonly the posterior aspect of the femur, sometimes with linear separation from the bone (the string sign). Usually well differentiated and slow-growing, and metastasizes late.
- **Periosteal osteosarcoma.** Uncommon variant. Presents as a poorly mineralized mass, extending from the surface of the bone. Usually intermediate grade (and prognosis). Radiographs demonstrate cortical erosion (periosteal surface) with 'sunray spicules' due to the periosteal reaction.
- **Telangiectatic osteosarcoma.** High-grade, aggressive variant. Prognosis and management similar to the classic intramedullary form. Usually presents in the metaphysis of long bones as a rapidly growing, painful, and lytic mass.

Clinical Presentation

Osteosarcoma presents with localized pain, and later a defined swelling may be palpable. An episode of trauma is often cited as the precipitating event by the patient.

Investigations

The common radiological features are demonstrated in Figure 20.17. The tumour is typically eccentrically placed in the metaphysis/proximal or distal diaphysis. Use of MRI is invaluable to identify the extent of intramedullary involvement, as well as soft

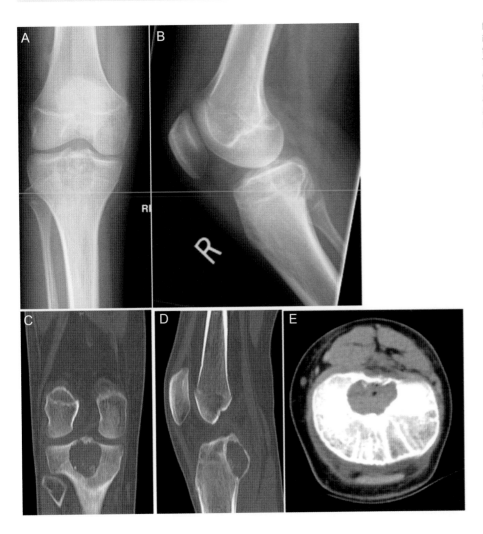

Figure 20.16 Chondroblastoma. They are typically located in the epiphyses, but as in this case, they may extend into the metaphyseal region. They are usually eccentric, involving less than half of the entire epiphysis. The lesion is rimmed by a sclerotic margin, and small punctate calcifications are present in the tumour. Commonly, the physis adjacent to the lesion is present at the time of diagnosis.

tissue extension and the proximity to neurovascular structures. The latter information will determine whether the tumour may be resected and limb salvage achieved.

Spiral chest CT is performed once the diagnosis is made. Pulmonary metastases measuring >2 mm in diameter are identified in up to 20% of cases. In the absence of metastases, 5-year disease-free survival is 60–80%. With pulmonary metastases, this falls to 0–40%, depending on the number of lesions. Bone metastases are generally not survivable.

A technetium-99m bone scan may be used to identify skip metastases and involvement elsewhere.

Blood tests do not help with the diagnosis, but elevated levels of alkaline phosphatase and lactate dehydrogenase have been associated with poorer prognosis. Levels normalize with successful treatment and rise in the event of recurrence.

Biopsy

A carefully planned biopsy should be performed by the treating surgeon. This confirms the diagnosis (Figure 20.18). A core-needle biopsy or an open biopsy may be performed. Standard principles are employed as follows.

- The surgeon performing the definitive procedure should perform the biopsy, following careful evaluation of the MRI scan.
- The biopsy tract should be fully excised at the time of the definitive surgery; thus, the tract will normally be in line with the planned extensile approach.
- Longitudinal incisions are mandatory in limbs. Fascial planes are not developed.
- Meticulous haemostasis is undertaken. If a drain is used, it should be in line with the incision, so that the tract is also excised.
- Uninvolved compartments should be avoided, if possible.
- Frozen section can be used to confirm that an adequate, viable sample has been taken.

Staging

Once the diagnosis is established, the tumour should be locally and systematically staged. The most useful local imaging modality is MRI. This is useful in identifying the extent of intramedullary and extracompartmental involvement, as well

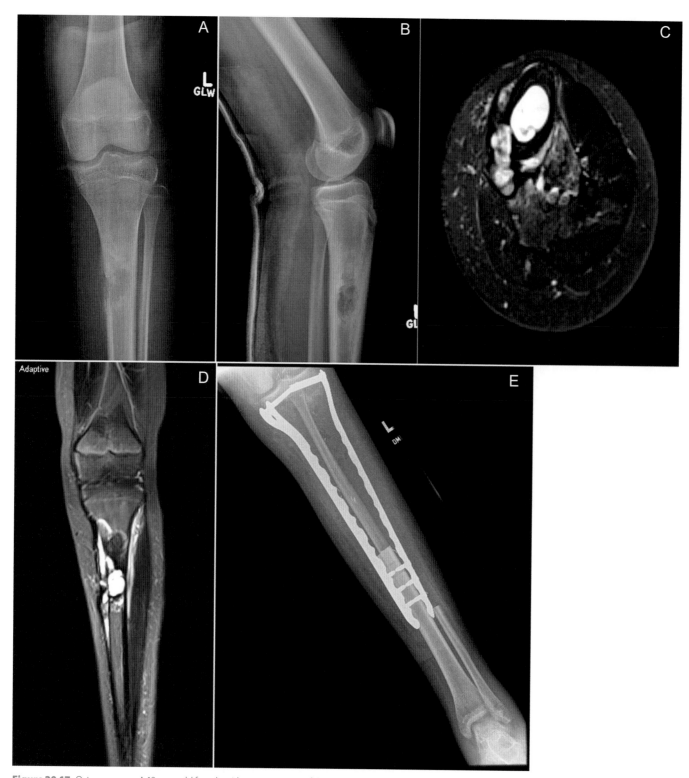

Figure 20.17 Osteosarcoma. A 13-year-old female with osteosarcoma of the proximal tibial diaphysis. A permeative lesion, eccentrically located in the proximal diaphysis, with cortical destruction and a wide zone of transition. Post-operative radiograph following wide excision and reconstruction with ipsilateral vascularized fibular graft.

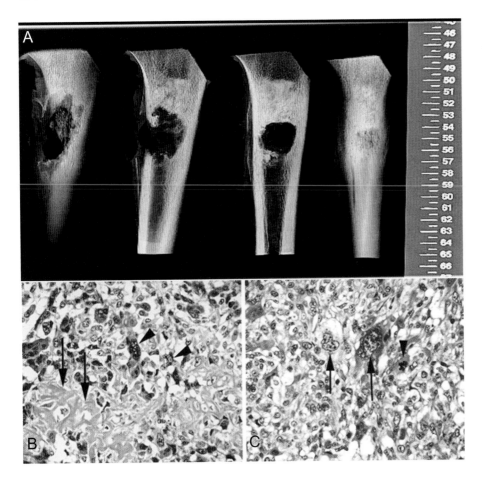

Figure 20.18 Osteosarcoma histopathology. (A) Lytic lesion and periosteal elevation clearly evident on radiograph of resected bone. (B) Photomicrograph of an osteosarcoma, showing pink, lace-like osteoid matrix (arrows) and significant atypia with numerous bizarre cells (arrowheads). (C) Photomicrograph of an osteosarcoma showing bizarre cells (arrows) and a mitotic figure (arrowhead). Haematoxylin and eosin, original magnification ×400.

as skip metastases along the bone. The proximity/involvement of neurovascular structures is seen, as well as the proximity to the physis/articular surface, to allow for surgical planning. Systemic staging is undertaken with chest CT and whole-body bone scanning.

Principles of Management

Management involves a multidisciplinary team, also including paediatric oncology, radiology, and pathology. Care is undertaken in specialist centres.

Prior to definitive surgical treatment, neoadjuvant chemotherapy is undertaken. Chemotherapy has been shown to markedly improve disease-free survival (survival was 10–15% despite amputation prior to the chemotherapy era in late 1970s). The commonly used regimen combines cisplatin, adriamycin, and methotrexate. This is typically given for an 11-week period prior to surgery, near the end of which an interval MRI scan is performed. With successful treatment, the soft tissue component and reactive oedema diminish in size. Histological analysis following tumour excision with >90% tumour necrosis is associated with a better prognosis.

Surgical treatment is tailored to the individual case (Figure 20.19). The primary consideration is resection with a safe, negative margin. Treatment options can be divided into limb-sparing and amputation. Amputation is generally reserved for cases:

- With neurovascular invasion/encasement
- Where a safe margin cannot be achieved
- When the circumferential tumour necessitates resection of numerous important tissues.

Where possible, the joint is preserved. This is based on whether the tumour extends beyond the physis or not. If not, a portion of the epiphysis with the articular surface is preserved, and intercalary reconstructive options include use of an autograft (e.g. vascularized fibula), allograft, or endoprosthesis to restore a gap in the bone. When the joint must be resected, reconstructive options include endoprosthesis, osteoarticular allograft, or rotationplasty in carefully selected and informed patients. An endoprosthesis preserves limb length and may be extendable during growth, but will require revision and limits activities. Rotationplasty radically alters the appearance and necessitates an external prosthetic, but is durable with any activity and usually does not require revision.

Ewing's Sarcoma

Ewing's sarcoma is the second commonest primary malignant tumour of bone in children and was first described by James Ewing in 1921. It is part of a family of small, round blue cell tumours, including primitive neuroectodermal tumours. The

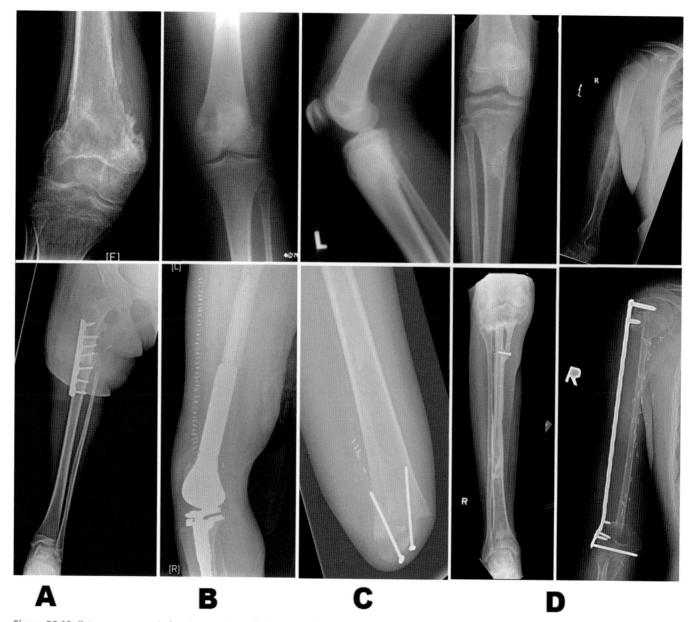

Figure 20.19 Osteosarcoma: surgical treatment options. (A) Excision and rotationplasty. (B) Endoprosthesis. (C) Amputation. (D) Excision and reconstruction using vascularized fibular graft.

cell of origin is unknown, but almost all Ewing sarcomas have rearrangements of *EWSR1* on chromosome 22, most commonly the t(11;22) translocation resulting in the *EWSR1::FLI1* fusion gene.

Location

Ewing's sarcoma commonly presents in the pelvis, femur, tibia, and proximal humerus (metaphyseal or diaphyseal).

Presentation

Ewing's sarcoma presents with localized pain and swelling. The swelling itself may be tender. The patient may be febrile, with raised inflammatory markers, but usually not until later in the disease process. Levels of lactate dehydrogenase may be raised and can be monitored to assess response to treatment.

Radiology

This is more commonly diaphyseal than in osteosarcoma. A substantial soft tissue mass is often seen. There may be a permeative lesion with a laminated periosteal reaction – described as an 'onion skin' appearance – but this is not always present. MRI is essential to quantify the level of medullary involvement and the presence of skip lesions (Figure 20.20). Systemic staging is undertaken with chest CT, whole-body bone scanning, and bone marrow aspiration in children. Bone biopsy typically

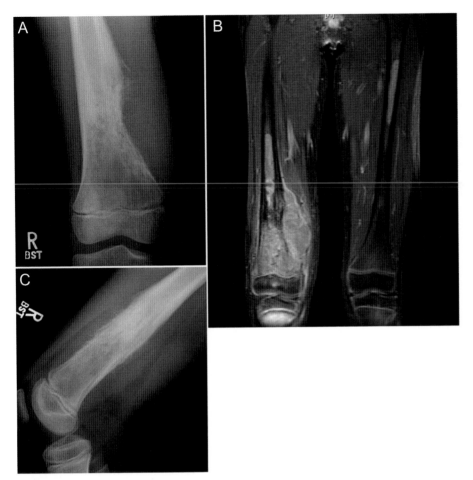

Figure 20.20 A 10-year-old boy with Ewing's sarcoma. Plain radiographs demonstrating a permeative lesion at the diaphyseal–metaphyseal junction, with cortical erosion, periosteal elevation, and 'sunray spicules'. A wide zone of transition is present with a substantial soft tissue component. MRI confirms soft tissue involvement and tumour spread to the proximal third of the medullary canal. The distal femoral epiphysis may be involved.

shows sheets of small, round blue tumour cells with a high nuclear-to-cytoplasmic ratio. The cytoplasm is scant and eosinophilic, and usually contains glycogen. The nuclei are round, with finely dispersed chromatin and one or more tiny nucleoli (Figure 20.21). Tumour markers are important for subclassification and guiding prognosis.

Treatment

Systemic chemotherapy is essential, and is given prior to (neoadjuvant), and following, local control, as with osteosarcoma, although the drugs are different. Surgery is preferred over radiotherapy for local control of resectable tumours because of a lower local recurrence rate. It is uncertain whether this alters survival. Occasionally, radiotherapy and surgery are combined for massive pelvic tumours.

Cycles of chemotherapy are given at 2- to 3-week intervals, lasting for 6–9 months. Vincristine, doxorubicin, and cyclophosphamide are used. Addition of ifosfamide and etoposide has been shown to improve outcome in non-metastatic disease. Four to six cycles are administered prior to surgical resection.

Surgery (with or without radiotherapy) results in better local control and possibly survival, compared to radiotherapy alone [29]. Radiotherapy alone may be considered in areas where reconstructive options are limited (e.g. acetabulum, bilateral sacrum) [30], but there is an associated risk of secondary malignancies [31, 32] and tumour recurrence. Surgical considerations are similar to osteosarcoma.

Prognosis

This is primarily affected by the presence or absence of metastatic disease. Following successful local control, a 5-year survival rate of 70% can be achieved. This reduces to 30% with metastases at presentation.

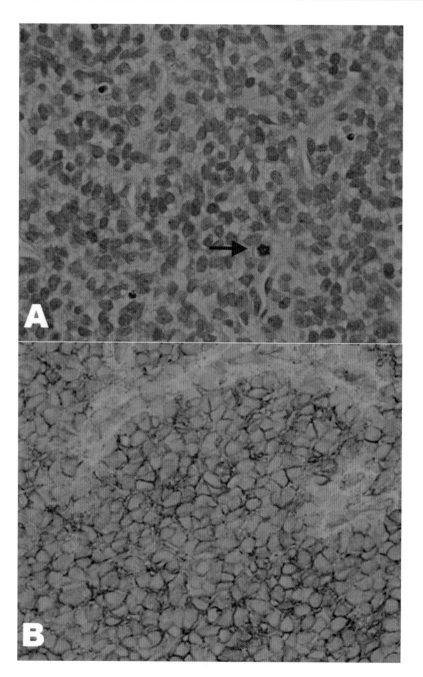

Figure 20.21 Ewing's sarcoma histopathology. (A) Sheet-like proliferation of small, round blue cells. The cells have vacuolar ('bubbly') cytoplasm and finely dispersed chromatin. No evidence of differentiation is seen. A mitotic figure is seen (arrow). Haematoxylin and eosin, original magnification ×600. (B) Immunohistochemical staining of CD99 showing a membranous pattern of positivity characteristic of Ewing's sarcoma. CD99 immunostain (Dako®) and haematoxylin counterstain, original magnification ×600.

Rhabdomyosarcoma

Rhabdomyosarcoma is the commonest soft tissue sarcoma in children. It can present anywhere in the body. There are two distinct forms that involve the extremities:

- **Embryonal rhabdomyosarcoma**: usually occurs in infants and young children. Has a more favourable outcome (5-year survival rate of 80%)
- **Alveolar rhabdomyosarcoma**: usually has a poorer prognosis and presents with a higher incidence of lymph node metastases. Associated with rearrangements involving *FOXO1* with either *PAX3* (t(2;13)) or *PAX7* (t(1;13)) (Figures 20.22 and 20.23).

Clinical Presentation

Rhabdomyosarcoma usually presents with a painless, firm deep soft tissue swelling. It may grow quite rapidly.

There is an increased prevalence of rhabdomyosarcoma with the following conditions: neurofibromatosis, Li–Fraumeni syndrome (mutation in the *p53* tumour suppressor gene), and Beckwith–Wiedemann syndrome.

Radiological Features

Plain radiographs are not usually helpful. MRI is the investigation of choice for diagnosis and surgical planning. CT chest is required to identify metastases. A bone scan, with or without

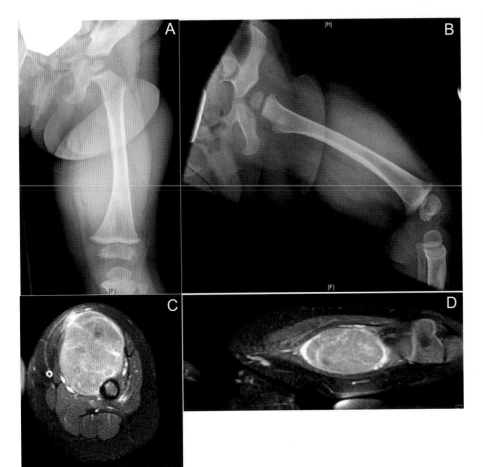

Figure 20.22 Alveolar rhabdomyosarcoma of the thigh in a 13-month-old girl. Soft tissue swelling is notable on the plain radiographs (A, B). MRI demonstrates a large, encapsulated soft tissue mass in the anteromedial thigh, abutting the proximal femur (C, D). Wide surgical excision was combined with adjuvant chemotherapy. A biopsy of the lesion was performed using standard principles. Fluorescence in situ hybridization (FISH) or reverse-transcriptase PCR can be used to identify the translocation.

bone marrow biopsy, may be performed to identify bone marrow involvement. Some authors recommend sentinel node biopsy, given the propensity for lymph node metastases in the alveolar variant.

Treatment

A multidisciplinary team approach is required. Combination treatment is given with chemotherapy, wide surgical excision (where possible), and possibly local radiotherapy. The chemotherapy regimen includes vincristine, cyclophosphamide, and actinomycin D. Treatment is stratified according to stage, node involvement, and histological type.

Prognosis

This varies according to the stage of disease, presence of metastases at diagnosis, and whether complete resection has been achieved. The overall survival rate is 74% without metastases, falling to 20–30% with metastases at presentation [33].

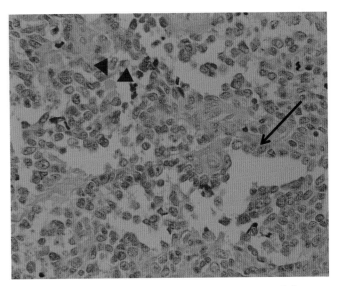

Figure 20.23 Photomicrograph of alveolar rhabdomyosarcoma. Cells are separated into vague nests by pink collagen and are discohesive ('falling apart') within the centre of the nests. Tumour cells line up along the collagen (arrow), and some show striated muscle differentiation in the form of pink cytoplasm (arrowheads). Haematoxylin and eosin, original magnification ×400.

References

1. Campanacci M, Capanna R, Picci P. Unicameral and aneurysmal bone cysts. *Clin Orthop Relat Res.* 1986;204:25–36.

2. Vayego SA, De Conti OJ, Varella-Garcia M. Complex cytogenetic rearrangement in a case of unicameral bone cyst. *Cancer Genet Cytogenet.* 1996;86(1):46–9.

3. Shindell R, Connolly JF, Lippiello L. Prostaglandin levels in a unicameral bone cyst treated by corticosteroid injection. *J Pediatr Orthop.* 1987;7(2):210–12.

4. McGlynn FJ, Mickelson MR, El-Khoury GY. The fallen fragment sign in unicameral bone cyst. *Clin Orthop Relat Res.* 1981;156:157–9.

5. Kaelin AJ, MacEwen GD. Unicameral bone cysts. Natural history and the risk of fracture. *Int Orthop.* 1989;13(4):275–82.

6. Wright JG, Yandow S, Donaldson S, Marley L. A randomized clinical trial comparing intralesional bone marrow and steroid injections for simple bone cysts. *J Bone Joint Surg Am.* 2008;90(4):722–30.

7. Alshryda S, Wright J. Evidence based treatment for simple bone cyst. In: Alshryda S, Huntley JS, Banaszkiewicz P, eds. *Paediatric Orthopaedics: An Evidence-Based Approach to Clinical Questions.* Cham: Springer; 2016. pp. 51–75.

8. Alshryda S, Howard JJ, Huntley JS, Schoenecker JG. *The Pediatric and Adolescent Hip: Essentials and Evidence.* Springer International Publishing; 2019.

9. Scaglietti O, Marchetti PG, Bartolozzi P. Final results obtained in the treatment of bone cysts with methylprednisolone acetate (depo-medrol) and a discussion of results achieved in other bone lesions. *Clin Orthop Relat Res.* 1982;165:33–42.

10. Docquier PL, Delloye C. Treatment of simple bone cysts with aspiration and a single bone marrow injection. *J Pediatr Orthop.* 2003;23(6):766–73.

11. Canavese F, Wright JG, Cole WG, Hopyan S. Unicameral bone cysts: comparison of percutaneous curettage, steroid, and autologous bone marrow injections. *J Pediatr Orthop.* 2010;31(1):50–5.

12. Hou HY, Wu K, Wang CT, Chang SM, Lin WH, Yang RS. Treatment of unicameral bone cyst: a comparative study of selected techniques. *J Bone Joint Surg Am.* 2010;92(4):855–62.

13. Rapp TB, Ward JP, Alaia MJ. Aneurysmal bone cyst. *J Am Acad Orthop Surg.* 2012;20(4):233–41.

14. Agaram NP, Bredella MA. Aneurysmal Bone Cyst. In: WHO Classification of Tumours: Soft Tissue and Bone Tumours. 5th Ed, IARC Press, 2020, pp 437–9.

15. Herring JA. *Tachdjians' Pediatric Orthopaedics*, 4th ed, Vol. 1. Philadelphia, PA: Saunders Elsevier; 2008.

16. Cottalorda J, Kohler R, Sales de Gauzy J, *et al.* Epidemiology of aneurysmal bone cyst in children: a multicenter study and literature review. *J Pediatr Orthop B.* 2004;13(6):389–94.

17. Oliveira AM, Hsi BL, Weremowicz S, *et al.* USP6 (*Tre2*) fusion oncogenes in aneurysmal bone cyst. *Cancer Res.* 2004;64(6):1920–3.

18. Leithner A, Lang S, Windhager R, *et al.* Expression of insulin-like growth factor-I (IGF-I) in aneurysmal bone cyst. *Mod Pathol.* 2001;14(11):1100–4.

19. Zenonos G, Jamil O, Governale LS, Jernigan S, Hedequist D, Proctor MR. Surgical treatment for primary spinal aneurysmal bone cysts: experience from Children's Hospital Boston. *J Neurosurg Pediatr.* 2012;9(3):305–15.

20. Gibbs CP, Jr., Hefele MC, Peabody TD, Montag AG, Aithal V, Simon MA. Aneurysmal bone cyst of the extremities. Factors related to local recurrence after curettage with a high-speed burr. *J Bone Joint Surg Am.* 1999;81(12):1671–8.

21. Weinstein LS, Shenker A, Gejman PV, Merino MJ, Friedman E, Spiegel AM. Activating mutations of the stimulatory G protein in the McCune-Albright syndrome. *N Engl J Med.* 1991;325(24):1688–95.

22. Yamamoto T, Ozono K, Kasayama S, *et al.* Increased IL-6-production by cells isolated from the fibrous bone dysplasia tissues in patients with McCune–Albright syndrome. *J Clin Invest.* 1996;98(1):30–5.

23. DiCaprio MR, Enneking WF. Fibrous dysplasia. Pathophysiology, evaluation, and treatment. *J Bone Joint Surg Am.* 2005;87(8):1848–64.

24. Rosenberg AE, Bloem JL, Sumathi VP. Fibrous Dysplasia. In: WHO Classification of Tumours: Soft Tissue and Bone Tumours. 5th Ed, IARC Press, 2020, pp 472–4.

25. Ahmed AR, Tan TS, Unni KK, Collins MS, Wenger DE, Sim FH. Secondary chondrosarcoma in osteochondroma: report of 107 patients. *Clin Orthop Relat Res.* 2003(411):193–206.

26. Busse M, Feta A, Presto J, *et al.* Contribution of EXT1, EXT2, and EXTL3 to heparan sulfate chain elongation. *J Biol Chem.* 2007;282(45):32802–10.

27. Schmale GA, Conrad EU, 3rd, Raskind WH. The natural history of hereditary multiple exostoses. *J Bone Joint Surg Am.* 1994;76(7):986–92.

28. Amary F, Bloem JL, Cleven AHG, Konishi E. Chondroblastoma. In: WHO Classification of Tumours: Soft Tissue and Bone Tumours. 5th Ed, IARC Press, 2020, pp 359-61.

29. Dunst J, Schuck A. Role of radiotherapy in Ewing tumors. *Pediatr Blood Cancer.* 2004;42(5):465–70.

30. Yock TI, Krailo M, Fryer CJ, *et al.* Local control in pelvic Ewing sarcoma: analysis from INT-0091–a report from the Children's Oncology Group. *J Clin Oncol.* 2006;24(24):3838–43.

31. Bacci G, Longhi A, Barbieri E, *et al.* Second malignancy in 597 patients with Ewing sarcoma of bone treated at a single institution with adjuvant and neoadjuvant chemotherapy between 1972 and 1999. *J Pediatr Hematol Oncol.* 2005;27(10):517–20.

32. Henderson TO, Whitton J, Stovall M, *et al.* Secondary sarcomas in childhood cancer survivors: a report from the Childhood Cancer Survivor Study. *J Natl Cancer Inst.* 2007;99(4):300–8.

33. Andrassy RJ, Corpron CA, Hays D, *et al.* Extremity sarcomas: an analysis of prognostic factors from the Intergroup Rhabdomyosarcoma Study III. *J Pediatr Surg.* 1996;31(1):191–6.

Chapter 21

Skeletal Dysplasia

Anish P. Sanghrajka and James A. Fernandes

Introduction

Skeletal dysplasia (SD) is a heterogenous group of inherited disorders characterized by abnormal growth of bone and/or cartilage, resulting in abnormal shape and size of the skeleton, spine, and/or head.

Making the Diagnosis

A multidisciplinary approach is necessary to diagnose and treat SD. This should include paediatricians, radiologists, geneticists, and orthopaedic surgeons. Other specialties, such as ophthalmology, renal, and cardiology, may get involved, depending on the type of dysplasia.

A thorough history and examination are essential, and often enough to establish the differential diagnosis.

- History should include:
  - o Antenatal/postnatal complications, including abortions and stillbirths
  - o Developmental history
  - o Past medical history, including:
    - □ Problems with eyes
    - □ Problems with hearing
    - □ Respiratory problems
  - o Family history.
- Examination should include:
  - o Standing height – most bone dysplasias cause short stature (defined as height that is less than the third percentile for the chronological age)
  - o Sitting height – this should be compared with standing height on growth charts to determine whether shortening is proportionate (trunk and limbs are short such as in mucopolysaccharidosis, spondyloepiphyseal dysplasia (SED)) or disproportionate (short limbs or trunk only such as in achondroplasia).
  - o Determining the pattern of limb shortening based upon the segment that is most affected (Table 21.1)

Table 21.1 Patterns of limb and trunk shortening

Pattern descriptor	Segment affected	Examples
Rhizomelic	Proximal (femur, humerus)	1. Achondroplasia (and hypochondroplasia, the rhizomelic type of chondrodysplasia punctata) 2. The Jansen type of metaphyseal dysplasia 3. SED congenita 4. Thanatophoric dysplasia 5. Diastrophic dysplasia 6. Congenital short femur
Mesomelic	Middle (forearm, leg)	1. Langer and Nievergelt types of mesomelic dysplasias 2. Robinow syndrome 3. Reinhardt syndrome
Acromelic	Distal (hand and fingers)	1. Acrodysostosis 2. Peripheral dysostosis
Micromelic	Entire limb	1. Achondrogenesis 2. Fibrochondrogenesis 3. Kniest dysplasia 4. Dyssegmental dysplasia 5. Roberts syndrome
Short trunk		3. Morquio syndrome 4. Kniest syndrome 5. Metatrophic dysplasia 6. SED 7. SEMD

Phocomelia is a rare congenital defect in which the hands are attached to short arms, or the feet to short legs. The term comes from *phoco* (meaning 'seal') and *melia* (meaning 'limb'), to indicate that a limb is like a seal's flipper, as in exposure of the developing fetus to thalidomide.
SED, spondyloepiphyseal dysplasia; SEMD, spondyloepimetaphyseal dysplasia.

- o Spinal examination – for any deformity (sagittal or coronal)
- o Lower limb alignment
- o Examination of each joint
- o Facies:
  - □ Forehead (e.g. frontal bossing in achondroplasia)
  - □ Trefoil (triangular) facies and blue sclerae in osteogenesis imperfecta
  - □ Eyes to assess for cataract and determine the interocular distance
  - □ Nasal bridge (e.g. depressed)
  - □ Dentition (abnormalities may indicate a collagenopathy)
- • Radiographs:
  - o Skeletal survey to establish:
    - □ Which bone(s) are affected
    - □ Which anatomical locations are affected (epiphysis, metaphysis, diaphysis)
    - □ Joint dislocations
  - o Images reviewed by a specialist paediatric, orthopaedic radiologist.
- • Genetic counselling and testing:
  - o Close liaison with the geneticist is vital. However, some understanding of terminology and its meaning is useful for the examination (and practice)
  - o Based on the history and clinical, radiological, and laboratory findings, a working diagnosis is made
  - o When a suspected diagnosis is obvious, such as achondroplasia or infantile cortical hyperostosis, specific gene(s) sequencing is requested – in these two examples, testing for *FGFR3* in achondroplasia and *COL1A1* in infantile cortical hyperostosis
  - o Most genetic centres compile several genes under one panel (e.g. skeletal dysplasia gene panel, neuromuscular diseases gene panel, epilepsy gene panel, etc.). These panels test for several genes that have been implicated in these problems – SD in our case. These panels differ

from one place to another, based on the incidence of various SD to strike a balance between testing affordability and diagnostic yield

- o If the above are negative or there is no clear clue on what the patient may have, whole exome sequencing (WES) or whole genome sequencing (WGS) may be requested. The former tests for aberrations of all exons in comparison to normal, whereas the latter tests for exons and introns. They are usually expensive but have higher diagnostic yields. Results from these are usually stored in a database and checked periodically (typically every 2 years) with new discoveries.

Classification of Bone Dysplasia

Thomas Fairbank was the first to classify SD in 1951 [1]. Philip Rubin refined Fairbank's classification by grouping the dysplasias according to the anatomical distribution of the abnormalities (Table 21.2) [2].

In more recent times, the International Skeletal Dysplasia Society has created a nosology classifying SD [3]. In the latest version from 2015, 436 different conditions were divided into 42 groups, defined by molecular, biochemical, and/or radiographic criteria. A total of 364 different genetic abnormalities have been identified to date. Some conditions have been grouped according to their common underlying gene or pathway (e.g. group 1 – *FGFR3* chondrodysplasia group), whereas other groups are based on localization of radiographic changes in specific bone structures (e.g. group 11 – metaphyseal dysplasias) or in the involved segment (e.g. group 17 – mesomelic and rhizomesomelic disorders). Details of this classification are beyond the exam requirement. However, in the following sections, we have provided a summary of the salient features of some of the individual dysplasias that we consider important for clinical practice and exams.

Achondroplasia

Achondroplasia is the commonest form of short stature, with an incidence of 1 per 10 000–100 000 live births.

Table 21.2 Rubin's classification of bone dysplasias

Location	Nature	Mechanism	Example
Epiphysis	Hypoplasia	Failure of articular cartilage	Spondyloepiphyseal dysplasia
		Failure of ossification centre	Multiple epiphyseal dysplasia
	Hyperplasia	Excess articular cartilage	Dysplasia epiphysealis hemimelica
Physis	Hypoplasia	Failure of proliferating cartilage	Achondroplasia
	Hyperplasia	Excess of hypertrophic cartilage	Enchondromatosis
Metaphysis	Hypoplasia	Failure to form primary spongiosa	Hypophosphatasia
		Failure to absorb primary spongiosa	Osteopetrosis
	Hyperplasia	Excessive spongiosa	Multiple exostosis
Diaphysis	Hypoplasia	Failure of periosteal bone formation	Osteogenesis imperfecta
	Hyperplasia	Excessive endosteal bone formation	Hyperphosphatasaemia

Basic Science

- Inherited as autosomal dominant, with complete penetrance.
- Ninety per cent of cases are due to spontaneous mutations, which have been linked with paternal age >36 years (suggesting the mutation occurs on the paternal rather than maternal chromosome).
- The risk of achondroplasia in offspring of two unaffected parents is 0.02%.
- The usual genotype for achondroplasia is heterozygous (the homozygous genotype is usually fatal in the neonatal period).
- The mutation is a glycine to arginine substitution in the gene encoding the fibroblast growth factor receptor 3 (*FGFR-3*) on chromosome 4p, resulting in inhibiting physeal chondrocyte proliferation, differentiation, and subsequent endochondral ossification.
- As the processes of intramembranous and periosteal ossification are unaffected, the clavicles and skull form normally, and whereas other long bones are shortened, they have a normal diameter.

Clinical Features

- Achondroplasia can be diagnosed using prenatal ultrasonography – short femora.
- The most noticeable clinical feature is disproportionate short stature with rhizomelia (Figure 22.1).
- The soft tissues of the limb, including the muscles, are relatively spared, giving the appearance that they are excessive for the length of the limbs. There is often also ligamentous laxity.
- The typical facies include frontal bossing, maxillary hypoplasia and a depression of the nasal bridge.
- There may be flexion contractures of the elbow, which can be the result of dislocation of the radial head.
- Relative shortening of the middle finger gives the appearance that all fingers are the same length ('starfish hand'). An abnormally increased separation of the middle and ring fingers gives the hand a 'trident' appearance.
- There is relative overgrowth of the fibula in relation to the tibia, believed to be the cause of tibia vara, genu varum and ankle varus.

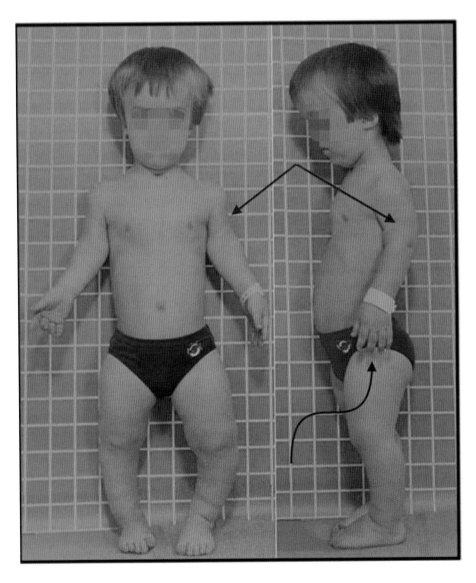

Figure 21.1 A child with classic features of achondroplasia, with a disproportionate short stature (the limbs are short, but the trunk is of normal height), rhizomelic shortening (short proximal segments, as indicated by straight red arrows), and trident hand (curved black arrow).

- Foramen magnum hypoplasia can cause craniocervical stenosis, which may cause hypotonia, sleep apnoea or even sudden death.
- Thoracolumbar kyphosis is commonly seen in infants, but usually resolves with growth and maturity as muscle tone improves.
- While stenosis of the spinal canal occurs in all patients with achondroplasia (secondary to thickening of the pedicles, hypertrophy of the facets and enlarged laminae), not all will develop symptoms due to this. Most of those who become symptomatic will do so by the third decade of life.

Radiographic Features

- The tubular bones (including those of the hands and feet) appear short, but with a relative increase in their density and diameter.
- The metaphyses are widened, with U- or V-shaped physes.
- The epiphyses are unaffected.
- Formed by intramembranous ossification, the pelvis appears broad and flat, with an inlet width that is greater than its depth ('champagne glass' pelvis):
  - o Squared-off iliac wings
  - o Flat horizontal acetabulum
  - o Markedly narrowed sacrosciatic notches

- o Relative overgrowth of the femoral greater trochanters, making the femoral neck appear to be in varus (but not true coxa vara).
- Premature fusion of the vertebral bodies with their arches results in increased narrowing of the spinal canal from L1 to L5. Radiographically, this is manifest by short, broad pedicles, with decreasing interpeduncular distances from L1 to L5 (as opposed to the widening that is usually seen in normal people).

Management

- The role of limb lengthening in achondroplasia is controversial. Unlike the congenital deficiencies, lengthening is tolerated very well in achondroplasia because of the relative excess of soft tissues.
- A single lengthening can achieve a 35% increase in the original bone length (7–15 cm). This does not result in a height within the normal range. Even after multiple staged lengthening of both femora and tibiae, achondroplasia patients still had a more negative body image than normal controls, leading many to question the benefits of such complex reconstruction.
- The lower limb angular deformities are rarely associated with degenerative changes in the knees, so surgery is

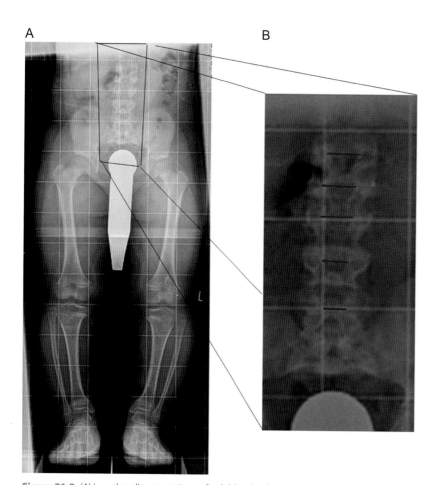
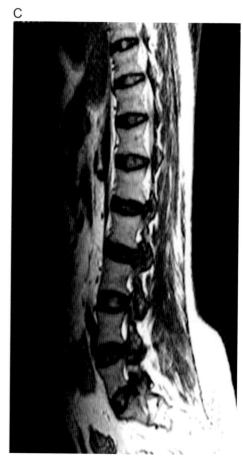

Figure 21.2 (A) Long leg alignment views of a child with achondroplasia. Notice the varus knees and ankles with joint laxity. (B) Spine radiograph showing decreasing interpedicular distance from top to bottom (normally should be increasing). (C) MRI of the spine showing canal stenosis, with very short pedicles.

recommended only for those with symptomatic or cosmetically unacceptable deformities.

- Spinal decompression may be required for those with symptomatic stenosis.
- Growth hormone has been shown to increase height in achondroplasia, but as it has a greater effect on the spine than on the lower limbs, it accentuates the disproportionate stature.
- VOXZOGO™ (vosoritide) has been approved recently by the Food and Drug Administration (FDA) and European Medicines Agency (EMA) for use to increase height in achondroplasia (5 years and older). It is given as an injection once a day. It is an analogue of C-type natriuretic peptide (CNP), so it may cause hypotension. In a multicentre randomized controlled trial, 60 patients were assigned to receive vosoritide, and 61 to receive placebo. After a 52-week trial, the adjusted mean difference in annualized growth velocity between the two groups was 1·57 cm per year in favour of vosoritide (95% confidence interval 1.22–1.93; two-sided $P <0.0001$) [4].

Hypochondroplasia

- Hypochondroplasia is a rare form of dwarfism resembling achondroplasia, but is less common and generally less severe.
- Hypochondroplasia and achondroplasia are allelic disorders, as both are the result of defects at the same gene locus (*FGFR-3* gene); the difference is the specific genetic mutation.
- Like achondroplasia, hypochondroplasia is inherited in an autosomal dominant fashion.
- Unlike achondroplasia, there is variability in the mutation that causes hypochondroplasia, and thus in the clinical expression. The clinical features are similar to those of achondroplasia, but milder, and may not be noticeable until later in childhood.

Pseudoachondroplasia

Unlike achondroplasia, pseudoachondroplasia (PSACH) affects the epiphyses and metaphyses. Those with the condition have short limbs and ligament laxity, and often develop premature osteoarthritis. The prevalence is 4 per 1 million.

Basic Science

- Although autosomal recessive forms are believed to exist, PSACH is usually transmitted as a dominant trait; both forms have mild and severe phenotypes.
- The defect affects the gene encoding cartilage oligomeric matrix protein (COMP), a large extracellular matrix protein expressed in cartilage, ligaments, and tendons.
- Mutations in the *COMP* gene result in intracellular retention of COMP within chondrocytes, which leads to:
  - o Premature cell death, resulting in decreased physeal growth

  - o A deficiency of extracellular COMP, which predisposes articular cartilage to degenerative changes.
- Similar mutations in the *COMP* gene are found in some forms of multiple epiphyseal dysplasia (MED).

Clinical Features

- Clinical features are not present at birth and become apparent in the first 3 years of life with rhizomelic shortening (Figure 21.3).
- Unlike achondroplasia, the skull and faces are unaffected. This helps to differentiate between the two conditions.
- Angular deformity of the lower limbs is a common feature, with both genu varum and valgum possible. There are often deformities in the distal femur, as well as in the proximal tibia.
- 'Windswept deformities' occur when genu valgum is present on one side and genu varum contralaterally (Figure 21.4).
- Ligamentous laxity associated with this condition can accentuate the deformities, which needs to be accounted for if considering corrective osteotomy.
- There is often incongruity between the femoral head, which is often flattened, and the acetabulum, which is often dysplastic.
- The epiphyseal deformities and joint incongruency often result in premature osteoarthritis.
- Odontoid hypoplasia, together with ligamentous laxity, can result in cervical atlantoaxial instability, which can cause symptoms ranging from increased fatigability to myelopathy.
- Radiographic investigations for C1–2 instability are therefore necessary in the preoperative assessment of any child.

Radiographic Findings

- Spine:
  - o Platyspondyly, with anterior beaking and irregular end plates
  - o Normal interpedicular distance
  - o Odontoid hypoplasia
  - o Atlantoaxial instability – may be seen on flexion–extension views.
- Extra-axial:
  - o Delayed ossification of the epiphyses
  - o Irregular and fragmented epiphyses, particularly affecting the hip/knee
  - o Synchronous and symmetrical involvement of the femoral epiphyses, without development of lucencies, differentiates this from Perthes' disease
  - o The femoral heads become flattened and enlarged, which may result in hip subluxation
  - o Knees can demonstrate varus or valgus malalignment.

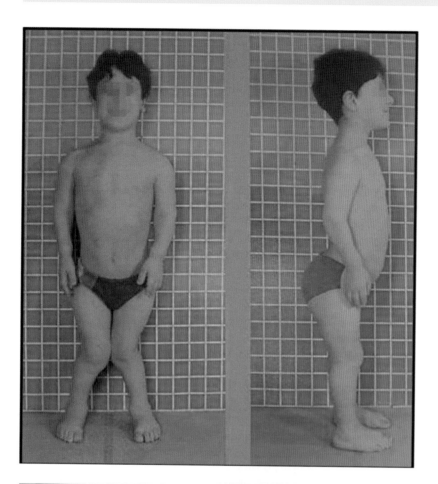

Figure 21.3 A child with pseudoachondroplasia showing a normal face and a disproportionate short stature (the limbs are short, but the trunk is of normal height).

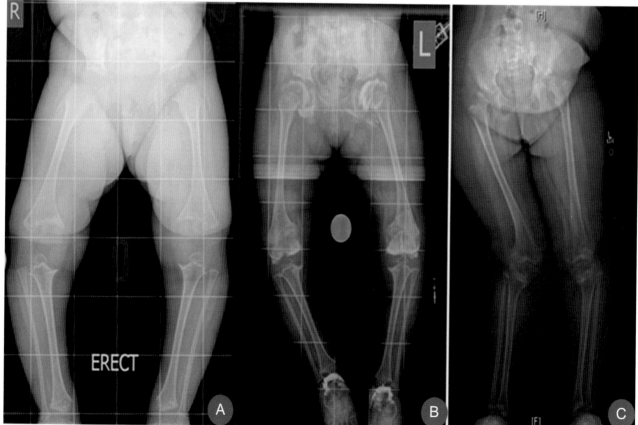

Figure 21.4 Radiological features of pseudoachondroplasia. (A, B) Irregular, flattened delayed epiphyses, delineated better with multiple arthrograms of the joint. (C) Image of another child, showing a windswept deformity.

Management

- Atlantoaxial fusion for cervical instability when present.
- Corrective osteotomies are usually required for lower limb malalignment.
- Valgus osteotomy of the proximal femur may improve both congruity of the joint and abductor function.
- Salvage acetabular augmentation (e.g. shelf) may improve femoral head coverage.
- Arthroplasty is technically demanding due to joint dysplasia and small bone sizes. Customized implants are usually required.

Spondyloepiphyseal Dysplasia

SED is a disproportionate short stature demonstrating progressive involvement of the spine and epiphyses of the long bones. The *congenita* (SEDC) type is present at birth, whereas the milder *tarda* (SEDT) type presents later in childhood.

Spondyloepiphyseal Dysplasia Congenita

Basic Science

- Caused by a mutation in the *COL2A1* gene, which encodes the α1 chain of type II procollagen.
- Inherited in an autosomal dominant fashion, but most cases are spontaneous mutations.

Clinical Features

- Short-trunk, rhizomelic, and mesomelic dwarfism
- Cervical spine instability (may cause myelopathy or respiratory problems)
- Wide-set eyes
- Barrel chest
- Hip flexion contractures with associated lumbar lordosis
- Waddling gait secondary to coxa vara
- Lower limb malalignment, usually genu valgum
- May have congenital talipes equinovarus (CTEV)
- The epiphyseal deformity predisposes to premature osteoarthritis
- Non-skeletal associations include:
  o Cleft palate
  o Myopia with retinal detachment
  o Cataracts
  o Deafness
  o Herniae
  o Nephrotic syndrome.

Radiographic Findings

(See Figure 21.5.)

- Delayed appearance of the epiphyses (femoral heads appear at age 5 years)
- Flattened, irregular epiphyses
- Platyspondyly, possibly with kyphoscoliosis

- Odontoid hypoplasia
- Atlantoaxial instability may be seen on flexion/extension views
- Coxa vara, if severe, may result in femoral neck discontinuity.

Management

- Posterior cervical fusion for atlantoaxial instability
- Scoliosis may require bracing, but the response is variable
- Consider proximal femoral valgus osteotomy if:
  o Progressive varus deformity
  o Neck shaft angle <100°
  o Hilgenreiner–epiphyseal angle is >60°
  o Fairbank's triangle present.
  (Note that proximal femoral valgus osteotomy will increase the genu valgum deformity.)
- Extension osteotomy of the proximal femur may be required for flexion deformities of the hips.
- Distal femoral varus osteotomies may be required for genu valgum.
- It is unclear whether corrective osteotomies prevent the development of degenerative joint disease. In one study, almost all patients with SED reported activity-related pain, even though half had undergone previous orthopaedic surgical procedures.

Spondyloepiphyseal Dysplasia Tarda

- SEDT usually presents in later childhood or adolescence with mild short stature or hip pain.
- Inheritance is X-linked recessive (*SEDL* gene) or autosomal recessive.
- Dysplasia of the femoral heads may be confused with Perthes' disease. Symmetrical, synchronous involvement of the hips, platyspondyly, and abnormalities of the other epiphyses help make the differentiation.
- Odontoid hypoplasia and consequent atlantoaxial instability may require posterior cervical fusion.
- Valgus proximal femoral osteotomy, with acetabular augmentation, aims to prevent premature arthritis, but outcomes remain unknown.
- Hip arthroplasty with custom implants may be required, even in early adult life.

Multiple Epiphyseal Dysplasia

MED was first described by Fairbank as dysplasia epiphysealis multiplex. It is characterized by a delay in appearance of the epiphyses, which, once formed, are irregular.

Basic Science

- Commonly autosomal dominant inheritance (rarely autosomal recessive).
- The predominant genetic mutation affects the *COMP* gene on chromosome 19 (similar to PSACH).

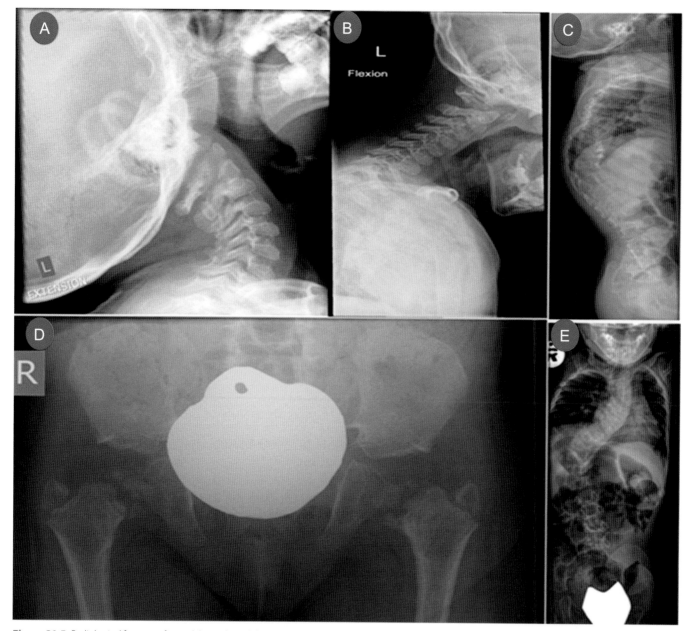

Figure 21.5 Radiological features of spondyloepiphyseal dysplasia. (A) and (B) are radiographs of a child with spondyloepiphyseal dysplasia congenita, demonstrating odontoid hypoplasia and subtle atlantoaxial instability. (D) is a radiograph of a pelvis showing delayed ossification and irregular epiphyses of the hips, with overgrown trochanters. Fairbank's triangle is present (more evident on the right) as a triangular metaphyseal fragment that is visible in the inferior part of the femoral neck; the fragment is surrounded by an inverted Y pattern. (C) and (E) show kyphoscoliosis with irregular vertebral epiphyses.

- The primary pathological abnormality in MED is irregular endochondral ossification of the epiphyses, with areas of degeneration. The articular cartilage becomes misshapen because of a lack of underlying osseous support.
- The femoral and humeral epiphyses are the most commonly affected, but the short tubular bones of the hands and feet may also be involved.

Clinical Features

- MED is not recognizable at birth and is often not diagnosed until adolescence.

- Presenting features can include:
  o Delayed walking
  o Pain
  o Limp and waddling gait
  o Joint stiffness or flexion contractures (especially the hips and knees)
  o Short stature
  o Genu varum/valgum
  o Short, stubby fingers and toes
  o Early osteoarthritis.

Radiographic Findings

(See Figure 21.6.)

- Delayed appearance of ossification centres, which, once apparent, are small and irregular.
- Reductions in epiphyseal and carpal heights can help make the diagnosis.
- Changes are most commonly seen in the proximal femur and need to be differentiated from bilateral Legg–Calvé–Perthes disease (LCPD). The following are suggestive of MED:
  - o Symmetrical, synchronous changes bilaterally
  - o Acetabular changes
  - o Absence of metaphyseal cysts (seen in LCPD)
  - o Epiphyseal irregularities in the knees/shoulders.
- Avascular necrosis of the femoral epiphysis can be seen in LCPD and MED, so neither MRI nor bone scanning can differentiate between the two conditions.
- Angular deformities, such as coxa vara or genu varum/valgum, may be present.
- The 'double-layered' patella may be seen on a lateral radiograph of the knee and is characteristic of MED.
- Short metacarpals and phalanges with irregular epiphyses.
- There may be mild vertebral end plate irregularities, but severe vertebral changes are not seen, differentiating MED from SED.

Management

- Physiotherapy to maintain joint range of motion.
- Although the radiographic changes are similar to those in LCPD, there is no evidence to support containment orthoses or surgery in MED.

- Painful hinge abduction may require proximal femoral valgus osteotomy.
- Corrective osteotomies of the femur may be required to correct lower limb malalignment.
- Osteoarthritis may require arthroplasty.

Diastrophic Dysplasia

'Diastrophic' is derived from the Greek word for 'twisted'. This condition is associated with severe short stature, rigid CTEV, scoliosis, and 'hitchhiker's thumb'.

Basic Science

- Autosomal recessive inheritance.
- The mutation affects the diastrophic dysplasia sulfate transporter (*DTDST*) gene on chromosome 5.
- Impaired function of the sulfate transporter ultimately leads to:
  - o Stunted endochondral growth
  - o Susceptibility of articular cartilage to early degenerative change.

Clinical Features

- This condition is easily diagnosed at birth by:
  - o The 'cauliflower ear'
  - o 'Hitchhiker's thumb' (Figure 21.7).
- The newborn child is very short-statured, with short limbs.
- A shortened, triangular first metacarpal causes radial subluxation of the metacarpophalangeal joint of the thumb, causing it to lie almost perpendicular to the index finger ('hitchhiker's thumb').
- The CTEV deformities are marked and rigid.

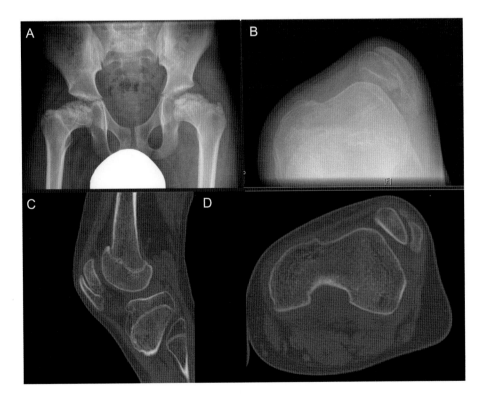

Figure 21.6 Multiple epiphyseal dysplasia. (A) A radiograph of the hips in a child with multiple epiphyseal dysplasia showing Legg–Calvé–Perthes disease-like appearance of the epiphysis. (B) Skyline view of the knee showing a dislocated patella, which also demonstrates the characteristic double-layered patella. (C, D) CT scans showing double-layered patella.

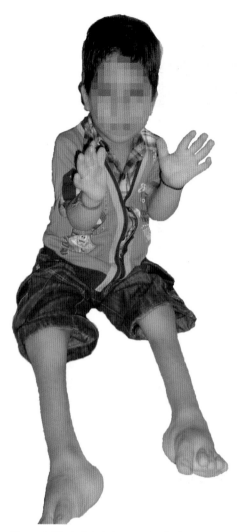

Figure 21.7 A clinical photograph of a diastrophic dwarf, with a 'hitchhiker's thumb'. Though not classical, note the club feet.

- Most patients have stiff joints, often with flexion contractures of the hips, knees, and elbows, but are ambulatory.
- Congenital dislocation of the hips in 25% of patients.
- Patellar and radial head dislocations are commonly seen.
- With increasing mobility, the child may develop kyphoscoliosis, which is often rigid and progressive.

Radiographic Features

(See Figure 21.8.)

- Delayed appearance of the epiphyses, which, once formed, are flattened and irregular
- Short, broad long bones with flared metaphyses
- Short, triangular first metacarpals and metatarsals
- A saucer-like indentation, often seen on the proximal femur
- Coxa vara
- Genu valgum.

Management

- Foot deformities are usually resistant to non-operative correction; nevertheless, Ponseti serial casting should be tried first. They may require open surgical release.
- Hip dislocations are teratologic, and whilst open reduction can be performed, pros and cons should be carefully balanced in non-walkers.
- Flexion contractures of the knee and hip may require soft tissue release, or even extension osteotomy.
- Severe and progressive spinal deformity may necessitate surgery during early childhood.

Chondrodysplasia Punctata

- This is a group of dysplasias characterized by multiple punctate calcifications within the unossified cartilage at the ends of the long bones, tarsal bones, pelvis, and vertebrae (Figure 21.9).
- These calcifications disappear within the first year of life, making early diagnosis important.
- The commonest form of this condition is Conradi–Hünermann syndrome, which is inherited as an X-linked dominant trait.
- There is a wide clinical spectrum, and clinical features include:
  o Short stature, possibly with rhizomelic limb shortening
  o Ichthyosiform erythroderma (dry, scaly skin)
  o Heart defects
  o Cataracts.

Metaphyseal Chondrodysplasia

- In this group of bone dysplasias, failure of normal mineralization of the zone of provisional calcification leads to widened physes and enlarged, cupped metaphyses (similar to rickets).
- The physeal pathology interferes with normal longitudinal bone growth, causing short stature and angular deformities (particularly coxa vara and genu varum).
- The epiphyses are spared, so arthritis is not common.
- There are several different types:
  o Jansen type:
    □ Rarest, but most severe type, usually apparent at birth
    □ Due to a mutation of the parathyroid hormone (PTH)/PTH-related peptide receptor gene
    □ Associated with severe hypercalcaemia and hypophosphatasia despite normal PTH levels
  o Schmid type:
    □ The commonest type of metaphyseal chondrodysplasia
    □ Autosomal dominant inheritance
    □ Genetic mutation on chromosome 6 (*COL10A1*) affects type X collagen

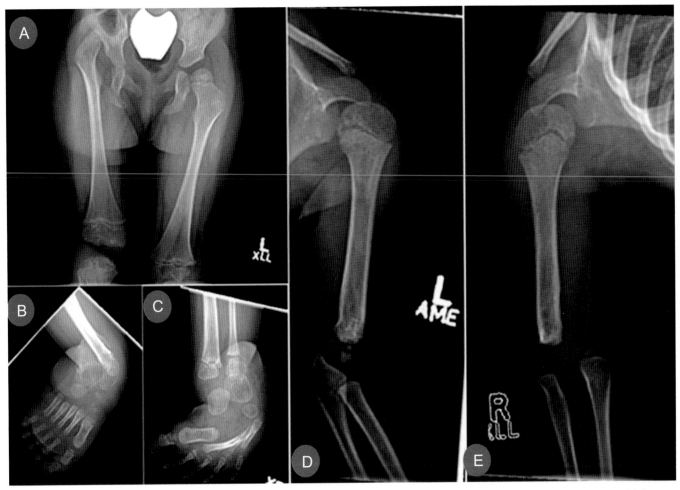

Figure 21.8 Radiological findings in diastrophic dysplasia. (A) Dislocated right hip with abnormal proximal and distal femoral epiphyses. (B, C) Severe club foot deformities. (D, E) Elbow contractures and radial head dislocation.

☐ Skeletal changes develop after weight-bearing at age 3–5 years.

Osteopetrosis

- Osteoclasts fail to resorb endochondral bone, whilst new bone formation continues, resulting in osteosclerosis.
- The resulting immature bone has fewer collagen fibrils, making it brittle ('marble bone'), and therefore susceptible to fracture.

Clinically, this results in:

- Deformity (i.e. coxa vara)
- Bone pain
- Osteomyelitis (commonly of the mandible)
- Pathological fractures (slow to heal).

Radiographic features include (Figure 21.10):

- Increased radio-opacity of the bones
- Loss of distinction between the cortex and the medullary canal
- 'Endobones', which are miniature radiodensities resembling tiny bones within the cortex of tubular bones; these are pathognomonic for osteopetrosis

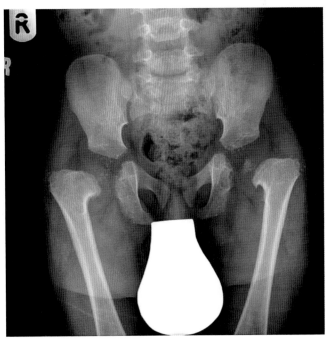

Figure 21.9 Chondrodysplasia punctata. Radiograph of an older child with Conradi–Hünermann syndrome with speckled ossification features of the right hip. This was associated with bilateral coxa vara.

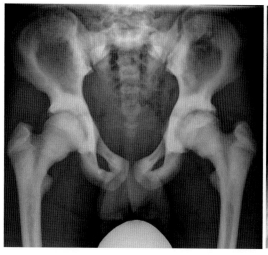
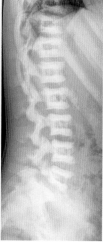

Figure 21.10 Osteopetrosis. There is increased radio-opacity of the bones, with loss of distinction between the cortex and the medullary canal. Note the 'Rugger jersey' spine, with zones of osteosclerosis adjacent to the vertebral end plates, and a radiolucent space centrally. Spondylolytic spondylolisthesis is noted at L5 seen as a feature in osteopetrosis.

- 'Rugger jersey' spine, with zones of osteosclerosis adjacent to the vertebral end plates, and a radiolucent space centrally

  There are two main types of osteopetrosis:

- Malignant osteopetrosis:
  o Autosomal recessive inheritance
  o Presents at birth or in early infancy
  o Additional clinical features include:
    □ Symptoms of pancytopenia, caused by obliteration of the bone marrow space by unresorbed bone
    □ Delayed dentition
    □ Blindness and deafness due to bony overgrowth of the cranial nerve foramina
  o This type is rapidly progressive and requires bone marrow transplantation in early childhood. If successful, the 5-year disease-free survival rate is over 70%. Osteosclerosis resolves, and normal bone marrow functioning and bone modelling resume.
- Benign osteopetrosis:
  o Autosomal dominant inheritance
  o About 40% of patients are asymptomatic and diagnosed incidentally
  o Two types:
    □ Type I – not associated with an increased fracture risk
    □ Type II – associated with mild anaemia and premature osteoarthritis
  o A small proportion of patients have osteopetrosis related to renal tubular acidosis, in which there is carbonic anhydrase deficiency.

Osteopoikilosis

- An autosomal dominant condition which is asymptomatic and requires no treatment.

- Characterized by clusters of 2- to 10-mm oval radiodensities within cancellous bone (Figure 21.11).
- Approximately 10% of patients have associated yellow subcutaneous nodules (the skin and bone changes together are called *dermatofibrosis lenticularis disseminata*).
- Osteopoikilosis may be confused with bone metastases; bone scans cannot differentiate between the two, as lesions may show increased or no uptake.
- Over time, the bone lesions may increase in size or regress and disappear.
- Malignant change, though rare, has been described.

Melorheostosis

- This rare dysplasia is not thought to be a genetic disorder.
- It is characterized by a 'flowing' hyperostosis of the cortex, the radiographic appearance of which has been likened to a candle with dripping wax (Figure 21.12).
- It may affect one bone (monosteotic), one limb, or multiple sites (polyosteotic).
- There are no reported cases of involvement of the skull or facial bones.
- It is associated with osteopoikilosis, neurofibromatosis, tuberous sclerosis, scleroderma, and rheumatoid arthritis.
- It usually presents in childhood or adolescence with bone pain and flexion tissue contractures.

Infantile Cortical Hyperostosis (Caffey's disease)

- Caffey's disease is a self-limiting condition mimicking infection.
- It usually presents before the age of 5 months with:
  o Fever and irritability

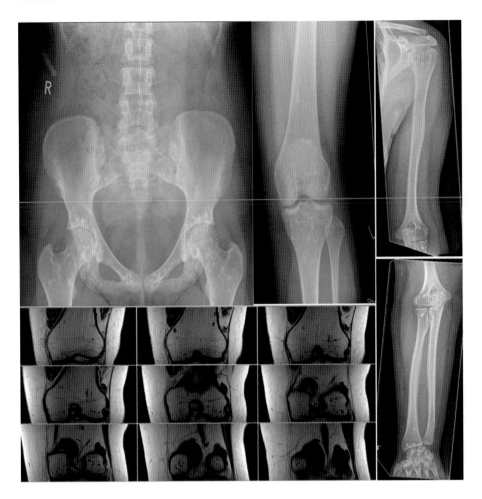

Figure 21.11 Osteopoikilosis. Plain X-rays and MRI scans showing numerous white densities of similar size spread throughout all the bones. Osteopoikilosis must be differentiated from osteoblastic metastases – it tends to present with larger and more irregular densities in less of a uniform pattern. Another differentiating factor is age, with osteoblastic metastases mostly affecting older people and osteopoikilosis found in people 20 years of age and younger.

o Localized deep soft tissue mass, most often over the mandible, but also frequently seen over the ulna, tibia, and clavicle

o Multifocal involvement – common

o Periosteal new bone formation over the diaphysis of the affected bone – demonstrated on radiographs

o Erythrocyte sedimentation rate and alkaline phosphatase levels may be elevated.

• The condition can occur in the prenatal period, and if occurring before 35 weeks' gestation, it can be fatal.

• Corticosteroids can be used in severe cases to treat acute systemic symptoms but do not affect the bony changes.

• Complete spontaneous recovery usually occurs within 6–9 months.

Cleidocranial Dysostosis

• A dysplasia of the bones formed by intramembranous ossification (including the clavicles, pelvis, and cranium).

• The pattern of inheritance is autosomal dominant, but a third of new cases are due to spontaneous mutations.

Clinical Features

• Often present before the age of 2 years and include the following:

• Hypoplasia or absence of one or both clavicles (the lateral end most commonly affected) (Figure 21.14)

• There may be similar underdevelopment of associated muscles (e.g. sternocleidomastoid and anterior deltoid)

• Abnormalities of the sternum, often with pectus excavatum

• Hypoplastic scapula, which may demonstrate winging

• Rarely, there may be upper limb pain or numbness due to irritation of the brachial plexus

• There are associations with syringomyelia and Wilms' tumour.

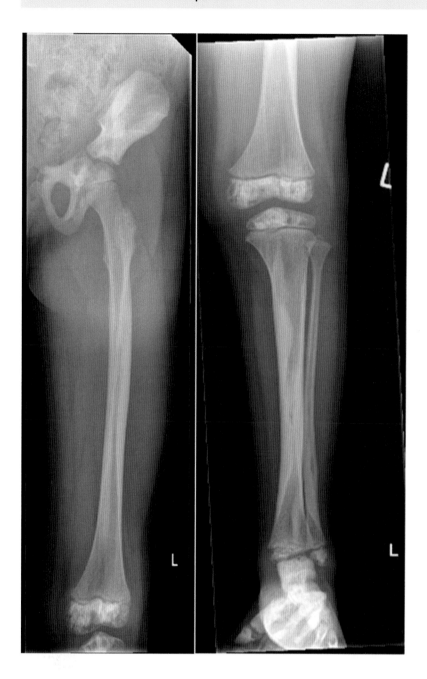

Figure 21.12 Melorheostosis. Notice thickening of the bony cortex resembling 'dripping candle wax'. In this patient, only the left side is involved.

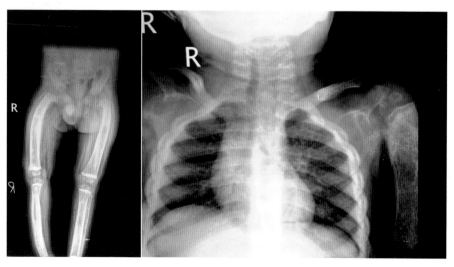

Figure 21.13 Infantile cortical hyperostosis. Radiographs showing infantile cortical hyperostosis as periosteal reactions and widening of bones seen in multiple segments. Other differential diagnoses need to be considered.

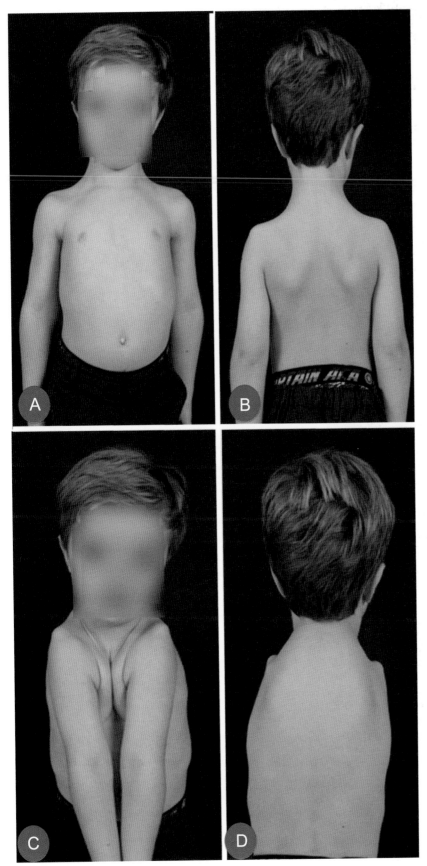

Figure 21.14 A child with cleidocranial dysostosis, with total absence of the clavicles. The patient is asymptomatic.

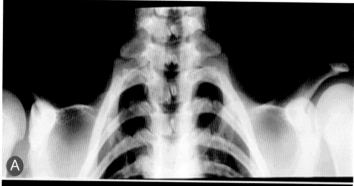

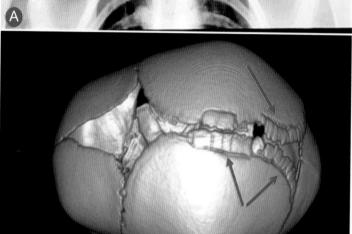

Figure 21.15 Cleidocranial dysostosis. (A) Radiograph showing absent clavicles. (B) A CT scan showing multiple wormian bones (red arrows).

Radiographic Features

- Hypoplastic/absent clavicle(s) (Figure 21.15)
- Multiple wormian bones in the skull
- Widened symphysis pubis and sacroiliac joints
- Coxa vara
- Scoliosis and spondylolysis
- Hypoplastic/absent terminal phalanges
- Increased length of the second metacarpals.

Orthopaedic Management

- Proximal femoral valgus osteotomy
- Excision of clavicular fragments to decompress the irritated brachial plexus
- Scapulothoracic arthrodesis for painful scapular winging
- Scoliosis treatment, as per adolescent idiopathic scoliosis.

References

1. Fairbank T. An atlas of general affections of the skeleton. By Sir Thomas Fairbank, D.S.O., O.B.E., M.S., Hon. M.Ch. (Orth.), F.R.C.S., Consulting Orthopaedic lSurgeon and Emeritus Lecturer in Orthopaedic Surgery, King's College Hospital. 7 × 10 ¼ in. Pp. 411 + xx, with 510 illustrations. 1951. Edinburgh: E. & S. Livingstone Ltd. 55s. *Br J Surg*. 1952;39(156):383.

2. Rubin P. Dynamic classification of bone dysplasias. *Acad Med*. 1964;39(11):1059.

3. Bonafe L, Cormier-Daire V, Hall C, *et al*. Nosology and classification of genetic skeletal disorders: 2015 revision. *Am J Med Genet Part A*. 2015;167A:2869–92.

4. Savarirayan R, *et al*. Once-daily, subcutaneous vosoritide therapy in children with achondroplasia: a randomised, double-blind, phase 3, placebo-controlled, multicentre trial. *Lancet*. 2020;396(10252):684–92.

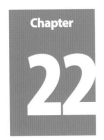

Metabolic Bone Disease

Richard Hutchinson, Mubashshar Ahmad, and Gavin DeKiewiet

Introduction

The key to understanding metabolic bone disease in children is to have a clear understanding of what bone is made of and how it grows at the physes. The structure of the physis is covered in detail in Chapter 25. An overview of the structure of bone and its role in calcium and phosphate homeostasis will be covered below.

Bone Structure

The extracellular matrix of bone can be divided broadly into two components:

- **Organic** (osteoid), 40% – mostly **type I collagen**
- Inorganic, 60% – mostly hydroxyapatite (HA) crystals.

In bone, type I collagen is formed by osteoblasts. Alpha 1 and 2 chains are produced under the influence of *COL1A1* and *COL1A2* genes, respectively. These chains then undergo two critical steps:

1. Hydroxylation
2. Triple helix formation.

Hydroxylation of lysine and proline amino acids, found along the α chains, occurs under the influence of hydroxylase enzymes. Vitamin C acts as a cofactor for these enzymes. Two α1 chains combine with one α2 chain to form the triple helix procollagen molecule. This molecule is then 'trimmed down' by peptidases into tropocollagen. At this point, the hydroxylated amino acids cause the formation of strong covalent bonds between tropocollagen molecules, in a process known as cross-linking, leading to formation of collagen fibrils. Collagen fibrils are then arranged in a quartered, staggered array pattern (Figure 22.1), with HA crystals settling between fibre ends. HA crystals form from calcium (Ca) and phosphate (PO_4) in the presence of the enzyme alkaline phosphatase (ALP) [1].

Any interruption to this complex process leads to bone that is more easily deformed or fractured. In growing bone, deficient or defective bone formation on the metaphyseal side of the physis can disrupt normal growth, resulting in short stature. Hence, plotting a child's height on a growth chart is an important part of clinical assessment when considering metabolic bone disease.

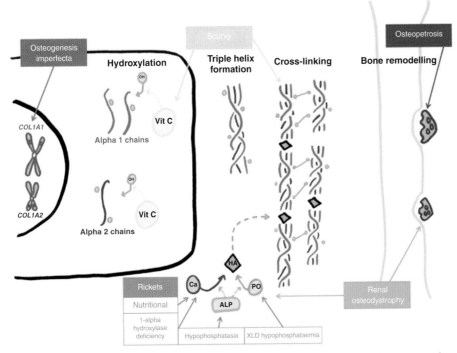

Figure 22.1 This figure gives an overview of how metabolic bone disease affects the different stages of bone formation and remodelling.

Calcium and Phosphate Homeostasis

- Ninety-eight per cent of the body's Ca, and 85% of its PO_4, is stored in bone, with only a small proportion present in blood.
- The bony skeleton acts as a reservoir of stored Ca and can be drawn upon to maintain serum Ca levels.
- Serum Ca plays vital roles in the clotting cascade and in maintaining cell function, nerve conduction, and muscle contraction.

Bone mineralization is regulated by both hormonal (e.g. vitamin D, parathyroid hormone (PTH)) and mechanical (via Wolff's law) factors. However, there is a hierarchy between these two factor groups. As Ca metabolism takes precedence, the hormonal effects will 'outdo' the mechanical ones. Hence, female amenorrhoeic runners get osteoporosis despite regular, significant mechanical forces applied across the bone [1].

Two hormones chiefly regulate serum levels of Ca and PO_4:

- Vitamin D
- PTH.

Vitamin D

There are two active forms of vitamin D: 1,25-dihydroxycholecalciferol (calcitriol) and 24,25-dihydroxycholecalciferol. The former is the most important for Ca homeostasis. The latter has a key role at the physis. Both are formed from pro-vitamins arising from two main sources:

- **Diet**:
  - ○ Vitamin D2 (ergocalciferol) and D3 (cholecalciferol)
  - ○ Sources: red meat, oily fish, and egg yolk
  - ○ Recommended daily intake in children: 400 IU
- **Liver + ultraviolet (UV) light**:
  - ○ 7-dihydrocholesterol produced in the liver and converted into vitamin D3 in the skin via UV light
  - ○ Melanin competes with 7-dihydrocholesterol – hence people who are heavily pigmented require longer exposure to UV light to produce an equivalent quantity of vitamin D.

These pro-vitamins are hydroxylated, first in the liver (forming 25-hydroxycholecalciferol) and then again in the kidney (forming either 1,25-dihydroxycholecalciferol or 24,25-dihydroxycholecalciferol). Vitamin D chiefly acts on the kidneys, bowel, and bone (Table 22.1).

Parathyroid Hormone

PTH is produced by the chief cells of the parathyroid glands in response to low serum Ca levels. Its production is inhibited by high serum Ca and vitamin D levels. PTH chiefly acts on the kidneys and bone (Table 22.1).

Teriparatide, a recombinant form of human PTH, has been used in the treatment of osteoporosis in adults. However, it is contraindicated in children due to its oncogenic potential.

Calcitonin

It is produced by C cells of the thyroid gland. Although the exact physiological function of calcitonin is unknown, it has a powerful inhibitory effect on osteoclasts, causing flattening of their ruffled border and withdrawal of osteoclasts from the bone surface. Salmon calcitonin is given intranasally as treatment for osteoporosis. In addition to inhibiting bone resorption, there is a significant analgesic effect, especially in osteoporotic patients with vertebral fractures.

Other hormones, including oestrogen, thyroxine, and corticosteroids, also play less significant roles in Ca homeostasis.

Bisphosphonates

Bisphosphonates have a very high affinity for bone mineral because they bind to hydroxyapatite crystals. Bisphosphonates are preferentially incorporated into sites of active bone remodelling, thus rapidly and specifically inhibiting bone resorption mediated by osteoclasts. This improves the existing bone microarchitecture and mineralization, and slows or prevents the progressive loss of structural elements. There are two classes of bisphosphonates:

1. Nitrogen-containing (etidronate) – not commonly used
2. Non-nitrogen-containing bisphosphonates (pamidronate, risedronate, alendronate, and zoledronate).

These two classes of bisphosphonates work differently in killing osteoclast cells. The commonest side effects of bisphosphonates are fever and myalgia. A rare, but significant, skeletal complication of bisphosphonate therapy is osteonecrosis of the jaw. This

Table 22.1 Quick reference guide showing the main sites of action and effects of vitamin D and PTH

	Sites of action	Action
Vitamin D	Bowel (small intestine)	↑ Ca absorption ↑ PO_4 absorption
	Bone (osteoblasts)	Stimulation of osteoclasts via RANK pathway (Figure 22.2)
	Kidney (distal convoluted tubule)	↑ Ca reabsorption
PTH	Bone (osteoblasts)	Stimulation of osteoclasts via RANK pathway, releasing Ca to circulation ↑ Ca
	Kidney (distal convoluted tubule)	↑ Ca reabsorption ↑ PO_4 excretion ↑ Vitamin D production

Ca, calcium; PO_4, phosphate; RANK, receptor activator of nuclear factor kappa B; PTH, parathyroid hormone.

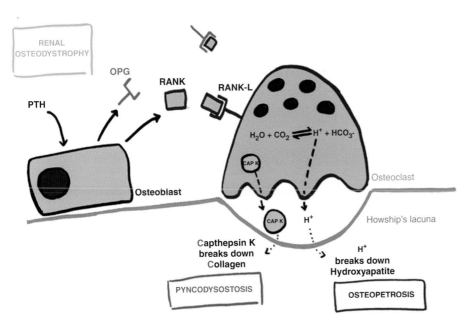

Figure 22.2 The receptor activator of nuclear factor kappa B (RANK) pathway is a key component of bone remodelling. Osteoblasts are stimulated to produce RANK, which binds to RANK ligand (RANK-L) on the surface of osteoclast precursors, stimulating osteoclast differentiation. RANK-L activation on mature osteoclasts stimulates bone resorption. Osteoprotegrin (OPG), also produced by osteoblasts, acts to regulate the RANK pathway by binding RANK. This figure also demonstrates the various points in bone remodelling affected by metabolic bone disorders.

occurs more commonly in patients with metastatic bone disease who receive monthly treatments.

Overview of Paediatric Metabolic Bone Disease

Paediatric metabolic bone disease can broadly be divided into three categories:

1. Mineral problems:
   a. Rickets
   b. Renal osteodystrophy (ROD)
   c. Osteopetrosis
2. Collagen problems:
   a. Osteogenesis imperfecta
   b. Scurvy
3. Both mineral and collagen problems:
   a. Osteoporosis.

As you will see below, all these conditions offer a great opportunity for FRCS examiners to ask basic science questions related to bone structure, remodelling, and Ca homeostasis (Figure 22.1). A quick reference guide briefly describing each condition, for that last-minute revision, is provided in Table 22.2.

Rickets

Rickets and osteomalacia share the exact same pathogenesis. However, they produce two very different clinical syndromes.

Rickets occurs when there is deficient mineralization of growing bone. In rickets, the cartilaginous matrix in the zone of provisional calcification (ZPC) is still replaced by osteoid, but there is insufficient production of HA crystals. This leads to the classical radiographic appearances of widened physes. Osteomalacia occurs due to deficient mineralization of mature trabecular and cortical bone [1].

Table 22.2 Quick reference guide giving brief descriptions of each of the metabolic bone conditions covered in this chapter

Condition	Brief description
Rickets	Deficient mineralization of growing bone
Osteomalacia	Deficient mineralization of mature bone
Renal osteodystrophy	• Hyperparathyroidism secondary to reduced phosphate excretion, leading to deficient mineralization and increased bone turnover • *Prolonged elevation of PTH eventually leads to downregulation of PTH receptors, resulting in low bone turnover (or adynamic renal osteodystrophy)*
Osteopetrosis	Abnormal bone sclerosis secondary to inability to break down hydroxyapatite crystals
Osteogenesis imperfecta	Genetically determined defect in type I collagen formation, leading to characteristic bone fragility; 90% result from defects in *COL1A1* or *COL1A2* genes
Scurvy	Nutritional deficiency in vitamin C resulting in deficient hydroxylation and subsequent failure of collagen cross-linking
Osteoporosis	Quantitative disorder of bone defined by reduced BMD and increased fracture risk

PTH, parathyroid hormone.

This means the main clinical features of rickets are deficient longitudinal growth and deformity. However, osteomalacia is characterized by symptoms of bone pain and fracture.

Clinical Features

- Short stature
- Genu varum/valgum
- Thickened wrists, elbows, and knees (Figure 22.3)
- Rachitic rosary (thickenings of the costochondral margins of the thorax described as looking like 'rosary prayer beads') (Figure 22.3)
- Harrison sulcus – forms at the lower border of the thoracic cage. Caused by deformation of the lower ribs due to breathing
- Kyphoscoliosis
- Plagiocephaly
- Frontal and parietal bossing
- Delayed appearance of 'milk teeth'.

Radiographic Features

- Widened physes
- Metaphyseal cupping (Figure 22.4)
- Looser zones ('pseudofractures') – transverse bands of unmineralized osteoid running perpendicular to the cortex
- Acetabular protrusion.

Normal bone mineralization requires sufficient levels of Ca and PO_4 in the presence of ALP. It can be useful therefore to separate the different causes of rickets according to these three factors. Table 22.3 shows the different types of rickets according to these criteria, as well as briefly describes the pathogenesis and medical treatment of each type. Surgical management in rickets is based on addressing the deformity, through guided growth or osteotomies, and treating pathological fractures.

Renal Osteodystrophy

In children with open physes, ROD can be thought of as 'renal rickets' accompanied by secondary/tertiary hyperparathyroidism. Like rickets, it leads to deficient mineralization, but additionally the failing kidneys also affect bone turnover and total bone volume.

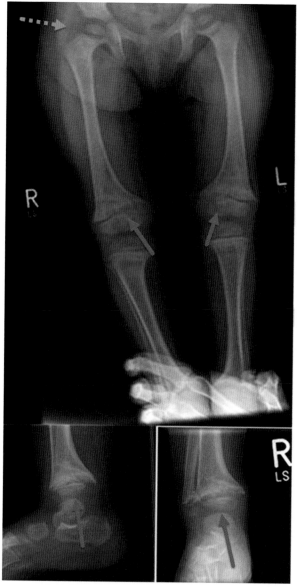

Figure 22.4 Widened physes and metaphyseal cupping (solid red arrows) classically seen in rickets. There is widening of the physes (dashed green arrow), which increases the risk of transphyseal fractures, including slipped upper femoral epiphysis.

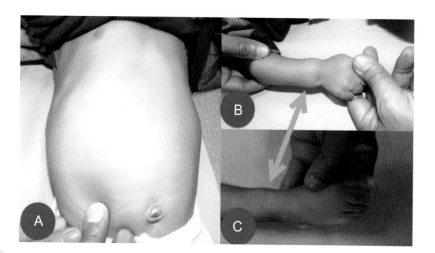

Figure 22.3 (A) Rachitic rosary (thickening of the osteochondral margins of the thorax described as looking like 'rosary prayer beads'; dashed red arrow). (B) and (C) show a thickened wrist and ankle, respectively.

Table 22.3 Brief overview of some of the more commonly asked causes of rickets

	Types of rickets	Inheritance pattern	Chromosome involved	Pathogenesis	Treatment
Low Ca	Nutritional rickets	–	–	Poor intake of Ca or vitamin D	Adequate vitamin D or Ca in diet
	1-α hydroxylase deficiency	AR	12	Unable to hydroxylate 25-cholecalciferol into active vitamin D in the kidney	Oral active vitamin D3
Low PO4	X-linked hypophosphataemia	XD	X (*PHEX* gene)	Renal PO_4 wasting Low serum PO_4 + hypercalcaemia	Oral PO_4 and active vitamin D3
Low ALP	Hypophosphatasia	AR	1 (*ALPL* gene)	ALP deficiency + hypercalcaemia	Treat hypercalcaemia Currently no reliable treatment for managing low ALP levels

Ca, calcium; AR, autosomal recessive; PO_4, phosphate; XD, X-linked dominant; ALP, alkaline phosphatase.

Pathogenesis

Chronic kidney disease (CKD) in children can be secondary to congenital (e.g. renal hypoplasia) or acquired (e.g. sickle cell disease leading to nephrotic syndrome) causes. PO_4 and Ca are both excreted via the kidney. In CKD, a reduction in functioning nephrons leads to reduced clearance of both Ca and PO_4. However, rising levels of serum PO_4 subsequently leads to a drop in the levels of free ionized Ca (as described in the paragraph below), which, in turn, stimulates PTH production, resulting in secondary hyperparathyroidism.

Increased PO_4 levels result in low serum free Ca levels via two pathways:

- PO_4 directly binds to free Ca in the bloodstream
- PO_4 stimulates fibroblast growth factor receptor 23 (FGFR-23) production by osteocytes, osteoblasts, and osteoclasts. FGFR-23 inhibits 1-α hydroxylase, which converts vitamin D into its active form. Reduction in vitamin D levels leads to reduction of both PO_4 and Ca absorption in the gut.

PTH tries to correct the hypocalcaemia by stimulating osteoblasts, which activate osteoclasts to break down bone (through the RANK pathway). This releases Ca into the bloodstream, but also releases PO_4. Normally, PTH would counteract this rise in PO_4 by increasing PO_4 excretion at the distal convoluted tubule. However, in the case of CKD, this cannot occur, leading to a decompensated PO_4 rise. This results in an unhealthy cycle of rising PO_4 levels, decreasing vitamin D levels, and rising PTH levels [2].

Initially, rising PTH levels result in a high bone turnover ROD. This leads to many of the orthopaedic manifestations associated with renal bone disease (e.g. osteitis fibrosa cystica). However, prolonged levels of high PTH can result in downregulation of PTH receptors in bone, eventually resulting in low bone turnover (or adynamic) ROD.

Osteitis Fibrosa Cystica

This describes the laying down of peritrabecular fibrous tissue in patients with ROD. This occurs as a result of high bone turnover. It can affect any bone and is the underlying cause of many classical radiological features such as brown tumours and pepper pot skull.

Clinical Features

Features of CKD in children include:

- Failure to thrive
- Delayed gross motor milestones
- Generalized listlessness/weakness
- Convulsions.

Orthopaedic features result from a combination of poor mineralization of bone (which produces similar features to rickets) and high bone turnover:

- Bone pain
- Short stature/growth retardation
- Angular deformities (e.g. genu varum/valgum)
- Scoliosis
- Slipped epiphyses – including slipped upper femoral epiphysis (SUFE; note that SUFE in ROD does not occur in the hypertrophic zone; instead the slip occurs at the junction of the ZPC and the primary spongiosa. Additional to slips of the upper femoral epiphysis, epiphysiolysis also occurs at other sites, for example, distal femur, proximal humerus, distal radius, distal ulna [3])
- Avascular necrosis
- Pathological fracture
- Myopathy.

Radiological Features

- Widened physes (without physeal cupping)
- Slipped epiphyses
- Osteopenia, thin cortices, indistinct trabeculae
- Ground-glass appearance of bone (due to laying down of fibrous tissue)
- 'Pepper pot' skull
- 'Rugger jersey' spine (this refers to the striped appearance of the vertebral bodies seen on sagittal views in both ROD

and osteopetrosis. In ROD, the lytic stripe represents poorly mineralized bone and the 'sclerotic' stripe represents normal bone. By contrast, the 'lytic' stripe in osteopetrosis is normal bone. The definition between the stripes is much sharper in osteopetrosis (Figure 21.10))

- Brown tumours (lytic lesions – can mimic metastases)
  - o Non-neoplastic masses of fibrous tissue, woven bone, and haemosiderin; the latter gives a classic macroscopic brown colour
- Subperiosteal resorption – classically of the metacarpals
- Soft tissue calcification.

Management

Medical management consists of:

- PO_4 binders – to reduce serum PO_4 levels
- Vitamin D and Ca supplementation
- Managing CKD – dialysis/transplant.

Surgical management demands a multidisciplinary team approach. These children are immunocompromised, especially if post-transplant. Surgical timing needs to be planned around dialysis or potentially holding off immunoregulating drugs (e.g. anti-tumour necrosis factor treatment). There also needs to be a clear plan regarding perioperative fluid balance.

Angular deformities can be treated by either guided growth or osteotomies (Figure 22.5) [4]. SUFE requires stabilization of the affected side, along with prophylactic pinning of the contralateral femur (Figure 22.6).

Osteopetrosis

Osteopetrosis is abnormal bone sclerosis secondary to inability to break down HA crystals.

Osteoclasts break down bone through the production of (Figure 22.2):

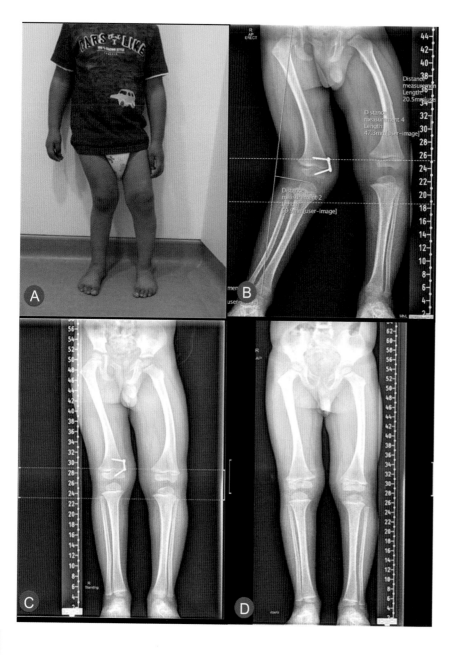

Figure 22.5 Use of guided growth (eight plates) to correct valgus deformity of the right lower limb.

Osteopetrosis occurs when osteoclasts are unable to transport H$^+$ into the lacunae. Pyncodysostosis occurs due to a deficiency in cathepsin K. Both lead to abnormal bone sclerosis.

Broadly speaking, osteopetrosis can be divided into two phenotypes:

- Malignant (autosomal recessive) form:
  o Usually diagnosed before the age of 1
  o Fatal in infancy secondary to pancytopenia, unless treated via bone marrow transplant
- Benign (autosomal dominant) form:
  o Normal lifespan
  o Does not require bone marrow transplant
  o The commonest form of benign osteopetrosis is called Albers–Schönberg disease.

Clinical Features

- Fractures:
  o Bone is much harder, but more brittle
- Osteomyelitis (especially mandibular osteomyelitis)
- Poor dentition
- Reduced intramedullary marrow space (therefore reduced red marrow):
  o Anaemia
  o Bleeding (thrombocytopenia)
  o Infection (leucocytopenia)
  o Hepatosplenomegaly due to increased extramedullary haematopoiesis
- Cranial nerve compression neuropathies:
  o Blindness (optic nerve compression)
  o Deafness (sensorineural)
    □ Conductive deafness (can also occur due to auditory ossicle involvement)
- Hypocalcaemia:
  o Ca 'locked away in bone'
  o Leads to seizures and tetany [5].

Radiological Features

- Sclerosis
- Loss of medullary canal (Figure 21.10)
- Rugger jersey spine
- Block metaphyses
- 'Bone within a bone'.
- Erlenmeyer flask femurs (Erlenmeyer flask deformities describe the characteristic 'chemistry flask' shape of the femurs seen in a number of conditions, including [6]: bone dysplasias (achondroplasia, metaphyseal dysplasia, osteopetrosis), lysosomal storage diseases (Gaucher/Niemann–Pick), haemoglobinopathies (sickle cell disease/thalassaemia), and fetal magnesium toxicity).

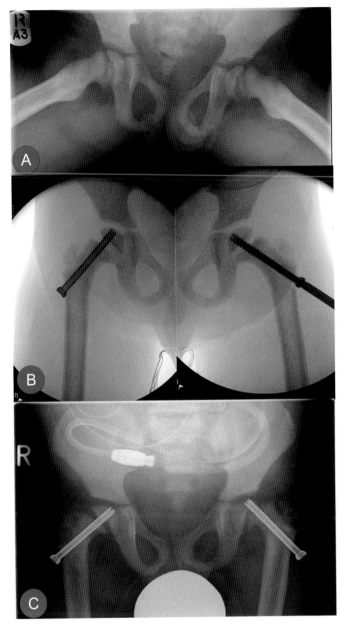

Figure 22.6 A child with renal osteodystrophy who developed bilateral slipped upper femoral epiphysis (A). It was stabilized with bilateral pinning in situ (B). However, both screws cut through, as the bones were very weak (C).

- Carbonic acid:
  o Carbonic anhydrase within osteoclasts catalyses the conversion of carbon dioxide (CO_2) and water (H_2O) into carbonic acid
  o Carbonic acid subsequently breaks down into bicarbonate (HCO_3^-) and protons (H$^+$)
  o H$^+$ are transported into Howship's lacunae, leading to acidification and breakdown of HA crystals
- Cathepsin K:
  o An enzyme produced by osteoclasts, which, when transported into Howship's lacunae, breaks down collagen.

Management

Malignant osteopetrosis requires bone marrow transplant in infancy. Interferon-gamma and calcitriol have been trialled as medical treatments aimed at increasing osteoclast function, with mixed results [5]. In orthopaedic practice, the main problems are dealing with fractures or implanting joint replacements in very abnormal bone.

Operating on osteopetrosis requires a multidisciplinary team approach, with involvement of paediatricians, and rigorous preoperative planning. Factors to consider include [7]:

- A high risk of drill breakage – consider diamond-tip drill bits, regular cooling of drills, multiple drill bits
- Contingency planning if hardware fails intraoperatively (e.g. advising parents that broken drill bits may need to be left in situ)
- Trying to avoid intramedullary devices
- Operating time which will be significantly increased
- Monitoring haemoglobin and platelet levels perioperatively, and being aware of an increased infection risk
- Fractures not remodelling in the same way as normal paediatric bone.

Scurvy

Scurvy occurs due to a nutritional deficiency in vitamin C (ascorbic acid). As described earlier, vitamin C acts as a key cofactor in hydroxylation and subsequent cross-linking of collagen [1].

Clinical Features

- Failure to thrive
- Spontaneous haemorrhage (with normal coagulation) – due to defective collagen in vascular structures:
  o Haemarthroses
  o Subperiosteal haemorrhage
  o Petechiae
  o Gum bleeding
  o Gastrointestinal tract bleeding
- Anaemia
- Poor wound healing
- Bone pain
- Fractures
- Scorbutic rosary (similar to rachitic rosary – see earlier).

Radiological Features

- Ongoing mineral deposition, despite compromised osteoid formation, leads to two classic X-ray signs:
  o Frankel's line – opaque white line at the ZPC
  o Wimberger's ring – opaque white line circumscribing secondary ossification centres.

- Osteopenia
- Metaphyseal spurs
- Metaphyseal corner fractures
- Periosteal reaction secondary to subperiosteal haematomas.

The features of multiple bruises, corner fractures, periosteal reactions, and malnourishment make scurvy a potential differential diagnosis in cases of suspected non-accidental injury (NAI) [8]. However, NAI is far commoner and carries significant mortality, so it must always be considered in the first instance.

Treatment

- Vitamin C replacement
- Ruling out NAI.

Osteoporosis

Unlike the conditions described above, the quality of collagen or mineralization is not affected in osteoporosis. Rather osteoporosis is an issue of bone quantity.

In adults, osteoporosis is defined as a bone mineral density (BMD) of at least 2.5 standard deviations (SDs) below peak bone mass. The BMD is calculated by dual-energy X-ray absorptiometry (DEXA), giving a T-score which compares the patient's BMD to that of a healthy 30-year-old sex- and ethnicity-matched patient. As children have not yet reached their peak bone mass, the T-score is not useful. The Z-score (i.e. the number of SDs above or below the mean BMD in an age-, sex-, and ethnicity-matched patient) eliminates the issue of age. However, we know that chronological age and skeletal age are not always equivalent (especially in children with chronic disease). Therefore, DEXA scan results cannot be relied upon in isolation.

Currently, paediatric osteoporosis is diagnosed if the child meets one of the following criteria [9]:

- Any vertebral fracture in the absence of local disease or high-energy trauma
- Two or more long bone fractures <10 years of age, with a Z-score <−2
- Three or more long bone fractures <19 years of age, with a Z-score <−2.

Causes

- Primary:
  o Idiopathic juvenile osteoporosis (very rare) (Figures 22.7 and 22.8)
- Secondary:
  o Limited mobility (e.g. cerebral palsy, Duchenne muscular dystrophy)
  o Iatrogenic (e.g. long-term steroid use)

Patient Information:

Name:	
Social Security No:	
Patient ID:	
Postal Code:	
Sex:	Male
Ethnicity:	White
Height:	136.4 cm
Weight:	40.6 kg
DOB:	01.05.1999
Age:	10
Menopause Age:	
Referring Physician:	

Scan Information:

Scan Date:	05 October 2009 - B1005090A
Scan Type:	f Left Hip
Analysis Date:	05.10.2009 13:18
Report Date:	05.10.2009 13:19
Institution:	CMMC NHS TRUST
Operator:	JA
Model:	Discovery A (S/N45335)
Comment:	
Software version:	12.6.1

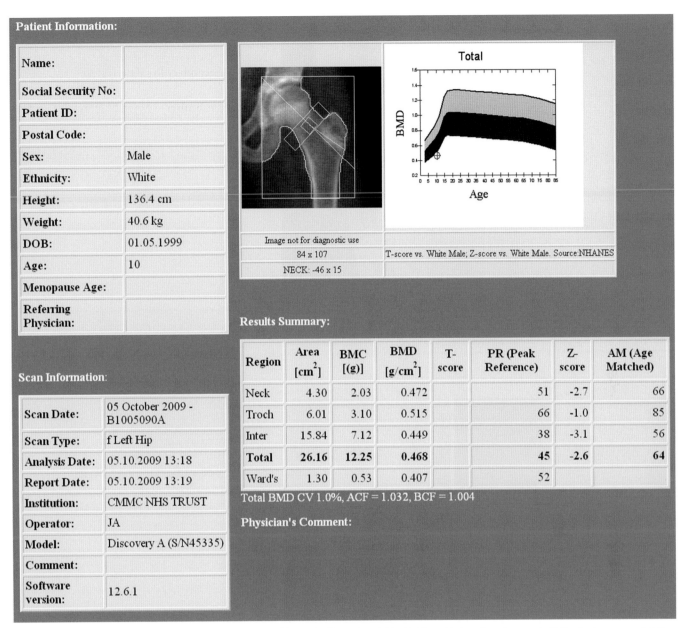

Image not for diagnostic use
84 x 107
NECK: -46 x 15

T-score vs. White Male; Z-score vs. White Male. Source:NHANES

Results Summary:

Region	Area [cm²]	BMC [(g)]	BMD [g/cm²]	T-score	PR (Peak Reference)	Z-score	AM (Age Matched)
Neck	4.30	2.03	0.472		51	-2.7	66
Troch	6.01	3.10	0.515		66	-1.0	85
Inter	15.84	7.12	0.449		38	-3.1	56
Total	**26.16**	**12.25**	**0.468**		**45**	**-2.6**	**64**
Ward's	1.30	0.53	0.407		52		

Total BMD CV 1.0%, ACF = 1.032, BCF = 1.004

Physician's Comment:

Figure 22.7 A dual-energy X-ray absorptiometry (DEXA) scan of the neck of femur in a child with idiopathic juvenile osteoporosis. Notice the low z-score (−2.6) and low bone density of 0.468 g cm⁻².

o Hormonal
o Anorexia nervosa.

Management

Medical treatment includes:
- Calcium and vitamin D supplementation
- Resistance exercises
- Bisphosphonates.

Surgical treatment includes:
- Fixing long bone fractures to allow early mobilization (Figure 22.9)
- Deformity correction
- Bracing for a short period to relieve back pain or for a long period to slow down deformity progression.

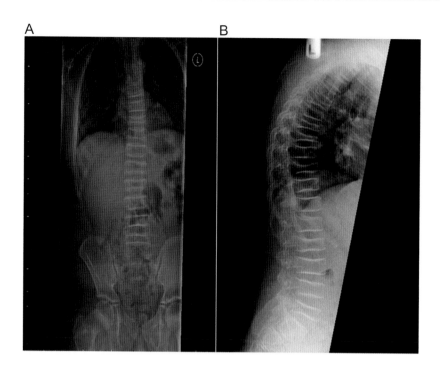

A B

Figure 22.8 A child with idiopathic juvenile osteoporosis, with multiple spontaneous vertebral fractures giving the classical cod fish appearance, with an anterior wedge fracture leading to thoracolumbar kyphosis.

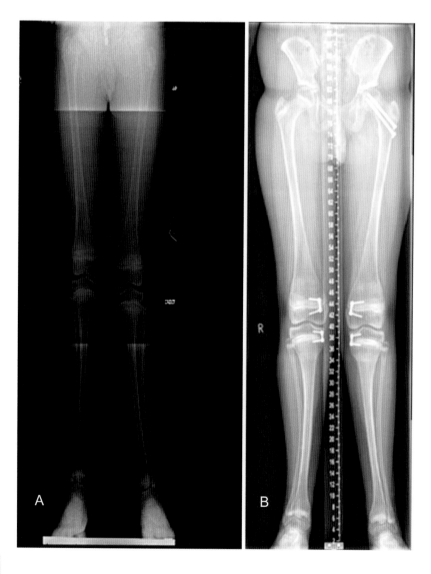

A B

Figure 22.9 X-rays of the same child illustrated in Figure 22.8 who developed a left neck of femur fracture, which was fixed with cannulated screws. He also underwent guided growth using eight plates over the medial distal femur and proximal tibia to correct valgus deformity of the knees. The lower screw could have been positioned in a better place (above the lesser trochanter) to reduce the risk of periprosthetic fracture, which is a real risk in these children.

References

1. Howard AW, Alman BA. Metabolic and endocrine abnormalities. In: Weinstein SL, Flynn JM, eds. *Lovell and Winter's Pediatric Orthopaedics*, 7th ed, Vol. 1. Philadelphia, PA: Lippincott Williams & Wilkins; 2014. pp. 140–76.

2. Wesseling-Perry K. Bone disease in pediatric chronic kidney disease. *Pediatr Nephrol*. 2013;28(4):569–76.

3. Mehls O, Ritz E, Krempien B, *et al.* Slipped epiphyses in renal osteodystrophy. *Arch Dis Child*. 1975;50:545–54.

4. Gigante C, Borgo A, Corradin M. Correction of lower limb deformities in children with renal osteodystrophy by guided growth technique. *J Child Orthop*. 2017;11:79–84.

5. Wu CC, Econs MJ, DiMeglio LA, *et al.* Diagnosis and management of osteopetrosis: consensus guidelines from osteopetrosis working group. *J Clin Endocrinol Metab*. 2017;102(9):3111–23.

6. Faden MA, Faden MA, Faden MA, *et al.* The Erlenmeyer flask bone deformity in skeletal dysplasias. *Am J Med Genet A*. 2009;149-A(6):1334–45.

7. Bhargava A, Vagela M, Lennox CME. 'Challenges in the management of fractures in osteopetrosis'! Review of the literature and technical tips learned from long-term management of seven patients. *Injury*. 2009;40:1167–71.

8. Paterson C. Multiple fractures in infancy: scurvy or nonaccidental injury? *Orthop Res Rev*. 2010;2:45–8.

9. Bachrach LK, Gordon CM. Bone densitometry in children and adolescents. *Pediatrics*. 2016;138(4):e20162398.

Chapter

23

Deformity Correction

Stan Jones, Farhan Ali, Anthony Cooper, and Alwyn Abraham

Introduction

A limb deformity can be defined as distortion from the normal form and this may be in the form of leg length discrepancy (LLD), angular deformity, rotational deformity, or a combination of these. Untreated substantive limb deformity can cause symptoms and affect limbs functions. An accurate assessment and appropriate treatment are the key to success in managing these patients.

Our understanding of assessment and management of deformity has progressed significantly in the last century. The concept of distraction histogenesis was pioneered by Professor Gavriil Ilizarov. He used circular external fixators to treat nonunions by compression. He noted that bone had formed at a fracture site after distraction when one of his patients misunderstood the instructions and turned the nuts in the wrong direction, lengthening the fracture site rather than compressing it. He called this 'distraction histogenesis' and he subsequently used it for limb lengthening.

Dror Paley deciphered the intuitive deformity assessment and planning undertaken by 'Ilizarov' surgeons and developed an easy and systematic approach to analysing lower limb deformity and planning treatment [1]. Dr Charles Taylor (with his brother Harold, an engineer) introduced the Taylor Spatial Frame (TSF), which was the first circular fixator combining hardware and software to accurately reduce fractures and correct bony deformities (Figure 23.1). It is based on the Stewart Gough platform principles where two platforms, one fixed (the base) and one mobile (the platform), are joined by six kinematic (adjustable) legs. The two platforms are replaced with rings and the legs are replaced with adjustable struts. Data on deformity descriptions and frame-mounting parameters are input to a computer program, producing a prescription to gradually adjust the struts which will correct the deformity.

When the TSF patency expired, three more similar devices were introduced into practice, with some extra useful features. These are the TrueLok Hexapod (TL-HEX) by Orthofix, Orthex by Orthopaediatrics, and the Multi-Axial correction system (MAX Frame) by DePuy Synthes (Figure 23.2).

 Video 23.1 What is a hexapod?

A   B

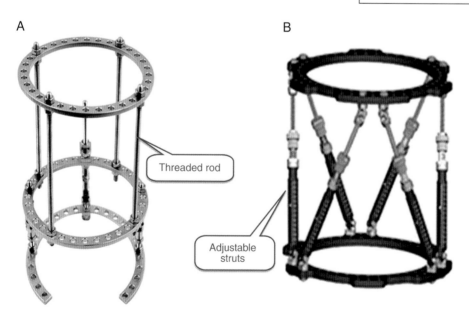

Threaded rod

Adjustable struts

Figure 23.1 The Ilizarov circular frame (A) in comparison to the Taylor Spatial Frame (TSF) (B). The TSF is based on the Stewart platform, with two rings and six legs (that is why it is also called a hexapod). The principle is extensively used in many industry fields (robotics, flight simulators, etc.). The TSF can correct multiple deformities simultaneously, using virtual hinges that the computer program creates, based on the input data. The Ilizarov frame can correct multiple deformities sequentially using physical hinges (hardware) that the surgeon puts in the right place at the right time. The latter makes Ilizarov less efficient and less accurate in correcting a complex deformity. However, for a simple deformity such as a short tibia, the Ilizarov frame is good and substantially cheaper.

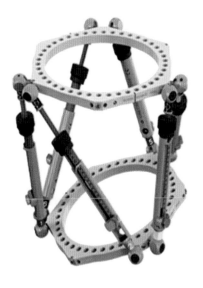
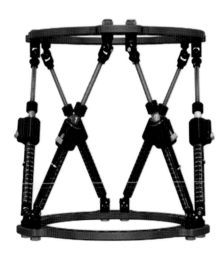
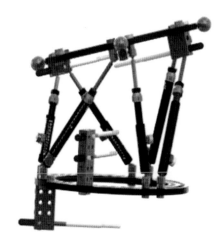

**TL-HEX
(Orthofix)**

**MAX Frame
DePuy Synthes**

**Orthex
Orthopaediatrics**

Figure 23.2 Newly introduced computerized circular frames.

Assessing Limb Deformity

History

Evaluation commences with a comprehensive history, in particular inquiring about any childhood illness, that is, meningitis, injury, or fracture and the family history of skeletal dysplasia. These may provide clues to the possible cause of the deformity. Where appropriate, the history should also focus on the underlying diagnosis; for example, a patient with achondroplasia may have sleep apnoea, whereas congenital pseudarthrosis of the tibia is most probably a feature of type I neurofibromatosis. The possible causes of limb deformities are listed in Table 23.1.

Clinical Assessment

This should include the following:

- General assessment
- Gait
- Limb assessment
- Neurovascular status.

General Assessment

Assess for abnormal height, limb asymmetry, enlarged tongue, and cutaneous manifestations such as café-au-lait spots and operative scars. Examine the footwear for any modifications.

Gait

The gait may reveal compensatory mechanisms such as circumduction, persistent flexion of the knee of a longer limb, or tiptoeing on the side of a shorter limb. For genu varum deformities, it is important to look for a lateral thrust at the knee, to give an idea of soft tissue laxity.

Limb Assessment

Measure the true length of each limb and segment, looking for any LLD and the site(s) of any difference. Assess the functional

Table 23.1 Possible causes of limb deformities

Causes	Examples
Congenital/genetic	1. Congenital femoral deficiency 2. Fibular hemimelia 3. Tibial pseudarthrosis 4. Posteromedial tibial bowing 5. Skeletal dysplasias (e.g. achondroplasia). Hemihypertrophy (Klippel–Trenaunay–Weber, Beckwith–Wiedemann, or idiopathic) 6. Osteogenesis imperfecta 7. Hemiatrophy syndromes, including club foot
Trauma	1. Malunited fractures 2. Overgrowth following a fracture 3. Physeal injury with growth arrest 4. Cozen fracture
Infection	1. Septic arthritis and osteomyelitis 2. Meningococcal sepsis involving growth plates
Neoplastic	1. Haemangiomas 2. Neurofibromatosis 3. Multiple hereditary exostosis 4. Fibrous dysplasia
Neuromuscular	1. Cerebral palsy 2. Spinal disorders
Inflammatory	1. Juvenile idiopathic arthritis (leads to overgrowth)
Miscellaneous	1. LCPD and AVN 2. SCFE 3. Blount's disease

LCPD, Legg–Calvé–Perthes disease; AVN, avascular necrosis; SCFE, slipped capital femoral epiphysis.

LLD by asking the patient to stand on graduated blocks placed under the shorter leg until the pelvis is level (see Chapter 2, Figure 2.13). Assess the rotational profile of the lower limbs (see Chapter 2 for details).

Assess the limb for any compensatory deformities; for example, a varus deformity at the ankle is compensated for by eversion at the subtalar joint and supination at the forefoot. If these compensating deformities are fixed, they would need to be addressed at the time of treatment (Figure 23.3).

Examine the joints above and below the deformity to rule out fixed contractures or joint instability. Uncorrected fixed joint contracture will lead to secondary deformities after surgery. For example, a patient with a recurvatum bony deformity of the ankle may also have a plantar flexion deformity of the ankle, and if this is not addressed at the time of surgery, it will lead to an equinus contracture of the ankle. In addition, joint instability may lead to subluxation or dislocation of the joint following deformity correction and lengthening.

Assess skin and soft tissue quality, paying attention to any scars and their relation to any potential future surgery and proximity to important structures.

Neurovascular Status

Neurovascular examination of the lower limbs and spinal examination complete the clinical evaluation. In children with hereditary multiple exostosis and achondroplasia, it is important to rule out spinal stenosis by examining for clonus, as neurological injury may develop following deformity correction by lengthening.

Radiological Assessment

- Standing long leg radiographs of both lower limbs, with an appropriate block under the short leg to level the pelvis, are the commonest way to measure the degree of angular deformity and LLD. The patellae should be 'neutral' (facing forward) and any physeal abnormality should be noted [2]. Long leg radiographs cannot inform rotational deformities.

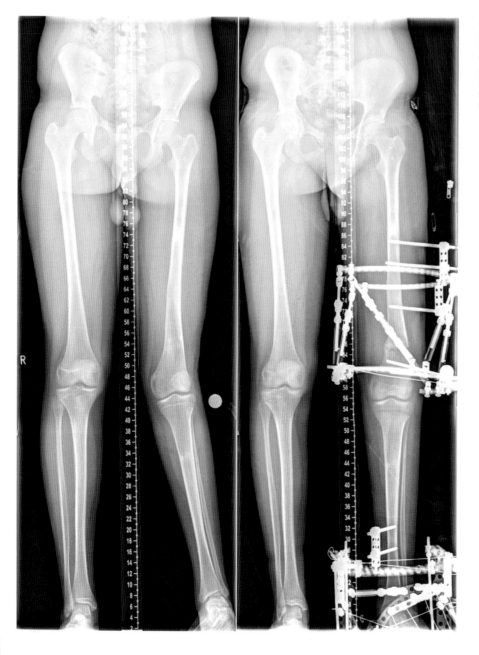

Figure 23.3 Distal femoral deformity with distal subtalar fixed deformity in a 14-year-old boy who had previous foot surgery presenting with genu valgum. He was noticed to have plantigrade feet, but with fixed supination. Isolated correction of the knee deformity would uncouple the foot deformity, so both were addressed together.

Table 23.2 Deformity description in the three standard planes

Planes	Angulation	Translation	Assessment[a]
Sagittal plane (S)	Procurvatum or recurvatum	Anterior or posterior	X-ray (lateral)
Coronal plane (C)	Varus or valgus	Medial or lateral	X-ray (anteroposterior)
Axial (A)	Internal or external	Short or long	Clinical or CT scan

[a] Assessing the magnitude of the deformity can be performed by using plain radiographs in the sagittal and coronal planes. However, in the axial plane, it can be assessed either clinically by comparing the direction of the feet in relation to the deformed limb or by performing CT to compare the rotation of the long bone condyles to each other.

- CT scans are also popular in assessing lower limb deformities, including the rotational profile.
- EOS is a low-dose three-dimensional imaging system that can assess bone geometry, including the rotational profile in various positions (such as sitting and standing). The high cost precludes its wide use.
- It may be necessary to estimate bone age. The left hand and wrist radiographs are the most often used to estimate bone age. This is particularly important if planning to correct the deformity using the technique of guided growth (epiphysiodesis).

Bone deformity is described as angulation or translation, or both, in each of the three planes of geometry, producing a matrix of all possible deformities (Table 23.2).

Steps for Radiological Assessment of Deformity (MAP the ABC)

1. **M**easure the mechanical axis (MA) deviation test: a line drawn from the centre of the femoral head to the centre of the ankle joint in the coronal plane should pass within zone 1 (see Chapter 6, Figure 6.10). This is usually about 8 mm from the centre of the knee joint.

2. Measure the joint orientation **A**ngles: the MA line connects the centre of the proximal joint to the centre of the distal joint. The anatomical axis (AA) line is the mid-diaphyseal line. The MA is a feature of the coronal plane only, whereas the AA line is used in the coronal and sagittal planes. The orientation of each joint can be measured using angles (called the joint orientation angle) created by the above-mentioned lines and the joint surface lines (JOLs). Figure 23.4 shows the standardized angle nomenclature: axis (m, mechanical; a, anatomical), side (M, medial; L, lateral), site (P, proximal; D, distal), and bone (F, femur; T, tibia). The mechanical lateral distal femoral angle (mLDFA) and mechanical medial proximal tibial angle (mMPTA) are around 87°, and the mechanical lateral proximal femoral angle (mLPFA) and mechanical lateral distal tibial angle (mLDTA) should be around 90°. The tibial MA and AA can be considered the same. The joint line convergence angle (JLCA) should be ≤2°; higher values may indicate abnormal laxity of the joint that has contributed to MA deviation (Figure 23.4).

3. **P**ick the deformed bone(s): determine if either the femur or the tibia, or indeed both bones, have deformity that has contributed to the MA deviation.

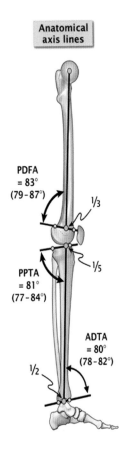

Figure 23.4 Lower limb alignment in the frontal and sagittal planes. Mechanical lateral proximal femoral angle (mLPFA), 90°; mechanical lateral distal femoral angle (mLDFA), 87°; mechanical lateral distal tibial angle (mLDTA), 89°; anatomical medial proximal femoral angle (aMPFA), 84°; anatomical lateral distal femoral angle (aLDFA), 81°. Note the difference of 7° between the anatomical and mechanical femoral angles, reflecting the angle between the femoral mechanical axis (MA) and the anatomic axis (AA). The tibial mechanical and anatomical angles are the same, because the axes are the same. In the sagittal plane angle, only the anatomical axis is used; this represents the mid-diaphyseal lines of the bones; these intersect the joint edge lines at the junction between the anterior third and the posterior two-thirds at the femur, the junction between the anterior fifth and the posterior four-fifths at the proximal tibia, and the junction halfway along the distal tibia.

399

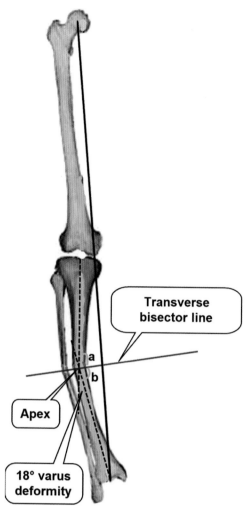

Figure 23.5 The apex (or CORA). This is the intersection point of the anatomical or mechanical axis when there is a deformity. A line passing through the apex divides the transverse angle into two equal angles (a and b).

4. **A**pex of the deformity (also known as CORA, which stands for the centre of rotation of angulation). The apex refers to the intersection point of the AA or MA when there is a deformity (Figure 23.5). A simple malunited fracture usually has one apex, but a bone with congenital bowing may have several apices. If the apex does not coincide with an obvious deformity, there may be another hidden deformity. An imaginary line that is drawn from the apex dividing the transverse angles (on either side of the apex) into two equal angles is called the transverse bisector line. Any point on this line can be used to realign the axes well – that is why it is called the axis of correction of angulation (ACA), and the chosen point is simply called the hinge point.

5. **B**one cuts (osteotomy): ideally the bone cut should go through the apex of the deformity; however, this is not always possible. The proximity of the apex to the joints and neurovascular structures, soft tissue problems, and the types of hardware fixation influence the optimal level of a corrective osteotomy. The surgeon cannot influence the apex but can control where the osteotomy and hinge points

are. Careful planning of the bone cut(s) and hinge point(s) in relationship to the apex is important for good correction. The following are useful rules (often called osteotomy rules):

a. Rule 1: when the osteotomy and hinge point are placed on the apex (or along the transverse bisector line), the two bony fragments are realigned without any coronal translation. If the hinge point is placed on the convex side of the deformed bone, opening wedge osteotomy occurs and the bone gets longer. If the hinge point is placed on the concave side, the two bony fragment ends jam unless a wedge is removed, resulting in shorter bone. If the hinge point is placed at the centre, a half-closing and half-opening wedge (neutral wedge) occurs (Figure 23.6).

b. Rule 2: if the osteotomy is done at a different level than the apex, then translation occurs.

c. Rule 3: if osteotomy is done at a different level than the apex, but the hinge is placed at the osteotomy site, the MA becomes parallel, whereas the AA becomes zigzagged (Figure 23.7).

6. **C**orrection: determine the optimal methods (acute or gradual) and the hardware to obtain the desired correction, that is, the fixator, nail, plate, or indeed a combination thereof [2].

Key Points: MAP the ABC

1. Measure the mechanical axis deviation.
2. Measure the joint orientation angles.
3. Pick the deformed bone(s).
4. Apex of the deformity.
5. Bone cut (osteotomy).
6. Correction.

Techniques to Correct Deformity

Acute Correction

Mild to moderate deformities can be corrected acutely and then stabilized using internal or external fixators. Acute correction should be avoided in deformities >30° because of the risk of neurovascular injury and compartment syndrome. Acute correction can be utilized to shorten, but not to lengthen, bones because of the risk of non-union.

Plate and screws are appropriate for periarticular deformities but are invasive. Intramedullary nailing is minimally invasive and useful in correcting diaphyseal and rotational deformities. The presence of the growth plate and remaining growth can influence the type of fixation (Figure 23.8).

Gradual Correction

Guided Growth

Bones grow longer through physes (growth plates). Each long bone has two physes, one at upper end and one at the lower end

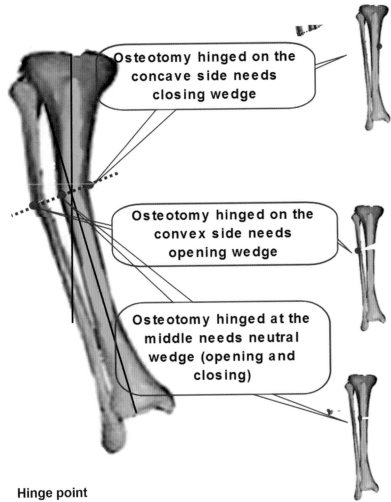

Osteotomy hinged on the concave side needs closing wedge

Osteotomy hinged on the convex side needs opening wedge

Osteotomy hinged at the middle needs neutral wedge (opening and closing)

● Hinge point

······· Transverse bisector line

Figure 23.6 Osteotomy rule 1. When the osteotomy and hinge point are placed on any point along the transverse bisector line, the two bony fragments are realigned without any coronal translation. If the hinge point is placed on the convex side of the deformed bone, opening wedge osteotomy occurs and the bone gets longer. If the hinge point is placed on the concave side, the two ends jam unless a wedge is removed, resulting in shorter bone. If the hinge point is placed at the centre, a half-closing and half-opening wedge (neutral wedge) occurs.

Figure 23.7 Osteotomy rule 3.

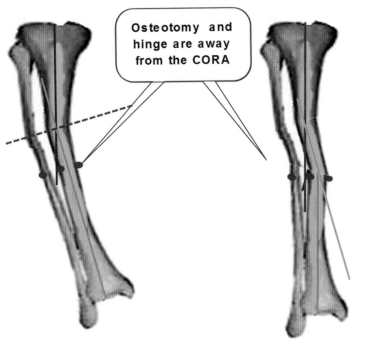

Osteotomy and hinge are away from the CORA

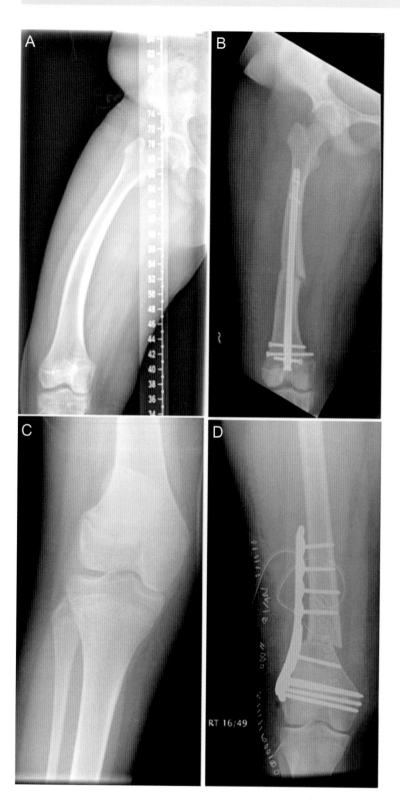

Figure 23.8 Acute deformity corrections. (A) and (B) show a femoral shaft varus deformity that was corrected using intramuscular nailing. (C) and (D) show a distal femoral valgus osteotomy that was corrected using a plate and screws. Notice the lateral translation of the distal femur because the osteotomy was made proximal to the apex.

(see Chapter 25, Figure 25.15). Heuter found that increased pressure across a physis inhibits growth, while decreased pressure promotes it. Volkmann reported that changing the compressive forces causes asymmetrical growth of a joint. These observations laid the ground for guided growth [3]. Therefore, inhibiting a whole physis results in shortening (this is known as epiphysiodesis). Inhibiting one side of a physis, whilst leaving the other side growing, results in the bone turning towards the inhibited side (this is called hemi-epiphysiodesis) (Figure 23.9).

Inhibition of growth can be temporary or permanent. Temporary epiphysiodesis is done using 8-plates (or similar tension band plates), whereas permanent epiphysiodesis may be done using a drill technique. The latter involves using a drill

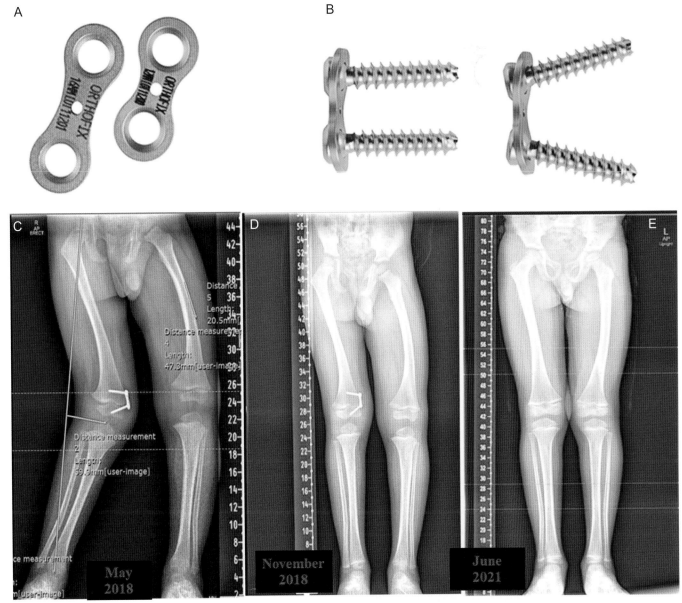

Figure 23.9 Guided growth. (A) shows 8-plates. The screws diverge with growth (B), indicating that the other side continues to lengthen. (C) and (D) show plain radiographs of a child with genu valgum of the right lower limb, which was treated with 8-plates. A complete correction was achieved (E).

to damage the growth plate. Through a small percutaneous incision, the drill bit is passed under X-ray screening through a single entry point on either side of the physis. Multiple passes in different directions, followed by curettage using a small curate, are usually enough to damage the physis permanently.

Distraction Osteogenesis

This utilizes the Ilizarov's principles to correct deformities using external fixators. These can be summarized as:

- Stable construct
- Low-energy osteotomy (preservation of blood supply)
- Latency period of 5–7 days to allow soft callus to form
- Distraction at a rate of 1 mm per day.

Traditionally, these have been achieved by external fixators (circular frames or monolateral fixator). However, lengthening

nails and plates have been introduced into practice and gaining popularity.

Monolateral Fixators

The commonest monolateral fixator in use is the Orthofix Limb Reconstruction System (LRS) (Figure 23.10).

Advantages: it is less bulky than a circular frame, which makes it more comfortable to patients with a femoral deformity. Based on careful selection of the pin site, it causes less interference with the joint range of motion.

Disadvantages: often rotational deformities are corrected acutely at the time of surgery. Generally, this is technically more challenging, with a lower margin of error, and has less manoeuvrability, as compared to a circular fixator. The number of fixation pins that can be used is limited, and it is more challenging to replace these should they get infected or become loose.

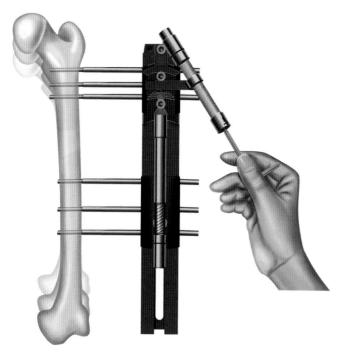

Figure 23.10 Monolateral external fixator (Limb Reconstruction System). This device can lengthen bones and can correct coronal malalignment (varus or valgus). Rotational deformity can be corrected acutely. The patient can sleep on their back or on the other side; something this can be awkward with a circular frame.

Circular Fixators

These are versatile deformity correction devices that can correct all aspects of deformity. They are broadly of two types:

- Traditional Ilizarov-type fixators (Figure 23.11)
- Computerized hexapod fixators.

Advantages: all aspects of deformity can be corrected gradually. They are mechanically more stable than monolateral fixators.

Disadvantages: fine wire fixation around the joints can cause patient discomfort and joint stiffness, and are prone to infection. Using half pins, in addition to wires, gives these fixators the advantages of monolateral fixators, with the versatility of circular fixators. They require some expertise, whilst the computerized hexapod fixators are expensive.

Lengthening Nails

Several nails have been introduced into practice. The commonest are Fitbone (Orthofix) and Precice nails (NuVasive). They work on similar telescoping principles when they receive activating signals. The former has an antenna which is implanted under the skin, and a wire that transfers the signal to the nail. This will make the girth of the limb less important when using the nail. However, extra care must be taken not to damage the antenna or wire during surgery. The Precice nail has rare earth magnets within its mechanism. An externally placed remote controller generates an electromagnetic field to turn the magnets, which, in turn, rotate the gear mechanism. There needs to be a distance of <5 cm between the control device and the nail for optimal function (Figure 23.12).

Advantages: comfort is the most important advantage of lengthening nails. It can be done with minimally invasive incisions.

Disadvantages: the technique is good for pure lengthening. Although some coronal and rotational deformities can be handled acutely during nail insertion, large deformities cannot be corrected. Nail lengthening is along the AA (not the MA). Although this does not matter in the tibia where both axes can be considered the same, it does matter in the femur where these axes diverge by around 7°. In effect, the knee is pushed in valgus during lengthening using a nail. As a rule of thumb, the MA moves laterally from the centre of the knee by 1 mm for each 1 cm lengthening. Tibial nails cannot be placed if the growth plates are open, and femoral nails in the younger child have a theoretical risk of avascular necrosis.

The size of the femoral canal is another important factor in using lengthening nails. To overcome this, growing plates have been introduced recently by NuVasive, but they are still being evaluated.

Key Points: Do Not Forget

- Deformity correction is a treatment requiring a multidisciplinary approach, with a motivated and *well-informed team, including the patient, parents, physiotherapist, nurses, clinical psychologist, and surgeon.*
- The frame lengthens the bone, and physiotherapy lengthens the muscles.
- Medical treatment can be a good option to correct deformity such as vitamin D supplementation in rickets, renal replacement in renal osteodystrophy, and vosoritide in achondroplasia.
- Do not confuse lengthening nails (Fitbone and Precice) with growing rods (Fassier–Duval and Sheffield rods). The former are used for lengthening bones, whereas the latter are meant to lengthen as bones grow.

Taylor Spatial Frame

The TSF was the first computerized hexapod fixator to be used in the UK and North America. A few more advanced frames have been introduced.

We focus here on the TSF to demonstrate the principles that underlie how computerized frames work.

To correct a deformity using a hexapod, the following are required:

1. The types and magnitudes of the deformity
2. The shape of the frame and its mounting parameters in relation to the bone (more specifically to the osteotomy)
3. Structures at risk (such as the common peroneal nerve when correcting a valgus leg)
4. The safe duration of deformity correction.

Whether it is a fracture or an osteotomy for deformity correction, there are two bony fragments: a proximal and a distal.

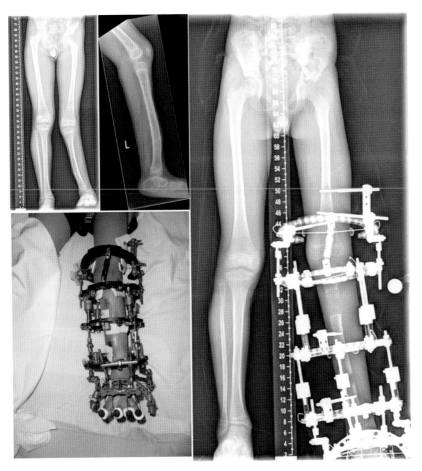

Figure 23.11 Fibular hemimelia deformity corrections using a multistack Ilizarov frame. The top two rings are to stabilize the knee joint during lengthening. These patients usually have no anterior cruciate ligament (evident by flattening of the tibial spine – confirmed on MRI). There is bifocal tibial lengthening proximally (ideal site) and at the apex of a lower tibial deformity (the surgeon used the deformity correction osteotomy to gain some length).

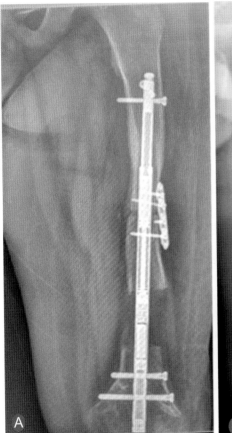
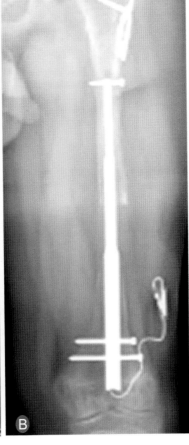

Figure 23.12 Lengthening nails. (A) shows the Precice nail used for lengthening a femur. There was a mid-shaft deformity which was corrected acutely before inserting the nail. (B) shows a Fitbone nail used for lengthening a femur. The antenna and wire must be handled with care to avoid damage.

In the language of hexapods, these become the 'reference' and 'moving' fragments. The surgeon can decide which bony fragment (i.e. proximal or distal) would become the reference fragment. Proximal referencing is when the proximal fragment is used as the reference fragment. The ring that is attached to the reference fragment is called the reference ring. Several factors are considered in choosing the reference fragment. In general, in non-unions or malunions with a short distal fragment, the attachment of the distal ring is more exactly determined in preoperative planning and surgery, and should be the referenced fragment rather than the longer proximal fragment.

The tip of the reference fragment is called 'the origin', whereas the tip of the moving fragment is called 'the reference'. The software creates a path to bring the corresponding point back to the origin.

Type and Magnitude of Deformity

There are six deformity measurements of the moving fragment, in relation to the reference fragment, to be identified (Figure 23.13 and Table 23.1):

1. AP view angulation (varus or valgus)
2. AP view translation (medial or lateral)
3. Lateral view angulation (procurvatum – apex anterior; or recurvatum – apex posterior)
4. Lateral view translation (anterior or posterior)
5. Axial view angulation (internal or external rotation)
6. Axial view translation (short or long).

Table 23.1 Deformity description in the three standard planes

Views	Angulation	Translation
AP	10° varus	8 mm medial
Lateral	12° apex anterior (procurvatum)	15 mm anterior
Clinical/CT scan	41° internal	10 mm long

Shape of Frame and Its Mounting Parameters to Bone

A simple TSF has two rings and six struts. Each ring is attached to a bony fragment. Theoretically, a ring can be mounted anywhere on the fragment, and provided the software knows the exact mounting parameters, correction can be achieved. However, in practice, we tend to mount the rings (particularly the reference ring) in a way to minimize mounting parameters, measurements, and errors. Rings should be mounted parallel to a nearby joint line, which is used as reference, and as close as possible to the origin. Although the mounting parameters of the reference ring only are important, it is good practice to mount both rings as if they were reference rings (to have the flexibility to use either as a reference ring if needed).

The reference ring carries what is called 'the master tab', which is the tab between strut number 1 and 2 that denotes the ring (and the frame) rotation. Ideally the ring should be mounted so that the reference ring rotation is 0°, that is, the master tab is in line with the patella or tibial tuberosity (not always possible) (Figure 23.14).

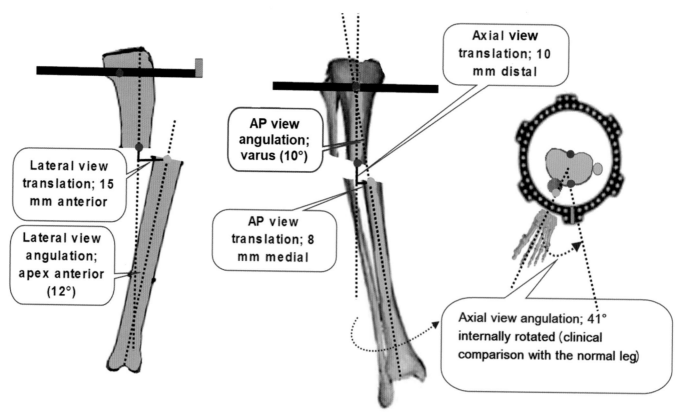

Figure 23.13 Deformity description in the Taylor Spatial Frame is illustrated. In this example, referencing is proximal. If distal referencing is used, the direction will be reversed, that is, medial becomes lateral and varus becomes valgus.

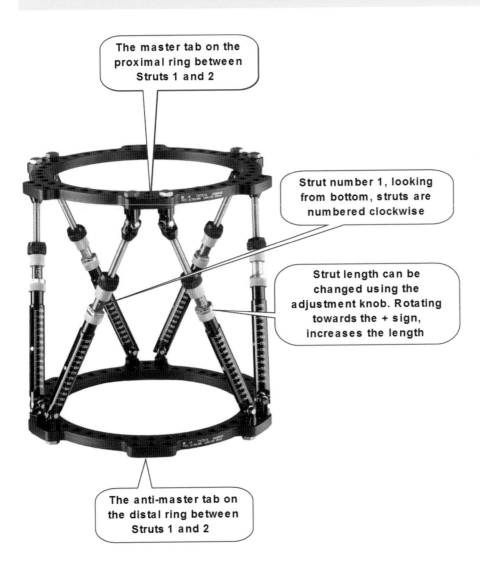

The master tab on the proximal ring between Struts 1 and 2

Strut number 1, looking from bottom, struts are numbered clockwise

Strut length can be changed using the adjustment knob. Rotating towards the + sign, increases the length

The anti-master tab on the distal ring between Struts 1 and 2

Figure 23.14 Taylor Spatial Frame: the proximal and distal full rings. Rings come in various sizes. Some are full ring, and some are part of a ring to allow for joint bending. Each hexapod has six adjustable struts. Struts come in four different sizes (extra small, small, medium, and large). Strut numbers are fixed, and mislabelling them results in problems.

The TSF software requires the following information about the frame:

1. The size and type of the proximal and distal rings
2. The size and length of each strut
3. The distance between the centre of the reference ring and the three planes (Figure 23.15).

A case study of deformity correction using the TL-HEX hexapod is shown in Videos 23.2 and 23.3.

 Video 23.2 Preoperative planning of tibia deformity using TL-HEX software.

 Video 23.3 Postoperative planning of tibia shaft deformity correction.

Key Points: Software Advances

Advancement in software capability automates most of the above measurements. However, it is important to understand the above principle to be able to converse with the software for optimal outcome.

Structures at Risk and Rate of Safe Distraction

Structures at risk (SAR) refer to important adjacent anatomical structures, such as nerve vessels, fragile wounds, or scars, that we do not want to get stretched or compressed fast. These need to be identified by providing their distance from the origin on three planes. Finally, the maximum safe distraction rate must be entered. One millimetre per day is generally accepted.

Leg Length Discrepancy

LLD is a frequent cause of parental anxiety. Twenty per cent of asymptomatic adults have an LLD averaging 5 mm. A variable amount of LLD has been implicated in the development of low back pain, sciatica, scoliosis, stress fractures, and plantar fasciitis. The evidence, however, is not compelling. A longer leg tilts the pelvis towards the short side, resulting in uncovering of the femoral head (long leg dysplasia) and this has been implicated with premature osteoarthritis.

Causes and evaluation are similar to other types of deformity; however, treatments merit special considerations, which are covered in this section. LLD is better tolerated by children, in comparison to other deformities, and shoe raises are acceptable

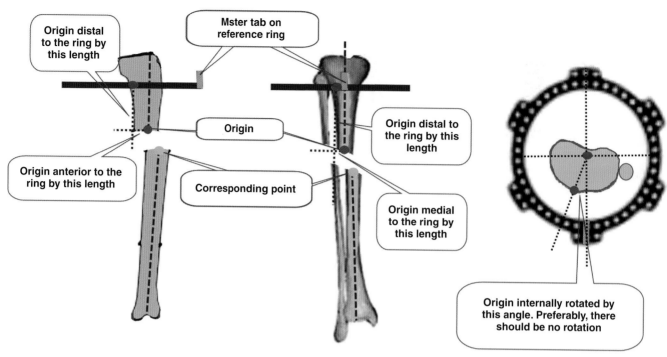

Figure 23.15 Mounting parameters for TSF. On the AP view, the origin (blue dot) is medial to the centre of the reference ring (red dot) by about 5 mm, and distal to the centre of the reference ring by 25 mm. On the lateral view, the origin is anterior to the centre of the ring by 8 mm, and distal to the ring by 20 mm. If the master tab is aligned with the patella or tibial tuberosity, the frame rotation would be 0°. In this example, the frame is externally rotated by 20°.

temporary treatment by parents until the optimal time for definitive correction.

The cause of LLD is important to predict the LLD at maturity, which is what matters. Shapiro [4] analysed 803 patients with LLD and demonstrated that not all discrepancies continue to increase at a constant rate with time. He described five basic patterns of LLD (Table 23.3 and Figure 23.16).

Predicting Leg Length Discrepancy

Being able to predict LLD at maturity is essential and helps one decide the best treatment option and when to intervene.

Methods available are:

1. The Menelaus method
2. The Green and Anderson growth remaining chart [5]
3. The Moseley's straight line graph
4. The Paley's multiplier method (and its phone app).

All these methods assume that there is a constant/linear rate of increase in LLD (Shapiro type I) and growth ends in girls at 14 years and in boys at 16 years. The multiplier phone app has become the commonest, although not necessarily the most accurate, method of predicting LLD at maturity and timing of epiphysiodesis in clinical practice. It is available for download from the following link: https://itunes.apple.com/us/app/multiplier/id460335161?mt=8.

We describe below these methods in brief.

The Menelaus Method

This method is also called the rule of thumb. By knowing how much each physis grows per year, one can predict the LLD that is

Table 23.3 Shapiro's five basic patterns of leg length discrepancy

Types	Description	Examples
I	Upward slope pattern; there is a consistent rate of growth inhibition of the shorter leg	Epiphyseal arrest, Ollier's disease, proximal femoral focal deficiency
II	Upward slope–deceleration pattern; the rate of growth inhibition decreases over time	Neuromuscular conditions
III	Upward slope–plateau pattern; after an initial constant growth inhibition, the legs grow at the same rate (plateau)	Overgrowth seen after femoral shaft fracture
IV	Upward slope–plateau–upward slope pattern; a constant rate of growth inhibition is interrupted by a period of growth at the same rate	Severe LCPD. There is initial shortening due to collapse of the femoral head that leads to LLD, which, after some time, increases again as a result of premature physeal arrest
V	Upward slope–plateau–downward slope; the slower-growing limb exhibits an initial growth deceleration, followed by symmetrical growth and finally increased growth, compared to the contralateral limb	Juvenile idiopathic arthritis due to overgrowth, then growth arrest

LCPD, Legg–Calvé–Perthes disease; LLD, leg length discrepancy.

caused by a damaged physis. Table 23.4 summarizes the average growth rate per year and the percentage contribution of various physes to yearly increase in height. The obvious concern is that these data have been drawn from published data which may not be applicable to individual patients.

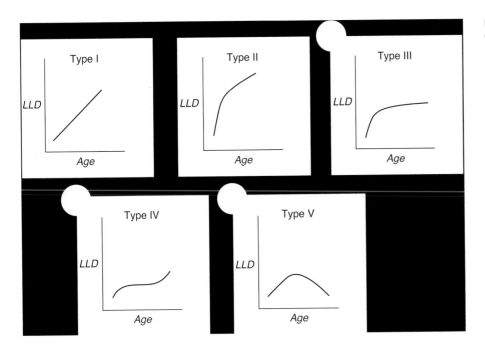

Figure 23.16 Shapiro's developmental patterns of leg length discrepancy.

Table 23.4 Contribution of various bones towards growth of the entire limb

	Lower limb			Upper limb	
Site	mm/year	% contribution	Site	mm/year	% contribution
Proximal femur	3	15	Proximal humerus	6	40
Distal femur	9	40	Distal humerus	2	10
Proximal tibia	6	30	Proximal radius	2	10
Distal tibia	5	15	Distal radius	6	40

The Green and Anderson Growth Remaining Chart

This predicts the growth remaining in the femur and tibia (of each limb – both the short and long ones), relative to the skeletal age of the patient (Figure 23.17). The skeletal age can be determined by taking wrist radiographs and comparing them to the Greulich and Pyle atlas.

The Moseley's Straight Line Graph

This method requires a special graph for each patient (Figure 23.18) and a number of radiological examinations (length of the normal leg and shorter leg, and skeletal age) on at least three different occasions over a period of time. With this information, an estimate of the time of skeletal maturity can be made. The projected LLD can then be derived by drawing a straight line for each leg through the measured points (Video 23.4). Using the reference slopes, one can then determine when epiphysiodesis can be done.

> **Video 23.4** Demonstration of how to use the Moseley's chart to predict leg length discrepancy at maturity.

Paley's Multiplier Method

Based on previous works, Paley *et al.* [6] introduced the multiplier method to estimate LLD and the patient's height at skeletal maturity. The group identified an arithmetic factor (called a multiplier) by dividing the femoral and tibial lengths at skeletal maturity by the femoral and tibial lengths at different ages, respectively. The length of each leg at skeletal maturity can be calculated by multiplying the current length by the appropriate multiplier for the subject's age and gender:

Mature (segment) length = present (segment) length × multiplier

The segment could be the tibia, the femur, or both, or the patient's height. There is a multiplier for every patient age. This multiplier varies according to sex and the cause of LLD (congenital or developmental). This was further developed into phone app(s). The Multiplier by the Rubin Institute for Advanced Orthopedics is the most widely used (Figure 23.19).

Treatment

The treatment objective is to achieve near-equal leg lengths at skeletal maturity without excessive risk, morbidity, or height reduction. The treatment algorithm generally used is depicted in Table 23.5. However, the clinician must assess each case based on its own merits. In paralytic cases such as cerebral palsy/myelomeningocele, it is advisable to leave the weaker limb slightly shorter, thus facilitating clearance of the foot in the swing phase of gait.

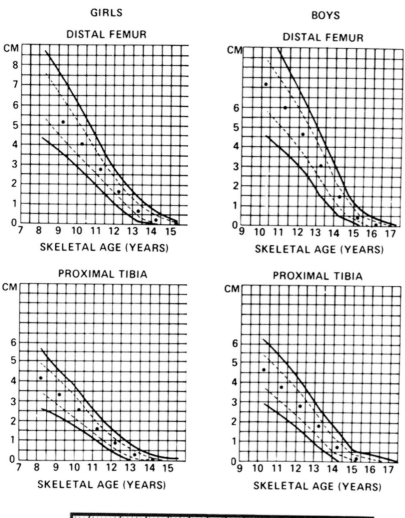

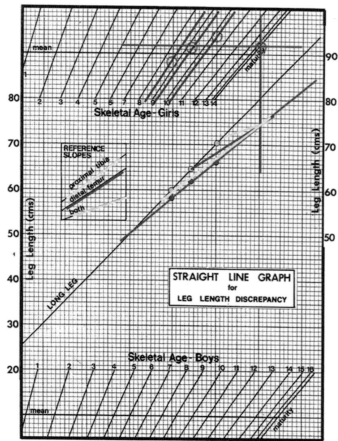

Figure 23.17 Green and Anderson graphs of growth remaining for girls and boys. Dashed lines, one standard deviation of the mean. Solid lines are two standard deviations of the mean.

Figure 23.18 Moseley's straight line method for predicting leg length discrepancy.

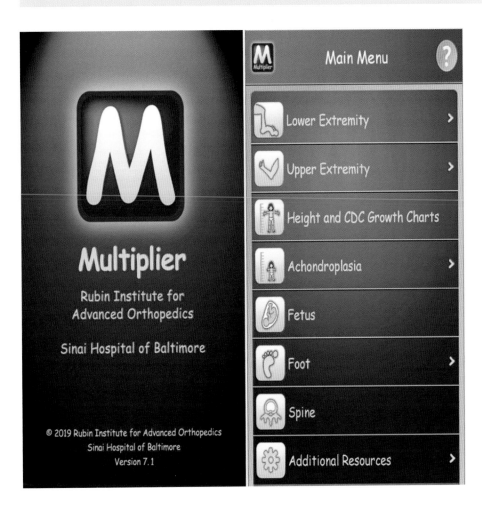

Figure 23.19 The Multiplier app, the start-up page, and the main menu.

Table 23.5 Recommended treatment options according to leg length discrepancy

Discrepancy	Treatment options
0–2 cm	No treatment if asymptomatic, shoe raise, epiphysiodesis
2–5 cm	Shoe raise, epiphysiodesis, limb lengthening, limb shortening
5–15 cm	Lengthening may be combined with epiphysiodesis or a shortening procedure
>15 cm	Lengthening + epiphysiodesis or shortening or ablative surgery and prosthetic use

Non-Operative

Shoe raises are not easily accepted by all patients and tend to be used as a short-term measure, especially for the younger child. A raise of up to 1 cm can be fitted inside the shoe, so it is not visible, whilst raises of >1 cm cause the shoe to come off during walking and are better fitted outside under the shoe heel.

Operative

Epiphysiodesis

Epiphysiodesis is the treatment of choice for smaller discrepancies (usually 2–5 cm) but may also be used in combination with other modalities for larger discrepancies.

The percutaneous drill technique (under X-ray guidance) is commonly used. This produces permanent physeal growth arrest and is important to time the surgery accurately by using the growth charts as previously described.

Epiphysiodesis may be undertaken using 8-plates/staples. The effect is reversible, and physeal growth resumes when the plates/staples are removed. This method is useful in situations when it is difficult to accurately predict the timing of epiphysiodesis or in the younger child.

Acute Bone Shortening

This is usually undertaken in the skeletally mature patient for discrepancies of 2–5 cm.

It has a lower complication rate, compared to lengthening procedures. Tibial shortening is undertaken less frequently than femoral shortening because it is technically more challenging and complications are more frequent, including vascular compromise and compartment syndrome.

Femoral shortening may result in an extensor lag due to quadriceps muscle weakening, and shortening should be limited to 10% or less of the original femoral length.

Short patients usually prefer lengthening to shortening.

Lengthening

This is usually done gradually using the distraction histogenesis principle described earlier.

Corticotomy for lengthening is done using a gigli saw or drill and osteotomes.

Distraction is usually started 5–7 days after surgery. Lengthening is at the rate of 1 mm per day, or slower if the regenerate is poor.

In the presence of significant acetabular dysplasia, the hip joint may subluxate during femoral lengthening and the dysplasia must be addressed surgically prior to lengthening.

In fibula hemimelia, the knee joint may be unstable and it is important to span the knee joint with the fixator during femoral lengthening to prevent knee subluxation/dislocation.

Complications of limb lengthening include pin site infection, osteomyelitis, wire breakage, poor regenerate formation, premature regenerate consolidation, neurovascular injury, joint stiffness, joint subluxation/dislocation, and regenerate fracture.

References

1. Paley D, Herzenberg JE. *Principle of Deformity Correction*, Vol. 2. Berlin: Springer; 2003.

2. Standard SC, Herzenberg JE, Conway JD, Siddiqui NA, McClure PK, Assayag MJ. *The Art of Limb Alignment*, 11th ed. Baltimore, MD: Rubin Institute for Advanced Orthopedics, Sinai Hospital of Baltimore; 2022.

3. Eastwood DM, Sanghrajka AP. Guided growth: recent advances in a deep-rooted concept. *J Bone Joint Surg Br.* 2011;93(1):12–18.

4. Shapiro F. Developmental patterns in lower-extremity length discrepancies. *J Bone Joint Surg Am.* 1982;64(5):639–51.

5. Anderson M, Green WT, Messner MB. Growth and predictions of growth in the lower extremities. *J Bone Joint Surg Am.* 1963;45-A:1–14.

6. Paley D, Bhave A, Herzenberg JE, Bowen JR. Multiplier method for predicting limb-length discrepancy. *J Bone Joint Surg Am.* 2000;82-A(10):1432–46.

Orthopaedic-Related Syndromes

Deborah M. Eastwood

Introduction

Many of the syndromes of 'orthopaedic interest' rely on the clinical skills of pattern recognition and some knowledge of genetics. Increasingly, in any given patient, the genotype can be mapped and the genetic mishap identified. However, whilst this does not always improve our understanding of the patient's phenotype, it can help our appreciation of which other systems are affected and perhaps in which way.

The autosomes and sex chromosomes are all 'divided' by the centromere into the short (p = *petit*) and long (q = next letter in the alphabet) arms. Some chromosomes contain a few big genes, and others contain lots of smaller genes. Depending on the importance of each gene, deletions, duplications, and trisomies may be associated with few clinical signs or problems that are incompatible with life. Each gene consists of nucleotides comprising a sugar, a phosphate, and a nitrogen-containing base. There are four such bases, and substitution of even a single base can have profound effects; for example, valine in the place of glutamic acid in the haemoglobin-beta gene on chromosome 11 will result in the autosomal recessive condition of sickle cell anaemia, assuming both maternal and paternal gene copies have the same substitution. In the autosomal dominant condition of achondroplasia, substitution of glycine with arginine in the fibroblast growth factor receptor-3 gene on the short arm of chromosome 4 results in an instantly recognizable phenotype.

Many mutations are de novo, rather than inherited, and thus whilst the family history is important, a negative history does not exclude a genetic disorder as the cause of the child's symptoms and signs. It is equally important to remember that many conditions, unlike achondroplasia, show significant phenotypic variation, even within a family.

This chapter discusses several syndromes of orthopaedic importance and highlights some principles which should be used when assessing any child, to ensure that a syndromic diagnosis is not overlooked. A holistic assessment is always important, and simply looking at the face and hands may give you valuable information.

Down Syndrome (Trisomy 21)

In Down syndrome, each person has three copies of chromosome 21: it is the commonest and the least severe of the three trisomies that survive until term; most trisomies are fatal in the antenatal period. Trisomy 21 along with trisomy 18 (Edward syndrome) and trisomy 13 (Patau syndrome) are all associated with significant difficulties and a reduced life expectancy.

The incidence of Down syndrome increases with advancing maternal age, but overall most children with this syndrome are born to younger mothers. Routine antenatal checks in the UK have traditionally used a 'combined serum screening test', which includes a maternal blood test and an ultrasound scan – the detection rate for trisomy 21 is 86%, and for Edward and Patau syndromes 80%. If the result of this test suggests the baby has a 'higher chance' of having Down syndrome, the family will be offered further testing, which may include an invasive diagnostic test such as chorionic villus sampling (CVS) between 11 and 14 weeks or an amniocentesis from 15 weeks onward. Both tests are associated with a small (<1%) chance of miscarriage. In the event of a positive test, families will be offered counselling and can opt to continue with the pregnancy or discuss a termination of the pregnancy.

More recently, a non-invasive prenatal test (NIPT) has become available. The NIPT uses the presence of circulating cell free DNA in the maternal blood to quantify the risk of these three trisomies. The sensitivity of this test is 100% for Down and Patau syndromes, and 92% for Edward syndrome. The test is also highly specific. As it is non-invasive for the fetus, there is no additional risk of miscarriage.

Children with Down syndrome have hypotonia and joint laxity, with delayed motor milestones. There are associated learning difficulties. Their hypermobility is often seen in the hip and ankle joints, which are not included in the Beighton scoring system, and thus if assessed by these criteria alone, children with Down syndrome may have low scores. Classically, there has been concern regarding the potential of C1–C2 instability, although most cases of instability are asymptomatic and only 1–2% of children develop symptoms (see Chapter 11, Figure 11.4). Flexible flat feet are almost universal in this population; symptoms usually respond to conservative measures. Many feet also develop hallux valgus.

The Hip

Hip instability is present in 1–7% of children. The natural history is often progressive, with hypermobility of the hip evolving to habitual, but often painless, dislocation, persistent subluxation, and/or fixed dislocation often with pain and loss of independent mobility [1]. Treatment focuses on reduction and stabilization of the hip joint and will vary with the patient's age and disease severity, but must take into account the associated anatomical abnormalities of the anteverted femur and **retroverted** acetabulum. Hip instability in Down syndrome

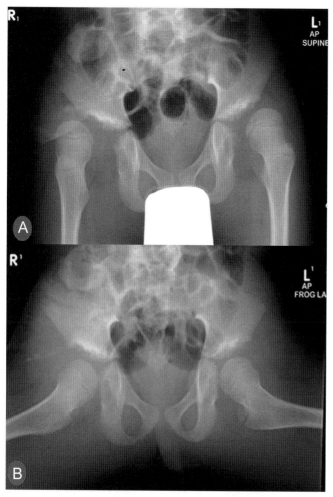

Figure 24.1 (A) AP supine and (B) frog lateral views of the pelvis of a 7-year-old boy with Down syndrome with subluxed, but reducible, hips.

may persist despite surgical intervention and it is a challenging condition to treat (Figure 24.1).

Children with Down syndrome are also at increased risk of developing Perthes' disease or slipped capital femoral epiphysis, when compared to the general population, but the incidence remains low at <1%.

The Knee

Patellofemoral instability is present in about 5% of cases, more commonly in girls/women. If symptomatic, surgical treatment may be warranted. Anterior knee pain and the feeling of instability can be disabling in this patient group who may have a limited ability to understand that the symptoms are not 'serious' and, for example, it is possible to function well despite these symptoms.

Scoliosis

A significant curve may develop in 6–8% of children, and this subgroup of patients have often undergone cardiac surgery in infancy. Bracing is often ineffective and surgical intervention may be required despite the relatively high complication rate associated with these procedures.

Inflammatory Arthropathy

Recent studies suggest there is an arthropathy associated with Down syndrome. Symptoms and signs are often not recognized, leading to a delay in diagnosis and more significant radiological changes at presentation. The fingers and wrists are frequently affected.

X-Linked Hypophosphataemic Rickets

Mutations in the *PHEX* gene on the X chromosome lead to unregulated production of fibroblast growth factor 23 (FGF-23), with urinary 'phosphate wasting' and hypophosphataemia, resulting in defective bone mineralization and poor tooth formation [2]. It is an X-linked dominant condition, so the female-to-male ratio should be close to 2:1. There is no evidence to support previous theories that females were less affected than males; any such differences seen in adult patients are more likely to be related to the effects of sex hormones and activity levels.

Clinical and radiological features are those of rickets, with the common finding of disproportionate short stature and lower limb deformity. Metaphyseal thickening is seen clinically around the fastest-growing physes, namely the distal femur, distal tibia, and distal radius, as well as the costochondral junctions which give rise to the rachitic rosary (and Harrison's sulcus) (see Chapter 22, Figure 22.3).

Prompt diagnosis and early medical treatment are the mainstays of management, and with healing of the rickets, there will be correction of lower limb deformity. Biochemically, at presentation, serum alkaline phosphatase (ALP) levels are high and phosphate levels low. Parathyroid hormone (PTH) levels should be measured regularly, as secondary hyperparathyroidism is common, partly as a result of the medication taken. In addition, tests such as serum ALP, calcium, and creatine levels, with urinary calcium/creatinine levels, are used to monitor treatment efficacy.

Until recently, phosphate supplements and high-dose calcitriol (the active form of vitamin D) were the mainstays of medical treatment – the medicines have an unpleasant taste and treatment compliance is often poor. More recently, burosumab, a fully human monoclonal immunoglobulin G1 (IgG1) antibody neutralizing FGF-23 has been approved for use. Early results of treatment in children suggest a significant improvement in physical ability and a significant reduction in patient-reported pain, fatigue, and functional disability.

Children present with a waddling gait, short stature, and limb deformity – this is usually symmetrical and may be either varus or valgus. Windswept deformities do occur. Torsional abnormalities are common. Patients commonly complain of muscle pain and weakness. There may be a history of dental pain and tooth abscesses.

With good medical management and compliance, the biochemical and radiological markers of rickets will improve. The limb deformities may improve for 12 months, once maximized medical management has been established. Residual deformity may require surgical treatment. Early, aggressive

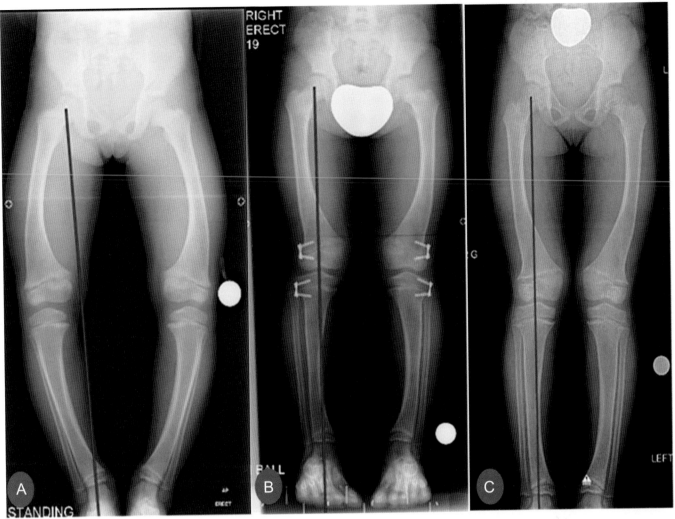

Figure 24.2 (A) Standing leg length radiograph. A girl aged 4 with X-linked hypophosphataemia and residual varus deformities despite 12 months of maximized medical care. The mechanical axis deviation for both legs (illustrated on her right) is significant. The metaphyses are cupped and flared, and the physes are widened. (B) Standing leg length radiograph. The patient was treated with the guided growth technique (plates across the distal femoral and proximal tibial physes), and after 12 months, her axes had corrected. (C) Standing leg length radiographs. Twelve months following plate removal, the patient's axes have remained good, but her rickets is still evident on X-ray.

surgery with osteotomies and internal or external fixation devices has been associated with high complication rates, and the current trend is to maintain limb alignment with guided growth techniques during childhood. Residual torsional and/or angular deformity can be corrected, if necessary, towards skeletal maturity (Figure 24.2). Bone metabolism and homeostasis are helped by prompt mobilization after surgery. Some patients develop scoliosis, and syringomyelia has been reported (Figure 24.3).

Neurofibromatosis

Neurofibromatosis type 1 (NF1) is the commonest of the three heterogenous conditions under the neurofibromatosis (NF) umbrella. The *NF1* gene is situated on chromosome 17 and normally functions as a tumour suppressor. The gene defect results in less suppression, and therefore, dysregulation of cell growth

and cell division is seen, with an increased risk of tumour (both benign and malignant) formation. The condition is associated with a variety of soft tissue and bony abnormalities. The phenotype is variable with café-au-lait spots and axillary freckling, frequently present by the age of 1 (Figure 24.4).

Benign neurofibromas are often visible and palpable in the subcutaneous tissues running in the line of the cutaneous nerves. Plexiform neurofibromas are larger and more complex (as their name implies) and these may undergo malignant transformation.

For the orthopaedic surgeon, the major causes of concern are the development of scoliosis and management of a tibial pseudarthrosis (dysplasia). Spinal deformity is common and may be dystrophic or non-dystrophic (see Chapter 10, Figure 10.9). The whole spine must be imaged carefully to exclude the presence of clinically silent intraspinal lesions. Dystrophic curves are often progressive, requiring aggressive operative management in childhood despite the increased risk of pseudarthrosis following spinal fusion.

Patients may have significant hypertension requiring appropriate medical management. In childhood, they are also at increased risk of developing low-grade gliomas, and thus headaches and visual disturbances are symptoms that must be taken seriously (Figure 24.5).

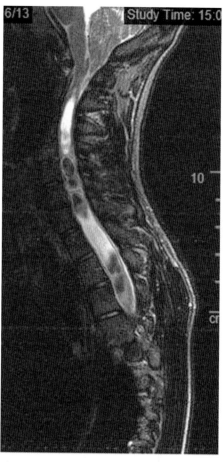

Figure 24.3 Sagittal MRI scan of a 12-year-old boy with X-linked hypophosphataemia, demonstrating low-lying cerebellar tonsils, compatible with a type 1 Chiari malformation and cervical syringomyelia.

Tibial Pseudarthrosis

This condition often presents in infancy as an apex anterolateral tibial bow prior to the development of a fracture. It is unclear what percentage of cases of tibial pseudarthrosis are NF1-positive, as routine genetic testing does not take place in the UK and the clinical phenotype may be otherwise mild. Recent studies would suggest up to 66% of cases are NF1-positive. In such patients, some researchers question the use of bone morphogenetic protein 2 (BMP 2) in obtaining bony union at the risk of stimulating tumour formation elsewhere. Bony changes may be present in other long bones (Figure 24.5) (see also Chapter 6, Figures 6.22 and 6.24).

Nail–Patella Syndrome

This autosomal dominant condition has characteristic clinical and radiographic features. The genetic defect is a loss-of-function mutation in the transcription factor LMXB1 on chromosome 4, which is responsible for normal development of the dorsal structures.

Almost all patients have abnormal fingernails and/or toenails, and many have small or absent patellae. Elbow dysplasia, particularly of the lateral aspect of the humerus and the radius, may be associated with dislocation of the radial head, cubitus valgus, and a flexion deformity. The iliac horns that are pathognomonic for this condition are present in up to 80% of patients. Although an interesting radiographic feature, the horns are usually asymptomatic. They may be palpable as exostoses arising off the posterior iliac wing. They are said to provide an origin for the gluteus medius muscles (Figure 24.6).

If patellofemoral instability is troublesome, treatment is guided by standard principles, ensuring that any underlying genu valgum is addressed concomitantly.

Glaucoma and renal failure are significant non-orthopaedic complications.

Kabuki Syndrome

A rare multisystem disorder with a genetic basis, and although two specific mutations have been identified, most cases are due to a de novo mutation. The facial features are distinctive but

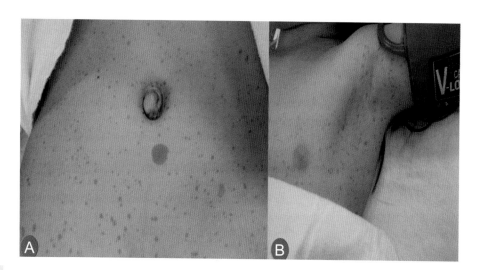

Figure 24.4 Café-au-lait spots (A) and axillary freckling (B) are considered as two criteria for diagnosing neurofibromatosis. Others include cutaneous neurofibromas, plexiform neurofibromas, optic glioma, Lisch nodules, distinctive bone lesions, and first-degree relatives with neurofibromatosis.

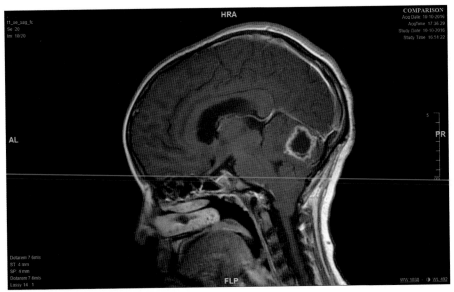

Figure 24.5 (A) Magnetic resonance scan showing a posterior fossa tumour in a child with neurofibromatosis type 1. Histology confirmed an astrocytoma. (B) Lateral radiograph of the left tibia of a girl aged 17, showing classical tibial bowing with pseudarthrosis. (C) AP radiograph of the forearm, showing extensive neurofibromatous involvement of the ulna.

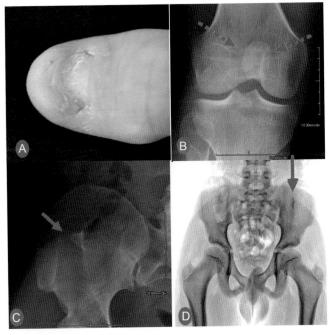

Figure 24.6 Nail–patella syndrome. (A) A photograph showing nail changes. (B) A plain knee radiograph showing a small patella with an irregular shape (dashed red arrows). (C) Pelvic radiograph – the solid red arrows point to the classic iliac horn (not as visible as people expect them to be). (D) Flexion deformity of the elbow and radial head dislocation. *Source:* https://en.wikipedia.org/wiki/Nail%E2%80%93patella_syndrome.

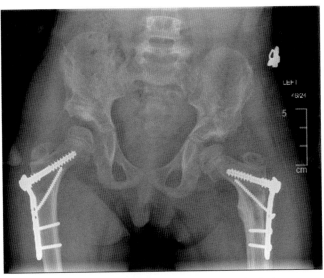

Figure 24.7 AP pelvic radiograph of a 6-year-old child with Kabuki syndrome who had residual dysplasia following closed reduction of bilateral developmental dysplasia of the hip. She underwent bilateral femoral and pelvic osteotomies to correct the bone shape and improve stability.

may only become apparent with growth. In keeping with many syndromes of orthopaedic significance, short stature, learning difficulties, and joint laxity are some of the common features, with hip dislocation being the most frequent indication for orthopaedic surgical intervention. As in all syndromes which feature joint laxity, correction of bony deformity is important (Figure 24.7).

Ehlers–Danlos Syndrome

This category includes syndromes with the common problems of disordered structure, production and/or processing of collagen leading to joint hypermobility, skin hyperextensibility, and tissue fragility. The 2017 revised classification identified 13 subtypes, with considerable phenotypic overlap. Firm diagnosis depends on molecular confirmation of the genetic variant. Several mutations are recognized in association with Ehlers–Danlos syndrome (EDS), either in collagen-encoding genes or in genes encoding collagen-modifying enzymes. Most frequently, the abnormality is with collagen type V (*COL5A1* or *COL5A2*) with an autosomal dominant inheritance. Rarely, a

COL1A1 mutation is identified and other genotypes have also been implicated.

The clinical criteria for the **hypermobile form of EDS (hEDS)** have been revised to allow better differentiation from other hypermobile syndromes. hEDS is the commonest subtype and although **no** genetic basis has been identified, it is considered to be autosomal dominant.

Classical EDS (cEDS) (autosomal dominant), **vascular EDS (vEDS)** (autosomal dominant), and **kyphoscoliotic EDS (kEDS)** (autosomal dominant) subtypes are all associated with extreme skin elasticity, joint hypermobility, and dislocations. Frequently, muscle hypotonia is associated with a delay in developmental motor milestones. The skin is fragile and bruises readily, so both traumatic and surgical scars are wide and atrophic. In vEDS, there is a risk of internal organ rupture/bleeding.

Physiotherapy and orthotics form the mainstays of orthopaedic treatment, with lifestyle advice as part of this multidisciplinary approach, which also concentrates on bone health and pain management. Surgery is an option for a select group of EDS patients with specific problems, but literature to support such interventions is very limited; stabilization of joints, particularly the feet, may be required, but recurrence rates are high, especially in the weight-bearing joints.

Pain is common and may not be related to the obvious clinical features of joint instability and muscle hypotonia; nerve entrapment syndromes should be considered.

Marfan Syndrome

Marfan syndrome is one of the commonest disorders of the connective tissues. It is caused by a mutation in the *FBN1* gene on chromosome 15, which is responsible for fibrillin 1 production, a component of the microfibrils in the extracellular matrix. Without fibrillin, connective tissues may be weak and, in effect, 'stretchy'. Mutation in fibrillin 1 results in dysregulation of the production of transforming growth factor (TGF) beta, a growth factor that instructs cells on 'how to behave'. Recent work suggests that medical treatments which reduce TGF beta levels may be beneficial.

The classic signs are disproportionate tall stature, with an arm span that exceeds the patient's height, arachnodactyly (spider fingers), a chest wall deformity which may be either pectus carinatum or pectus excavatum, and ocular lens dislocations. Mitral valve lesions and aortic aneurysms (with or without dissection) are common. Marfan syndrome has an autosomal dominant inheritance pattern, but 25% of cases are due to a de novo mutation. Extreme fatigue and orthostatic complaints are frequent symptoms (Figure 24.8).

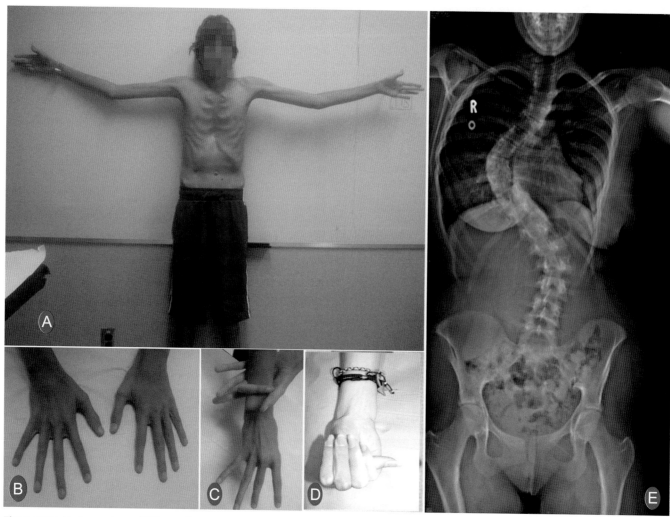

Figure 24.8 Marfan syndrome. (A) The arm length is typically greater than the height, and elbow extension <170°, with pectus excavatum. (B) Arachnodactyly (long, slender fingers). (C) Overlap of the little finger and the thumb when clasping the wrist. (D) Steinberg sign: the thumb extends beyond the ulnar border of the palm when held in a fist. (E) Scoliosis and protrusio acetabuli.

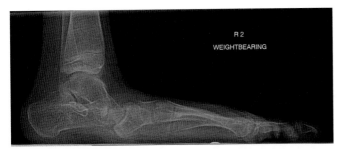

Figure 24.9 Lateral weight-bearing radiograph of the foot of a 10-year-old girl with Marfan syndrome. Note the length of the foot and the significant hindfoot valgus (no subtalar joint visible), as well as the subluxed talonavicular joint.

The main orthopaedic concern is scoliosis, which affects approximately 60% of patients. Most curves remain small, but the curve may be rapidly progressive and resistant to bracing when it presents a challenge for the surgeon and multidisciplinary team. There is also a high incidence of dural ectasia, which may be associated with back and leg pain. Surgery is associated with high complication rates.

Protrusio acetabuli is present in 25% of cases and may be associated with symptomatic early degenerative change.

As with EDS, many patients with Marfan syndrome have significant levels of chronic pain at multiple sites. Planovalgus feet are common and often troublesome (Figure 24.9).

Stickler Syndrome (Hereditary Arthro-ophthalmopathy)

This syndrome also includes a group of conditions with characteristic features associated with connective tissue disorders, leading to multisystem problems. As its name implies, it too is a genetic condition. Several gene mutations have been identified, and most are autosomal dominant in inheritance, with phenotypic variation.

Clinically, the child is often wearing both hearing aids and glasses, and has a notably flat mid face due to poor development of the maxilla and nasal bridge. The Pierre Robin sequence (cleft palate, micrognathia, and glossoptosis – a tongue that is further back than normal) may also be present. The presence of these mid-facial anomalies may require careful anaesthetic assessment prior to any surgery.

Orthopaedically, joint laxity is the main feature, with flat feet and uncomfortable hips being common symptoms. Valgus slips of the capital femoral epiphyses and protrusio have both been reported as a cause of hip pain (Figure 24.10). Scoliosis is not uncommon and is managed in keeping with routine principles.

Larsen Syndrome

This syndrome is characterized by ligamentous laxity and joint dislocation often present at birth. The 'full house' presentation would include dislocated hips and knees, with club foot deformities. The elbow joints may also be affected. The common genetic abnormality affects the *FLNB* gene, which makes the protein filamin B. It is associated with an autosomal dominant inheritance.

Early surgical management is often required to reduce and stabilize the joints. As the child grows, the short stature becomes

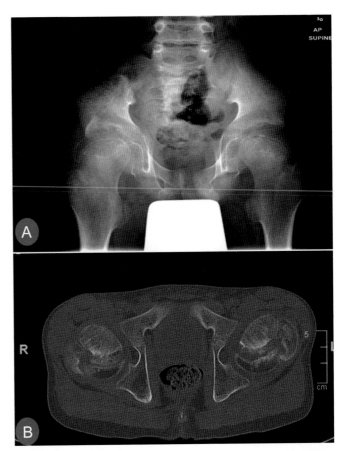

Figure 24.10 (A) AP radiograph of the pelvis of a boy aged 11 under regular follow-up for Stickler syndrome who presented with increasing ex-toeing and stiff hips with limited flexion. Imaging confirmed chronic valgus slips of both femoral epiphyses. (B) CT scan demonstrating posterior displacement of the femoral epiphyses.

obvious, and scoliosis and cervical kyphosis and instability may develop. A 'double' calcaneus with two ossification centres may be an interesting finding on X-ray (Figure 24.11).

Lysosomal Storage Disorders

The lysosome can be considered as the cell's 'recycling centre' where enzymatic degradation of unwanted/waste materials takes place. In this group of inherited disorders, various enzymes are missing and hence there is a build-up of waste products in **all** cells, leading to multiorgan damage and dysfunction. Enzyme replacement therapy (ERT) and/or haematopoietic stem cell transplant (HSCT) are used increasingly, but never a 'cure' for all aspects of the multisystemic condition.

This group includes conditions such as the mucopolysaccharidoses (MPS), Fabry disease, Gaucher disease, and Batten disease. Many are autosomal recessive.

Mucopolysaccharidoses

Dysostosis multiplex is the phrase used to describe the widespread skeletal changes found in MPS conditions where instability and subluxation of the upper cervical spine, thoracolumbar kyphosis, joint contractures or joint laxity, knock knees, and dysplastic, subluxed hips are common. The cartilaginous hip often looks better than the ossified hip and may influence

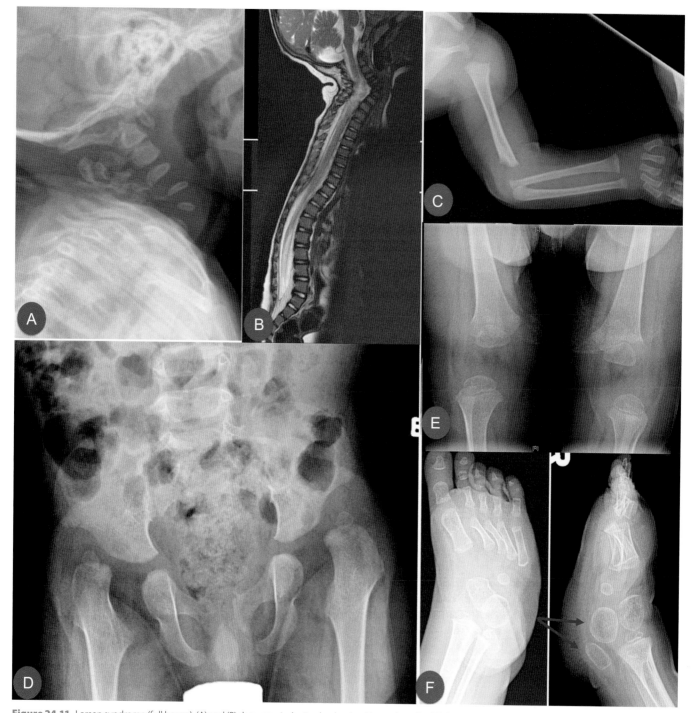

Figure 24.11 Larsen syndrome (full house). (A) and (B) show cervical spine kyphosis with myelopathy. (C) shows elbow dislocation. (D) shows bilateral hip dislocations. (E) shows bilateral knee subluxation. (F) shows a partially corrected club foot; the two red arrows point to the double ossification centre in the calcaneus.

surgical reconstruction (Figure 24.12). Guided growth is useful for correcting genu valgum (genu varum does not occur).

Many patients have neurophysiological changes in keeping with carpal tunnel syndrome, although the child may be asymptomatic or unable to describe their symptoms. Carpal tunnel decompression is helpful.

Symptoms of carpal tunnel syndrome in children include clumsiness, poor motor skills, and finger biting. Any child with

symptoms of carpal tunnel syndrome should be considered to have MPS until proven otherwise – some phenotypes are mild.

Gaucher Disease

Gaucher disease is a rare condition (which has never been encountered by the author) that seems to gain undue prominence at the time of exams. The adult-onset form (type 1) is the commonest, presenting with bone pain, fatigue, anaemia, and

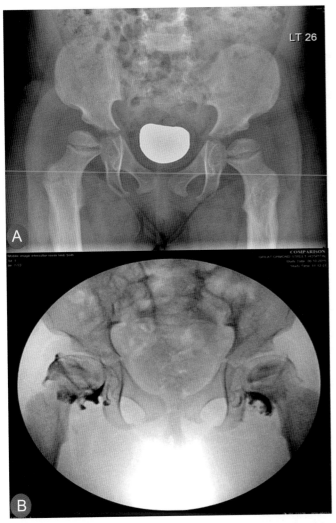

Figure 24.12 (A) AP pelvic radiograph of a child with mucopolysaccharidosis, showing abnormalities in both the femoral head and acetabular rim which are well formed. (B) Arthrograms of the same hips confirming that the cartilaginous femoral heads and the cartilaginous acetabulum are well formed, but not ossified.

Amyloplasia

Amyloplasia is the commonest form of AMC. The phenotype is characteristic with deformities that are often symmetrical (both left to right and upper to lower limbs) and more severe distally than proximally. Muscle strength, rather than range of joint movement, may be the key determinant of function and outcome.

Distal Arthrogryposis

Many of the distal arthrogrypotic subtypes demonstrate an autosomal dominant inheritance pattern, but with phenotypic variation. As the name implies, it is the distal joints that are affected. Congenital talipes equinovarus (CTEV) and congenital vertical talus (CVT) foot deformities are common; however, as the deformities are non-idiopathic, outcomes from the standard Ponseti or reverse Ponseti treatment programmes are not as reliable, and surgery may be required to obtain or maintain a plantigrade foot position. Some subtypes are eponymous such as Freeman–Sheldon and Beal syndromes.

Pterygia Syndromes

In affected children, there are soft tissue webs crossing the flexor aspect of joints (particularly the elbow and the knee) which add significantly to the joint contractures. The surgeon must remember that the web is not the only, or indeed the main, reason why the joint is contracted, and thus release on its own can be disappointing. The nerves crossing the flexor aspects of the joints may be out of position, and instead of lying close to the bone, they are close to the hypoteneuse of the web and hence surgical release of the web may not achieve much improvement in the deformity as the nerve is unable to stretch acutely.

The 'Overgrowth Syndromes'
PIK3CA-Related Overgrowth Spectrum (PROS)

This term describes a group of rare disorders that are associated with localized areas of overgrowth which can affect various tissue types. All have a mutation in the *PIK3CA* gene, affecting the AKT/mTOR pathway which is involved in the control of growth (Figure 24.13) [3]. Many mutations are mosaic. Modern treatments include drugs such as sirolimus (initially used as an anticancer drug) to limit cell growth, but there are side effects and regular haematological monitoring is required.

For the orthopaedic surgeon, most problems are soft tissue-related, with excessive vascular, lymphatic, and lipomatous tissue infiltrating the muscles, bones, and joints, causing pain and affecting function, with significant cosmetic implications. Multidisciplinary management is essential, with careful counselling prior to any surgical procedure, to ensure that patient/family expectations match those of the surgeon.

Klippel–Trenaunay syndrome, **Proteus syndrome**, **Proteus-like syndrome**, and **CLOVES syndrome** (congenital, lipomatous overgrowth with vascular malformations, epidermal naevi, and spinal or skeletal abnormalities) are now all recognized to be part of the PROS spectrum, with different tissues involved in different patients at different times and to different extents (Figure 24.14). Vascular malformations that extend into the joints often lead to recurrent bleeds and early degenerative change (Figure 24.15).

hepatosplenomegaly. Intravenous ERT or oral substrate reduction therapy (SRT) reduces symptoms and improves quality of life.

Arthrogryposis Multiplex Congenita

The term arthrogryposis means curved and hooked joints, and is therefore simply a description of the physical appearance. As the full term arthrogryposis multiplex congenita (AMC) implies, joint contractures are multiple (by definition, two or more joint contractures in two or more body areas) and present from birth, but are not usually genetic in origin. A key feature is that none of the musculoskeletal tissues around the contracted joint are normal, and thus a normal joint with normal function cannot be achieved with any form of treatment – either surgical or conservative: both the parents and clinicians must be aware of this, so that realistic treatment goals can be set. A multidisciplinary team is essential in the management of these complex cases.

Currently, there are several hundreds of recognized disorders that may present with arthrogryposis, and perhaps the simplest way of subdividing these is on the basis of whether or not the neurological examination is normal.

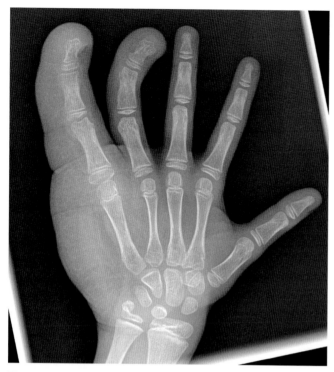

Figure 24.13 AP radiograph showing the non-dominant hand of an 8-year-old boy with PIK3CA-related overgrowth and macrodactyly of his fourth and fifth fingers. The soft tissue bulk prevents distal and proximal interphalangeal joint movement.

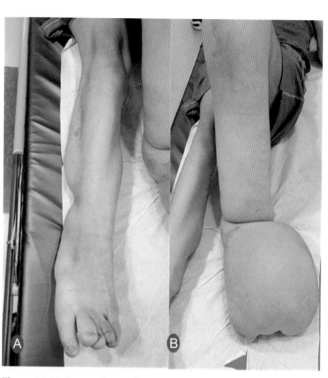

Figure 24.14 Proteus-like syndrome involving various tissues and parts of the body.

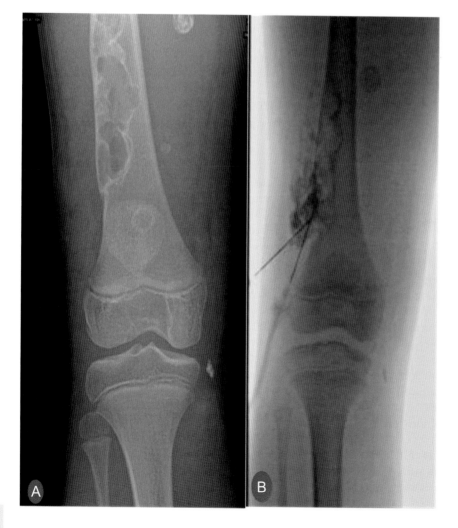

Figure 24.15 (A) AP radiograph of the distal femur of a 9-year-old child with an extensive vascular malformation. This is present in the femur, as shown by the lytic area in the diaphysis of the femur and there are multiple phleboliths in the soft tissues. (B) AP image taken during sclerotherapy of the vascular malformation.

References

1. Maranho DA, Fuchs K, Kim Y-J, Novais EN. Hip instability in patients with Down syndrome. *J Am Acad Orthop Surg* 2018;26(13):455–62.

2. Haffner D, Emma F, Eastwood DM, *et al.* Clinical practice recommendations for the diagnosis and management of X-linked hypophosphataemia. *Nat Rev Nephrol.* 2019;15(7): 435–55.

3. Keppler-Noreuil KM, Rios JJ, Parker VE, *et al.* PIK3CA-related overgrowth spectrum (PROS): diagnostic and testing eligibility criteria, differential diagnosis, and evaluation. *Am J Med Genet A.* 2015;167A(2):287–95. k

Miscellaneous Paediatric Orthopaedic Conditions

Ben Marson and Kathryn Price

Introduction

This chapter covers several conditions that have featured in previous exams but do not fit neatly in other chapters, including non-accidental injury, bladder exstrophy, osteogenesis imperfecta (OI), physis and physeal fractures, toe walkers, and others.

Non-accidental Injury

Background

Ambrose Tardieu first reported non-accidental injury (NAI) in 1860, noting the correlation between cutaneous lesions, fractures, subdural haematomas, and death [1]. Caffey again highlighted the association between long bone fractures and subdural haematomas in 1946 [2]. However, it was Henry Kempe who raised the profile of NAI in 1962 when he coined the term 'battered-child syndrome' [3]. He described the association between multiple fractures, subdural haematomas, failure to thrive, soft tissue swelling or bruising, and sudden unexplained death. He also highlighted the importance of situations in which the type or degree of injury did not correlate with the history. The US Child Abuse Prevention and Treatment Act (CAPTA) defines child abuse and neglect as:

> Any act or failure to act resulting in imminent risk of death, serious physical or emotional harm, sexual abuse or exploitation of a child by a parent or caretaker who is responsible for a child's welfare.

Child abuse is commoner than most would expect; it is estimated that 7% of children suffer serious physical abuse. Studies suggest that 25% of fatally abused children had been seen recently by a healthcare provider [4].

Predisposing Factors

It has been speculated that all that is required for child abuse to occur are:

- A child with provocative qualities
- A carer with a psychological predisposition for violence
- A stressor.

This means that NAI can be seen in any walk of life at any time. There are common predisposing risk factors, as shown in Table 25.1.

Injury Patterns

Pathognomonic injuries for NAI are rare, only accounting for approximately 5–10% of cases. Classic injuries seen in abuse are:

- Metaphyseal fractures (corner or bucket handle types) – twisting injury sustained at the level of the physis requiring holding the limb tight above and below the joint. Bucket handle fractures are essentially the same as corner fractures, but the avulsed bone fragment is larger and seen 'en face' as a bucket handle (Figures 25.1 and 25.2)
- Posterior rib fractures – in the absence of cardiopulmonary resuscitation or a major incident such as a road traffic accident, rib fractures are extremely rare. Children have a very compliant rib cage, so a huge amount of force is required to break a rib (Figure 25.3)
- Multiple fractures at different stages of healing (Figure 25.4).

The commonest sign of physical abuse in children is skin lesions. These can take the form of multiple bruises of different ages, particularly in areas not overlying bony prominences.

Table 25.1 Common predisposing risk factors for non-accidental injuries

Child qualities	Carer qualities	Social factors
• First-born child	• Young	• Financial difficulties
• <3 years	• Low social class	• Loss of a job
• Premature babies	• Single parent	• Divorce or separation
• Children with disabilities	• Previous history of abuse or domestic violence	• Social isolation
• Unplanned pregnancies	• Unemployment	• Bereavement
• Multiple births	• Drug and alcohol abuse	
• Stepchildren	• Mental illness	

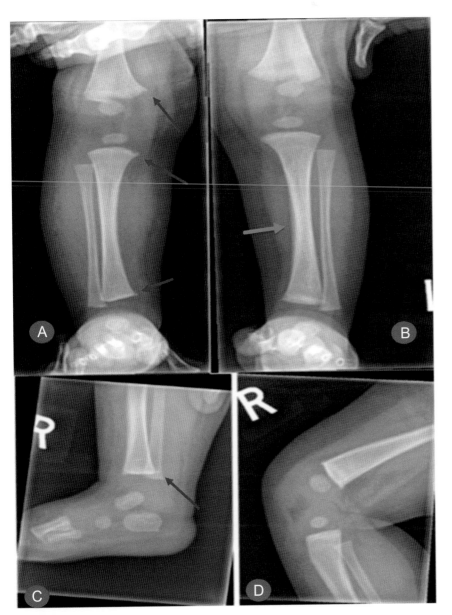

Figure 25.1 Corner fractures occur when a small piece of bone is avulsed due to shearing forces on the fragile growth plate, and are seen as a small piece at the corner fracture of the metaphysis (red arrows). They are often subtle, even on high-quality radiographs. In this child, there is also an unexplained periosteal reaction (blue arrow) on the left leg.

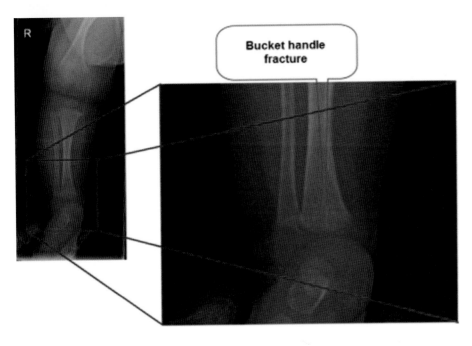

Bucket handle fracture

Figure 25.2 Bucket handle fractures are essentially the same as corner fractures.

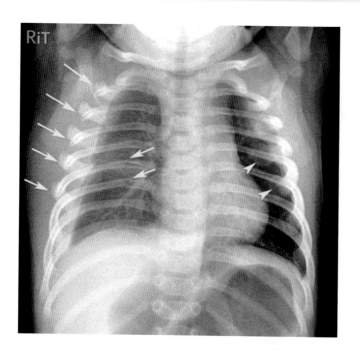

Figure 25.3 Chest radiograph showing multiple rib fractures (yellow arrows). Rib fractures have a very high specificity for non-accidental injury (NAI) in the absence of a history of major trauma such as a road traffic accident. In this child with proven NAI, there were multiple rib fractures at different healing stages – see callus formation on the left side (arrowheads), but absent on the right.

Classic sites for bruising are finger marks around the upper arms or throat, black eyes, and bruises around the ears, back, or genitalia. Bite marks and burns may also be seen (Figure 25.5).

The commonest fractures seen are spiral long bone fractures affecting the humerus, femur, and tibia. Digit fractures are common but are frequently missed. Long bone fractures commonly occur accidentally in children, so we rely on inconsistencies in the history to raise suspicion of NAI. The commonest factors to identify in the history are listed below:

- Ambulatory status – spiral long bone fractures are classic toddler's injuries as they learn to stand and walk. In children who are not yet walking, there is a high association with NAI
- Fracture not in keeping with the reported mechanism of injury – that is, spiral fracture reported as a direct blow
- Fracture magnitude in excess of what would be expected – significantly displaced or comminuted fractures in young children require a lot of energy due to plasticity of their bones
- Delayed presentation – buckle fractures will commonly present late due to their stable nature and lack of physical signs. Unstable complete fractures will cause pain and instability, and should be obviously apparent immediately. Failure to bring a child with an obvious injury for medical assessment should raise suspicion
- Differing stories or changing stories – there may be different accounts of the injury from different family members. Frequently where abuse has occurred, the family will change the story as time progresses in an attempt to explain the injury
- Attendance at multiple units with different injuries to avoid detection
- Recurrent failures to bring the child for review or recurrent cancellations of appointments.

Clinical Assessment

Careful, detailed documentation is absolutely essential in suspected cases of NAI. It can be extremely difficult to distinguish a deliberate from an accidental injury, and often it is only inconsistencies in the history that reveal the underlying problem. A careful history must be taken, detailing the events leading to the injury. Very close attention must be paid to the timing of events. Delayed presentation is very common in NAI. It is also important to get a clear story relating to the mechanism of injury, so that this can be compared with injury patterns. In NAI, there is commonly a discrepancy between the type or degree of injury sustained and the suggested mechanism. It is also vital to record any unusual behaviour on the part of the child or carer, and ideally in older patients, to obtain a history directly from the child.

A careful past medical and developmental history needs to be obtained and documented. It can be very important to note previous injuries, as well as any family history of multiple fractures that suggests an underlying condition such as OI. Achievement of developmental milestones is important, particularly the ambulatory status. For children who are ambulatory, the likelihood of fractures being due to NAI is markedly reduced.

It is important to examine the presenting injury carefully, with meticulous documentation of findings. In suspected cases of NAI, it is vital to examine the whole child thoroughly, looking for other injuries, in particular skin lesions. Multiple injuries at various stages of healing are strongly associated with NAI. All injuries must be catalogued, including the site, size, and colour of any skin lesions, for comparison later. Ideally, clinical photographs should be taken from two different views for adequate documentation. Similarly, any fractures must be clearly documented, including fracture site, presumed mechanism of injury, level of displacement, and stage of healing. Any abnormal family dynamics or impressions from the admitting team need to be recorded carefully.

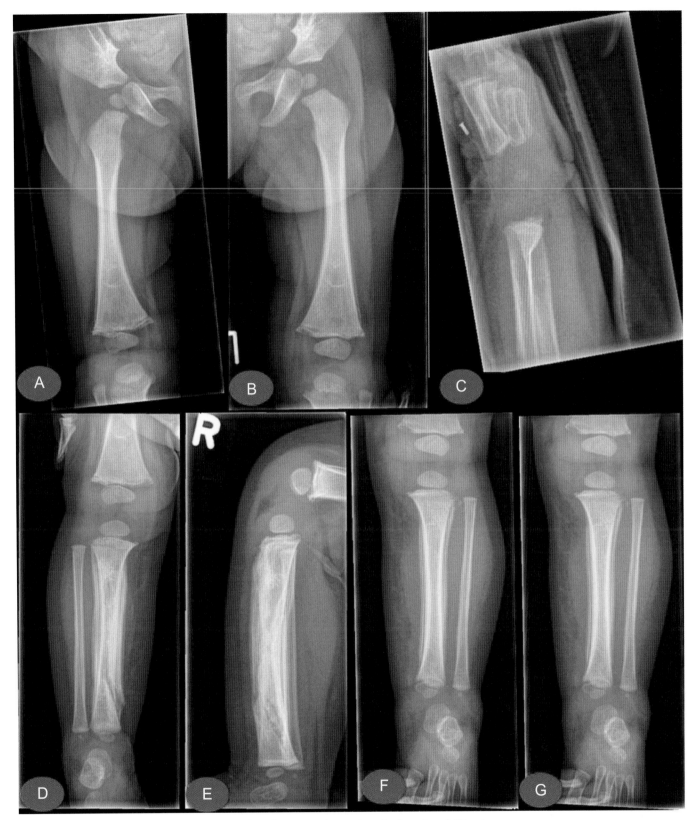

Figure 25.4 This young child presented with multiple bone fractures, with extensive callus formation of different ages.

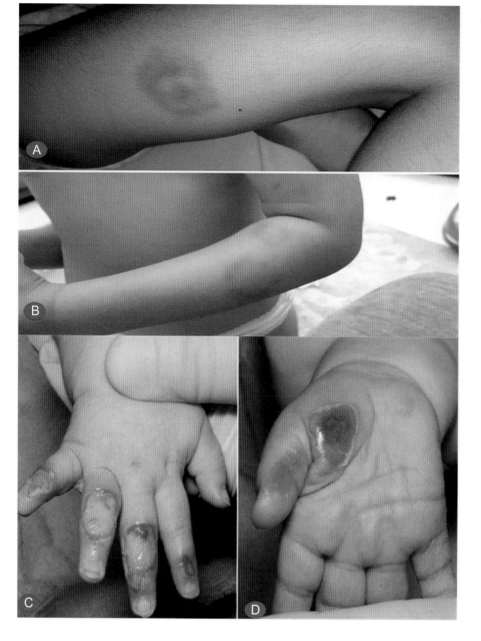

Figure 25.5 Skin injuries are valuable clues to the possibility of non-accidental injuries. Multiple bites of different ages (A, B) or burns in unexplained areas (C, D) are shown.

Radiological Assessment

Radiological assessment is necessary for all identified injuries. Fracture type and stage of healing can be very helpful in corroborating a history or refuting it. Radiological dating of injuries is not an exact science but is very helpful in allowing one to date injuries roughly (Table 25.2). Interval radiographs are required to ensure that no non-displaced fractures are missed and to date events more accurately.

Standards for radiological investigations of suspected NAI were published by the Royal College of Radiologists and the Royal College of Paediatrics and Child Health in March 2008.

In children under 2 years with suspected NAI, a full skeletal survey is indicated. This must be discussed among senior members of the child medical protection team, as it involves lots of radiation exposure. This involves the following series of images:

Table 25.2 Average time until appearance of radiological signs of healing

Signs	Average time to appearance on X-rays
Resolution of soft tissues	4–10 days
Subperiosteal new bone formation	10–14 days
Loss of fracture line delineation	14–21 days
Soft callus formation	14–21 days
Hard callus formation	21–42 days
Remodelling	1 year

1. CT head
2. AP chest
3. Oblique left ribs
4. Oblique right ribs

5. AP abdomen and pelvis
6. Lateral spine
7. PA both hands
8. PA both feet
9. AP both humeri
10. AP both forearms
11. AP both femurs
12. AP both tibia and fibula.

In children older than 2 years, this should be guided by the history and physical examination. A skeletal survey for NAI is different from a skeletal survey performed for other conditions such as dysplasia or neoplasia. The latter needs one side only.

Although bone scanning has been used as an alternative to skeletal survey for injuries, it may miss metaphyseal lesions due to increased uptake in that region. Moreover, spinal fractures and old or new injuries may not show up on the bone scan. For these reasons, it is not commonly employed. CT head identifies subtle skull fractures but also looks for intracranial

haemorrhages (Figure 25.6). Ophthalmology review to look for retinal haemorrhages is recommended.

Differential Diagnosis

- OI: mild forms of OI may present with multiple fractures occurring at low levels of trauma; many children will have white sclerae and show no other signs. Family history and skin testing can be helpful in making this diagnosis. Wormian bones are commonly seen on skull X-ray.
- Accidental trauma: the majority of injuries that occur because of abuse are the same as those that occur accidentally. The history and ambulatory status are extremely important in differentiating between the two.
- Normal variants: nutrient vessels, metaphyseal beaking, and physiological subperiosteal new bone formation (SPNBF) can all be confused with fractures. Physiological SPNBF is seen in 30–50% of children between 1 and 6 months of age, usually involves the tibia and femur, never extends to the metaphysis, and very rarely exceeds 2 mm; it is indistinguishable from fracture healing on X-ray.

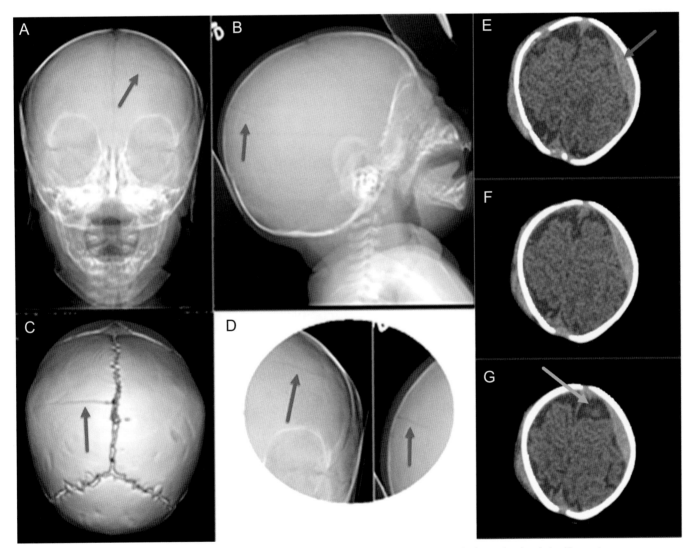

Figure 25.6 A child who presented with skull fracture from NAI. (F) and (G) show an extradural haematoma (red arrow) and a subdural haematoma (green arrow).

- Obstetric trauma: these fractures will usually have signs of healing by 11 days after birth and are associated with difficult births and large babies.
- Skin disorders: impetigo and blue spots can be confused with skin lesions but should be documented in the red book from the newborn examination.
- Haematological conditions: myelodysplasia, leukaemia, and other bleeding disorders may present with easy bruising and fractures.
- Infection: osteomyelitis may present with a periosteal reaction and a limp, and can be confused with healing fractures.
- Other rare diagnoses: rickets, scurvy, vitamin A intoxication leading to raised intracranial pressure, Caffey disease (also called infantile cortical hyperostosis – a rare, benign proliferating bone disease affecting infants), copper deficiency, skeletal dysplasias.

Management

The most important aspect of managing NAI is in identifying it. If there is any suspicion of NAI, then the child should be admitted directly to a place of safety. The paediatric and safeguarding teams should be notified, and social services informed. The decision to do skeletal surveys and further investigation is made after assessment by the multidisciplinary team, including paediatrics and orthopaedics.

Reporting suspected NAI is a legal and ethical requirement. The consequences of failing to identify and report abuse are high. The re-injury rate of battered children is between 30% and 50%, and the risk of death between 5% and 10% [5].

Bladder Exstrophy

Background

Bladder exstrophy is a congenital condition, affecting approximately 1 in 10 000–50 000 live births. It is part of a wider spectrum of anomalies affecting closure of the anterior abdominal wall, ranging from epispadias at one end to cloacal exstrophy at the other (Table 25.3).

Classical bladder exstrophy is characterized by failure of closure of the anterior abdominal wall, resulting in pelvic diastasis and an open bladder. It is believed that bladder exstrophy is caused by failure of the cloacal membrane to be reinforced by ingrowth of the mesoderm. It is more commonly seen in boys than girls, with a ratio of 2.5:1, and carries a 1 in 100 risk of occurrence in subsequent pregnancies.

Studies of the pelvis by CT and MRI and dissection of anatomic specimens showed that in classic exstrophy, the pubic bones are foreshortened by about one-third, the iliac wings are normal in size but externally rotated by approximately 13°, and the acetabula are retroverted but femoral version is normal. The sacroiliac joints are also externally rotated, and the pelvis is angled caudally. The bladder itself is small and fibrotic, and the external genitalia are hypoplastic. In cloacal exstrophy, there may be absence, hypoplasia, or asymmetry of the sacroiliac joint, as well as dislocation of the hips. Spina bifida is commonly associated with cloacal dystrophy [6] (Figure 25.7).

Radiographic Features

The pubic bones are foreshortened by about one-third and separated by about 4–5 cm at birth (normal being 1 cm) and increases with age (the differential diagnosis is cleidocranial dysplasia). The iliac bones are of normal size, but externally rotated. The acetabula are retroverted, but rarely dysplastic (Figure 25.8).

Natural History

Patients with bladder exstrophy do not commonly develop orthopaedic issues requiring surgery. They have normal athletic capabilities and are not increasingly affected by hip osteoarthritis, despite the acetabular retroversion. Pelvic osteotomy is usually only indicated if needed as part of a urological reconstruction procedure.

Children can have marked external rotation affecting their gait, but this typically resolves over time without surgical intervention. Patients may present with patellofemoral instability due to their abnormal rotational profile, but this rarely requires surgery. The only other common orthopaedic manifestation is sacroiliac joint pain [6].

Treatment

The treatment objective in bladder exstrophy is urological reconstruction, commonly obtained in staged procedures. The priorities are to close the bladder, gain continence, reconstruct the genitalia, and achieve an acceptable appearance. Pelvic osteotomy may be required to assist with the urological reconstruction.

Various surgical techniques have been recommended, each with pros and cons. In 1958, Schultz described a posterior pelvic osteotomy 2 weeks before closure of bladder exstrophy in a 2-year-old boy. Being posterior and with the bone being thick, the osteotomy was associated with blood loss and high complication rates. Salter used his innominate osteotomy (anterior) for bladder exstrophy in 1974. It was easier and most surgeons are familiar with the technique; however, as it passes between the two attachments of the inguinal ligament, the neurovascular structures are often compressed during the closure. In

Table 25.3 Spectrum of bladder exstrophy

Condition	Genitalia	Bladder	Hindgut	Pubic symphysis	Others
Epispadias	Open	Intact	Intact	Diastasis common	Rare
Classic bladder exstrophy	Open	Open	Intact	Wide diastasis common	Rare
Cloacal Exstrophy	Open	Open	Open	Wide diastasis common	Renal, musculoskeletal, spinal, and neural anomalies in 50%

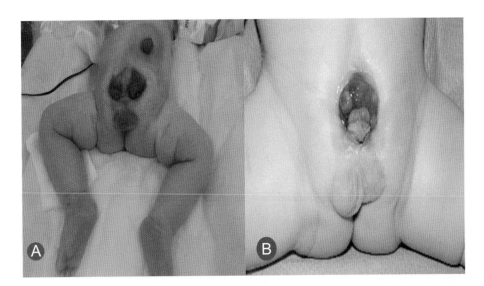

Figure 25.7 (A) is a clinical picture of a patient with cloacal exstrophy, who had had ileostomy shortly after birth and came for definitive surgical correction. (B) is a clinical picture of a patient with classic bladder exstrophy, with no need for ileostomy.

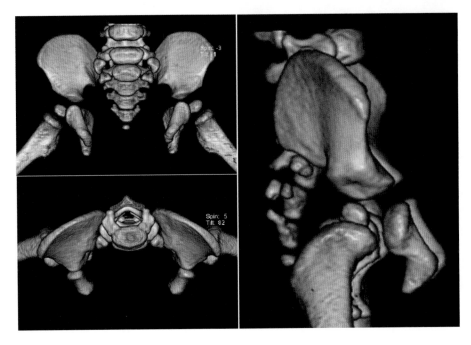

Figure 25.8 CT scan showing bladder exstrophy. Notice the foreshortened and separated pubic bones and both acetabula which are retroverted.

1994, the diagonal osteotomy was introduced to overcome Salter osteotomy shortfall. This starts just before the inguinal ligament. Sponseller popularized the combined osteotomy. The Manchester Children Group modified the combined osteotomy into Y pelvic osteotomy to reduce the risk of damaging the sacroiliac joint (Figure 25.9).

The osteotomized pelvis is usually immobilized using external fixation with post-operative mermaid dressing for 4–6 weeks. However, immobilization using traction only (i.e. without an external fixator) is also used (Figure 25.10).

Complications occur in approximately 4% of cases, including wound infection, dehiscence, and neurovascular symptoms.

Osteogenesis Imperfecta

Background

OI is a genetic disorder of connective tissue, resulting in defective type I collagen metabolism. Type I collagen is the commonest protein in bone and a major structural component of bone, tendons, and ligaments. This molecule is a tightly wound triple helix, which relies on having glycine as every third amino acid in the chain to maintain its structure. Defects may be quantitative or qualitative. Quantitative defects result in lower levels of structurally normal collagen, whilst qualitative defects occur when glycine residues are substituted for other amino acids, leading to unfolding of the triple helix. The severity of the phenotype is dependent on the location of the defect in the collagen molecule, with more severe phenotypes being associated with abnormalities near the N-terminal of the chain [5, 7].

OI affects 1 in 15 000–20 000 live births. More than 90% of cases are caused by mutations in the *COL1A1* and *COL1A2* genes. The *COL1A1* gene is located on chromosome 7q, whilst *COL1A2* is found on chromosome 17q. Diagnosis can be made in most cases by culturing skin fibroblasts to analyse the type I collagen or by isolating DNA from white cells to identify the *COL1A1* and *COL1A2* genes.

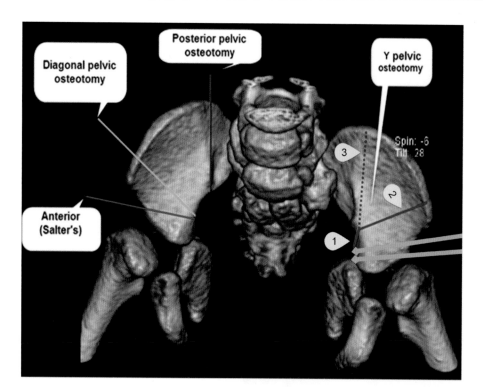

Figure 25.9 Pelvic osteotomies that are used in bladder exstrophy. The Y pelvic osteotomy involves the Smith–Peterson approach to the hip, with insertion of two pins (grey arrows) in the supra-acetabular areas. The stem of the Y is done first (marked 1), then followed by a diagonal osteotomy from just behind the anterior superior iliac spine to the Y stem. These are full osteotomies. The third osteotomy involves the inner table of the iliac wing and goes parallel to the sacroiliac joint.

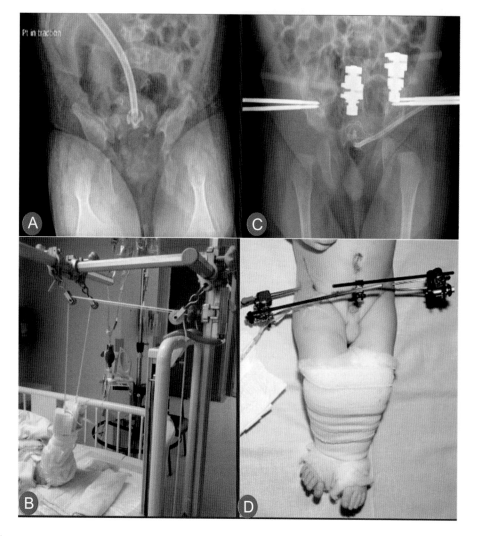

Figure 25.10 (A, B) Pelvic osteotomy was performed with post-operative traction; no fixation was used. (C, D) Pelvic osteotomies were immobilized using external fixators and mermaid bandage (the authors' preferred option).

Approximately 10–15% of cases do not have the classic mutations in collagen and will not be identified by these tests. This means that a positive test for OI confirms the diagnosis, but a negative test does not exclude it. Bone markers are normal, apart from alkaline phosphatase level, which is elevated because of increased bone turnover.

Classification

The best-known classification of OI is the Sillence classification, which divides patients into four groups based on clinical features. Fifteen additional groups of patients have subsequently been identified (currently up to type XIX), which do not fit within this traditional model. There is no defect in type I collagen in these conditions (Table 25.4).

Presentation

Children may present to the orthopaedic department with bone pain, muscle weakness, or ligamentous hyperlaxity. Patients have thin, translucent skin, with easy bruising and subcutaneous haemorrhages. They may have blue sclerae and dentinogenesis imperfecta (fragile, opalescent teeth) (Figure 25.11). There is an increased tendency to develop hernias, and any surgical scars are likely to be wide. It is common to present with presenile hearing loss starting in the patient's twenties, and there is frequently a history of excessive sweating, owing to the hypermetabolic state.

Children with type I OI may present with a couple of fractures in childhood. This is the commonest type of OI and also the mildest. Children will classically have blue sclerae and may have very few symptoms. By the time they reach skeletal maturity, bone quality tends to have improved and they may have very few issues in adulthood.

Type II OI is fatal, either in utero or in the perinatal period.

Type III OI is the most severe survivable form of the condition. Children are typically born with significant bowing affecting all four limbs. This bowing is always purely in the sagittal plane and is typically in the region of 90° for each long bone. The patients fracture their limbs very frequently with minimal force and are at risk of developing progressive deformity after any malunion. They commonly have associated learning disabilities and hearing issues, and are very prone to developing scoliosis. These children commonly sustain birth injuries which are commonly mistaken for NAI.

Type IV lies between type I and type III in severity. There is definitely an increased risk of fracture, in comparison to the normal population, but patients do not get progressive bowing of the limbs unless this is in relation to poorly managed fractures.

The only clinically relevant type in the additional groups is type V. These children develop ossification of the interosseous membrane in the forearm, with radial head dislocation, and are prone to developing hypertrophic callus formation.

Table 25.4 Sillence classification for osteogenesis imperfecta

Type	Subtypes	Teeth	Sclera	Clinical features	Prognosis
I	IA	Normal	Blue	Autosomal dominant, mildest form of OI with less severe fragility fractures, short stature	Normal life expectancy
	IB	Dentinogenesis imperfecta	Blue	Less severe fragility fractures, short stature	Normal life expectancy
II	II	Normal	Blue	Autosomal recessive and autosomal dominant, the worst type, associated with perinatal death	Perinatal or early infant death
III	III	Dentinogenesis imperfecta	Bluish at birth, white by puberty	Autosomal recessive and autosomal dominant, the worst survivable type. Progressive deformity, multiple fractures, scoliosis, severe limitation of function	Will usually require wheelchair, premature death
IV	IVA	Normal	White	Autosomal dominant, fragility fractures, short stature, moderate deformity of long bones, kyphoscoliosis	Fair
	IVB	Dentinogenesis imperfecta	White	Fragility fractures, short stature, moderate deformity of long bones, kyphoscoliosis	Fair

Beyond Sillence classification

V	Autosomal dominant, moderate to severe bone fragility, accounting for 4–5% of cases of OI. Patients develop calcification of the interosseous membrane of the forearm, with severe restriction of hand movement and dislocation of the radial head. They may develop hyperplastic callus formation after minor trauma, fractures, or surgery. This can be extremely difficult to differentiate from osteosarcoma
VI	Radiologically mimic rickets, with Looser zones commonly seen; however, the growth plate is not involved in OI and biochemistry is normal
VII	Autosomal recessive, affecting specific communities such as those of Native American, Northern Quebec, or Irish descent. There is a mutation affecting chromosome 3, leading to bone fragility and rhizomelic limb shortening. There is no discernible defect in type I collagen in this condition. Recent advances have linked this type to *CRTAP/LEPRE1* genes [8]; treatment targeting these defects is ongoing

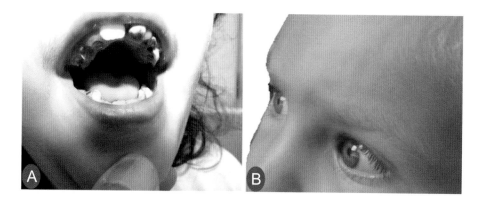

Figure 25.11 (A) shows a child with dentinogenesis imperfecta. (B) shows blue sclerae in a patient with OI.

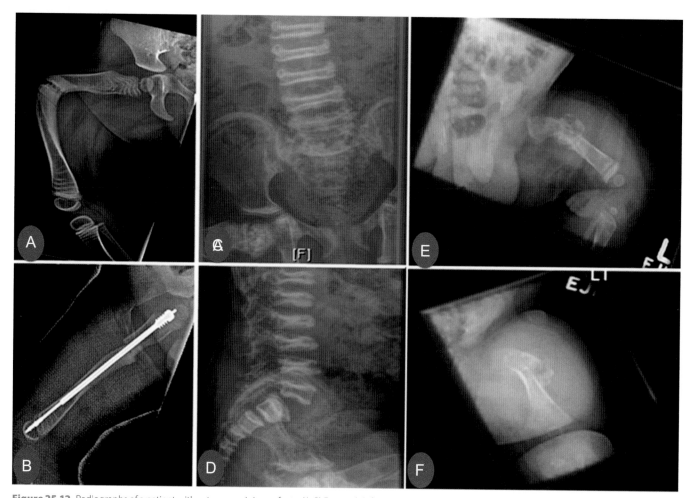

Figure 25.12 Radiographs of a patient with osteogenesis imperfecta. (A, B) Femoral deformity and fracture treated with a growing rod (Fassier–Duval rod). Notice the transverse sclerotic lines associated with pamidronate treatment. (C, D) Platyspondyly and biconcave vertebrae. (E, F) Hyperplastic callus formation.

As fractures heal, there may be a very florid healing response, which can be easily mistaken for an osteosarcoma. It is important that the family is warned about this condition early in childhood.

Inheritance was felt to be autosomal dominant for types I and IV, and autosomal recessive for types II and III. This has been contested recently. Severity is not predictable. The level of disability of the parent will not necessarily be similar for children.

Medical Management

There is no specific therapy for the underlying cause of OI, but various therapies have been tried to treat the consequences. Growth hormone has been used in the past, with little success, and there is some evidence that mesenchymal stromal cell transplant may partially correct the OI phenotype. This is an area of research for the future but is not widely used therapeutically at this time.

Bisphosphonates are the mainstay of medical therapy. These drugs inhibit osteoclastic resorption of bone, thus inhibiting bone resorption and increasing bone mass. They reduce bone turnover rates and increase the bone mineral density. In some cases, this has been shown to reduce the occurrence of fractures, but this has not been the case in other series. Bisphosphonates have also been shown to improve muscle strength and mobility and to give a sense of well-being. They are particularly effective when used in children under the age of 3 years. For those with the more severe types of OI, early administration of bisphosphonates can help to reduce the occurrence of the severe phenotypes.

The commonest regime reported is three-monthly cycles of intravenous pamidronate. For each cycle of bisphosphonate therapy, a classic transverse line of sclerosis is seen on radiographs, allowing monitoring of growth between cycles (Figure 25.12). Radiographs will usually show equally spaced transverse lines moving away from the physis in each long bone.

Side effects of bisphosphonates include an influenza-like reaction after the first pamidronate infusion, with vomiting, fever, and a rash. This can be associated with a transient decrease in serum calcium levels, and a transient increase in parathyroid hormone secretion. Jaw osteonecrosis is a rare, but serious, complication. There is delayed healing after osteotomies, but no delay in fracture healing unless the fracture is atypical. The bone can become brittle with bisphosphonate use, and this can make the child more prone to bending-type fractures in some cases.

'Can the bone be stronger, but more brittle?' is a common basic science question. Increased bone matrix mineralization found in OI will result in a higher bone matrix elastic modulus, and therefore in ultimate strength, but in less ability for plastic deformation and less energy absorption (less area under the stress strain graph).

Fracture Management

Fractures in children with OI will heal at a similar rate to fractures in normal children. The problem is that fractures still heal with weak OI bone. Due to the increased risk of fractures in these children, it is best to avoid malunion wherever possible. Any angulation in the bone will cause a stress-riser and potentially cause further fractures. Early weight-bearing is important to try to maintain as much bone stock as possible, as disuse osteopenia is a significant problem in this group.

The majority of fractures in these children can still be treated non-operatively in plaster. If there is going to be a prolonged period of non-weight-bearing, then surgical fixation is preferable to allow earlier mobilization. If fixing a fracture in an OI patient, the method should be modified, where possible, to protect the whole bone. Techniques such as plating will leave a stress-riser in the bone and likely lead to periprosthetic fractures. Intramedullary nailing provides fracture fixation and minimizes the risk of refracture.

Deformity Correction

For those children with type III OI, they are typically born with significant bowing of the femur, tibia, fibula, humerus, and forearm. They are unable to stand with these deformities and will therefore need corrective surgery to allow mobilization.

Due to the severity of the bowing, multiple osteotomies are commonly required in order to get a nail down the intramedullary canal. Children with OI bleed significantly, making this a very major procedure in small children. Growing rods, such as the Faisser–Duval or Sheffield rods, are used to allow fixation of the osteotomies and provide longer-term protection for the limb. The growing rods are anchored in the epiphyses at either end of the bone and can telescope as the child grows. Typically, the rods will need to be exchanged twice during their childhood, ultimately being changed to solid adult-style nails (Figures 25.13 and 25.14).

This surgery will typically be carried out as a staged procedure. The surgeon can either do one leg at a time or do both femurs, followed by both tibias. Post-operative immobilization is necessary, as growing rods have no rotational stability. It is not uncommon for the child to sustain a fracture of the unfixed bones during the post-operative period.

Children with type III OI have multiple medical comorbidities. It is not appropriate to put them through this major surgery, unless they are going to have ambulatory potential. When the child looks like they are trying to get themselves moving, this is the time to plan the intervention.

Straightening the long bones and fixing them with growing rods have the following benefits:

- Straightening the bone, which removes the stress-riser
- Having an intramedullary rod which protects against recurrent fractures
- Allowing weight-bearing, which further increases the bone quality further.

Spinal Involvement

Scoliosis occurs in 40–100% of cases of OI as a result of ligamentous laxity and multiple spinal wedge fractures. The severity of the scoliosis is related to the severity of the bone fragility, with six or more biconcave vertebrae indicating the potential for development of severe kyphosis. Curves <50° should be observed for progression. Bracing has been attempted in some cases but can lead to severe rib fractures and does not commonly prevent progression. Patients with curves >50° usually require surgical fixation, with posterior segmental fixation usually sufficient. During any surgical procedure, there is a high risk from anaesthesia and also from excessive bleeding.

Spondylolisthesis and basilar impression may also be seen. In basilar impression, the relatively soft bone of the foramen magnum migrates into the posterior cranial fossa. The upper cervical spine compresses the spinal cord, leading to headaches, facial spasm, numbness, bulbar palsy, and long tract signs.

Physis and Physeal Injuries
Introduction
The paediatric skeleton is different from the adult skeleton because the bones are more elastic and have growth plates (physes). In comparison to bone, the relative strength of the physis changes with age, becoming weaker as the child grows; hence

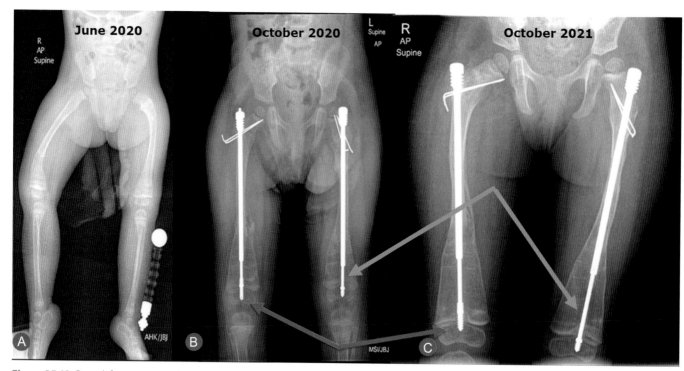

Figure 25.13 Bone deformities preclude ambulation and risk further fractures. The Fassier–Duvall (FD) growing rod is the most commonly used (www.pegamedical.com) to correct these deformities, whilst allowing for growth. It has two sliding parts: a thin male part and a large female part. It does not protect the femoral neck. Adding fine K-wires will protect the neck partially. During follow-up, it should be checked that telescoping of the nail is happening (green arrows) and the ends are still anchored to the epiphyses. On the right side, the male part seems to be moving away from the physis, so it may need changing.

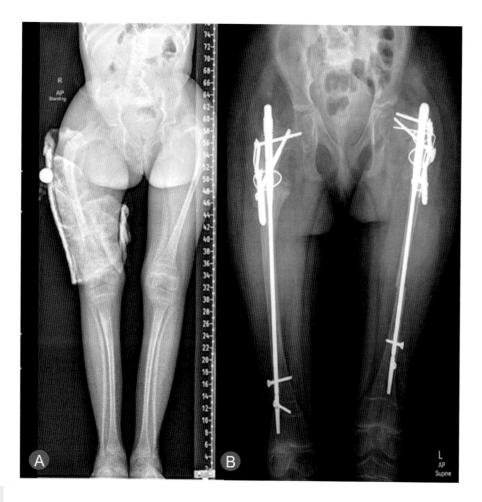

Figure 25.14 A child with osteogenesis imperfecta, with substantive proximal femoral deformity that precluded mobility and was associated with recurrent fractures. She was treated with deformity correction using the GAP nail from Pega Medical. This nail provides more robust fixation around the neck, but it does not expand with bone growth; the size is usually bigger than the Fassier–Duval rod.

physeal injuries are commoner in the adolescent group. The physis can be injured in many ways:

- Directly – fracture involving the physis
- Fracture elsewhere in a limb segment (the result of ischaemia)
- Infection
- Bone cyst
- Tumour
- Irradiation
- Repetitive stress (sports injury).

An understanding of the anatomy and physiology of the physis is important to help one understand, and thus manage, these injuries properly.

The Physis

Histologically, the physis consists of chondrocytes surrounded by an extracellular matrix (Figure 25.15). The chondrocytes are arranged in columns along the longitudinal axes of the respective bones directed towards the metaphysis where endochondral ossification takes place.

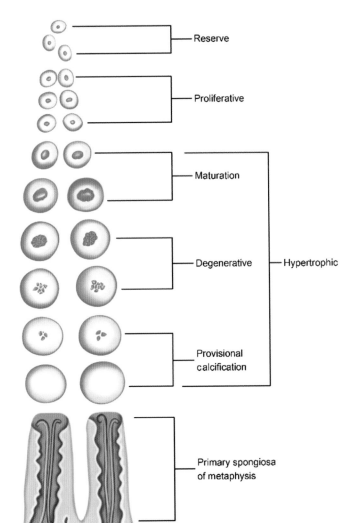

Figure 25.15 Zones of the physis.

The physis is divided into four zones:

1. Reserve zone
2. Proliferative zone
3. Hypertrophic zone
4. Zone of endochondral ossification (in the primary spongiosa of the metaphysis).

The reserve and proliferative zones have an abundance of extracellular matrix and thus resist shear forces easily. The hypertrophic zone has significantly less extracellular matrix, compared to the reserve and proliferative zones, and is therefore the weakest zone. It is believed that most physeal injuries occur in this zone, although any zone may be involved in high-energy injuries.

In the hypertrophic zone, chondrocytes increase in size, accumulate calcium in their mitochondria, and degenerate. In addition, oxygen tension becomes progressively lower as cells pass through this zone. The zone is further subdivided into three zones:

1. Maturation
2. Degeneration
3. Provisional calcification.

The **groove of Ranvier** at the periphery of the physis contains an active group of chondrocytes and contributes to lateral growth (width) of the physis.

The physis is encircled by the **perichondrial ring of LaCroix**. This is a dense fibrous continuation of the periosteum and provides strong mechanical support at the bone/physis interface.

The physis of long bones, such as that of the distal femur, has an undulating pattern with mamillary processes. These features provide greater shear strength.

Blood supply of the growth plate is provided by:

1. Epiphyseal vessels
2. Metaphyseal vessels
3. Vessels from the perichondrial ring of LaCroix.

The epiphyseal vessels are the main source of blood supply. However, in the physis of the proximal femur and proximal humerus where the epiphysis is covered fully by articular cartilage, the main source of vascularity is the metaphyseal vessels.

The blood supply to these physes can be significantly compromised in severe physeal injuries that cause epiphyseal separation.

Physeal Injuries

Eighteen per cent of all fractures in children are physeal. Boys are affected more than girls, and the phalanges are most commonly involved. Over the years, various classification systems based on radiographs have been described such as Salter–Harris [9], Ogden [10], and Peterson [11] (see Chapter 9, Figure 9.3). The Salter–Harris classification based on five fracture patterns is the most widely used. This classification not only helps guide the choice of treatment, but also predicts the prognosis.

Type 1

This is characterized by separation of the epiphysis from the metaphysis. These fractures are rare and are observed most frequently in infants, involving the proximal or distal humerus and the distal femoral physes. A slipped upper femoral epiphysis (SUFE) can be regarded as a type 1 injury (see Chapter 4, Figure 4a.4). Radiographs of undisplaced type 1 fractures look normal, except for soft tissue swelling; hence careful examination of the limb is required. Ultrasound, MRI, or arthrography may be required to confirm the diagnosis. The aim of treatment is to maintain satisfactory alignment of the epiphysis and metaphysis. Prognosis is generally excellent.

Type II

The fracture line extends across the physis and exits through the metaphysis (Thurstan Holland fragment) at the opposite end of the fracture (see Chapter 9, Figure 9.3). This is the commonest Salter–Harris fracture pattern. The treatment of choice for displaced fractures is careful, gentle closed reduction and immobilization, although occasionally a flap of the periosteum may be entrapped between the epiphysis and the metaphysis, blocking reduction. This requires careful surgical exploration to remove the entrapped periosteum. Prognosis is good.

Type III

The fracture line extends through the physis and epiphysis, creating an intra-articular injury, for example, Tillaux fracture of the ankle (see Chapter 9, Figure 9.8). These fractures are usually the result of high-energy injuries and thus have a risk of growth disturbance and deformity due to physeal damage.

Anatomical open reduction and stabilization with screws are usually required to restore articular congruency. It is advisable to avoid penetration of the joint and physis with the screws, wherever possible.

Type IV

The fracture line extends from the metaphysis, crosses the physis, and goes into the epiphysis (Figure 25.16).

This fracture pattern is frequently seen around the medial malleolus but may occur in other physes. Anatomical reduction and adequate stabilization with screws, etc. are required. If treated properly, the prognosis is good.

Type V

Type V is described as a compression injury to the physis. Initial radiographs are usually normal, and these injuries are recognized in hindsight when an angular deformity or a leg length discrepancy due to physeal fusion develops some time later. A classic example is a recurvatum deformity due to growth arrest affecting the proximal tibial physis.

Complications

Complications associated with physeal fractures are no different to that of other fractures, except for the complication of physeal growth arrest which may lead to angular deformity or limb length inequality.

The type and severity of deformity will depend upon:

1. Which physis is affected (from worst to best: distal femur, distal tibia, proximal tibia, and distal radius)
2. The extent and types of physeal injury (from worst to best: Salter–Harris IV > III > I > II)
3. The cause of physeal injury (infection worse than trauma)
4. The size of the physeal bar (the larger, the worse: >50% of the surface area of the physis, 30–50%, and <30%)
5. The site of the physeal bar (peripherally located bars are easier to excise than central or linear ones – Figures 25.16 and 25.17, respectively)
6. The time lapse since injury
7. The skeletal maturity of the patient.

Identification of the type of growth disturbance is important, as surgery may be required to correct deformity or to prevent it from developing further. In addition to plain radiographs, MRI and CT are usually required to define the size and position of a bony bar.

Treatment options are:
- Observation
- Completion of a partial arrest by epiphysiodesis
- Physeal bar resection
- Correction of angular deformity or leg length inequality.

Observation is an acceptable option if the physeal bar involves the whole physis and the predicted limb length discrepancy or angular deformity at skeletal maturity is acceptable. This is usually the case in older children approaching maturity.

Completion of a partial arrest by drill epiphysiodesis is usually undertaken for eccentric bars to prevent deformity from worsening. Additional surgery may be required in these cases to correct deformities that are present at the time.

Resection of a physeal bar is usually undertaken if significant growth remains (>2 years) and the bar is <30% of the surface area of the physis.

Identifying the full extent of the bar intraoperatively can be challenging. Intraoperative CT, MRI, or intraosseous endoscopy have been utilized. Following bar resection, it is advisable to fill the space created with autologous fat or poly-methylmethacrylate to prevent re-formation of the bar (Figure 25.17).

Angular deformity can be corrected acutely using standard osteotomy techniques or the technique of distraction osteogenesis. The choice of technique depends on the surgeon's expertise, age of the patient, and severity of the deformity.

Toe Walking

Toe walking is defined as the inability to make heel contact with the floor during the initial stance phase of the gait cycle and the absence of full foot contact with the ground during the remainder of the stance phase of the gait cycle. The forefoot engages in most of floor contact throughout the gait cycle.

Four clinically distinctive groups have been recognized, as detailed below.

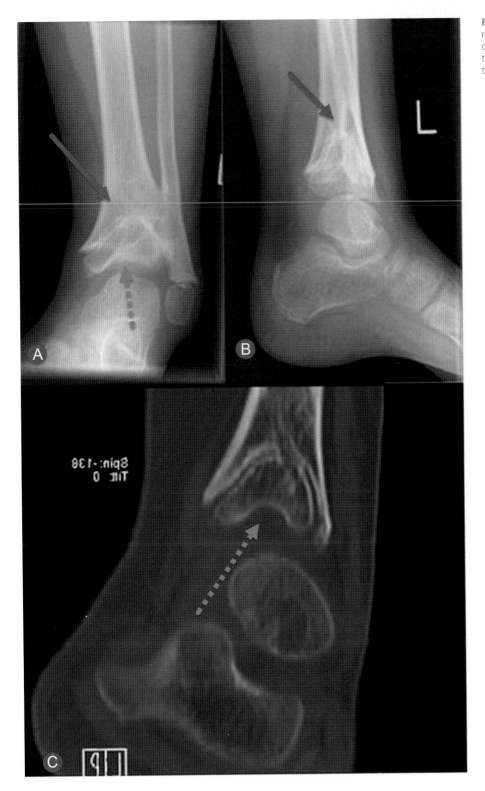

Figure 25.16 Central physeal arrest (solid red arrow). These arrests cause intra-articular deformity (dashed blue arrow). Therefore, treatment should be initiated promptly, even if this means total epiphysiodesis.

Group 1: Early Learning Stage

This is common when children start walking. It is intermittent and rarely continues beyond the second year of life. Examination often is completely normal. There is no tightness in the tendo Achilles and the child is neurologically normal. Assurance is the only thing required in this group. Sometimes, wearing boots force the patient to walk on heels.

Group II: Neuromuscular Conditions

Several neuromuscular conditions cause toe walking. Sometimes, toe walking is the very first presentation of conditions such as cerebral palsy and Duchenne muscular dystrophy. Neurological examination is often abnormal, although subtle. That is why referring these children to a neurologist is recommended.

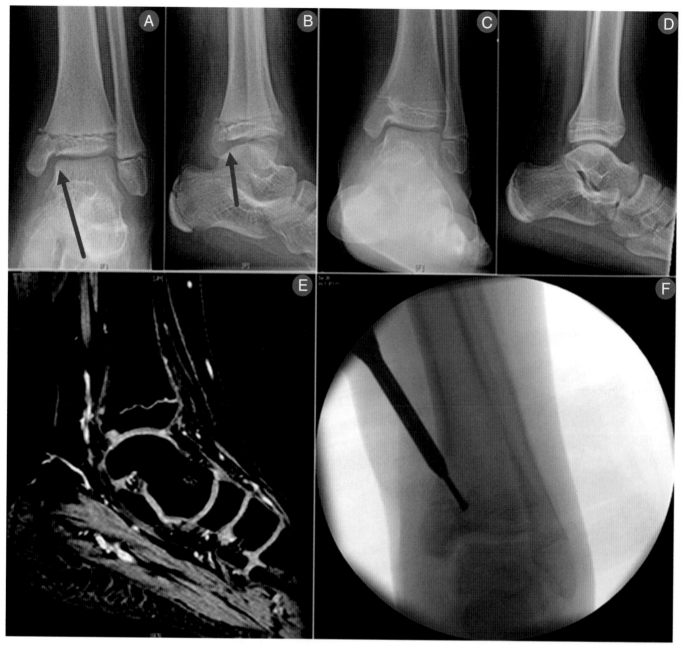

Figure 25.17 Peripheral physeal arrest. These radiographs show a Salter–Harris type IV fracture of the ankle in an 8-year-old boy, which was treated non-operatively with a cast, with subsequent development of peripheral physeal arrest and distal tibial varus deformity. A bar resection was undertaken, and the area packed with fat.

Group III: Children Who Have Learning Difficulties or Autism

This group of patients often walk high on their toes (Figure 25.18). The forefoot is often wide and thick, whereas the heel is small and smooth. A history of learning behaviour is often present (although some parents deny or do not accept it). A history of speech delay and swallowing difficulty is common. Initially, the tendo Achilles is normal, with no tightness, but later becomes tight. This group is the most challenging to treat. Behavioural and sensory physiotherapy is the mainstay of treatment. Serial casting if the tendo Achilles is tight, followed by temporary ankle–foot orthosis to break the habit of toe walking, can be useful. Surgical lengthening of the tendo Achilles when tight is very unpredictable, as it is the result of toe walking, rather than the cause.

Group IV: Idiopathic Toe Walker

As the name implies, no cause can be found in these children other than a short tendo Achilles. If it is minor shortening, physiotherapy and serial casting are very successful. Otherwise, lengthening of the tendo Achilles is very successful.

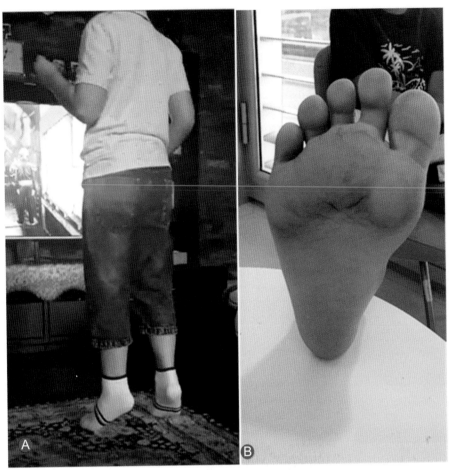

Figure 25.18 Group III toe walkers. They usually walk high on their toes, more than could be explained by the length of the tendo Achilles. Frequently, they can stand with their heels on the floor. Their forefeet are wide and thick, whereas the heel is small and smooth.

Lumbosacral Agenesis

Background

Lumbosacral agenesis is the congenital absence of one or more lumbar vertebra, with partial or complete absence of the sacrum. This is an uncommon condition, with an incidence of 1 in 25 000 live births. Cases may be associated with neural deficiency (compromise affecting the cauda equina or exiting nerve roots at the level of the deficiency) or frank myelomeningocele (Figure 25.19).

Lumbosacral agenesis is associated with maternal diabetes and insulin use during pregnancy. However, the precise aetiology is unknown.

Clinical Features

The deformity and disability caused by lumbosacral agenesis are very variable, and functional outcome depends on the degree of spino-pelvic stability and neural function. Typically, the upper limbs are unaffected, but hip dysplasia and lower limb contractures are common. Abnormalities in the lower gastrointestinal and urinary tracts are frequently seen.

Classification

Guille *et al.* developed a classification system to predict the walking potential for children with lumbosacral agenesis.

- Type A children have a spine that articulates in the midline of the pelvis, with low instability and good walking potential if there is no myelomeningocele.
- Type B children have a spine that articulates away from the midline, with less stability.
- Type C children have a spine that does not articulate with the pelvis at all.

In a series of six patients with type B or C agenesis and myelomeningocele, only one patient was ambulant indoors [12].

Management

Surgical management of lumbosacral agenesis is controversial, with variable management of contractures and spino-pelvic instability. The presence of a myelomeningocele is associated with poor function.

Surgical options include fusion of the spine to the pelvis to improve core stability and function. Management of lower limb issues for those with neural compromise should follow

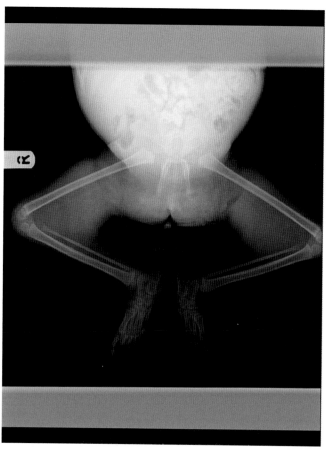

Figure 25.19 A child with lumbosacral agenesis. Notice the small lower limbs, knee contractures, and dysplastic pelvis and hips.

the principles that guide management of children with spina bifida.

Sclerotome Subtraction and Thalidomide

A sclerotome has been defined as a longitudinal band of skeletal tissue that is supplied by one segmental spinal nerve. They underlie the myotomes and dermatomes, and have been implicated in reduction deformities of the limbs such as following thalidomide exposure [13].

Thalidomide alters the development of the limb bud in humans (but not in rodents) at days 20–36 post-conception through causing apoptosis of the apical ectodermal ridge (AER). The AER forms the tip of the limb buds and is the area from which the limb grows and develops, much like the physis in bone growth. Complete removal of the AER results in amelia where there is complete failure of development of a limb. Partial destruction of the AER results in phocomelia where there is partial lack of development of a limb. This deficiency typically involves the radial aspect of the upper limb (with malformation of the thumb and first two fingers) and the tibial side of the lower limb. Thalidomide exposure is also associated with malformation of structures of the head and neck, particularly ear and facial development.

The molecular activity of thalidomide inhibits the usual cell survival pathways of WNT/β-catenin and Akt by suppression of fibroblast growth factor 8 and 10. This is caused by a range of mechanisms, including increasing oxidative stress, anti-angiogenesis, and downregulation of the cell maintenance proteasome [13].

References

1. Tardieu A. Etude médico-légale sur les sévices et mauvais traitements exercés sur des enfants. *Annales d'hygiène publique et de médecine légale*. 1860;13:361–98.

2. Caffey J. Multiple fractures in the long bones of infants suffering from chronic subdural hematoma. *Am J Roentgenol Radium Ther*. 1946;56(2):163–73.

3. Kempe CH, Silverman FN, Steele BF, Droegemueller W, Silver HK. The battered-child syndrome. *JAMA*. 1962;181:17–24.

4. Lucas DR, Wezner KC, Milner JS, *et al*. Victim, perpetrator, family, and incident characteristics of infant and child homicide in the United States Air Force. *Child Abuse Negl*. 2002;26(2):167–86.

5. Herring JA. *Tachdjians' Pediatric Orthopaedics*, 5th ed. Philadelphia, PA: Saunders Elsevier; 2014.

6. Kantor R, Salai M, Ganel A. Orthopaedic long-term aspects of bladder exstrophy. *Clin Orthop Relat Res*. 1997(335):240–5.

7. Sponseller PD, Ain MC. The skeletal dysplasias. In: Weinstein SL, Flynn JM, eds. *Lovell and Winter's Pediatric Orthopaedics*, 7th ed. Philadelphia, PA: Lippincott Williams & Wilkins; 2014. pp. 117–217.

8. Baldridge D, Schwarze U, Morello R, *et al*. *CRTAP* and *LEPRE1* mutations in recessive osteogenesis imperfecta. *Hum Mutat*. 2008;29(12):1435–42.

9. Salter R, Harris W. Injuries involving the epiphyseal plate. *J Bone Joint Surg Am*. 1963;45A:587–622.

10. Ogden JA. Injury to the growth mechanisms of the immature skeleton. *Skeletal Radiol*. 1981;6(4): 237–53.

11. Peterson CA, Peterson HA. Analysis of the incidence of injuries to the epiphyseal growth plate. *J Trauma*. 1972;12(4):275–81.

12. Guille JT, Benevides R, DeAlba CC, Siriram V, Kumar SJ. Lumbosacral agenesis: a new classification correlating spinal deformity and ambulatory potential. *J Bone Joint Surg Am*. 2002;84(1):32–8.

13. Knobloch J, Jungck D, Koch A. The molecular mechanisms of thalidomide teratogenicity and implications for modern medicine. *Curr Mol Med*. 2017;17(2):108–17.

Index